Mental Health Intervention and Treatment of First Responders and Emergency Workers

Clint A. Bowers
University of Central Florida, USA

Deborah C. Beidel
University of Central Florida, USA

Madeline R. Marks
University of Central Florida, USA

A volume in the Advances in Psychology, Mental Health, and Behavioral Studies (APMHBS) Book Series

IGI Global
DISSEMINATOR OF KNOWLEDGE

Published in the United States of America by
IGI Global
Medical Information Science Reference (an imprint of IGI Global)
701 E. Chocolate Avenue
Hershey PA, USA 17033
Tel: 717-533-8845
Fax: 717-533-8661
E-mail: cust@igi-global.com
Web site: http://www.igi-global.com

Library of Congress Cataloging-in-Publication Data

Names: Bowers, Clint A., editor. | Beidel, Deborah C., editor. | Marks, Madeline R., 1990- editor.
Title: Mental health intervention and treatment of first responders and emergency workers / Clint A. Bowers, Deborah C. Beidel, and Madeline R. Marks, Editors.
Description: Hershey, PA : Medical Information Science Reference (an imprint of IGI Global), [2020] | Includes bibliographical references.
Identifiers: LCCN 2019010657| ISBN 9781522598039 (hardcover) | ISBN 9781522598046 (ebook)
Subjects: | MESH: Emergency Responders--psychology | Occupational Health | Mental Disorders--diagnosis | Mental Disorders--therapy
Classification: LCC RC480.6 | NLM WA 290 | DDC 616.89/025--dc23 LC record available at https://lccn.loc.gov/2019010657

This book is published in the IGI Global book series Advances in Psychology, Mental Health, and Behavioral Studies (APMHBS) (ISSN: 2475-6660; eISSN: 2475-6679)

British Cataloguing in Publication Data
A Cataloguing in Publication record for this book is available from the British Library.

For electronic access to this publication, please contact: eresources@igi-global.com.

Advances in Psychology, Mental Health, and Behavioral Studies (APMHBS) Book Series

Bryan Christiansen
Global Research Society, LLC, USA
Harish C. Chandan
Argosy University, USA

ISSN:2475-6660
EISSN:2475-6679

Mission

The complexity of the human mind has puzzled researchers and physicians for centuries. While widely studied, the brain still remains largely misunderstood.

The **Advances in Psychology, Mental Health, and Behavioral Studies (APMHBS)** book series presents comprehensive research publications focusing on topics relating to the human psyche, cognition, psychiatric care, mental and developmental disorders, as well as human behavior and interaction. Featuring diverse and innovative research, publications within APMHBS are ideally designed for use by mental health professionals, academicians, researchers, and upper-level students.

Coverage

- Human Interaction
- Human Behavior
- Cognition
- Substance Abuse
- Addiction
- Psychiatry
- Trauma & Stress
- Neurological Disorders
- Eating Disorders
- Treatment & Care

IGI Global is currently accepting manuscripts for publication within this series. To submit a proposal for a volume in this series, please contact our Acquisition Editors at Acquisitions@igi-global.com or visit: http://www.igi-global.com/publish/.

The Advances in Psychology, Mental Health, and Behavioral Studies (APMHBS) Book Series (ISSN 2475-6660) is published by IGI Global, 701 E. Chocolate Avenue, Hershey, PA 17033-1240, USA, www.igi-global.com. This series is composed of titles available for purchase individually; each title is edited to be contextually exclusive from any other title within the series. For pricing and ordering information please visit http://www.igi-global.com/book-series/advances-psychology-mental-health-behavioral/110200. Postmaster: Send all address changes to above address.

Titles in this Series

For a list of additional titles in this series, please visit:
https://www.igi-global.com/book/mental-health-intervention-treatment-first/223949

The Psychology and Dynamics Behind Social Media Interactions
Malinda Desjarlais (Mount Royal University, Canada)
Information Science Reference • © 2020 • 477pp • H/C (ISBN: 9781522594123) • US $195.00

Multifaceted Approach to Digital Addiction and Its Treatment
Bahadir Bozoglan (IF Weinheim Institute for Systemic Education and Development, Germany)
Information Science Reference • © 2019 • 388pp • H/C (ISBN: 9781522584490) • US $225.00

Media Models to Foster Collective Human Coherence in the PSYCHecology
Stephen Brock Schafer (Pacific Rim Enterprises, USA)
Information Science Reference • © 2019 • 307pp • H/C (ISBN: 9781522590651) • US $195.00

Developing and Sustaining Play Therapy Clinics
Erin M. Dugan (LSU Health New Orleans, USA) Krystal Vaughn (LSU Health New Orleans, USA) and Kellie Camelford (LSU Health New Orleans, USA)
Medical Information Science Reference • © 2019 • 316pp • H/C (ISBN: 9781522582267) • US $265.00

Ethical Problem-Solving and Decision-Making for Positive and Conclusive Outcomes
Penelope D. Keough (National University, USA)
Information Science Reference • © 2019 • 326pp • H/C (ISBN: 9781522575825) • US $195.00

Chronic Stress and Its Effect on Brain Structure and Connectivity
Ana Starcevic (University of Belgrade, Serbia)
Medical Information Science Reference • © 2019 • 318pp • H/C (ISBN: 9781522575139) • US $225.00

Analyzing the Role of Cognitive Biases in the Decision-Making Process
Verónica Juárez Ramos (International University of Rioja, Spain)
Information Science Reference • © 2019 • 262pp • H/C (ISBN: 9781522529781) • US $190.00

The Mental Health Effects of Informal Caregiving Emerging Research and Opportunities
Debra Gavin Ware (Argosy University, USA) and Tarnue Johnson (Argosy University, USA & Kirkwood Community College, USA)
Medical Information Science Reference • © 2019 • 131pp • H/C (ISBN: 9781522574521) • US $195.00

IGI Global
DISSEMINATOR OF KNOWLEDGE

701 East Chocolate Avenue, Hershey, PA 17033, USA
Tel: 717-533-8845 x100 • Fax: 717-533-8661
E-Mail: cust@igi-global.com • www.igi-global.com

List of Reviewers

Tore Aune, *Norwegian University of Science and Technology, Norway*
Jenna Beltramo, *University of Central Florida, USA*
Emily Bernstein, *University of Central Florida, USA*
Brian Bunnell, *University of South Florida, USA*
Janis Cannon-Bowers, *Cannon-Bowers Consulting, Inc., USA*
Jeffrey Cassisi, *University of Central Florida, USA*
Matt Cook, *University of Central Florida, USA*
Annelise Cunningham, *University of Central Florida, USA*
Michael Dunn, *University of Central Florida, USA*
Ashley Hinch, *University of Central Florida, USA*
Kristin Horan, *University of Central Florida, USA*
Steve Jex, *University of Central Florida, USA*
Rabekah Kanefsky, *University of Central Florida, USA*
Matthew Kramer, *University of Central Florida, USA*
Michelle Lilly, *Northern Illinois University, USA*
Brandon Matsumaya, *University of Central Florida, USA*
Krystal Morrison, *University of Central Florida, USA*
Sandra Neer, *University of Central Florida, USA*
Kim Neisler, *University of Central Florida, USA*
Amie Newins, *University of Central Florida, USA*
Emily Ross, *University of Central Florida, USA*
Jessica Ruiz, *University of Central Florida, USA*
Mindy Shoss, *University of Central Florida, USA*
Brittany Stephenson, *University of Central Florida, USA*
Jamie Striler, *University of Central Florida, USA*
Benjamin Trachik, *Walter Reed Army Institute of Research, USA*
Tamra Wiggins, *Harford County Emergency Services, USA*

Table of Contents

Detailed Table of Contents

For law enforcement agencies and the mental health professionals who serve them, one question is always foremost: How can we provide the right services to improve officers' wellbeing? These decisions are typically made without any data about what officers want. This chapter details one agency's attempt to solicit such feedback with an anonymous online survey about mental health and overall wellness. A brief background describes the context of the survey, which occurred at the same time as other mental health initiatives in the department. The authors discuss the choices involved in developing and promoting the survey, in hopes that readers will make better informed choices should they survey their own first responders. The survey results are reviewed, many of which (including the high response rate) were surprising, and the changes the department has begun to make in response to this feedback. The responses from 14 other public safety agencies throughout Virginia are also summarized.

First responders maintain strong marriages in spite of the potential negative impact of multiple stressors including schedule conflicts, financial strain, and the threat of illness, disability, and death. Patterns of thought and behavior that are beneficial at work, such as vigilance, rapidly establishing control, and shutting off emotional responding cause problems at home, particularly when intensified by trauma. Excessive belief in a partner's heroism and the choice by some responders of dependent romantic partners cause other problems, as does the sometimes culturally sanctioned practice of coping through alcohol use or sexual encounters. Shifts in perspective that reframe common concerns more positively are offered. Departments are encouraged to increase efforts to support spouses and marriages, given the importance of close relationships to health.

First responders are exposed to many potentially traumatic events throughout their careers. Given the risk of adverse mental and physical health outcomes secondary to frequent trauma exposure, access to culturally-sensitive, evidence-informed early intervention is paramount. Critical Incident Stress Management (CISM) and components therein (e.g., Critical Incident Stress Debriefing, peer support) represent the most commonly utilized early interventions within first responder organizations. Limited research has evaluated these models, and evaluation of early interventions presents many challenges due to characteristics of first responder cultures and organizational demands and constraints. Psychological First Aid (PFA) is a widely endorsed and promising evidence-informed early intervention model grounded in research on trauma recovery and resilience. This chapter examines the theoretical underpinnings and core actions of PFA and describes the potentially diverse applications of PFA within first responder organizations and concludes by discussing recommendations and future directions.

Chapter 9
The HEROES Project: Building Mental Resilience in First Responders 154
Alex R. Thornton, Indiana University, Kelley School of Business, USA
Daniel M. Blumberg, Alliant International University, USA
Konstantinos Papazoglou, Yale School of Medicine, USA
Luciano Giromini, University of Turin, Italy

The chapter introduces the HEROES Project, an online training resource that develops mental resilience. The goal is to provide the reader with insight into a resource that can be used as an adjunct to employee assistance programs, critical incident stress debriefing, and counseling. The HEROES Project is the first virtual training course that combines the therapeutic tools of clinical and organizational psychology and provides first responders access to a self-driven wellness program. This respects many first responders' preference for anonymous and private self-care, while the autonomous nature of the training reinforces for all first responders that they are ultimately responsible for maintaining their own wellness.

Chapter 10
Disaster Responder Self-Care, Self-Compassion, and Protective Factors: A Pilot Study on Responders' Resilience and Competence 169
Gargi Roysircar, Antioch University New England, USA
Allyssa M. Lanza, Psychological Solutions, USA
Marie F. Macedonia, Antioch University New England, USA

The study examined the relationships among resilience, self-care, self-compassion of first responders. In addition, the study assessed the contributions of protective and risk factors to responders' resilience and disaster response competencies. Five research hypotheses and three research questions were examined with Pearson r correlations, multiple regressions, one t-test, one MANOVA, and post hoc tests, showing significant and meaningful results. In addition, the internal consistency reliabilities of the DRCQ scales were investigated which were strong to very strong. It was hypothesized and shown that there were significant positive relationships among self-care, self-compassion, and resilience. A second hypothesis was retained that the two dimensions of self-care (i.e., self-care practices and physical safety) were predictors of self-compassion. Responders who consciously observed self-care practices fostered and strengthened self-compassion and vice versa.

Peer support, as part of a recovery-oriented approach to treatment, is a valuable resource across various clinical and nonclinical populations. Specifically, in fire service, peer support may bridge the gap between firefighters' behavioral health needs and access to professional services. The current chapter summarizes the literature on peer support utility, presents data on barriers to treatment, and describes the roles clinicians can fill in partnering with fire service peer support to enhance the quality and reach of behavioral health services offered to fire service personnel. Finally, future research directions are outlined to continue the conversation about how to improve collaborations between peer supporters, clinicians, and others working to support the needs and strengths of firefighters.

In this chapter, the authors draw upon a review of the empirical and theoretical literature, as well as their extensive experience developing interventions among law enforcement officers, to provide a commentary on the needs of first responder training. The chapter begins by outlining the need for intervention, highlighting the severe consequences experienced by first responders as a result of their occupational stressors. The chapter then offers a review of the potential structure and timing of first responder training. Finally, specific psychophysiological mechanisms to be targeted during training are reviewed, including summaries of the relevant evidence base supporting their utility.

Mental health professionals are only recently beginning to understand the risks for stress-related disorders experienced by first responders. For example, it is clear that first responders are at increased risk for Post-Traumatic Stress Disorder. Unfortunately, clinicians currently have a limited repertoire with which to treat these disorders. Treatments for PTSD have been developed for use with military patients, for the most part. It is not clear that these treatments are appropriate, and effective, for first responders. In this chapter, the authors describe a pilot study designed to evaluate whether one specific treatment approach creates similar clinical outcomes for first responders as have been observed for a military sample. The results indicate that clinical outcomes for first responders were nearly identical as those obtained with military personnel. The results are discussed in terms of future directions for research in this area.

First responders, including Emergency Medical Services personnel and firefighters, support community members in times of crisis. When responding to emergencies, first responders often experience both direct and vicarious trauma. Over time, the pace and intensity of a career as a first responder leads to poor health habits and high risk for mental health issues including posttraumatic stress disorder. Due to concern about peer perception and mental health stigma, these professionals are less likely to seek mental health supports to manage and process trauma. This chapter explores Narrative Therapy as an ideal option for mental health treatment of first responder trauma, providing a collaborative approach to therapy using the natural coping strategy of storytelling.

Improving the opportunities for enhanced health and wellness in first responders has gained national attention in recent years. Employers and other stakeholders striving to improve employee utilization of available resources will need to increase transparency in the process and improve understanding between first responders and clinicians. One potential process, early warning systems (EWS) are primarily designed to alert management to an at-risk employee. However, the continuing goal of any effort should be to identify and remedy any employee issue before the employee exhibits the predetermined number of events that trigger an early warning alert. Although many organizations are adopting an EWS by either choice or mandate, they are largely separate and distinct from the agency's health and wellness programming. Administrators are not only unsure of what data to consider, but also what to do when an alert is activated. Ideally, agencies move toward early intervention systems that themselves are conceptualized within the larger framework of wellness programming.

The chapter describes a replicable and innovative approach designed to assist first responder communities through the mental health challenges they face in their personal and professional lives. The First Responder Assistance Program (FRAP) strives to create a healthy environment, through a unified structure, three tiered organizational and relational intervention approach, inclusive of peer support, peer chaplaincy support, and clinician involvement. The FRAP Model establishes a direct correlation between organizational wellness, and the individual health of its members. It emphasizes a "top to bottom" organizational intervention, with the understanding that no matter how much help is provided to the individual, the environment must be addressed in order to obtain sustainable results. It stresses a "holistic" approach to healing with a focus on post traumatic growth and the systematic building of individual and organizational resilience.

Preface

The editors of this book all work for UCF RESTORES, a treatment and research center at the University of Central Florida dedicated to stress and trauma-related illnesses. Prior to June of 2016, we were primarily focused on military trauma--while we had done some work with first responders, we were hardly "experts" in the field. However, on the morning of the Pulse nightclub shooting here in Orlando, we were called to provide care to the hundreds of first responders that were involved in the tragedy. Since that day, we have treated or trained well over one thousand first responders. We have also consulted with many departments, giving advice on everything from peer support training, to assessment of trauma-related injuries, to organizational policies regarding mental health.

Like most social scientists that work with first responders, in the beginning we were largely uninformed about the depth and breadth of stressors that are encountered by these employees. We spent hours at fire stations, dispatch centers, and on police ride-alongs. At the same time, we reviewed the research literature in this area and became acutely aware of the relatively small collection of researchers working in this critical area. We also familiarized ourselves with best practices in treatment for these groups, again discovering that there was much work to be done. Finally, we learned that the resources to help these heroes are simply inadequate. From research to treatment to prevention, there is simply insufficient resources to take care of the men and women who risk their lives to protect us.

All of that said, the goal of the present book was simply to create a resource that would allow therapists, managers, and researchers to quickly come "up-to-speed" in the current thinking on matters related to first responder mental health. We recruited experts in the field to write chapters, and we're grateful for their participation. We also received excellent chapters from the open call that made us aware of issues we hadn't even considered. All in all, we believe that the book will be a great help to anyone who hopes to participate in this emerging area of treatment and research.

ORGANIZATION OF THE BOOK

The first section of the book relates to informing clinicians and policy-makers about the unique mental health issues confronted by first responders. Many of the issues related to this population are reviewed in Chapter 1 by Mills, Milloy, and Carson. These researchers conducted a survey of a large police department. Similar to other studies, they found that a substantial portion of their sample reported symptoms of mental illness. Their data also highlight the reluctance than officers have in seeking support. An interesting aspect of this chapter is that the authors detail how their department responded to the findings.

These responses could serve as a model for other departments struggling to figure out how to improve mental health policies.

Another finding of interest is that the stressors endured by first responders are likely to add challenges to their marriage. In Chapter 2, Lisa Garmezy discusses the unique factors that therapists should understand when working with these couples. These include not only the occupational stressors associated with the job, but the beliefs that spouses may have about first responders, the role of co-workers in the coping process, and issues related to substance abuse and infidelity. The author offers importance guidance for the therapists and the departments that are trying to support these marriages.

It is also generally accepted that first responders are at risk for substance abuse. In Chapter 3, Lia Smith and her colleagues from the University of Houston review the recent literature in this area. They also describe the complex relationship between trauma, PTSD, and substance abuse. They describe important considerations for clinicians working with this group. They also provide guidance for researchers working in this area.

Females were once a rarity among first responders, but their numbers are increasing steadily. In Chapter 4, Brittany Hollerbach describes several unique factors that should be considered when attempting to understand the stressors confronted by female first responders. This include issues such as bullying/harassment; reproductive health, inadequate equipment, and several other concerns. This chapter should be enlightening to administrators, first responders, and clinicians.

Dispatchers are often the "forgotten heroes" among first responders. However, we are beginning to understand the unique, and significant, stressors endured by this population. The final two chapters of this section elucidate the challenges confronted by this group of professionals. In the first of these, Isabel Gardett and her colleagues from the International Academies of Emergency Dispatch describe the job demands of the dispatcher position and the manner in which each demand might influence the employee's mental health. In the following chapter, Michelle Lilly and colleagues review the research related to mental illness in these employees. They describe the implications of the research for both prevention and treatment in this group.

Because first responders are at such high risk for negative health outcomes, it is understandable that social scientists have explored preventative strategies. Section Two of this book includes chapters that discuss a variety of prevention approaches. In Chapter 7, Arble and Arnetz provide a review of the theoretical and empirical factors related to preventative interventions with first responders. They describe the challenges associated with primary prevention in this population. They also provide a review of the existing empirical data related to interventions such as mindfulness. They describe how an intervention developed in Sweden was adapted for a large urban police force. These may applicable to other departments as they struggle with the issue of prevention.

Jeffrey Mitchell is one of the most renowned scholars in the area of first responder mental health. His Critical Incident Stress Management program is regarded as the "industry standard" in the area of responding to trauma. In Chapter 8, Dr. Mitchell describes the development and expansion of this program over the years. He describes the essential elements of a successful program, and reviews the research associated with CISM outcomes. Finally, he describes the role of Critical Incident Stress Debriefing in the overall crisis management process.

Psychological First Aid (PFA) is another popular prevention intervention following exposure to severe stressors. In Chapter 9, Brucia and colleagues review the theory that underlies the PFA approach. Specific elements of the PFA intervention are described. They also discuss some "lessons learned" in implementing this approach within first responder organizations.

Developing resilience in at-risk personnel has been a popular primary prevention approach in a variety of stressful occupations. In Chapter 10, Renee Kosor and her colleagues describe an online tool that they have developed to apply this approach to first responders. The authors describe how they've developed the online program and share feedback and results that they've collected from this novel tool.

As first responders are becoming involved in peer support and other paraprofessional approaches, it is important that they also attend to their own psychological needs. In Chapter 11, Gargi Royriscar and her colleagues from Antioch University provide results from a study on these topics that was conducted with disaster response workers. The authors describe how self-care behaviors may protect against vicarious trauma. They also provide interesting directions for studying these issues among first responders.

Section 3 is focused on issues related to the treatment of first responders. One unique factor in treating first responders is that they may have had a quasi-therapeutic relationship with a peer supporter before seeking formal treatment. In Chapter 12, Dobani and her colleagues describe the challenges and opportunities arising from this situation. They also provide some interesting case studies to illustrate their points.

Although there are, certainly, evidence-based treatments for PTSD, most of these treatments have not been validated for use with first responders. In Chapter 13, we present results from a study done at UCF RESTORES that evaluated PTSD outcomes in first responders treated with Trauma Management Therapy. The results indicate that the effects of the therapy are equally positive for first responders as previously observed in a military sample. The authors describe how the therapy might be further optimized for this sample.

Another therapeutic approach that might be useful with first responders is narrative therapy. In Chapter 14, DeDiego and her colleagues describe the rationale underlying this approach and the elements that comprise effective narrative therapy. They also provide a case study that demonstrates how this approach can be used to meet the special challenges associated with first responders.

The final section of the book is dedicated to consideration of the organizational factors that may facilitate, or hamper, mental health among first responders. The first chapter of this section, written by Alex Thornton and colleagues, describes an innovative "early warning system" to identify at-risk first responders. Given the high-risk factors in this population, this type of system offers the promise of identifying symptomatic personnel so that they can receive treatment as soon as possible. This chapter includes discussion of not just the assessment portion, but the interventions that might be responsive to identified issues.

The chaplaincy plays a critical role in supporting mental health in many departments. However, it is not always clear how best to integrate the chaplain's role in the larger organizational framework. In Chapter 16, Chaplain Mario Gonzalez and his colleagues discuss the issues related in integrating the many facets of behavioral health care into the workings of a large fire department. They discuss a comprehensive model designed to organize the many facets of a comprehensive behavioral health program into a package that is easily deployable in departments.

Finally, in Chapter 17, Chief Kim Neisler and her colleagues consider the implementation of mental health programs from the manager's perspective. They describe important considerations for ensuring that an appropriate standard of care is articulated and achieved when dealing with the variety of mental health issues that might emerge among first responders.

All told, we believe that these chapters provide a comprehensive review of issues that must be considered, current best practices, and future directions for social scientists conducting research in this topic. We hope that this volume calls attention to this critical area and inspires therapists, managers, and researchers to continue to build upon this current knowledge base.

Chapter 1
Assessing Needs: Using a Wellness Survey to Guide Interventions

Colby Mills
Fairfax County Police Department, USA

Jill Milloy
Fairfax County Police Department, USA

Jaysyn Carson
Fairfax County Police Department, USA

ABSTRACT

For law enforcement agencies and the mental health professionals who serve them, one question is always foremost: How can we provide the right services to improve officers' wellbeing? These decisions are typically made without any data about what officers want. This chapter details one agency's attempt to solicit such feedback with an anonymous online survey about mental health and overall wellness. A brief background describes the context of the survey, which occurred at the same time as other mental health initiatives in the department. The authors discuss the choices involved in developing and promoting the survey, in hopes that readers will make better informed choices should they survey their own first responders. The survey results are reviewed, many of which (including the high response rate) were surprising, and the changes the department has begun to make in response to this feedback. The responses from 14 other public safety agencies throughout Virginia are also summarized.

INTRODUCTION

For law enforcement agencies and the mental health professionals who serve them, one question is always foremost: how can we provide the right services to improve officers' well-being? Agency leaders must struggle to apportion their limited budgets in the most efficient manner possible; psychologists struggle to advise their agencies about what will do the most good for the greatest number. These decisions are

DOI: 10.4018/978-1-5225-9803-9.ch001

typically made without any data about what officers want. Officers, meanwhile, know what they want but do not feel empowered to speak up: not only is there stigma about asking for help, there is also typically no reliable way to give such feedback.

This chapter details one agency's attempt to solicit such feedback with an anonymous online survey about mental health and overall wellness. A brief background describes the context of the survey, which occurred at the same time as other mental health initiatives in the Department. The authors discuss the choices involved in developing and promoting the survey, in hopes that readers will make better informed choices should they survey their own first responders. The survey results are reviewed, many of which (including the high response rate) were surprising, and the changes the Department has begun to make in response to this feedback. The responses from fourteen other public safety agencies throughout Virginia who decided to conduct the survey themselves are also summarized.

BACKGROUND

The Fairfax County Police Department (FCPD) is a large suburban agency outside the nation's capital. Approximately 1,400 officers police a county of 1.4 million residents, supported by approximately 300 civilian personnel.

FCPD is fortunate to have the budget to provide a wide variety of supportive resources to its officers and staff. A robust and well-trained Peer Support program includes approximately 50 officers spread throughout the agency, and there is a Police Chaplain assigned to every station and specialty unit. The County also provides an Employee Assistance Program to all county employees. Finally, FCPD contracts with a small group of police psychologists to provide comprehensive services: therapy, trainings, 24/7 critical incident response, and annual wellness checks. The supportive resources, known collectively as Incident Support Services (ISS), share a commander and often respond to critical incidents together. A separate psychologist conducts FCPD's pre-employment screenings and fitness for duty evaluations. The department's leaders, from the Chief down, are progressive in their thinking and supportive of mental health services.

Like most agencies, however, FCPD has known its share of tragedy. The Department has suffered from 15 suicides of active and retired officers in the last 30 years, five of which were in the last six years. Finally, in August 2017, an officer died by suicide in the parking lot of the station where he worked. Amid the shock and grief throughout the agency, many individuals felt called to act. For example, the Chief of Police began speaking openly at roll calls and to other agencies about trauma, making unprecedented individual efforts to destigmatize the effects of trauma and the benefits of seeking help.

The Department approved the survey in early 2018 as part of a coordinated response to an officer's death by suicide. The overall goals were to raise awareness and reduce stigma about psychological health, trauma, and suicide. A team of Peer Support officers and psychologists, including the three authors, developed and promoted an educational video ("Consequences of the Badge") that featured sworn personnel from local public safety agencies speaking openly about their intensely personal experiences with trauma and with their own suicidal ideation. Peer Support and two of the psychologists presented the video at every roll call throughout the Department. The survey was developed and conducted during this time period, which may help explain the high response rate (see below).

ISS leaders also realized that preventing the next tragic death would require officers' feedback. The agency needed to know what they needed and what obstacles stood in their way of seeking help and enjoying good health. Since supportive services are only one part of a much larger picture, officers would also be asked how they thought their agency could improve their health.

The survey had three goals. The first was to take a "snapshot" of officers' overall well-being and how it could be improved. Second, the authors intended to use these results to advocate for changes within the agency: not only to the supportive services, but throughout the Department. The Chief of Police provided his enthusiastic support and was receptive to making any necessary changes. As the survey evolved, the authors realized that they could also use the results to educate: the Department could show its "snapshot" to others, provide factual information about the health and needs of one agency, and demonstrate some of the many ways that the stressors of police work take their toll on officers.

DESIGN

The design team consisted of the three authors, along with input from the commander of Incident Support Services. Rather than use an existing survey, the authors designed the survey organically, with an eye toward the individual needs and culture of this Department. Academic rigor was intentionally sacrificed in favor of making the survey user-friendly and as relevant as possible to the potential respondents. At the time, the authors were focused exclusively on taking an internal 'snapshot' of the well-being of our own personnel; there was no expectation that other agencies would adopt the survey for their own use. The authors developed questions about how the unique stressors of an FCPD career are affecting officers' health and what might help improve their health.

The authors were also thoughtful about what *not* to ask, even in an anonymous survey. They abstained from questions that seemed too intrusive or clinical in nature, or that might be perceived as making a respondent easy to personally identify. Officers were asked for only one piece of demographic data (length of time with the department) and were asked about problems or negative changes rather than symptoms or diagnoses (e.g., "have you experienced anxiety" instead of "have you been diagnosed with an anxiety disorder"). The lone exception was Posttraumatic Stress Disorder, which seems to carry slightly less stigma than other diagnoses and which this agency had directly addressed with the video and roll call training.

The bulk of the survey consisted of twenty checkbox-style questions about psychological and physical health. The survey questions are listed in Appendix 1. Topics included a variety of responses to stress, whether cumulative or critical, including experiences that are common in those who suffer from Posttraumatic Stress Disorder or vicarious trauma (e.g., hypervigilance). The authors asked respondents about their physical health, both at the start of their career and now. Because sleep problems are endemic among public safety (Rajaratnam et al., 2011), there were questions about quality and quantity of sleep. The authors also asked about seeking help for psychological injuries, including any perceived obstacles to doing so.

The survey included three questions about suicide, a topic that is still (sadly) difficult to discuss openly. The question about suicidal ideation was preceded by a "warmup" question ("Have you ever known a coworker who has had suicidal thoughts?"). The authors hoped that this question would be a transition into a difficult topic and perhaps make it easier for officers to endorse their own suicidal thoughts. For those who endorsed suicidal thoughts, there was a follow-up question about how recent those thoughts were.

The survey ended with three open textbox questions about how to improve health and quality of life in the Department. Respondents were asked what they could do for themselves, what they would like their immediate supervisor to do for them, and how they felt the agency could help them. The authors hoped that the textbox format would allow respondents to raise issues and concerns that had not been addressed elsewhere, and to make suggestions that might improve the Department and the well-being of all officers.

SOLICITING RESPONSES

Police officers often have a tenuous relationship with psychologists and others who serve them in a supportive capacity. Trained to be strong, stoic, and independent, they may feel some understandable reluctance to accept help or to allow someone else access to their private thoughts and emotions. Knowing this, the authors assumed that a survey sent out by the supportive personnel would be unlikely to yield results. Just as important was the need to ensure the officers' confidentiality.

To address the first issue, Lt. Carson approached the employee groups, who agreed to send it out with their blessing. The heads of the employee groups sent out a letter to all officers (members and non-members alike), endorsing the survey and encouraging officers to respond. The employee groups served as custodians of the survey: this was intended to promote trust among officers, and also offered an extra protection against the results being subject to the Freedom Of Information Act (FOIA).

The authors chose to ensure confidentiality by means of anonymity. We used SurveyMonkey (www.surveymonkey.com), a web-based survey engine that does not track individual respondents. Since SurveyMonkey is widely used, most potential respondents would likely be aware of the anonymity it offered and might feel more at ease that their responses would not be used to single them out or damage their careers in any way.

When the authors have presented the results in any form, they have taken further steps to ensure confidentiality. Whenever the survey results have been presented (to FCPD's commanders, to educate other agencies, etc.), they have been shown in aggregate form only. The textbox responses have only been presented in terms of general trends or categories of responses: no individual responses have been quoted or released.

An important drawback to anonymity was that the authors would have no means to offer support to respondents who endorsed serious difficulties such as recent suicidal ideation. It was decided (not without some reservations!) that the benefits of anonymity outweighed the potential costs.

RESULTS

The survey was posted online for three weeks. The heads of the employee groups, along with Lt. Carson, announced its release and sent periodic reminders to all personnel in the agency. The authors anticipated the standard response rate for internal Department surveys, anecdotally ten to fifteen percent, and were astonished to find that approximately 350 people, or 24% of sworn officers, had completed the survey *in the first 24 hours*. By the time the survey closed, there were 847 respondents, or 57% of sworn personnel.

Demographics: As noted, the only demographic data captured was number of years with the Department. The results formed a rough bell curve, from new officers (five years or less on) to very experienced officers (25 or more years on). Almost half (49%) of the respondents had been with the Department for eleven to twenty years at the time of the survey.

Psychological Health: Respondents endorsed a variety of problems. The most frequently reported difficulties were increased cynicism (85%), anxiety (71%), and insomnia (69%). Many respondents (62%) endorsed hypervigilance. Approximately half (48%) reported feeling more irritable or agitated. 42% endorsed increased alcohol use, compared to a much lower number reporting increased use of pain medications (7%). Very few respondents (4%) reported having been diagnosed with PTSD, although nearly half (49%) believed they suffered from reactions to potentially traumatic events. Most respondents (75%) believed their attitude or outlook has deteriorated during their police career and that their loved ones would agree (79%).

Occupational Stress: 87% of officers indicated that their careers are stressful. Only 11%, however, attributed their stress to critical or potentially traumatizing one-time incidents, such as an officer-involved shooting. 40% listed day-to-day stress as most stressful, and 35% said that day-to-day work issues create just as much stress as critical incidents.

Suicide: 37% of those surveyed reported knowing a coworker who had disclosed suicidal ideation; 13% endorsed suicidal ideation of their own. Of those, relatively few endorsed recent thoughts: only 2% of total respondents endorsed ideation within the last month.

Seeking Support: A longstanding concern among professionals who support first responders is their unwillingness to seek assistance when needed. Although most respondents reported that they had changed for the worse, often in a variety of ways, only a quarter of them (26%) had ever sought any form of Departmental support. When asked why they had not sought help, most said they wanted to handle their difficulties themselves (65%). There was also significant concern about negative consequences at work (35%). Most of those who did seek support found it helpful (77%).

Sleep: The majority of respondents (63%) report getting five to six hours of sleep per night, on average. Only 24% endorsed a healthy amount of sleep (seven or more hours per night). When asked if they had ever been diagnosed with a sleep disorder, however, the vast majority (85%) had not.

Physical Health: Respondents rated their physical health as either excellent (58%) or good (33%) when their careers began. By comparison, their current physical health had deteriorated, with most responses in the good (40%) or average (30%) categories. Over the course of their careers, the percentage of those who rated their physical health as poor rose from 1% to 11%.

Textbox Responses: In order to code responses, the authors developed categories that seemed to encompass the range of responses for each question and then coded each response accordingly.

Regarding what they could do to improve their own health, about half of the responses (48%) concerned physical health. The most common responses involved exercising more or losing weight. Some respondents also mentioned cutting back on alcohol use. A minority (14%) mentioned psychological support, either psychotherapy or Peer Support—notably, some officers asked for mandatory psychological wellness checks. A quarter of respondents (27%) said their best solution was to quit or retire. (If all 227 of these officers were to act on their desires, that would constitute a loss of more than three thousand years of collective law enforcement experience!)

When asked how their immediate supervisors could help them, approximately half of the respondents (48%) had no suggestions. Some made positive remarks about their supervisors. The most frequent request was for supervisors to change specific behaviors or personal qualities (25%). One frequent request was not to be micromanaged, a well-known pet peeve among officers.

Regarding the agency, responses varied more widely. Roughly a third of respondents wanted their leaders to change their personal qualities (e.g., showing more integrity or compassion) or specific behaviors (e.g., advocate for staff's needs). Another quarter (23%) wanted leaders to decrease their stress by addressing their pay and benefits. 13% wanted leaders to increase supportive resources; a similar number responded with "Nothing" or "I don't know".

DISCUSSION OF FCPD RESULTS

The survey responses appear to be reasonably representative of this Department. The high response rate, coupled with the years of experience of most of the respondents, suggest that the responses paint an accurate picture of officers' overall well-being. Part of the reason for the high response rate may have been the roll-call trainings and the "Consequences of the Badge" video. The video and Department-wide discussions of psychological wellness may have encouraged officers to express their thoughts and opinions in the survey.

The results provide further confirmation that most officers endorse being affected for the worse by their job, yet are generally not willing to seek help. Despite high self-reported levels of anxiety, insomnia, and hypervigilance, officers generally have not sought support because they wanted to "tough it out" or feared damage to their careers. Most respondents acknowledged that they are not who they used to be, either in physical or emotional terms. When asked how they could improve their own health, however, most officers focused on improving their physical health rather than seeking emotional support.

Some results ran contrary to conventional wisdom. Despite the focus within police culture on critical incident stress, our respondents endorsed day-to-day organizational stress as being more impactful. Also, although officers had considerable feedback for the agency in general, approximately half of them had no complaints and sometimes even praise for their immediate supervisors. There is some support in the research literature for generally positive views of immediate supervisors (Mastrofski, Rosenbaum, & Fridell, 2011). A meta-analysis of police leadership in the United Kingdom also suggests, as our officers indicated, that leaders' degree of genuine concern for their officers is linked to the officers' psychological health (Campbell & Kodz, 2011).

Some results were also substantially different from findings reported in the research literature. At 4%, the rate of self-reported PTSD diagnoses were well below typical research estimates of PTSD among police, which generally fall in the range of 8 to 18% (Hartley, Sarkesian, Violanti, Andrew, & Burchfiel, 2013) and even as high as 32% (Asmundsen & Stapleton, 2008). One possible explanation for the disparity is the methodology: this survey asked officers to volunteer whether they had ever been formally diagnosed with PTSD, while most research studies use screening measures such as the PTSD Checklist (Blevins et al., 2015) to assess rates of probable PTSD. In the current survey, a "yes" response also depends on the officer not only being diagnosed, but actually seeking out a mental health professional in the first place.

The design and implementation of this survey appeared to have benefits and limitations. Protecting anonymity and securing the endorsement and cooperation of the employee groups helped yield a high response rate. The survey also struck a careful balance between keeping the survey short and assessing a wide range of topics regarding officers' health. The survey gathered valuable feedback and suggestions, which FCPD leaders are using to make changes that should benefit all officers (see below). These results have also established a baseline from which to evaluate the success or failure of those changes.

The potential limitations are many: as noted earlier, the survey was not designed as a rigorous research instrument. While most respondents are probably sworn officers, the decision was made not to ask about the respondent's status. In addition, all data are self-reported, and there is no way to verify the rates of negative experiences against any objective standards, such as diagnostic interviews. As with most surveys, this one is also open to the bias of self-selection: officers who feel healthy may have been less likely to complete the survey, and officers with greater stress or impairment may have been more motivated to complete it.

FCPD CHANGES IN RESPONSE TO SURVEY RESULTS

Before the survey even launched, the Department had already committed to respond quickly to the results. It was crucial to make changes that addressed officers' concerns, could be implemented quickly to indicate respect for the officers' feedback, and just as importantly, to offer relief to officers. Other identified changes were more complex and would be implemented over time. Changes were organized into six categories: Policy, Leadership, Training, Physical Health, Safety Nets, and Programs.

Policy: Importantly, some of the immediate and significant changes were in the "Policy" category. It was clear that the level of officers' stress needed immediate attention. The authors believed that the high rates of reported problems (e.g., hypervigilance, anxiety, irritability and agitation) are related to the stress of the job and the repeated exposure to potentially traumatic events (PTEs), with half of the respondents endorsing they suffered from exposure to PTEs. From experience, we knew that the impact of their job was not only affecting the officers' psychological health, but for some, their behavior and work performance. As already noted, the survey intentionally did not try to "diagnose" officers, but many of the responses frequently endorsed by officers could be related to repeated exposure to PTEs. Many go untreated because they are fearful of the stigma attached to seeking treatment and fear of being found not fit for duty.

The survey results demanded policy and cultural shifts. The impact of underlying job-related factors demonstrated in the survey could not be ignored. The goals (and hurdles) were to reduce stigma so that officers would proactively come forward for help; look at behavioral and work performance problems to see if there were job-related causes; and when appropriate, offer treatment diversion and a temporary reassignment, sometimes delaying an imminent Internal Affairs investigation. Obviously, when infractions are involved, there are exceptions dependent upon the degree or nature of the problem when officers would not have the option to choose the treatment diversion.

To reduce stigma, ISS personnel had attended all roll calls to show the Consequences of the Badge video, and publicly shared and discussed the survey results in an attempt to "normalize" the impact on law enforcement. Public forums led to discussions in which senior officers were willing to discuss the impact of the job, making it less stigmatizing for younger officers to seek support.

In addition to reducing stigma, policy changes were implemented to change the Department's responses to behavioral and performance problems, including behavior that required referral to Internal Affairs (IA). Commanders are now more likely to consider the potential causes of these behaviors, not just the behaviors themselves. If stress or trauma seems to be underlying an officer's problem behaviors (and depending on the nature of the infraction), he or she might be given the opportunity to seek mental health treatment, be reassigned to a temporary step-down assignment or injury leave instead of a fit for duty evaluation, or to choose treatment diversion versus an IA investigation. The agency is treating psychological injuries more like physical injuries.

In addition to these changes, policies were also introduced to address exposure to trauma. All supervisors are now tasked with documenting potentially traumatic incidents in case an officer develops posttraumatic symptoms in the future. While making these changes, however, the authors learned that this would not be enough: officers diagnosed with PTSD were ineligible for benefits through worker's compensation unless they also sustained a physical injury during the critical incident. In response, a Departmental workgroup (including the authors) has drafted a legislative bill that would cover PTSD in first responders irrespective of physical injury. This would be a presumption bill similar in many ways to laws in Florida and Arizona. Although the bill has considerable support in Virginia's General Assembly, it has yet to be passed.

Leadership: Although many responses regarding supervisors were positive, critiques of leaders tended to focus on their behaviors and personal qualities, including their leadership skills. A few of the changes to be implemented will be additional mandatory leadership training, increasing the time and grade requirements for promotion, and the use of 360° assessments.

Trainings: The Department is selecting (or developing in-house) more trainings to improve officers' psychological health. Topics include resilience, mindfulness, and the Stress First Aid (Watson et al., 2013) model. The Department is also changing aspects of its tactical training: squads will trained as teams to improve morale and performance, and reality-based training in the field will be used more frequently. In addition, officers who are returning to their assignments (e.g., following injury leave or intensive psychological treatment) will be exposed to stress inoculation training to insure successful return to their assignment.

Physical Health: A wellness coordinator has been assigned to specifically address the needs of officers. A nutritionist will be added to the team because many officers expressed concern about their diet and physical health, as well as a sleep specialist given the number of officers who are getting inadequate sleep.

Safety Nets: Creating safety nets was a natural follow-up to policy changes. They included instituting regular wellness checks, enhancing the early warning system, and encouraging officers to self-report problems or come forward with concerns about fellow officers.

Psychological wellness checks were requested by many survey respondents. They were made mandatory for two reasons: to insure compliance and to reduce the stigma of meeting with a police psychologist. Anecdotally, most officers seem to enjoy the interview, and it has even seemed to build a bond between the psychologists and the officers--demystifying some of what happens in conversations with psychologists. As part of informed consent, officers are notified that their attendance will be tracked but that no other details of the conversation will be released (with the standard exceptions to confidentiality). They are frankly advised that "showing up for the interview" met the criteria for attendance even if they chose not to participate and that the content of the conversation would not be shared with the department. Officers are educated that the wellness check is to provide confidential feedback about their current psychological health (not to assess job performance or fitness for duty). These initial checks will form a baseline from which to provide ongoing feedback about officers' psychological health over time.

Another aspect of the safety net was enhancement of the early warning system to monitor officers' behaviors. It is designed to alert supervisors when there is an escalation with an officer's behavior so that supervisors can address the problem before it worsens. FCPD uses a computerized early warning system, which now sends notifications about "flagged" officers to the ISS Director for triage and assistance.

Much effort was also put into encouraging officers to come forward if they were struggling, without fear of negative impact to their careers. They would not be at risk of losing their job or assignment, but rather would be assessed for needed support, whether it be a temporary reassignment or mental health support. Officers would also be encouraged to come forward if they were concerned about their peers and the department would respond as compassionately and confidentially as possible. The police culture has a quick and reliable grapevine, and word is beginning to spread that officers are being treated compassionately and returning to (or remaining on) duty while undergoing treatment.

Programs: Program development was also an area in which some immediate changes were implemented. FCPD's robust ISS was further strengthened. Lt. Carson, who had established credibility as a Peer Support Commander for many years, has now become the ISS Director and reports directly to the Chief. Some of his new duties are to manage program development, write policy changes, and spearhead changes in the law.

Immediate changes include educating spouses/significant others about law enforcement stress and asking them to complete a survey about their own well-being. Long-term goals include building a wellness center that would serve all local first responders. These centralized services may include additional clinicians, a psychiatrist for medication evaluations, a sleep specialist, exercise and nutrition training, as well as alternative therapies such as acupuncture.

In summary, the Department appreciated the candor of the survey responses and is responding with immediate and long-ranging changes to improve officer well-being. To assess the impact of these changes, a follow-up officer survey is planned.

VIRGINIA PUBLIC SAFETY: AGGREGATE RESULTS

As word spread about the FCPD survey, fourteen other public safety agencies across Virginia decided to adopt the survey for themselves and were gracious enough to share their results. Below are general trends from the survey responses of 3,430 first responders, including FCPD. Results discussed here include fire departments, public safety communications agencies, and law enforcement agencies (police and sheriffs). At the time of publication, several other agencies are conducting the survey or considering doing so. Below are general similarities and differences across the three public safety branches, summarized in Figure 1.

Demographics: Demographic data was roughly similar: most of the respondents had at least six years' experience. Respondents included 2,731 from law enforcement agencies, 584 from fire departments, and 115 from public safety communication agencies. Therefore, these results are more representative of law enforcement officers than of firefighters, rescue personnel, or dispatchers.

Psychological Health: As with FCPD, the most frequently reported difficulties were increased cynicism, anxiety, and insomnia. Anxiety was especially consistent, being reported at rates of 66 to 72%

Figure 1.

	Police (n = 2,731)	Fire & Rescue (n = 584)	P.S. Communication (n = 115)
More confrontational	24	33	22
More irritable/agitated	52	67	65
More cynical	81	66	79
Depression	41	46	49
Anxiety	71	66	72
Need for an antidepressant	18	15	28
Increased alcohol use	43	43	25
Increased pain medication	10	13	14
Flashbacks/nightmares	27	27	9
Insomnia	67	90	75
Avoiding trauma reminders	21	25	26
Hypervigilance	67	47	59
Shutting down/withdrawal	43	38	44
Suicidal ideation	14	18	26

across all three public safety branches. Irritability/agitation was also endorsed at high rates. 25% of dispatchers endorsed increased alcohol use; the percentage of police and firefighters was identical at 43%.

Suicide: Responses varied widely across public safety branches. The percentage of those who reported knowing a coworker with suicidal ideation varied from 28% (dispatchers) to 45% (firefighters). The percentages of respondents who endorsed suicidal ideation of their own ranged from 14% among police to 26% among dispatchers.

Seeking Support: Results here were generally similar to FCPD's results. When asked why they had not sought help, most (over 60%) said they either wanted to handle their difficulties themselves or did not consider their problems to be very important. There was also significant concern about negative consequences at work. Very few respondents said that help was unavailable (10% or less across all three branches).

Sleep: Across all agencies, the majority of respondents report getting five to six hours of sleep per night. As with the FCPD results, only a minority (25% or less) endorsed an appropriate amount of sleep. This was especially pronounced among firefighters: only 6% endorsed getting seven or more hours of sleep, and nearly 40% reported getting four hours or less.

Textbox Responses: Responses are available from a handful of the above agencies across all three branches. The results so far are generally similar to those from FCPD. When asked what they can do for themselves, the vast majority endorse improving their fitness and/or diet. Approximately half of all respondents did not have any criticism of their immediate supervisors; those who did frequently mentioned the supervisor's personal qualities or undesirable behaviors such as micromanaging. Responses regarding what they expect from their agencies tended to revolve around the behaviors or personal qualities of the agency's leaders. One notable difference was in the desire to quit or retire: FCPD's rate of 27% was substantially higher than other agencies, whose rates were generally 10 to 15%.

SUMMARY AND FUTURE DIRECTIONS

The results across all three branches of public safety suggest many more similarities than differences. All reported high rates of anxiety, cynicism, and irritability, and very few personnel get an appropriate amount of sleep. 25% or more drink more alcohol than they used to. And although help was usually available, many have not sought it out, either because they did not consider their needs important or because they wanted to "tough it out" on their own.

The results regarding suicide are alarming. Nearly half of firefighters have known a coworker with suicidal thoughts; a quarter of dispatchers have contemplated suicide themselves. The elevated rates of suicidal ideation reported here are generally consistent with other results regarding public safety personnel (Carleton et al., 2018) and are low by some estimates, particularly for firefighters (Stanley et al., 2015). In an era in which deaths by suicide routinely outnumber line-of-duty deaths (Heyman, Dill, & Douglas, 2018), these results add more evidence that suicide prevention efforts are crucial in public safety agencies.

The authors hope that readers will come away from this chapter with a more detailed understanding of the sources of officers' stress, how stress can manifest, and how officers want to address these problems. Perhaps these results will match your own perceptions of law enforcement; perhaps you were surprised by some of them. This discussion is intended to deepen the reader's awareness about what might be affecting any public safety member with whom you work.

Readers are also encouraged to improve on the methodology described here. As noted earlier, the authors developed this survey to fit the unique culture of FCPD and assumed the results would be primarily for internal use. It was not expected that other agencies would adopt it at all, let alone "as is", and we were surprised (happily) by the opportunity to examine aggregate data from across multiple agencies and thousands of respondents. Perhaps others with more expertise in clinical research will be able to design and conduct similar surveys that are more rigorous and reliable.

Just as individuals may experience growth in response to grief and trauma, so too may agencies. FCPD is sadly not unique in having suffered the tragedy of officer suicide, nor is it the only agency to have responded with growth amid the pain and loss. The overwhelming number of thoughtful responses to this survey, the agency's swift efforts to change for the better, and the survey itself are signs of post-traumatic growth in the wake of a death by suicide. In closing, the authors hope that this survey offers something useful to clinicians whose agencies are either grieving their own tragedy or seeking to prevent the next one.

REFERENCES

Asmundson, G. J., & Stapleton, J. A. (2008). Associations between dimensions of anxiety sensitivity and PTSD symptom clusters in active-duty police officers. *Cognitive Behaviour Therapy*, *37*(2), 66–75. doi:10.1080/16506070801969005 PMID:18470738

Blevins, C. A., Weathers, F. W., Davis, M. T., Witte, T. K., & Domino, J. L. (2015). The posttraumatic stress disorder checklist for DSM-5 (PCL-5): Development and initial psychometric evaluation. *Journal of Traumatic Stress*, *28*(6), 489–498. doi:10.1002/jts.22059 PMID:26606250

Campbell, I., & Kodz, J. (2011). What makes great police leadership? What research can tell us about the effectiveness of different leadership styles, competencies and behaviours. A Rapid Evidence Review. *National Policing Improvement Agency*, *11*, 1–27.

Carleton, R. N., Afifi, T. O., Turner, S., Taillieu, T., LeBouthillier, D. M., Duranceau, S., ... Hozempa, K. (2018). Suicidal ideation, plans, and attempts among public safety personnel in Canada. *Canadian Psychology*, *59*(3), 220–231. doi:10.1037/cap0000136

Hartley, T. A., Sarkisian, K., Violanti, J. M., Andrew, M. E., & Burchfiel, C. M. (2013). PTSD symptoms among police officers: Associations with frequency, recency, and types of traumatic events. *International Journal of Emergency Mental Health*, *15*(4), 241. PMID:24707587

Heyman, M., Dill, J., & Douglas, R. (2018). *The Ruderman White Paper on Mental Health and Suicide of First Responders*. Ruderman Family Foundation.

Mastrofski, S. D., Rosenbaum, D. P., & Fridell, L. (2011). *Police supervision: A 360-degree view of eight police departments*. National Police Research Platform.

Rajaratnam, S. M., Barger, L. K., Lockley, S. W., Shea, S. A., Wang, W., Landrigan, C. P., ... Epstein, L. J. (2011). Sleep disorders, health, and safety in police officers. *Journal of the American Medical Association*, *306*(23), 2567–2578. PMID:22187276

Stanley, I. H., Hom, M. A., Hagan, C. R., & Joiner, T. E. (2015). Career prevalence and correlates of suicidal thoughts and behaviors among firefighters. *Journal of Affective Disorders*, *187*, 163–171. PMID:26339926

Violanti, J. M., Robinson, C. F., & Shen, R. (2013). Law enforcement suicide: A national analysis. *International Journal of Emergency Mental Health and Human Resilience*, *15*(4), 289–297. PMID:24707591

APPENDIX 1

List of FCPD Survey Questions

1. How many years have you been with the Department?
    - 0-5 years
    - 6-10 years
    - 11-15 years
    - 16-20 years
    - 21-25 years
2. Do you think working in law enforcement (public safety) has changed your attitude?
    - Definitely for the better
    - Maybe a little better
    - Not at all
    - Maybe a little worse
    - Definitely for the worse
3. Do those close to you (spouse, best friend, etc.) think that you have changed?
    - Definitely for the better
    - Maybe a little better
    - Not at all
    - Maybe a little worse
    - Definitely for the worse
4. If you have changed for the worse, in what way?
    - More confrontational
    - More irritable/agitated
    - More cynical
    - More withdrawn
    - Depressed or anxious
5. Does this profession affect your family/personal life?
    - Yes, for the better
    - Yes, for the worse
    - Not really
6. Do you share your work experiences with your spouse/significant other?
    - Yes, fully
    - Yes, but not too graphic
    - Sometimes
    - Never
    - N/A
7. Do you think working in the Public Safety field has caused any of the listed concerns?
    - Depression
    - Anxiety
    - Need for an antidepressant
    - Increased alcohol use
    - Increased pain medication use

8. Do you experience any of the following from working in the Public Safety field?
    - Flashbacks or nightmares
    - Lack of sleep
    - Avoiding reminders of critical events
    - Feeling hypervigilant or overly watchful
    - Shutting down or being withdrawn
9. Do you think you suffer from reactions to traumatic events?
    - Definitely
    - Probably, but not sure
    - I don't think so
    - No
10. Have you ever been formally diagnosed with Posttraumatic Stress Disorder?
    - Yes, job-related
    - Yes, not job-related
    - I was diagnosed with something different, not PTSD
    - No
11. Have you ever sought SUPPORT services: Chaplains, Peer Support, Psychologists, or Employee Assistance Program?
    - Yes, and it helped
    - Yes, but it didn't help
    - No
12. If you wanted help but DIDN'T seek it, why not? Check all that apply:
    - Stigma/felt "weak" or embarrassed
    - Work might find out
    - I couldn't find the help I needed
    - Other people told me not to
    - I wanted to handle it on my own
    - I didn't think it was a big deal
13. What's most stressful about your job?
    - Critical incidents I've handled
    - Day-to-day stress
    - Both are equally stressful
    - My job really isn't stressful at all
14. Have you ever known a coworker who has had suicidal thoughts?
    - Yes
    - No
15. Have you ever had thoughts about wanting to die, that others would be better off without you?
    - Yes
    - No
16. When was the most recent time you had any suicidal thoughts?
    - Within the last week
    - Within the last month
    - Within the last year
    - Not in more than a year
    - Never

17. How was your physical health when your career began?
    - Excellent
    - Good
    - Average
    - Poor
18. How is your current physical health?
    - Excellent
    - Good
    - Average
    - Poor
19. How many hours of sleep (on average) do you get on a worknight?
    - 8+ hours
    - 7-8 hours
    - 5-6 hours
    - 3-4 hours
    - Less than 3 hours
20. Have you been formally diagnosed with a sleep disorder (apnea, shift work disorder, etc.)?
    - Yes
    - No

APPENDIX 2

Table 1. Percentages of negative experiences from public safety personnel in (14 agencies)

Chapter 2
Swimming Upstream:
The First Responder's Marriage

Lisa Berg Garmezy
Independent Researcher, USA

ABSTRACT

First responders maintain strong marriages in spite of the potential negative impact of multiple stressors including schedule conflicts, financial strain, and the threat of illness, disability, and death. Patterns of thought and behavior that are beneficial at work, such as vigilance, rapidly establishing control, and shutting off emotional responding cause problems at home, particularly when intensified by trauma. Excessive belief in a partner's heroism and the choice by some responders of dependent romantic partners cause other problems, as does the sometimes culturally sanctioned practice of coping through alcohol use or sexual encounters. Shifts in perspective that reframe common concerns more positively are offered. Departments are encouraged to increase efforts to support spouses and marriages, given the importance of close relationships to health.

INTRODUCTION

The influential assumption that first responders have higher divorce rates than the general population is widespread. Available evidence suggests that on the contrary, police and fire marriages are more stable than those of the general population. The rate of divorce was 16.4% in the general population in the 2000 census, but 14.1% for firefighters, 15.0% for police, and 23.9% for dispatchers (McCoy and Aamodt, 2010). Rates for police first-line supervisors and detectives were under thirteen percent, and for first-line fire supervisors, under nine percent. Jahnke (2015) reviewed 2008 data showing that 33% of married U. S. adults had experienced at least one divorce: Her sample of 1456 firefighters found 24.4% of married men and 27.3% of married women had experienced at least one previous divorce. Among all sample respondents, single and married, twenty percent of men and forty percent of women had been divorced.

Responders are typically hired with clean records concerning violence, substance abuse, and legal trouble, increasing their likelihood of showing emotional stability and staying married. Law enforcement officers, but not other responders, take pre-employment psychological examinations to assess

DOI: 10.4018/978-1-5225-9803-9.ch002

their stability. Marital satisfaction is attainable, although career-related stress and negative patterns of interaction, like strong currents, threaten to push couples apart.

This chapter focuses on common challenges to responder marriages and other relationships, although for brevity the terms spouse and marriage are used throughout. Unrealistic initial expectations, career-related stressors, and acquired patterns of thought and behavior that support functioning at work but prove ineffective or harmful at home are examined. These issues are not present in all marriages or relationships, and where present, may be highly significant or minor. Practical recommendations for clinicians and departments follow. Commonalities are emphasized; space does not permit addressing important differences between and within subgroups, e.g., firefighters tend to be a younger population than police officers. It should be noted that the scant research and clinical literature on responder relationships often focuses on white male responders with female spouses who are not first responders themselves. The material here may be less relevant to other pairings.

EXPECTATIONS OF A HERO

In healthy responder marriages, support and respect are mutual. Spouses take genuine pride in the responder's career and are glad he or she has meaningful work, while their efforts are valued in return. Career-related stressors are accepted in light of the responder's altruism and personal fulfillment and the couple's civic-mindedness. In fact, cognitive dissonance theory predicts that the more the career negatively impacts couple or family life, the more family members will value it, in order to rationalize their loved ones' continued involvement. This is especially true for the half of firefighters who are volunteers, who take on the risks and unpredictable call-ups without the justification of a paycheck. To the extent that responders engage in altruistic activities at considerable risk to themselves, they are legitimately heroes (Patton, Smith, & Lilienfeld, 2018).

All responder relationships must respond to a question: Are responders selfless public servants with superhuman courage or ordinary men and women doing a difficult job? An exaggerated belief in the responder's heroism sets up expectations that his or her work is more important than the spouse's, and that his or her needs will be more important as well. It also suggests that invulnerable heroes will bear burdens silently and alone, as is celebrated in the cultural narrative surrounding heroes (Zuckerman, 2015). Both parties in these relationships may expect the spouse to take a secondary role in fighting the couple's battles.

In fact, a conspiracy of silence characterizes many responder marriages. Both responder and spouse protect each other by failing to disclose their fears about the career. Responders also shield civilian family members from graphic details of their work. They are protecting themselves as much as their spouses, by keeping the home a sanctuary that is untouched by violence, loss and death. Regrettably, the omissions often create a gap between the partners.

In contrast, colleagues become a second family. The shared experience and camaraderie of the police or fire station is attractive to job-seekers. Once the career begins, peers buffer the impact of stress and trauma (Bohl-Penrod & Clark, 2017). Meyer, et al. (2012) found the presence of social support (likely to be emotional and instrumental) and other factors, not level of exposure to potentially traumatic events, seemed to determine the development of PTSD in firefighters. Like other traumatized groups, each responder profession experiences "shared stress," defined as "the feeling that you have to manage everything within our own community because you don't know what you'll encounter in society at large" (DeAngelis, 2019).

The same vital connections with peers can undermine marriages. Traditionally, these male-dominated professions have been influenced by a "fraternity culture" that condones coping with stress in unhealthy ways, notably drinking and casual sexual encounters (S. Buser, personal communication, Jan. 25, 2019). This may be more pronounced in the firehouse. Nationally, twelve to thirteen percent of police officers are women while only seven percent of the fire service is made up of women.

In a subset of dysfunctional relationships, responders and people in need of rescue feel a mutual attraction based in excessive expectations of heroism on the part of the responder. Here, the responder takes the role of a strong competent problem solver, i.e., a Rescuer, who joins with a weaker, less competent partner who may have been found on-duty. The dependence of the rescued person gratifies the emotional needs of the Rescuer and assures him or her that the partner will stay. Needy citizens of both genders embrace responders as symbols of safety and stability, choosing a "Wonder Woman" or knight in shining armor. Some citizens take seriously the bumper sticker, "Feel safe--sleep with a cop."

While relationships based on this imbalance are mutually satisfactory at first, the passage of time exposes a flawed foundation (Lamia & Krieger, 2009). If the rescued partner outgrows the pattern and the Rescuer supports the partner's growth, the marriage can continue on a stronger footing. Should a chronic mental health problem underlie the rescued person's crisis, with, for example, poor judgment or the tendency to idealize relationship partners as symptoms, an essentially healthy Rescuer is likely to become dissatisfied. Alternatively, a Rescuer with an anxious attachment style or low self-esteem who is unwilling to forego the adulation may discourage the spouse's growth or seek a new partner who will be appropriately grateful for his or her help.

This lens for examining the first responder's marriage fits loosely within the theoretical framework of cognitive-behavioral therapy. Valuing service to others is the responder's schema, or way of viewing and organizing the world. The expectation that heroism or masculinity means limited emotional responsiveness is a second schema that may be present. In faltering marriages involving a Rescuer, the belief that one's partner cannot manage his or her own life unassisted is a core belief supporting the first schema. Schemas and core beliefs shape perceptions, attitudes, expectations and behavior, at times to the detriment of the relationship (Dattilio, 2010). To a great extent, we see what we expect to see.

COMMON CAREER STRESSES

From the first day on the job, first responders face occupational stress, reviewed elsewhere in this volume, compounding the pressure of premarital expectations and the everyday difficulties of making marriage work. Foremost on the list of stressors is the threat of danger and disability, reflected in a mother's lament on Facebook that each time her eleven-year-old son was called to the school office he thought his firefighter father had died.

All first responders risk their health on a daily basis. Contagion and violence on the job is an issue for police, EMTs and paramedics. Less directly, chronic sleep disturbance is linked to cardiovascular disease and depression and has other detrimental effects on health; decreased alertness impairs functioning on the road and elsewhere (Hall, Brindle, & Buysse, 2018). Shift work is considered probably carcinogenic and has an established link to breast cancer (Hansen, 2017). The link between exposure to toxins in smoke and some firefighter cancers is so strong that these are now considered line-of-duty deaths, outnumbering traditional line-of-duty deaths. Firefighters also have higher rates of deaths due to cardiac disorders compared to the general population (Henderson, Van Hasselt, LeDuc, & Couwels, 2016). Suicide rates, higher among police than firefighters, exceed those of the general population in both groups, and in both groups are more frequent than line-of-duty deaths (Henderson, Van Hasselt, LeDuc, & Couwels, 2016; Violanti, 2010). This litany of vulnerabilities introduces a frightening expectation of a curtailed lifespan, and brings the stresses of caregiving, grief and loss into responder communities.

As readers are aware, shiftwork and missed holidays and special occasions play havoc with personal lives. For spouses, attending gatherings unaccompanied or dismissing "outside" friendships can cause sadness or isolation. Husbands and wives cope alone with crises from broken bones to national disasters. Schedules put satisfying sexual relationships at risk; spouses eventually lose patience with being woken in the middle of the night for sex when a full day's activities await. One bright spot is that parents can sometimes be more available to school-aged children than employees with nine-to-five schedules, but this possibility may increase the stress of work-family balance, recently shown to be significant in both sexes (Schockley, DeNunzio, Shen, Arvan, & Knudsen, 2017).

As in all professions, a stressful shift can heighten reactivity to ordinary adverse experiences at home (Neff & Karney, 2009). After double shifts or multiday on-duty periods, exhaustion may be present on both sides, since spouses must manage childcare and household duties alone. As the fire season appears to be lengthening, wildland firefighters may be deployed for a few days to several months. Longer deployments require periods of adjustment. Spouses may be reluctant to resume previous roles after developing new competencies or spheres of influence, such as budgeting, and shifts in responsibilities may occur. Resentment about absences can mar reunions.

Financial problems are a common marital stressor. Responders, particularly in single-earner families, typically work overtime or second jobs to supplement their median annual incomes of $62,960 for police officers, $49,080 for firefighters, and $33,380 for a combined group of paramedics and EMTs (Bureau of Labor Statistics, 2017). Many couples adopt lifestyles that depend on the extra funds, resulting in financial hardship when the supplemental income is lost due to injury or other reasons. In a destructive cycle, some families seem to feel that the responder's long hours at work justify excessive spending, then compensate for absences with more spending, yielding higher bills and still longer hours. When young wives ask how to support their newly minted responders, a strong answer is, "Make a family budget and stick to it."

Responders who are female, who are people of color, or who belong to marginalized communities have additional challenges. They may face harassment or exclusion by peers, a lack of positive supervision, salary inequality, and other forms of discrimination. The LGBTQ community serves in many places without legal protection or ready access to support. Women may feel they have to prove themselves over and over to citizens and coworkers; they face unique career and health concerns when pregnant. Responders of color may feel the tension of divided loyalties when civilian and responder cultures clash, as has happened after the fatal shootings of unarmed Black male civilians. Most first responders feel they live in a fishbowl, judged by their neighbors, their departments, the media, and citizens with cell phones cameras at the ready.

Volunteers or civilian paraprofessionals may be less exposed to these stressors and to potentially traumatic events, but also less prepared and supported when critical incidents do occur, such as when a dispatcher feels guilty after sending a responder to an injury-causing call. Their marriages are also vulnerable to the disruptions described.

BRINGING THE JOB HOME

Over the years, these jobs seem to change people. On the plus side, first responder cultures cultivate greater appreciation for truthfulness, loyalty, duty, leadership, and honor. Other changes are less desirable. While basic personality traits may be unchanged, as Gerber and Ward's 2011 review of literature on police officers concluded, accumulated negative experiences are likely to alter beliefs, attitudes and actions. Burnout, the decreased empathy due to psychological exhaustion and organizational dissatisfaction seen in some human service professionals is an example of one such cluster of changes that may impact first responders (Cieslak, et al., 2014).

Professional and personal accounts agree that responder marriages are threatened by "bringing the job home," or acting toward one's spouse and family as one acts toward citizens or colleagues while on-duty (e.g., Gagliano & Gagliano, 2018, Kirschman, 2004, and White and Honig, 1995). Kirschman, Kamena and Fay (2014) write that "the police officer's paradox" is that skills that are essential to the job are potentially damaging to relationships. The points below highlight the most relevant aspects of job spillover.

Unlike earlier work, Marier and Moule (2018) found that police officers developed cynicism. When an officer interrupts a sexual assault in progress and finds that the perpetrator is his own parish priest, as happened in Houston, his worldview is altered. Responders need reasonable skepticism. Moving beyond skepticism to develop negative expectations of others as a result of experience may be adaptive on the job, e.g., by improving adherence to safety protocols. Spouses, however, wonder what happened to the sweet, helpful partners they married; they are appalled if the lack of trust extends to them without cause.

Second, the need for rapid decision-making on-duty leads to a habit of dichotomous black-and--white thinking—something is good or bad, useful or not. In relationships, Dattilio (2010) identifies this as a cognitive distortion which discards important information and is not conducive to nuanced discussions or compromise. At home, for example, a responder whose spouse questioned a minor parenting decision could conclude, "She doesn't need my input on the kids."

Third, vigilance on the job is indispensable. Usually vigilance is so ingrained that it is never fully turned off, e.g., a responder is likely to automatically note the location of emergency exits in a restaurant, or avoid crowds, to the frustration of family members. The high level of physiological arousal required for sustained attention and readiness to respond lingers after a shift, particularly after a difficult shift, and can affect relationships. The responder is likely to feel keyed up, on edge, irritable or impatient, or on occasion, elated at surviving; he or she may seek sex as a path to relaxation. Hypervigilance refers to an unchanging and excessive elevated level of arousal, reactivity, and monitoring of the environment for threats. Responders often medicate this exhausting state with alcohol.

Last, suppressing feelings is appropriate at work but damaging at home. Regehr, Goldberg and Hughes (2002) quote a paramedic as saying, about a victim's mother, "You got to really concentrate on blocking her out because her emotions may affect yours." A practice of turning off emotional responses to keep the job at bay backfires when spouses want empathy and intimacy. Spouses' daily problems are also dwarfed by on-duty incidents: A firefighter who recently handled the burned body of a child may have difficulty caring about office politics. This lack of responsiveness leads Gagliano (2014) to write of the chronic emotional neglect of the firefighter's wife. If interpreted as rejection or indifference, it will lower marital satisfaction.

The overwhelmed responder who cannot empathize to meet a spouse's (normal) emotional needs, because of the difficulties of one shift or decades, is likely to withdraw. He or she may also withdraw when stressed, believing that the spouse will not understand or should not be burdened, or that it is important to conform to a hero stereotype. The withdrawal can infuriate the spouse who may perceive the responder, already frequently unavailable, as selfish or withholding. Typically, the spouse tries harder to engage the responder, who may become more determined to resist these attempts. The responder reacts by seeking greater emotional distance from the spouse, and the demand-withdrawal cycle repeats and escalates (Ross, Karney, Nguyen, & Bradbury, 2018). The responder's genuine need for emotional and physiological separation between work and the shift must be accounted for in working to alter this demand-withdrawal pattern, as discussed below.

CONTROL AND AGGRESSION

Perhaps more than the other changes in behavior, the first responder's practice of quickly taking control is essential at work but has far-reaching negative consequences at home. Control efforts can reflect a Rescuer's presumption that the less competent spouse should defer to his or her leadership, or more commonly, simply result from job spillover. On the job, but not at home, noncompliance cannot be tolerated. Responders are desensitized to aggression and trained to take orders without question; family members are not. The intimidation tactics that facilitate control on-duty—barking orders, name-calling, the invasion of personal space and so on—can be upsetting or frightening to civilian spouses and children. Deliberately or unwittingly, responders' behavior can come to resemble a list of warning signs of emotional abuse. It will be interpreted as hostile by partners.

The reliance on control, coupled with an awareness of danger honed by seeing broken bodies on a regular basis, may lead to overprotection of spouses or children and/or adopting an authoritarian parenting style. Vigilant or hypervigilant (a difficult line to draw), a responder may be loath to grant developing children and teens the increased independence they seek, leading to resentment and resistance. Black-and-white thinking can lead to castrophizing transgressions on the part of a child or adolescent.

Parent-child power struggles are exacerbated when the responder's attempted solution is becoming still more authoritarian. Successful parents come to understand that in these conflicts, "If you lose you lose, and if you win you lose," as the short-term "win" teaches obedience without decision-making skills and jeopardizes the relationship. Marital problems develop when spouses consistently take opposing positions on child-rearing. More often, the nonresponder becomes the "softer," more flexible parent, although a reluctance to discipline on the part of frequently absent responders is also seen. Further problems develop when one partner attempts to mediate the other's parent-child conflicts and is unhappily unable to fully support either partner or child. When rules vary according to the responder's presence or absence, conflict, disappointment and stress can build.

Factors such as the expectation of obedience, a habit of intimidation, and the desensitization to violence in interpersonal interactions appear to contribute to higher rates of intimate partner violence (IPV) in first responders. Stinson and Liederbach's (2013) analysis of previous research suggests that a greater amount of exposure to violence on the job causes greater "authoritarian spillover," i.e., use of coercive tactics at home, which increases the risk of violence. Estimates are that police officers perpetrate intimate partner violence at a rate two-and-a-half times greater than that of the general population (National Center for Women in Policing, 2018). In a 1991 survey of law enforcement officers, forty percent reported violent behavior with their partners; less than ten percent did so a decade later (Stinson & Liederbach, 2013). Along with shifting cultural norms, the difference may be due to a 1996 prohibition on owning firearms by anyone convicted of a misdemeanor crime of domestic violence.

Because it means the certain loss of a law enforcement career and compromises other responder careers, both parties will be reluctant to disclose IPV. (Clients have expressed that reporting a minor incident seems too vindictive.) The abused partner may also be silenced by threats, fear of retaliation, fear of being outed in closeted same-sex partners, or by the anticipation of unfair treatment by the responder's cohort in the justice system. The therapist's initial assessment should include exploration of aggression in the relationship, e.g., questions about having to physically restrain the partner "for her own good." Safety planning, when needed, is complicated by the constant presence of weapons and responders' access to information unavailable to the public, such as the location of shelters.

TRAUMA AND ITS AFTERMATH

Some of the most serious problems of responder marriages are mutually reinforcing. Trauma experiences increase the likelihood of alcohol abuse or dependence (Smith, et al., 2018). In turn, the IPV discussed above increases in the presence of alcohol abuse or dependence (McCrady & Epstein, 2015). These problems, which also develop in the absence of trauma, are addressed elsewhere in this volume. Their impact on children increases parental distress, at times triggering further maladaptive behavior.

Exposure to potentially traumatic events is universal in this population; paramedics in particular see a constant stream of severe injuries and death. The cumulative stress of repeated empathic contacts with victims leads to vicarious (cumulative) or secondary (sudden-onset) trauma after witnessing the traumatic experiences of others (Cieslak, et al., 2014; Rzeszutek, Partyka, & Golab, 2015). Both can lead to negative emotion, avoidance of reminders, withdrawal, hyperarousal, re-experiencing of the trauma, a sense of a foreshortened future, and other symptoms. Less frequently, responders experience primary trauma when they see a colleague injured or killed or when they fear for their own lives or the lives of those close to them. In these cases, it is the spouse that is likely to suffer vicarious or secondary trauma. Conn (2018) reports that two unpublished doctoral dissertations found secondary trauma symptoms in first responder wives, with a correlation to alcohol use and reported distress.

Trauma on the job impacts responders differently. After a critical incident, some responders will be resilient, showing no impact on functioning, and some will experience temporary symptoms of anxiety, guilt, anger and so on, or develop an Acute Stress Disorder which resolves in less than thirty days. Some will experience enduring emotional disturbance. Estimated rates of posttraumatic stress disorder (PTSD) in firefighters vary from 4.2% to 30% (Meyer, et al., 2012); Benedek, Fullerton and Ursano (2007) found 13% to 18% rates one to four years following a disaster. In police, estimates of PTSD in active-duty officers range from seven to nineteen percent (Conn, 2018). Trauma need not lead to a trauma-related diagnosis: major depression, substance abuse disorders, and other diagnoses are also seen. Extreme overprotectiveness may hide a generalized anxiety disorder, and hypervigilance may lead to obsessive behavior.

To an extent, the changes referred to above as job spillover parallel diagnostic criteria for PTSD, although symptom severity differs. Hypervigilance is a symptom of PTSD, as are negative beliefs and expectations about the world. If an adaptive ability to shut off emotions hardens into an inability to experience a full range of positive emotions, this is also a symptom. Another PTSD criterion, the avoidance of trauma cues, is not typically seen, but when trauma is job-related, avoidance is difficult to manage. In short, many responders meet some but not all criteria for a PTSD diagnosis or experience symptoms that cannot be diagnosed as PTSD because the problems are not sufficiently dysfunctional (Conn, 2018).

The impact on spouses of subclinical posttraumatic stress or "walking PTSD" may resemble the impact of the full syndrome, again with less severity. Mansfield, Schaper, Yanagida and Rosen (2014) found severe PTSD symptoms were linked to relationship dissatisfaction and reports of IPV in veterans' spouses. Subjects described the veterans as poor communicators who were "emotionally distant and easy to anger." This led to stress, sadness, isolation, and anger for the wives, who requested more spouse and family support services.

Alcohol Use

As noted earlier, alcohol is a time-honored way of dealing with potentially traumatic work experiences; physical injury puts responders at risk for opioid abuse as well (Schlosser & McAleer, 2017). Haddock et al. (2012) found that among 656 male subjects, nine percent of professional and ten percent of volunteer firefighters had driven while intoxicated in the previous thirty days. More recent work found a 4.3% rate of the same behavior in female firefighters, and a correlation between more years in the career and excessive drinking (Haddock, Poston, Jahnke & Jitnarin, 2017). This is alcohol consumption at a level that jeopardizes employment and family stability. Far greater numbers of responders use alcohol at lower but still harmful levels. Kirschman, Kamena and Fay (2014) report research showing first responders do not have a higher rate of alcohol dependency but do binge drink more than other professions.

A literature review by Rodriguez, Overup and Neighbors (2013) noted that spouses of individuals with alcohol problems report "elevated rates of anxiety, depression, and somatic concerns, as well as decreased levels of marital satisfaction," along with higher rates of mood disorders and physical and emotional abuse. They note that alcohol problems and relationship problems occur and reoccur in a chicken-and-egg "feedback loop," in which drinkers underestimate the harm alcohol use does to marital adjustment.

Unhealthy coping behaviors exist because they mitigate problems. In couples seeking treatment for alcohol abuse-related issues, "Every couple enters treatment with mixed feelings about change" (McCrady & Epstein, 2015). Positive experiences with alcohol, attachment to drinking friends, and tacit or explicit knowledge of how alcohol smooths marital interactions and socializing may decrease one or both partner's motivation for the drinking to stop. Spouses who are part of the responder community in two-career couples or by extension may ignore negative consequences of drinking longer than other partners.

When emotional numbness has become too ingrained or interaction patterns are too rigid, substance use can allow access to constricted emotions or disinhibit behavior, facilitating communication and assertiveness in the marriage (McCrady & Epstein, 2015). Drinking to facilitate sex may be seen among "rescued" wives—dysfunctional spouses who chose partners willing to prop them up—or others with a sexual abuse history. In other responders, drinking blurs negative emotions and memories, constituting part of a demand-withdrawal cycle.

To reduce or abstain from alcohol use or other problem behaviors, therapists recommend habit change and eliminating environmental cues. This modification is difficult to achieve, e.g., firefighters must continue to live with drinkers. Responders may be concerned that colleagues will be less available for life-saving back-up if they socialize together less, a possibility that must be weighed against imminent loss of the marriage and possible eventual job loss.

Betrayal and Infidelity

No review of responders' marriages would be complete without addressing a second maladaptive coping strategy, sexual encounters. Infidelity occurs in between twenty to forty percent of U. S. marriages (Marin, Christensen, & Atkins, 2014). Although no data exist, responders report that it is frequent. Like drinking, distracting extramarital affairs with "uniform junkies" can be used to numb oneself or cut through numbness. Each shift is likely to bring encounters with citizens who romanticize the work of the responder. No one is tied to a desk. Boredom is rampant. Colleagues, unlike many spouses, have common interests and shared experiences. Moreover, people do not become first responders unless they are willing to take risks.

Betrayal has special significance to this population, and in an Us vs. Them world, police officers at least, may already feel betrayed by a public they feel undervalues their service (White & Honig, 1995). Given the cynicism and dichotomous thinking of responders, truth-telling is essential. Any deviation from the truth shifts perception of the teller from trustworthy to completely untrustworthy. An acutely painful breaking of trust can be perceived in a spouse's "likes" on social media, flirting, emotional affair, or even deceptions about spending. Perceived betrayals can then be used to justify affairs that are often in part retaliatory. Other roots of unfaithfulness may lie in the custom of concealing harsher aspects of one's working life. The gap between actual activities and what is reported to a trusting spouse may begin a pattern of deception, including hiding substance use.

After an affair or other transgression, the presumed hero's fall from grace can be devastating. Responders often become depressed when they realize too late that a fling that meant little cost them the family life they held dear. When an affair is disclosed during marriage counseling, if the couple can disregard skeptics, they can consciously rebuild their relationship: in the general population, the majority of couples with this history remain married at five-year follow-up (Marin, Christensen, & Atkins, 2014).

At the end of a responder marriage, black-and-white thinking is likely to obscure any good qualities in the ex, to the detriment of co-parenting. As with any divorce, partners need to establish healthy boundaries and shield children from conflict. Adjustment becomes more complicated if the responder and the ex continue to interact in a shared workplace or a shared set of community gathering places.

BUILDING BETTER CONNECTIONS

Those wishing to support first responders' marriages can do so by showing how attitudes, beliefs and behaviors that are beneficial on the job can cause problems at home, a concept that is readily grasped. Initial expectations and the downside of putting someone on a pedestal must be examined without denigrating the genuine sacrifices made by responders and their families. In marriages involving a Rescuer who was attracted to a spouse's neediness, the Rescuer must become more trusting and less protective as the rescued partner takes on more independent functioning.

The hero myth and responder cultures can sabotage intimacy and rob the responder of needed support, by prohibiting vulnerability and discouraging emotional expression. Violanti (2014) found officers valued postcritical incident counseling sessions because they liked the result when they opened up to spouses, as recommended in the sessions. The relative value of peer versus family support remains an open question for research.

When responder couples recognize the pressures on their marriages that will push them apart if they do not "swim upstream," they can join together to actively work on improving the relationship, setting aside the assumption that lasting happiness should be effortless. Time spent with people with rewarding marriages, for example through participation in a faith community, will support this effort.

Where problems such as the overuse of alcohol or substances, pathological overeating, hypersexuality or gambling are identified, the probability that these behaviors are a way of coping with trauma or some other undiagnosed mental health problem should be considered. The behavior is unlikely to cease until underlying disorders are treated and alternative constructive ways of coping are established. Responders can and do handle stress, including posttraumatic stress, with professional help, spirituality, athleticism, creative pursuits, and time in nature.

Healing the Breach

In counseling, spouses can explore their initial expectations, noting early assumptions about strength and competence, and examine their disappointments. Training in communication skills will facilitate articulating needs and concerns, emphasizing the validity of both partners' agendas. It makes explicit the idea that the courtesies that smooth interactions on-duty should be used at home. Going forward, "sharing the headlines" of shifts, without gritty details, is encouraged, to ensure that the spouse is knowledgeable about the responder's world. Transparency usually quiets worries about attractive work partners.

Consistent with the present discussion of arousal and hypervigilance, a critically important skill for this population is emotional self-regulation, through relaxation, deep breathing or other techniques such as those used in dialectical behavior training (Dimeff & Koerner, 2007). These may be particularly important when the responder's session is scheduled shortly before, shortly after, or during a shift. Work on the marriage is advanced when each partner assumes some responsibility for his or her level of arousal—breaking out of an "all or nothing" pattern--and is able to self-soothe as needed. Apps developed for veterans, e.g., *Breathe2Relax* are helpful, portable, and carry credibility in this population. Cognitive behavioral therapy for anger reduction is useful; responders may be more willing to admit this problem than others. Training in parenting and problem-solving skills offers neutral guidelines to replace doing things "his way" or "her way."

The cognitive behavior therapy model (Dattilio, 2010) offers techniques for restructuring styles of thinking and beliefs that prevent couples from moving forward. One of these is learning to view a concern from a different frame of reference. A sampling of reframes that have proved valuable, at least in defusing initial tension, is listed below.

- Coming to see the responder's overprotectiveness as fear for a beloved family, rather than a need to control, and understanding that the fear is entirely consistent with his or her experience of the world as a dangerous place.
- Coming to see suspiciousness of the spouse as a reflex based in distrust of others, not the spouse, since infidelity is ubiquitous in the responder's environment. Threat detection easily becomes a threat in itself.
- Viewing the responder's enthusiasm about his colleagues/friends and desire to be with them as a conduit to life-saving social support rather than a frivolous or questionable use of time. The responder's natural tendency to affiliate is a coping strength.

- Recognizing some withdrawal on the part of the responder as a needed form of decompression or self-care, rather than selfishness or rejection. Respect for the responder's work must extend to respect for what he or she does to stay emotionally grounded. Couples can be counseled to build "reentry" time into their schedules, e.g., a minimum of thirty minutes for the responder to physically and psychologically separate from work during which no demands are presented by the civilian spouse. Educating couples about demand-withdrawal cycles, a universal problem, is helpful.
- Viewing a degree of emotional numbing and excessive vigilance as understandable sequelae of the job, "outsourcing" the blame to traumatic experiences instead of attributing it to character flaws in the responder.
- Understanding that a traditional head-of-the-household role includes accepting influence from the spouse.
- Recognizing that spouses' past hurtful behavior was not maliciously intended but resulted from a lack of understanding of partner needs shaped by poor communication on both sides. In other words, couples who find therapy useful—and the majority do—come to view their partners' poor behavior in the past as more ignorant than mean-spirited.

A last shift in perspective is offered, because readers may bristle at the use of the term *rescuer* in a somewhat pejorative manner. Berne's (1985) Parent-Adult-Child transactional analysis offers different vocabulary to describe a similar pattern. In his framework, the responder plays the part of authoritative and at times authoritarian and nurturing Parent, in contrast to the naïve, playful, at times irresponsible Child, or Spouse. When the Parent gets more parental or critical or authoritative, e.g., in insisting on adherence to a limited budget, the Child gets more rebellious or dismissive of the Parent's input, and vice versa. The P-A-C formulation reminds the client of the first rule for healing marriages: Begin with yourself, that is, shift into dependable Adult mode.

As the list of reframed perceptions suggests, improving relationships takes work on both sides. Core beliefs about a spouse's competence or emotional responsiveness tend to calcify over the years. Lasting change is not always possible, and the choice by a Rescuer of a partner with a history of trauma or poor decisions may make it elusive. Unfortunately, couples do not always enter treatment at the point in time when both are ready to change and both firmly wish to stay married.

Working with responder couples requires examining one's own biases, positive or negative, about first responders. The therapist should also monitor his or her personal reaction to a responder's subtle, unintentional or overt attempts at control during sessions. As the therapist reigns in job spillover behaviors, he or she will need to address any perception of alliance with the spouse against the responder. Sensitivity to the meaning of independence, power, and gender roles in different cultures must be maintained while helping to modify schema and behavior that the clients themselves have identified as contributing to their unhappiness. The therapist should be prepared to support same-sex or mixed-sex marriages and to respect conservative views, e.g., on a daughter's sexuality. Last, the therapist must be a source of appropriate referrals as many cases involving trauma, violence or addiction require specialists in these areas.

Couples' therapists are probably more likely than individual therapists to hear unfiltered accounts of misconduct on the part of responder. When a therapist is integrated into a responder department or community and his or her income depends on the allegiance of that community, the therapist may hesitate to damage the relationship by reporting abuse, initiating an involuntary hospitalization for a suicidal client, or in other ways. As an example, in Houston a responder was found guilty of embezzling more than $600,000 from union funds over seven years. Had he confessed while in therapy, the therapist could not have reported the crime without risking his or her license. The limits of confidentiality must be crystal clear to all concerned. The perception that it will be maintained in every instance except as mandated by state law is critical to responders' utilization of mental health services. Trust can be fragile.

The Department's Role

In part, improving responder marriages requires changing aspects of the occupational cultures surrounding these professions. They often embrace traditional masculinity which has been shown to discourage help-seeking and normalize risky behavior such as excessive drinking (Pappas, 2019). Seeking mental health services is stigmatized. Leadership can promote self-care and seeking professional help, and ease access to qualified therapists whose knowledge of responder stress is bolstered by ride-alongs and participation in other department events. Professional services should be complemented by continuously available peer-support teams and chaplaincy services. Discussion of the impact of responder stress on family life is appropriate in training academies and periodically throughout the responder's career.

Trainees and veterans should be encouraged to retain interests and friendships outside the first responder world, which enhance coping by offering affirmation for those who lack acceptance at work, diversified social support, and positive experiences in the community to partially balance negative on-duty experiences. This also prepares the responder for eventual retirement, when responders whose identity centers on the career and colleagues may be particularly vulnerable to depression.

Departments are encouraged to sponsor programs to strengthen family life for couples or spouses alone, such as the Houston Police Department's voluntary classes on Stepfamily Living, and the Mesquite, Texas Healthy Marriage and Family Project (Garmezy & Cummins, 2000; Westphal, 2009). Presentations can normalize predictable stressors of the career, such as self-blame on the part of firefighters, jumpstarting discussions of these topics. Moreover, they can educate, offer support and publicize resources regarding career-related concerns such as secondary trauma and more universal relationship concerns. Less formally, family open houses, recreational events, ceremonies, and spouse groups all help to build social networks. When spouses feel they, too, gain a welcoming second family via the responder's career, they will be better positioned to withstand the career stressors that change their lives, and to help responders withstand them. In law enforcement, proactive communication with spouses following critical incidents can be considered a best practice (e.g., Usher, Friedhoff, Cochran, & Pandya, 2016).

Supporting marriage and social connections, including among spouses, promotes employee wellness. Research underscores the links between social support and improved health and between strong marriages and better health outcomes, including decreased absenteeism (Johnson, 2012; Schetter, 2017). The first responder professions stand out as a bastion of connectedness at a time when the hazards of isolation and aloneness in contemporary society are increasingly recognized. It is cause for optimism that healthy marriages are likely to indirectly decrease employees' vulnerability to the depression, alcoholism, and other concerns that arguably are as much a part of responder culture as the acquired "job tools" described here.

In conclusion, an observation from a divorced former client could be broadcast in training academies everywhere. After his second wife left, the officer commented, "You might as well keep the one you have because they're all the same." He was right; they are. All expect emotional support and all expect that their needs as well as their partners' needs will be met.

Most responder marriages fulfill these hopes. The survival of these relationships in the currents that swirl around them is a tribute to the strength and resilience of responders and the people they marry.

ACKNOWLEDGMENT

The support of S. J. Buser, Ph.D., Clinical Director, Houston Fire Department CISM Team, is gratefully acknowledged.

REFERENCES

Benedek, D. M., Fullerton, C., & Ursano, R. (2007). First responders: Mental health consequences of natural and human-made disasters for public health and public safety workers. *Annual Review of Public Health*. doi:10.1146/annurev.publichealth.28.021406.144037 PMID:17367284

Berne, E. (1985). *Games people play: The basic handbook of transactional analysis*. New York: Ballantine Books.

Bohl-Penrod, N. K., & Clark, D. W. (2017). Peer support in public safety organizations. In C. L. Mitchell & E. H. Dorian (Eds.), *Police psychology and its growing impact on modern law enforcement* (pp. 237–251). Hershey, PA: IGI Global.

Bureau of Labor Statistics, U. S. Department of Labor. (2017). *Occupational outlook handbook*. Retrieved from http://bls.gov

Cieslak, R., Luszczynska, A., Shoji, K., Douglas, A., Melville, E., & Benight, C. C. (2014). A meta-analysis of the relationship between job burnout and secondary traumatic stress among workers with indirect exposure to trauma. *Psychological Services*, *11*(1), 75–86. doi:10.1037/a0033798 PMID:23937082

Dattilio, F. M. (2010). *Cognitive-behavioral therapy with couples and families: A comprehensive guide for clinicians*. New York: Guilford Press.

DeAngelis, T. (2019). The legacy of trauma. *Monitor on Psychology*, *50*, 36–43.

Dimeff, L. A., & Koerner, K. (2017). *Dialectical Behavior Therapy in clinical practice: Applications across disorders and settings*. New York: Guilford Press.

Gagliano, A. (2014). *Why women leave*. Retrieved from http://fireengineering.com

Gagliano, A., & Gagliano, M. (2018). *Challenges of the firefighter marriage*. Tulsa, OK: Fire Engineering Books & Videos.

Garmezy, L. B., & Cummins, V. L. (2000). *Preventing police stress through co-training of officers and spouses*. Poster session presented at the meeting of the American Psychological Association, Washington, DC.

Gerber, G. L., & Ward, K. C. (2011). Police personality: Theoretical issues and research. In J. Kitaeff (Ed.), *Handbook of police psychology* (pp. 421–436). New York: Routledge.

Haddock, C. K., Jahnke, S. A., Poston, W. S., Jitnarin, K., Kaipust, C. M., Tuley, B., & Hyder, M. L. (2012). Alcohol use among firefighters in the Central United States. *Occupational Medicine*, *62*(8), 661–664. doi:10.1093/occmed/kqs162 PMID:23064207

Haddock, C. K., Poston, W. S., Jahnke, S. A., & Jitnarin. (2017). Alcohol use and problem drinking among women firefighters. *Women's Health Issues, 27*, 632-638. Retrieved from http://whijournal.com

Hall, M. H., Brindle, R. C., & Buysse, D. J. (2018). Sleep and cardiovascular disease: Emerging opportunities for psychologists. *The American Psychologist*, *73*(8), 994–1006. doi:10.1037/amp0000362 PMID:30394778

Hansen, J. (2017). Night shift work and risk of breast cancer. *Current Environmental Health Reports, 4*, 325-339. Retrieved from http://ncbi.nlm.nih.gov doi/ doi:10.100740572-017-0155-y

Henderson, S. N., Van Hasselt, V. B., LeDuc, T. J., & Couwels, J. (2016). Firefighter suicide: Understanding cultural challenges for mental health professionals. *Professional Psychology, Research and Practice*, *47*(3), 224–230. doi:10.1037/pro0000072

Jahnke, S. A. (2015). Firefighter divorce: 3 important facts. *FireRescue1*. Retrieved from http://firerescue1.com

Johnson, M. D. (2012). Healthy marriage initiatives: On the need for empiricism in policy implementation. *The American Psychologist*, *67*(4), 296–308. doi:10.1037/a0027743 PMID:22468785

Kimbrel, N. A., Steffen, L. E., Meyer, E. C., Kruse, M. I., Knight, J. A., Zimering, R. T., & Gulliver, S. B. (2011). A revised measure of occupational stress for firefighters: Psychometric properties and relationship to posttraumatic stress disorder, depression and substance abuse. *Psychological Services*, *8*(4), 294–306. doi:10.1037/a0025845

Kirschman, E. (2004). *I love a fire fighter: What the family needs to know*. New York: Guilford Press.

Kirschman, E., Kamena, M., & Fay, J. (2014). *Counseling cops: What clinicians need to know*. New York: Guilford Press.

Lamia, M. C., & Krieger, M. J. (2009). *The White Knight Syndrome: Rescuing yourself from your need to rescue others*. Oakland, CA: New Harbinger Publications.

Mansfield, A. J., Schaper, K. M., Yanagida, A. M., & Rose, C. S. (2014). One day at a time: The experiences of partners of veterans with posttraumatic stress disorder. *Professional Psychology, Research and Practice*, *45*, 488–495.

Marier, C. J., & Moule, R. K. (2018). Feeling blue: Officer perceptions of public antipathy predict police occupational norms (Abstract). *American Journal of Criminal Justice*, advance online publication. Retrieved from http://link.springer.com

Marin, R. A., Christensen, A., & Atkins, D. C. (2014). Infidelity and behavioral couple therapy: Relationship outcomes over 5 years following therapy. *Couple & Family Psychology*, *3*, 1–12.

McCoy, S. P., & Aamodt, M. G. (2010). A comparison of law enforcement divorce rates with those of other occupations. *Journal of Police and Criminal Psychology*, *25*, 1–16.

McCrady, B. S., & Epstein, E. E. (2015). Couple therapy and alcohol problems. In A. S. Gurman, J. L. Lebow, & D. K. Snyder (Eds.), *Clinical Handbook of Couple Therapy* (5th ed.; pp. 555–584). New York: Guilford.

Meyer, E. C., Zimering, R. T., Daly, E., Knight, J., Kanholz, B. W., & Gulliver, S. B. (2012). Predictors of posttraumatic stress disorder and other psychological symptoms in trauma-exposed firefighters. *Psychological Services*, *9*, 1–15. PMID:22449083

National Center for Women and Policing. (2018). *Police family violence fact sheet*. Retrieved from http://www.womenandpolicing.com/violencefs.asp

Neff, L. A., & Karney, B. R. (2009). Stress and reactivity to daily relationship experiences: How stress hinders adaptive processes in marriage. *Journal of Personality and Social Psychology*, *97*(3), 435–450. doi:10.1037/a0015663 PMID:19686000

Pappas, S. (2019). APA issues first-ever guidelines for practice with men and boys. *Monitor on Psychology*, *50*, 34–39.

Patton, C. L., Smith, S. F., & Lilienfeld, S. O. (2018). Psychopathy and heroism in first responders: Traits cut from the same cloth? *Personality Disorders*, *9*, 354–368. PMID:29120196

Rodriguez, L. M., Overup, C. S., & Neighbors, C. (2013). Perceptions of partner's problematic alcohol use affect relationship outcomes beyond partner self-reported drinking: Alcohol use in committed romantic relationships. *Psychology of Addictive Behaviors*, *27*, 627–638. PMID:23438240

Ross, J. M., Karney, B. R., Nguyen, T. P., & Bradbury, T. N. (2018). Communication that is maladaptive for middle-class couples is adaptive for socioeconomically disadvantaged couples. *Journal of Personality and Social Psychology*; advance online publication. doi:10.1037/pspi0000158 PMID:30321045

Rzeszutek, M., Partyka, M., & Golab, A. (2015). Temperament traits, social support, and secondary traumatic stress disorder symptoms in a sample of trauma therapists. *Professional Psychology, Research and Practice*, *46*(4), 213–220. doi:10.1037/pro0000024

Schetter, C. D. (2017). Moving research on health and close relationships forward—a challenge and an obligation: Introduction to the Special Issue. *The American Psychologist*, *72*(6), 511–516. doi:10.1037/amp0000158 PMID:28880098

Schlosser, L. Z., & McAleer, G. (2017). *Opioid use disorders among police and public safety personnel: What law enforcement leaders need to know*. Retrieved from: http://www.policechiefmagazine.org/opioid-use-among-police-personnel/?ref=279dcb8fe44480f796646d6de97346de

Schockley, K. M., DeNunzio, M. M., Shen, W., Arvan, M. L., & Knudsen, E. A. (2017). Disentangling the relationship between gender and work-family conflict: An integration of theoretical perspectives using meta-analytic methods. *The Journal of Applied Psychology*, *102*(12), 1601–1635. doi:10.1037/apl0000246 PMID:28749157

Smith, L. J., Paulus, D. J., Gallagher, M. W., Norman, S. B., Tran, J. K., & Vujanovic, A. A. (2018). Perceived stress and probable alcohol misuse in firefighters: The role of posttraumatic stress. *International Journal of Stress Management*; advance online publication. doi:10.1037tr0000118

Stinson, P. M., & Liederbach, J. (2013). *Fox in the henhouse: A study of police officers arrested for crimes associated with domestic or family violence.* Bowling Green State University Criminal Justice Faculty Publications. Retrieved from https://scholarworks.bgsu.edu/crim_just_pub/6

Usher, L., Friedhoff, S., Cochran, S., & Pandya, A. (2016). *Preparing for the unimaginable: How chiefs can safeguard officer mental health before and after mass casualty events.* Washington, DC: U. S. Department of Justice Office of Community Oriented Policing Services.

Violanti, J. M. (2010). Police suicide: A national comparison with firefighter and military personnel. *Policing: An International Journal of Police Strategies & Management, 33*(2), 270–286. doi:10.1108/13639511011044885

Violanti, J. M. (2014). *Dying for the job: Police work exposure and health.* Springfield, IL: Charles C. Thomas.

Westphal, G. (2009). Law Enforcement Healthy Marriage and Family Project. *The Police Chief, 76*, 48–50.

White, E. K., & Honig, A. L. (1995). Law enforcement families. In M. I. Kurke & E. M. Scrivner (Eds.), *Police psychology into the 21st century* (pp. 189–206). Hillsdale, NJ: Lawrence Erlbaum Associates.

ADDITIONAL READING

Ashton, A., Lillis, R., & Ramirez, W. (2018, August 6). 249 nights away at California fires: Firefighter families cope with a 'new normal.' *The Sacramento Bee.* Retrieved from http://www.sacbee.com

Carpenter, B., Gillepsie, D., & Jorge, R. (2019). *Developing firefighter resiliency.* Tulsa, OK: Fire Engineering Books & Videos.

Jahnke, S. A., Poston, W. S., Jitnarin, N., & Haddock, C. K. (2018). Maternal and child health among female firefighters in the U.S. *Maternal and Child Health Journal, 22*(6), 922–931; advance online publication. doi:10.100710995-018-2468-3 PMID:29423588

Kiecolt-Glaser, J. K. (2018). Marriage, divorce, and the immune system. *The American Psychologist, 73*(9), 1098–1108. doi:10.1037/amp0000388 PMID:30525786

Lanza, A., Roysircar, G., & Rodgers, S. (2018). First responder mental healthcare: Evidence-based prevention, postvention, and treatment. *Professional Psychology, Research and Practice, 49*(3), 193–204. doi:10.1037/pro0000192

Neria, Y., DiGrande, L., & Adams, B. G. (2011). Posttraumatic stress disorder following the September 11, 2001, terrorist attacks: A review of the literature among highly exposed populations. *The American Psychologist, 66*(6), 429–446. doi:10.1037/a0024791 PMID:21823772

Wile, D. B. (2008). *After the honeymoon: How conflict can improve your relationship* (rev. ed.). Oakland, CA: Collaborative Couple Therapy Books.

Chapter 3
Posttraumatic Stress and Alcohol Use Among First Responders

Lia J Smith
University of Houston, USA

Maya Zegel
University of Houston, USA

Brooke A. Bartlett
University of Houston, USA

Antoine Lebeaut
University of Houston, USA

Anka A Vujanovic
University of Houston, USA

ABSTRACT

Developing research suggests that the co-occurrence of posttraumatic stress disorder (PTSD) and alcohol use disorder (AUD) is a significant clinical concern across first responder populations. This comorbidity is difficult to treat and marked by a more costly, complex, and chronic clinical course when compared to either disorder alone. Significant associations between PTSD/AUD comorbidity and various psychological, behavioral, and physical health outcomes among first responder samples have been documented. This chapter provides a theoretical framework and empirical review of the literature relevant to PTSD/AUD in the context of firefighter, police, and other first responder populations (e.g., emergency medical technicians). Future directions, utilizing varied methodologies and assessment tools, and focusing upon varied first responder populations are enumerated to build upon this preliminary, yet clinically meaningful, empirical foundation. This research domain has great potential to inform specialized, evidence-based clinical care for first responders.

DOI: 10.4018/978-1-5225-9803-9.ch003

INTRODUCTION

The co-occurrence of posttraumatic stress disorder (PTSD) and alcohol use disorder (AUD) is an increasingly significant clinical concern across first responder populations (e.g., firefighters, police officers, rescue workers; Chopko, Palmieri, & Adams, 2013; Harvey et al., 2016; Ménard & Arter, 2013; Paulus, Vujanovic, Schuhmann, Smith, & Tran, 2017). While the PTSD/AUD comorbidity is well-established and highly prevalent among both the general population and military veterans (e.g., Fuehrlein et al., 2016; Grant et al., 2015; Kessler, Chiu, Demler, & Walters, 2005; Milliken, Auchterlonie, & Hoge, 2007; Pietrzak, Goldstein, Southwick, & Grant, 2011), our understanding of PTSD/AUD among first responders is much more limited. Broadly, across populations, both research and clinical practice have demonstrated that PTSD/AUD is difficult-to-treat and marked by a more costly, complex, and chronic clinical course when compared to either disorder alone (e.g., McCauley, Killeen, Gros, Brady, & Back, 2012; Mills, Teesson, Ross, & Peters, 2006; Schafer & Najavits, 2007; Vujanovic, Bonn-Miller, & Petry, 2016). Among first responder populations, available literature suggests that first responders may use alcohol to cope with PTSD-related symptomatology (Simons, Gaher, Jacobs, Meyer, & Johnson-Jimenez, 2005; Smith, Gallagher, Tran, & Vujanovic, 2018; Tomaka, Magoc, Morales-Monks, & Reyes, 2017). Further, emergent literature suggests that PTSD/AUD has important clinical implications among first responders due to documented associations with various mental health concerns (e.g., depression and suicidality; Chopko et al., 2013; Pietrzak et al., 2012; Violanti, 2004), behavioral health issues (e.g., sleep disturbance; Yun, Ahn, Jeong, Joo, & Choi, 2015), and occupational problems (e.g., occupational stress, critical incidents, work productivity; Chopko et al., 2013; Kim, Park, & Kim, 2017; Ménard & Arter, 2013, 2014).

Available research among first responders suggests that PTSD and AUD symptoms are both highly prevalent. This extant research also underscores the potential clinical relevance of this comorbidity, although epidemiological studies documenting actual prevalence rates within first responder populations are lacking. Building upon our understanding of the PTSD/AUD comorbidity among first responders can inform evidence-based prevention and intervention efforts. While attention to first responders has increased in recent years, several methodological challenges and gaps exist, which warrant future scientific attention. Thus, the objective of the current chapter is to provide a clinically-informed theoretical framework and summary of the literature regarding of PTSD/AUD among first responders. Current methodological limitations will be enumerated and future directions will be discussed to propel this domain of inquiry further and to advance evidence-based mental health services for first responders.

BACKGROUND

First responders represent an at-risk population with regard to alcohol misuse and AUD (e.g., Jones, 2017). Among firefighters, for example, nearly half report current excessive alcohol use (i.e., 3 or more drinks per occasion) and one-third report past-month heavy episodic drinking (i.e., 5 or more drinks per occasion; Haddock, Day, Poston, Jahnke, & Jitnarin, 2015). Lifetime AUD prevalence rates are substantial among firefighters, with approximately 47% reporting a lifetime AUD (North, Tivis, McMillen, Pfefferbaum, Spitznagel, et al., 2002), which is significantly higher than the 29.1% lifetime AUD prevalence documented in the general population (Grant et al., 2015). Further, among urban police officers, 18.1% of men and 15.9% of women report experiencing adverse consequences from alcohol use (e.g., driving while intoxicated, occupational problems), with 7.8% of the sample meeting criteria for lifetime AUD (Ballenger et al., 2011). Overall, the prevalence of alcohol misuse and AUD symptoms among first responders underscores the importance of better understanding factors related to alcohol use among this unique population.

PTSD symptomatology provides an important avenue to better understand alcohol use among first responders. Indeed, by virtue of their careers, first responders are particularly at-risk for exposure to traumatic events and PTSD symptomatology (e.g., Jones, 2017). Duty-related trauma exposure has been estimated to be as high as 91.5% among firefighters (Meyer et al., 2012) and 94% among paramedic trainees (Fjeldheim et al., 2014). Furthermore, research among police officers has found that those within small and midsize departments had an average exposure rate of 188 work-related potentially traumatic events over the course of their careers (Chopko, Palmieri, & Adams, 2015). The estimated prevalence of current (i.e., present in the past month) PTSD among first responders varies widely. For example, estimates among firefighters range from 8% (Del Ben, Scotti, Chen, & Fortson, 2006) to 22.2% in the United States ([US]; Corneil, Beaton, Murphy, Johnson, & Pike, 1999), depending upon the assessment methods utilized and samples studied. Estimates also suggest that 21% of emergency medical personnel (EMS) and paramedics (Jones, 2017) and 24% of police officers meet diagnostic criteria for current PTSD (Fox et al., 2012). General US population estimates, in contrast, have reported that the 12-month prevalence of PTSD is 4.7% and lifetime prevalence is 8.3% (Kilpatrick et al., 2013). Many more first responders may also suffer from subclinical PTSD, which is associated with similar levels of impairment as diagnostic PTSD in general population samples (e.g., Bergman, Przeworski, & Feeny, 2016; Pietrzak et al., 2011; Zlotnick, Franklin, & Zimmerman, 2002).

While PTSD/AUD remains understudied among first responders, mounting work has evaluated the associations between PTSD and AUD symptoms among first responders with attention to psychological mechanisms underlying and related to this association (e.g. Chopko et al., 2013; Harvey et al., 2016; Ménard & Arter, 2013; Paulus et al., 2017; Wagner, Heinrichs, & Ehlert, 1998). Across studies, the self-medication model of PTSD/AUD comorbidity has been highlighted, positing that first responders with PTSD symptomatology may be at a heightened risk for alcohol misuse and AUD due to a tendency to use alcohol as a means of coping with negative affect (Khantzian, 1999; Ménard & Arter, 2013; Simpson, Stappenbeck, Luterek, Lehavot, & Kaysen, 2014; Smith et al., 2018; Tomaka et al., 2017). Despite the focus on the self-medication model of comorbidity, it is important to note that other trajectories may also be pertinent to understand PTSD/AUD among first responders. For example, AUD might lead to greater off-hours drinking behavior among first responders, which may in turn lead to increased risk of non-duty-related trauma exposure (e.g., motor vehicle accidents, physical violence). Alternatively, AUD and PTSD may develop concurrently following trauma exposure (e.g., Murphy, Beaton, Pike, & Johnson, 1999). Given the clinical complexity of PTSD/AUD comorbidity, it is important to better understand this relationship within specific first responder populations.

MAIN FOCUS OF THE CHAPTER

Empirical Research in Firefighters Populations

Empirical research among firefighters has exploded within the past few years, facilitating increased understanding of PTSD/AUD associations in this vulnerable population. Most of the work in this area has been limited to the documentation of positive associations between PTSD symptoms and alcohol use, using survey-based cross-sectional designs (e.g., Ci, Lan, Zhang, Zhou, & De, 2015; Smith et al., 2011; Stanley, Boffa, Hom, Kimbrel, & Joiner, 2017). However, an increasing number of studies have focused on specific alcohol- and PTSD-related outcomes, as enumerated below.

Alcohol outcomes. Studies examining alcohol outcomes, specifically, have found evidence for heavy alcohol use throughout various firefighter populations. For example, within a sample of male urban firefighters (*N* =2,707), 30% met criteria for *Diagnostic and Statistical Manual of Mental Disorders* (4th ed; *DSM-IV*) probable alcohol dependence (RAPS4; Cherpitel, 2000). This study further demonstrated that higher levels of depression were positively correlated with alcohol-related outcomes for firefighters with lower, but not higher, levels of PTSD symptoms (Paulus et al., 2017). Longitudinal research conducted prospectively over 3 years demonstrated that PTSD symptoms predicted a greater number of alcoholic drinks consumed per week among firefighters recruited from seven US cities (Gulliver et al., 2018). Furthermore, associations have been documented between PTSD symptom severity and probable alcohol misuse (Smith et al., 2018) as well as increased alcohol use problems, as based upon self-report screening measures (Chang et al., 2016; Kim et al., 2017; Kim, Park, & Kim, 2018). Heavy alcohol use has also been evidenced within firefighter subgroups, such as women firefighters (*N* =1,913), with findings indicating that women firefighter 'problem drinkers' (score of ≥2 on the CAGE; O'Brien, 2008) were 2.5 times more likely to report symptoms of PTSD than non-problem drinkers (Haddock, Poston, Jahnke, & Jitnarin, 2017). Additionally, longitudinal work in urban fire departments (*N* = 188), conducted prospectively across two years (Murphy et al., 1999), found a positive correlation between PTSD 'caseness' (IES score of ≥ 26; Horowitz, Wilner, & Alvarez, 1979) at baseline and self-reported drinking problems at two year follow-up.

Two studies to date have examined the association between the factor structure of PTSD symptom clusters and alcohol outcomes in racial/ethnic minority populations of firefighters. First, Arbona and Schwartz (2016) evaluated the *DSM-IV* dysphoria model of PTSD symptoms (i.e., re-experiencing, avoidance, dysphoria, and hyperarousal; Simms, Watson, & Doebbeling, 2002) among Hispanic male career firefighters (*N* = 551) and found that the dysphoria symptom cluster, indexed via the PTSD Checklist (Weathers, Litz, Herman, Huska, & Keane, 1993), showed the strongest correlation with *DSM-IV* alcohol abuse/dependence (*r* = .37), indexed via the RAPS4 (Cherpitel, 2000). Further, when controlling for marital status, PTSD re-experiencing and dysphoria symptom clusters contributed unique variance to *DSM-IV* alcohol abuse/dependence (Arbona & Schwartz, 2016). Relatedly, among African-American male firefighters from the same fire department, Arbona, Fan, and Noor (2016) demonstrated that each PTSD symptom cluster in the dysphoria model had low magnitude (*r* = .20 - .29) significant correlations with *DSM-IV* alcohol abuse/dependence, also indexed via the RAPS4 (Cherpitel, 2000).

To date, three studies have examined alcohol use motives, broadly, among firefighters (North, Tivis, McMillen, Pfefferbaum, Cox, et al., 2002; Smith et al., 2018; Tomaka et al., 2017). These studies have demonstrated that drinking to cope with negative affect is associated with greater PTSD symptomatology (Smith et al., 2018; Tomaka et al., 2017) and functional impairment (North, Tivis, McMillen, Pfefferbaum, Cox, et al., 2002). In addition, coping-oriented alcohol use motives were found to mediate, or account for, the association between PTSD symptoms and problem drinking (Tomaka et al., 2017).

PTSD outcomes. Several studies investigating PTSD/AUD associations among firefighters have focused upon PTSD-related outcomes. Much of this work has studied firefighter populations exposed to the World Trade Center disaster on 9/11/2001 (i.e., 9/11; Berninger, Webber, Cohen, et al., 2010; Berninger, Webber, Niles, et al., 2010; Chiu et al., 2011; Soo et al., 2011). For example, a study examining firefighters ($N = 5,656$) exposed to 9/11 demonstrated that an increase in alcohol use in the immediate aftermath of the disaster was associated with probable current PTSD, as indexed by the PTSD Checklist (PCL) for *DSM-5* (PCL-5; Blevins, Weathers, Davis, Witte, & Domino, 2015), and delayed onset of probable PTSD 1.6-3.8 years following 9/11 (Berninger, Webber, Niles, et al., 2010). Furthermore, an analysis of retired firefighters exposed to 9/11 ($N = 1,915$) demonstrated that depression mediated the association between alcohol use and PTSD (Chiu et al., 2011). Overall, results from these studies suggest that firefighters may use alcohol as a means of coping with distress.

Clinical correlates. Several studies discussed above have demonstrated that depression symptomatology may be a clinical correlate relevant to both PTSD and alcohol use among firefighters (e.g., Arbona & Schwartz, 2016; Chiu et al., 2011; Lima Ede, Assuncao, & Barreto, 2015; Paulus et al., 2017), as consistent with literature on general population samples (e.g., Lee, Liverant, Lowmaster, Gradus, & Sloan, 2014; Murphy et al., 2013; Weinberger, Maciejewski, McKee, Reutenauer, & Mazure, 2009). In addition, Martin and colleagues (2017) examined male urban firefighters ($N = 2,883$) and found that alcohol dependence, indexed via self-report, was indirectly related to suicide risk through severity of depression and posttraumatic stress. Finally, sleep disturbance has been found to moderate, or exacerbate, the association between PTSD symptom severity and both alcohol use severity alcohol use coping motives among firefighters (Smith et al., 2018). This is an important avenue for further study given that irregular sleep schedules and overnight shifts may lead to chronic sleep disturbance in firefighters.

Empirical Research in Police Populations

Research relevant to PTSD/AUD associations among police populations, as compared to firefighter populations, is scant. Much of the work among police officers has been focused upon documenting average PTSD symptom levels and alcohol use rates (e.g., Fox et al., 2012; Violanti et al., 2011). Similar to the research among firefighter populations, published studies among police (enumerated below) have largely been limited to the documentation of associations between PTSD symptoms and alcohol use, using survey-based cross-sectional designs.

Alcohol outcomes. Studies focused on associations between PTSD symptomatology and alcohol use outcomes are limited. Broadly, PTSD symptoms have been related to number of daily alcoholic drinks (e.g., McCanlies, Mnatsakanova, Andrew, Burchfiel, & Violanti, 2014) and probable alcohol problems (e.g., Chopko, Facemire, Palmieri, & Schwartz, 2016; Chopko, Palmieri, & Facemire, 2014; Mumford, Taylor, & Kubu, 2015; Pietrzak et al., 2012). Building upon these associations, a cross-sectional study of urban police officers ($N = 747$) found that higher PTSD severity was related to greater probability of lifetime alcohol-related problems, but not to current alcohol use (i.e., prior week alcohol consumption and past month binge drinking; Ballenger et al., 2011). Additionally, a study examining police from 13 different countries ($N = 1,453$) found that the interaction of more severe critical (i.e., traumatic) incidents and increased PTSD symptom severity predicted heightened problematic drinking for men, but not women, police officers (Ménard & Arter, 2014). Finally, a study examining police officers in a mid-western state (N = 193) found that greater PTSD avoidance symptoms, specifically, were related to the alcohol dependence and hazardous use but not harmful use (Chopko et al., 2013).

To date, one study has examined alcohol use motives among police officers (Ménard & Arter, 2013). This study (N = 750) demonstrated significant positive bivariate associations between problematic alcohol use and *DSM-IV* PTSD symptom severity. Further, negative coping strategies demonstrated direct and indirect associations with problematic alcohol use and *DSM-IV* PTSD symptom severity through critical incident severity.

PTSD outcomes. There is a paucity of research examining associations between alcohol use and PTSD-related outcomes among police officers. One study (Inslicht et al., 2010) utilized a prospective longitudinal design to follow urban police officers (N = 278) from academy training through the following 12 months of service. Here, family history of substance use, including alcohol, increased the risk for experiencing greater peritraumatic distress during critical incident exposure which, in turn, increased the risk for developing symptoms of PTSD among police officers.

Clinical correlates. Clinical correlates of PTSD/AUD-relevant associations among police officers have also been understudied, and existing work has focused almost exclusively on suicidal ideation. First, in an examination of Northeastern police offices in the US (N = 115), the comorbid risk of PTSD and problematic alcohol use increased the odds of suicide ideation by a factor of 10 (Violanti, 2004). However, in another report, PTSD symptoms and problematic alcohol use were not significantly associated with suicidal ideation, with only depression emerging as a significant predictor of suicidal ideation among Midwestern police offices in the US (N=193; Chopko et al., 2014). Notably, all studies were cross-sectional and utilized self-report measures of the variables of interest.

Empirical Research in Other First Responder Populations

Research relevant to PTSD/AUD associations among other first responder populations is significantly limited. This work has frequently been cross-sectional in nature and often groups together various first responder populations, such as trained volunteers, emergency healthcare providers, psychosocial healthcare providers (e.g., religious counselors, social workers), and civilian rescue workers alongside firefighters and police officers into heterogeneous samples. Much of this work has documented significant positive associations between PTSD symptom levels and alcohol use (Bogstrand, Skogstad, & Ekeberg, 2016), possible alcohol problems (Bromet et al., 2016; Yip, Zeig-Owens, Webber, et al., 2016), and alcohol use coping motives (Stewart, Mitchell, Wright, & Loba, 2004). Overall, similar to work focused on firefighter and police officer populations, high rates of PTSD and alcohol use were noted descriptively (e.g., Carleton et al., 2018; Osofsky et al., 2011; Yip, Zeig-Owens, Hall, et al., 2016). As described below, few articles have examined associations between alcohol use and PTSD outcomes in other first responders. No published studies to date have documented PTSD symptoms with regard to alcohol use outcomes or examined clinical correlates of PTSD/AUD among other first responder populations.

PTSD outcomes. First, among American Red Cross workers who responded to 9/11, changes in alcohol use following disaster response use was associated with all *DSM-IV* PTSD symptom cluster severity; and elevated alcohol use severity was associated specifically with *DSM-IV* PTSD avoidance and hyperarousal symptom severity (Simons et al., 2005). Additionally, in a large study of nationally registered emergency medical technicians and paramedics, alcohol use severity was positively related to PTSD symptom severity, particularly for those endorsing higher chronic stress and critical incident stress (Donnelly, 2012). Finally, one study to date examined the association between the factor structure of

PTSD symptom clusters and alcohol use outcomes in first responders, broadly. Specifically, Ruggero et al. (2013) evaluated the *DSM-IV* dysphoria model of PTSD symptoms (i.e., re-experiencing, avoidance, dysphoria, and hyperarousal; Simms et al., 2002) among 9/11 responders ($N = 954$) and found that the PTSD avoidance symptom cluster, indexed via the PCL, showed the strongest association with *DSM-IV* alcohol abuse (Ruggero et al., 2013).

SOLUTIONS AND RECOMMENDATIONS

There is increasing recognition of the prevalence and clinical significance of PTSD/AUD associations among first responder populations. The emergent literature has consistently confirmed positive associations between PTSD symptom severity and alcohol use severity, with limited research documenting associations between PTSD symptom severity and alcohol use coping motives, specifically. This literature suggests that first responders experiencing elevated PTSD symptoms may be at risk for problematic alcohol use, and conversely, that first responders presenting with alcohol use problems may also have heightened PTSD symptoms. It is important to build upon this important literature in order to inform specialized, evidence-based interventions tailored to the unique needs of first responders.

The extant research is limited in several key ways that should be addressed by future work in order to promote a more clinically meaningful understanding of PTSD/AUD comorbidity among first responders. First, extant research has utilized primarily cross-sectional designs, restricting our ability to formulate conclusions about temporality or causality. Relatedly, most studies have relied almost exclusively on self-report indices of PTSD and alcohol use. More concentrated research efforts are needed, utilizing longitudinal designs as well as interview-based and experimental measures to better understand associations between PTSD and AUD symptomatology. Second, more representative national and international samples are needed in order to inform the external validity of findings. With representative samples, researchers will be able to more conclusively determine prevalence rates of diagnostic and subclinical PTSD and AUD as well as to evaluate similarities and differences in functioning and clinical outcomes of clinical versus subclinical symptom ranges. Similarly, exploring racial/ethnic and gender differences in PTSD/AUD associations among first responders will be crucial to enhancing our understanding of the manifestations of this comorbidity across unique segments of the population. Third, the literature has inconsistently assessed trauma exposure per *DSM* criteria, a necessary element to diagnosing and understanding PTSD reactions. Notably, trauma assessment among first responders may require unique approaches as this population may come to normalize their traumatic event exposure, therefore limiting their reporting of events labeled as "traumatic." Describing events more specifically (e.g., flood or hurricane versus 'natural disaster') may aid in more accurate assessments of potentially traumatic experiences. Finally, first responders are often contacted for participation in research studies within their places of work. This may lead to biased and/or under-reporting, and therefore, researchers may consider contacting first responders in forums unrelated to work to improve validity of responses.

FUTURE RESEARCH DIRECTIONS

Future research directions and opportunities are wide and vast. We foresee several areas of inquiry, in addition to those already discussed above, with important implications for first responder populations. First, research examining similarities and differences between various first responder populations with regard to PTSD/AUD symptomatology would elucidate if there are distinct and/or overlapping treatment needs across first responders. Few studies have examined between-group comparisons and this work has largely been limited to descriptive analyses (i.e., mean differences). Second, while emerging research has documented positive associations between PTSD symptom severity with coping-oriented alcohol use (Ménard & Arter, 2013; North, Tivis, McMillen, Pfefferbaum, Cox, et al., 2002; Smith et al., 2018; Stewart et al., 2004; Tomaka et al., 2017), this area of work remains scant. Future work may expand upon these initial studies and contribute vital knowledge about *why* and *in what contexts* first responders consume alcohol in order to inform alcohol reduction intervention and prevention programs. Third, additional research examining associations between PTSD/AUD and relevant clinical correlates (e.g., depression, suicidality, sleep disturbance, occupational outcomes) is needed. More advanced, rigorous study of such correlates can facilitate our understanding of the complex interplay of such factors in the etiology, maintenance, or exacerbation of PTSD/AUD in first responders. This line of work can also inform intervention and prevention efforts for high risk behaviors, such as suicidal behavior or driving while intoxicated. Fourth, studying first responder 'culture' is important for better understanding the potential impact of professional identity and mental health-related stigma on emotional awareness and communication as well as treatment initiation (Hom, Stanley, Ringer, & Joiner, 2016). Finally, examining moderators and mediators of PTSD/AUD associations (e.g., sleep disturbance, emotion regulation) will increase our understanding of transdiagnostic and biopsychosocial processes underlying this complex interplay of symptoms to inform treatment programming for first responders.

Clinical Considerations

The extant literature on this topic presents clinically-relevant implications for treatment-seeking first responders who present with elevated levels of PTSD and AUD symptomatology. First, comprehensive screening and assessment of PTSD and AUD among first responders is essential for appropriate treatment planning. Clinicians should assess for PTSD among first responders with AUD and screen for AUD among those presenting with trauma-related concerns. Second, assessment of commonly co-occurring conditions (e.g., depression) and behaviors (e.g., sleep disturbance, suicidality) is imperative for intervening effectively and preventing harm. Third, it is important for clinicians working with first responders to be aware of the potential impact of mental health stigma on symptom reporting, treatment-seeking, and treatment completion (Hom et al., 2016). Fourth, increased clinical attention should be given to unique first responder sub-populations (e.g., women, volunteers, sexual minorities, cultural subgroups) that may experience increased stress, discrimination, and harassment compared to their peers. Fifth, web-based interventions have great potential to increase access to mental health services for first responders living in rural areas, completing long shifts, and/ or working multiple jobs. Web-based interventions and telehealth services can dramatically improve dissemination and implementation efforts for evidence-based interventions among first responders. Finally, extant integrated, evidence-based interventions for PTSD/AUD can be adapted for first responders. For example, Concurrent Treatment of PTSD and Substance

Use Disorders Using Prolonged Exposure (COPE; Back et al., 2015) can provide an excellent integrated treatment avenue for addressing PTSD and AUD and can be employed among first responder populations.

CONCLUSION

Taken together, extant literature suggests that both PTSD and AUD as well as the PTSD/AUD comorbidity are significant concerns across first responder populations. More methodologically rigorous research is needed among larger and more representative populations to evaluate the development, maintenance, and treatment of PTSD/AUD among first responder populations. To create effective and engaging prevention and intervention clinical resources targeting PTSD/AUD within this unique and vulnerable population, we need to seek greater understanding of not only the risk factors associated with mental health concerns among first responders, but also the strength and resilience factors that may mitigate the development of PTSD/AUD. It is imperative that increased research attention is given to this vulnerable population characterized by stress and danger for the service of others.

This research received no specific grant from any funding agency in the public, commercial, or not-for-profit sectors.

REFERENCES

Arbona, C., & Schwartz, J. P. (2016). Posttraumatic stress disorder symptom clusters, depression, alcohol abuse, and general stress among Hispanic male firefighters. *Hispanic Journal of Behavioral Sciences*, *38*(4), 507–522. doi:10.1177/0739986316661328

Back, S. E., Foa, E. B., Killeen, T. K., Mills, K. L., Teesson, M., Dansky Cotton, B., & Brady, K. T. (2015). *Treatments that work. Concurrent treatment of PTSD and substance use disorders using prolonged exposure (COPE): Therapist guide*. New York, NY: Oxford University Press.

Ballenger, J. F., Best, S. R., Metzler, T. J., Wasserman, D. A., Mohr, D. C., Liberman, A., ... Marmar, C. R. (2011). Patterns and predictors of alcohol use in male and female urban police officers. *The American Journal on Addictions*, *20*(1), 21–29. doi:10.1111/j.1521-0391.2010.00092.x PMID:21175917

Bergman, H. E., Przeworski, A., & Feeny, N. C. (2016). Rates of subthreshold PTSD among U.S. military veterans and service members: A literature review. *Military Psychology*, *29*(2), 117–127. doi:10.1037/mil0000154 PMID:28630531

Berninger, A., Webber, M. P., Cohen, H. W., Gustave, J., Lee, R., Niles, J. K., ... Prezant, D. J. (2010). Trends of elevated PTSD risk in firefighters exposed to the World Trade Center disaster: 2001-2005. *Public Health Reports*, *125*(4), 556–566. PMID:20597456

Berninger, A., Webber, M. P., Niles, J. K., Gustave, J., Lee, R., Cohen, H. W., ... Prezant, D. J. (2010). Longitudinal study of probable post-traumatic stress disorder in firefighters exposed to the World Trade Center disaster. *American Journal of Industrial Medicine*, *53*(12), 1177–1185. PMID:20862700

Blevins, C. A., Weathers, F. W., Davis, M. T., Witte, T. K., & Domino, J. L. (2015). The Posttraumatic Stress Disorder Checklist for DSM-5 (PCL-5): Development and initial psychometric evaluation. *Journal of Traumatic Stress*, *28*(6), 489–498. doi:10.1002/jts.22059 PMID:26606250

Bogstrand, S. T., Skogstad, L., & Ekeberg, O. (2016). The association between alcohol, medicinal drug use and post-traumatic stress symptoms among Norwegian rescue workers after the 22 July twin terror attacks. *International Emergency Nursing*, *28*, 29–33. doi:10.1016/j.ienj.2016.03.003 PMID:27068750

Bromet, E. J., Hobbs, M. J., Clouston, S. A., Gonzalez, A., Kotov, R., & Luft, B. J. (2016). DSM-IV post-traumatic stress disorder among World Trade Center responders 11-13 years after the disaster of 11 September 2001 (9/11). *Psychological Medicine*, *46*(4), 771–783. doi:10.1017/S0033291715002184 PMID:26603700

Carleton, R. N., Afifi, T. O., Turner, S., Taillieu, T., Duranceau, S., LeBouthillier, D. M., ... Asmundson, G. J. G. (2018). Mental disorder symptoms among public safety personnel in Canada. *Canadian Journal of Psychiatry*, *63*(1), 54–64. doi:10.1177/0706743717723825 PMID:28845686

Chang, J. H., Kim, D., Jang, E., Park, J. E., Bae, H., Han, C. W., & Kim, S. H. (2016). Reliability and validity of the Korean version of the Symptom Checklist Post Traumatic Stress Disorder Scale. *Journal of Korean Medical Science*, *31*(5), 777–782. doi:10.3346/jkms.2016.31.5.777 PMID:27134501

Cherpitel, C. J. (2000). A brief screening instrument for problem drinking in the emergency room: The RAPS4. Rapid Alcohol Problems Screen. *Journal of Studies on Alcohol*, *61*(3), 447–449. doi:10.15288/jsa.2000.61.447 PMID:10807217

Chiu, S., Niles, J. K., Webber, M. P., Zeig-Owens, R., Gustave, J., Lee, R., ... Prezant, D. J. (2011). Evaluating risk factors and possible mediation effects in posttraumatic depression and posttraumatic stress disorder comorbidity. *Public Health Reports*, *126*(2), 201–209. PMID:21387950

Chopko, B. A., Facemire, V. C., Palmieri, P. A., & Schwartz, R. C. (2016). Spirituality and health outcomes among police officers: Empirical evidence supporting a paradigm shift. *Criminal Justice Studies*, *29*(4), 363–377. doi:10.1080/1478601X.2016.1216412

Chopko, B. A., Palmieri, P. A., & Adams, R. E. (2013). Associations between police stress and alcohol use: Implications for practice. *Journal of Loss and Trauma*, *18*(5), 482–497.

Chopko, B. A., Palmieri, P. A., & Adams, R. E. (2015). Critical incident history questionnaire replication: Frequency and severity of trauma exposure among officers from small and midsize police agencies. *Journal of Traumatic Stress*, *28*(2), 157–161. doi:10.1002/jts.21996 PMID:25808672

Chopko, B. A., Palmieri, P. A., & Facemire, V. C. (2014). Prevalence and predictors of suicidal ideation among U.S. law enforcement officers. *Journal of Police and Criminal Psychology*, *29*(1), 1–9.

Ci, S., Lan, Y., Zhang, Q., Zhou, D., & De, J. (2015). Analysis of posttraumatic stress disorder in rescuers and firefighters. *Zhonghua Lao Dong Wei Sheng Zhi Ye Bing Za Zhi*, *33*(6), 448–450. PMID:26653381

Corneil, W., Beaton, R., Murphy, S., Johnson, C., & Pike, K. (1999). Exposure to traumatic incidents and prevalence of posttraumatic stress symptomatology in urban firefighters in two countries. *Journal of Occupational Health Psychology*, *4*(2), 131–141. doi:10.1037/1076-8998.4.2.131 PMID:10212865

Del Ben, K. S., Scotti, J. R., Chen, Y. C., & Fortson, B. L. (2006). Prevalence of posttraumatic stress disorder symptoms in firefighters. *Work and Stress*, *20*(1), 37–48.

Donnelly, E. (2012). Work-related stress and posttraumatic stress in emergency medical services. *Prehospital Emergency Care*, *16*(1), 76–85. doi:10.3109/10903127.2011.621044 PMID:22128908

Fjeldheim, C. B., Nothling, J., Pretorius, K., Basson, M., Ganasen, K., Heneke, R., ... Seedat, S. (2014). Trauma exposure, posttraumatic stress disorder and the effect of explanatory variables in paramedic trainees. *BMC Emergency Medicine*, *14*(11), 1–7. PMID:24755358

Fox, J., Desai, M. M., Britten, K., Lucas, G., Luneau, R., & Rosenthal, M. S. (2012). Mental-health conditions, barriers to care, and productivity loss among officers in an urban police department. *Connecticut Medicine*, *76*(9), 525–531. PMID:23155671

Fuehrlein, B. S., Mota, N., Arias, A. J., Trevisan, L. A., Kachadourian, L. K., Krystal, J. H., ... Pietrzak, R. H. (2016). The burden of alcohol use disorders in US military veterans: Results from the National Health and Resilience in Veterans Study. *Addiction (Abingdon, England)*, *111*(10), 1786–1794. doi:10.1111/add.13423 PMID:27061707

Grant, B. F., Goldstein, R. B., Saha, T. D., Chou, S. P., Jung, J., Zhang, H., ... Hasin, D. S. (2015). Epidemiology of DSM-5 Alcohol Use Disorder: Results from the National Epidemiologic Survey on Alcohol and Related Conditions III. *Journal of the American Medical Association Psychiatry*, *72*(8), 757–766. PMID:26039070

Gulliver, S. B., Zimering, R., Knight, J., Morissette, S., Kamholz, B., Meyer, E., ... Kimbrel, N. (2018). Tobacco and alcohol use among firefighters during their first 3 years of service. *Psychology of Addictive Behaviors*, *32*(3), 255–263. doi:10.1037/adb0000366 PMID:29771556

Haddock, C. K., Day, R. S., Poston, W. S., Jahnke, S. A., & Jitnarin, N. (2015). Alcohol use and caloric intake from alcohol in a national cohort of U.S. career firefighters. *Journal of Studies on Alcohol and Drugs*, *76*(3), 360–366. PMID:25978821

Haddock, C. K., Poston, W. S. C., Jahnke, S. A., & Jitnarin, N. (2017). Alcohol use and problem drinking among women firefighters. *Women's Health Issues*, *27*(6), 632–638. PMID:28822615

Harvey, S. B., Milligan-Saville, J. S., Paterson, H. M., Harkness, E. L., Marsh, A. M., Dobson, M., ... Bryant, R. A. (2016). The mental health of fire-fighters: An examination of the impact of repeated trauma exposure. *The Australian and New Zealand Journal of Psychiatry*, *50*(7), 649–658. doi:10.1177/0004867415615217 PMID:26607303

Hom, M. A., Stanley, I. H., Ringer, F. B., & Joiner, T. E. (2016). Mental health service use among firefighters with suicidal thoughts and behaviors. *Psychiatric Services (Washington, D.C.)*, *67*(6), 688–691. doi:10.1176/appi.ps.201500177 PMID:26927574

Horowitz, M., Wilner, N., & Alvarez, W. (1979). The Impact of Event Scale: A measure of subjective stress. *Psychosomatic Medicine*, *41*(3), 209–218. PMID:472086

Inslicht, S. S., McCaslin, S. E., Metzler, T. J., Henn-Haase, C., Hart, S. L., Maguen, S., ... Marmar, C. R. (2010). Family psychiatric history, peritraumatic reactivity, and posttraumatic stress symptoms: A prospective study of police. *Journal of Psychiatric Research*, *44*(1), 22–31. PMID:19683259

Jones, S. (2017). Describing the mental health profile of first responders: A systematic review. *Journal of the American Psychiatric Nurses Association*, *23*(3), 200–214. doi:10.1177/1078390317695266 PMID:28445653

Kessler, R. C., Chiu, W. T., Demler, O., & Walters, E. E. (2005). Prevalence, severity, and comorbidity of twelve-month DSM-IV disorders in the National Comorbidity Survey Replication (NCS-R). *Archives of General Psychiatry*, *62*(6), 617–627. doi:10.1001/archpsyc.62.6.617 PMID:15939839

Khantzian, E. J. (1999). *Treating addiction as a human process*. Northvale, NJ: Jason Aronson.

Kilpatrick, D. G., Resnick, H. S., Milanak, M. E., Miller, M. W., Keyes, K. M., & Friedman, M. J. (2013). National estimates of exposure to traumatic events and PTSD prevalence using DSM-IV and DSM-5 criteria. *Journal of Traumatic Stress*, *26*(5), 537–547. doi:10.1002/jts.21848 PMID:24151000

Kim, J. I., Park, H., & Kim, J. H. (2017). The mediation effect of PTSD, perceived job stress and resilience on the relationship between trauma exposure and the development of depression and alcohol use problems in Korean firefighters: A cross-sectional study. *Journal of Affective Disorders*, *229*, 450–455. doi:10.1016/j.jad.2017.12.055 PMID:29331707

Kim, J. I., Park, H., & Kim, J. H. (2018). Alcohol use disorders and insomnia mediate the association between PTSD symptoms and suicidal ideation in Korean firefighters. *Depression and Anxiety*, *35*(11), 1095–1103. doi:10.1002/da.22803 PMID:30028563

Lee, D. J., Liverant, G. I., Lowmaster, S. E., Gradus, J. L., & Sloan, D. M. (2014). PTSD and reasons for living: Associations with depressive symptoms and alcohol use. *Psychiatry Research*, *219*(3), 550–555. doi:10.1016/j.psychres.2014.06.016 PMID:24984579

Lima Ede, P., Assuncao, A. A., & Barreto, S. M. (2015). Prevalence of depression among firefighters. *Cadernos de Saude Publica*, *31*(4), 733–743. PMID:25945983

McCanlies, E. C., Mnatsakanova, A., Andrew, M. E., Burchfiel, C. M., & Violanti, J. M. (2014). Positive psychological factors are associated with lower PTSD symptoms among police officers: Post Hurricane Katrina. *Stress and Health*, *30*(5), 405–415. doi:10.1002mi.2615 PMID:25476965

McCauley, J. L., Killeen, T., Gros, D. F., Brady, K. T., & Back, S. E. (2012). Posttraumatic stress disorder and co-occurring substance use sisorders: Advances in assessment and treatment. *Clinical Psychologist*, *19*(3), 1–27.

Ménard, K. S., & Arter, M. L. (2013). Police officer alcohol use and trauma symptoms: Associations with critical incidents, coping, and social stressors. *International Journal of Stress Management*, *20*(1), 37–56. doi:10.1037/a0031434

Ménard, K. S., & Arter, M. L. (2014). Stress, coping, alcohol use, and posttraumatic stress disorder among an international sample of police officers: Does gender matter? *Police Quarterly*, *17*(4), 307–327. doi:10.1177/1098611114548097

Meyer, E. C., Zimering, R., Daly, E., Knight, J., Kamholz, B. W., & Gulliver, S. B. (2012). Predictors of posttraumatic stress disorder and other psychological symptoms in trauma-exposed firefighters. *Psychological Services*, *9*(1), 1–15. doi:10.1037/a0026414 PMID:22449083

Milliken, C. S., Auchterlonie, J. L., & Hoge, C. W. (2007). Longitudinal assessment of mental health problems among active and reserve component soldiers returning from the Iraq war. *Journal of the American Medical Association*, *298*(18), 2141–2148. doi:10.1001/jama.298.18.2141 PMID:18000197

Mills, K. L., Teesson, M., Ross, J., & Peters, L. (2006). Trauma, PTSD, and substance use disorders: Findings from the Australian National Survey of Mental Health and Well-Being. *The American Journal of Psychiatry*, *163*(4), 652–658. PMID:16585440

Mumford, E. A., Taylor, B. G., & Kubu, B. (2015). Law enforcement officer safety and wellness. *Police Quarterly*, *18*(2), 111–133.

Murphy, J. G., Yurasek, A. M., Dennhardt, A. A., Skidmore, J. R., McDevitt-Murphy, M. E., MacKillop, J., & Martens, M. P. (2013). Symptoms of depression and PTSD are associated with elevated alcohol demand. *Drug and Alcohol Dependence*, *127*(1-3), 129–136. PMID:22809894

Murphy, S. A., Beaton, R. D., Pike, K. C., & Johnson, L. C. (1999). Occupational stressors, stress responses, and alcohol consumption among professional firefighters: A prospective, longitudinal analysis. *International Journal of Stress Management*, *6*(3), 179–196. doi:10.1023/A:1021934725246

North, C. S., Tivis, L., McMillen, J. C., Pfefferbaum, B., Cox, J., Spitznagel, E. L., ... Smith, E. M. (2002). Coping, functioning, and adjustment of rescue workers after the Oklahoma City bombing. *Journal of Traumatic Stress*, *15*(3), 171–175. doi:10.1023/A:1015286909111 PMID:12092908

North, C. S., Tivis, L., McMillen, J. C., Pfefferbaum, B., Spitznagel, E. L., Cox, J., ... Smith, E. M. (2002). Psychiatric disorders in rescue workers after the Oklahoma City bombing. *The American Journal of Psychiatry*, *159*(5), 857–859. doi:10.1176/appi.ajp.159.5.857 PMID:11986143

O'Brien, C. P. (2008). The CAGE questionnaire for detection of alcoholism: A remarkably useful but simple tool. *Journal of the American Medical Association*, *300*(17), 2054–2056. doi:10.1001/jama.2008.570 PMID:18984895

Osofsky, H. J., Osofsky, J. D., Arey, J., Kronenberg, M. E., Hansel, T., & Many, M. (2011). Hurricane Katrina's first responders: The struggle to protect and serve in the aftermath of the disaster. *Disaster Medicine and Public Health Preparedness*, *5*(S2Suppl 2), S214–S219. doi:10.1001/dmp.2011.53 PMID:21865490

Paulus, D. J., Vujanovic, A. A., Schuhmann, B. B., Smith, L. J., & Tran, J. (2017). Main and interactive effects of depression and posttraumatic stress in relation to alcohol dependence among urban male firefighters. *Psychiatry Research*, *251*, 69–75. doi:10.1016/j.psychres.2017.02.011 PMID:28189939

Pietrzak, R. H., Goldstein, R. B., Southwick, S. M., & Grant, B. F. (2011). Prevalence and Axis I comorbidity of full and partial posttraumatic stress disorder in the United States: Results from Wave 2 of the National Epidemiologic Survey on Alcohol and Related Conditions. *Journal of Anxiety Disorders*, *25*(3), 456–465. doi:10.1016/j.janxdis.2010.11.010 PMID:21168991

Pietrzak, R. H., Schechter, C. B., Bromet, E. J., Katz, C. L., Reissman, D. B., Ozbay, F., ... Southwick, S. M. (2012). The burden of full and subsyndromal posttraumatic stress disorder among police involved in the World Trade Center rescue and recovery effort. *Journal of Psychiatric Research*, *46*(7), 835–842. doi:10.1016/j.jpsychires.2012.03.011 PMID:22464942

Ruggero, C. J., Kotov, R., Callahan, J. L., Kilmer, J. N., Luft, B. J., & Bromet, E. J. (2013). PTSD symptom dimensions and their relationship to functioning in World Trade Center responders. *Psychiatry Research*, *210*(3), 1049–1055. PMID:24064462

Schafer, I., & Najavits, L. M. (2007). Clinical challenges in the treatment of patients with posttraumatic stress disorder and substance abuse. *Current Opinion in Psychiatry*, *20*(6), 614–618. PMID:17921765

Simms, L. J., Watson, D., & Doebbeling, B. N. (2002). Confirmatory factor analyses of posttraumatic stress symptoms in deployed and nondeployed veterans of the Gulf War. *Journal of Abnormal Psychology*, *111*(4), 637–647. doi:10.1037/0021-843X.111.4.637 PMID:12428777

Simons, J. S., Gaher, R. M., Jacobs, G. A., Meyer, D., & Johnson-Jimenez, E. (2005). Associations between alcohol use and PTSD symptoms among American Red Cross disaster relief workers responding to the 9/11/2001 attacks. *The American Journal of Drug and Alcohol Abuse*, *31*(2), 285–304. doi:10.1081/ADA-47937 PMID:15912717

Simpson, T. L., Stappenbeck, C. A., Luterek, J. A., Lehavot, K., & Kaysen, D. L. (2014). Drinking motives moderate daily relationships between PTSD symptoms and alcohol use. *Journal of Abnormal Psychology*, *123*(1), 237–247. doi:10.1037/a0035193 PMID:24661174

Smith, B. W., Ortiz, J. A., Steffen, L. E., Tooley, E. M., Wiggins, K. T., Yeater, E. A., ... Bernard, M. L. (2011). Mindfulness is associated with fewer PTSD symptoms, depressive symptoms, physical symptoms, and alcohol problems in urban firefighters. *Journal of Consulting and Clinical Psychology*, *79*(5), 613–617. doi:10.1037/a0025189 PMID:21875175

Smith, L. J., Gallagher, M. W., Tran, J. K., & Vujanovic, A. A. (2018). Posttraumatic stress, alcohol use, and alcohol use motives in firefighters: The role of sleep disturbance. *Comprehensive Psychiatry*, *87*, 64–71. doi:10.1016/j.comppsych.2018.09.001 PMID:30219373

Smith, L. J., Paulus, D. J., Gallagher, M. W., Norman, S. B., Tran, J. K., & Vujanovic, A. A. (2018). Perceived stress and probable alcohol misuse in firefighters: The role of posttraumatic stress. *International Journal of Stress Management*; Advance online publication. doi:10.1037tr0000118

Soo, J., Webber, M. P., Gustave, J., Lee, R., Hall, C. B., Cohen, H. W., ... Prezant, D. J. (2011). Trends in probable PTSD in firefighters exposed to the World Trade Center disaster, 2001-2010. *Disaster Medicine and Public Health Preparedness*, *5*(S2Suppl 2), S197–S203. doi:10.1001/dmp.2011.48 PMID:21900417

Stanley, I. H., Boffa, J. W., Hom, M. A., Kimbrel, N. A., & Joiner, T. E. (2017). Differences in psychiatric symptoms and barriers to mental health care between volunteer and career firefighters. *Psychiatry Research*, *247*, 236–242. doi:10.1016/j.psychres.2016.11.037 PMID:27930964

Stewart, S. H., Mitchell, T. L., Wright, K. D., & Loba, P. (2004). The relations of PTSD symptoms to alcohol use and coping drinking in volunteers who responded to the Swissair Flight 111 airline disaster. *Journal of Anxiety Disorders*, *18*(1), 51–68. PMID:14725868

Tomaka, J., Magoc, D., Morales-Monks, S. M., & Reyes, A. C. (2017). Posttraumatic stress symptoms and alcohol-related outcomes among municipal firefighters. *Journal of Traumatic Stress*, *30*(4), 416–424. PMID:28699663

Violanti, J. M. (2004). Predictors of police suicide ideation. *Suicide & Life-Threatening Behavior*, *34*(3), 277–283. doi:10.1521uli.34.3.277.42775 PMID:15385182

Violanti, J. M., Slaven, J. E., Charles, L. E., Burchfiel, C. M., Andrew, M. E., & Homish, G. G. (2011). Police and alcohol use: A descriptive analysis and associations with stress outcomes. *American Journal of Criminal Justice*, *36*(4), 344–356.

Vujanovic, B.-M., Bonn-Miller, M. O., & Petry, N. M. (2016). Co-occurring posttraumatic stress and substance use: Emerging research on correlates, mechanisms, and treatments-Introduction to the special issue. *Psychology of Addictive Behaviors*, *30*(7), 713–719. doi:10.1037/adb0000222 PMID:27786510

Wagner, D., Heinrichs, M., & Ehlert, U. (1998). Prevalence of symptoms of posttraumatic stress disorder in German professional firefighters. *The American Journal of Psychiatry*, *155*(12), 1727–1732. doi:10.1176/ajp.155.12.1727 PMID:9842783

Weathers, F., Litz, B., Herman, D., Huska, J., & Keane, T. (1993). *The PTSD Checklist (PCL): Reliability, validity, and diagnostic utility.* Paper presented at the Annual Convention of the International Society for Traumatic Stress Studies, San Antonio, TX.

Weinberger, A. H., Maciejewski, P. K., McKee, S. A., Reutenauer, E. L., & Mazure, C. M. (2009). Gender differences in associations between lifetime alcohol, depression, panic disorder, and posttraumatic stress disorder and tobacco withdrawal. *The American Journal on Addictions*, *18*(2), 140–147. PMID:19283566

Yip, J., Zeig-Owens, R., Hall, C. B., Webber, M. P., Olivieri, B., Schwartz, T., ... Prezant, D. J. (2016). Health conditions as mediators of the association between World Trade Center exposure and health-related quality of life in firefighters and EMS workers. *Journal of Occupational and Environmental Medicine*, *58*(2), 200–206. doi:10.1097/JOM.0000000000000597 PMID:26849265

Yip, J., Zeig-Owens, R., Webber, M. P., Kablanian, A., Hall, C. B., Vossbrinck, M., ... Prezant, D. J. (2016). World Trade Center-related physical and mental health burden among New York City Fire Department emergency medical service workers. *Occupational and Environmental Medicine*, *73*(1), 13–20. doi:10.1136/oemed-2014-102601 PMID:25876606

Yun, J. A., Ahn, Y. S., Jeong, K. S., Joo, E. J., & Choi, K. S. (2015). The relationship between chronotype and sleep quality in Korean firefighters. *Clinical Psychopharmacology and Neuroscience*, *13*(2), 201–208. doi:10.9758/cpn.2015.13.2.201 PMID:26243849

Zlotnick, C., Franklin, C. L., & Zimmerman, M. (2002). Does "subthreshold" posttraumatic stress disorder have any clinical relevance? *Comprehensive Psychiatry*, *43*(6), 413–419. doi:10.1053/comp.2002.35900 PMID:12439826

ADDITIONAL READING

Back, S. E., Brady, K. T., Sonne, S. C., & Verduin, M. L. (2006). Symptom improvement in co-occurring PTSD and alcohol dependence. *The Journal of Nervous and Mental Disease*, *194*(9), 690–696. PMID:16971821

Back, S. E., Foa, E. B., Killeen, T. K., Mills, K. L., Teesson, M., Dansky Cotton, B., & Brady, K. T. (2015). *Treatments that work. Concurrent treatment of PTSD and substance use disorders using prolonged exposure (COPE): Therapist guide*. New York, NY: Oxford University Press.

Back, S. E., Killeen, T., Badour, C. L., Flanagan, J. C., Allan, N. P., Ana, E. S., ... Brady, K. T. (2019). Concurrent treatment of substance use disorders and PTSD using prolonged exposure: A randomized clinical trial in military veterans. *Addictive Behaviors*, *90*, 369–377. PMID:30529244

Carleton, R. N., Afifi, T. O., Turner, S., Taillieu, T., Duranceau, S., LeBouthillier, D. M., ... Asmundson, G. J. G. (2018). Mental disorder symptoms among public safety personnel in Canada. *Canadian Journal of Psychiatry*, *63*(1), 54–64. PMID:28845686

Chopko, B. A., Palmieri, P. A., & Adams, R. E. (2013). Associations between police stress and alcohol use: Implications for practice. *Journal of Loss and Trauma*, *18*(5), 482–497.

Jones, S. (2017). Describing the mental health profile of first responders: A systematic review. *Journal of the American Psychiatric Nurses Association*, *23*(3), 200–214. doi:10.1177/1078390317695266 PMID:28445653

Jones, S., Nagel, C., McSweeney, J., & Curran, G. (2018). Prevalence and correlates of psychiatric symptoms among first responders in a southern state. *Archives of Psychiatric Nursing*, *32*(6), 828–835. doi:10.1016/j.apnu.2018.06.007 PMID:30454624

Katz, C. L., Jutras-Aswad, D., Kiliman, M., Pilatowicz, I., Akerele, E., Marrone, K., & Ozbay, F. (2012). Alcohol use in Polish 9/11 responders: Implications for cross-cultural treatment. *Journal of Psychiatric Practice*, *18*(1), 55–63. doi:10.1097/01.pra.0000410989.46346.14 PMID:22261985

KEY TERMS AND DEFINITIONS

Alcohol Use Disorder: A pattern of problematic alcohol use leading to clinically significant impairment or distress, as manifested by symptoms such as failure to fulfill major role obligations, alcohol craving, and recurrent alcohol use in physically hazardous situations (e.g., while driving).

Comorbidity: The presence of one of more mental health conditions occurring at the same time.

Posttraumatic Stress Disorder: A mental health problem that some people develop after experiencing or witnessing a violent or life-threatening event, like combat, physical assault, natural disasters, transportation accidents, or sexual or physical abuse or assault.

Problematic Alcohol Use: A drinking pattern that results in significant and recurrent adverse consequences.

Specialized Evidence-Based Interventions: Mental health interventions that have been developed and/or modified through research for the needs of unique populations.

Transdiagnostic: Beliefs, behaviors, or patterns of emotional responding that are associated with various mental health conditions and may be implicated in their development, maintenance, or treatment.

Trauma: Exposure to an event, such as actual or threatened death, serious injury, or sexual violence through direct experience, witnessing an event occurs to others, learning that an event occurred to a close family member or friend, or repeated occupational exposure to details of events.

Chapter 4
Unique Job Roles and Mental Health Risk Factors Among Emergency Dispatchers

Isabel Gardett
International Academies of Emergency Dispatch, USA

Edward Trefts
International Academies of Emergency Dispatch, USA

Christopher Olola
https://orcid.org/0000-0003-2250-5096
International Academies of Emergency Dispatch, USA

Greg Scott
International Academies of Emergency Dispatch, USA

ABSTRACT

Emergency medical, fire, and police dispatchers are often called the first, first responders. Working in emergency communication centers, they are the first point of contact with medical, fire, and law enforcement resources and the first point of access to public health and public safety systems for millions of callers each year. Emergency dispatchers face unique risks to their mental health, and the roles and responsibilities specific to their work produce stressors not synonymous with those encountered by other first responders and emergency workers. Yet relatively little research has been done to understand the specific mental health concerns of this vital and often overlooked segment of the emergency services profession. The aim of this chapter is to provide an overview of the job-specific tasks and work characteristics that make the emergency dispatcher's job qualitatively different from the jobs of other emergency workers and first responders, then discuss the unique mental health risks associated with their work.

DOI: 10.4018/978-1-5225-9803-9.ch004

INTRODUCTION

Emergency medical, fire, and police dispatchers are often called the *first*, first responders (Clawson, Dernocoeur, & Murray 2015). They are the first point of contact with medical, fire, and law enforcement resources and the first point of access to the public health and public safety systems for tens of millions of callers each year. However, the work of emergency dispatchers differs significantly from that of other first responders and emergency workers. Emergency dispatchers handle situations of equal emotional weight to those encountered by first responders—including medical emergencies, structure fires, motor vehicle crashes, domestic violence, and the whole long list of human tragedies—but must do so remotely. Being removed from the scene might seem to make their job easier or less stressful, but the opposite is often the case.

Significant research has demonstrated that field responders experience very high levels of stress (McQuerry, Giano, & Merten, 2018), burnout (Boland et al., 2018; Khatiban, Hosseini, Bikmoradi, Roshanaei, Karampourian, 2015; Mitani, Fujita, Nakata, & Shirakawa, 2006), suicide (Carleton et al., 2018b), post-traumatic stress disorder (PTSD) (Berger et al., 2012; Carlier, Lamberts, & Gersons, 1997; Fullerton, Ursano, & Wang, 2004; Haugen, Evces, & Weiss, 2012), and other mental health effects (Carleton et al., 2018a) from repeatedly responding to and managing others' trauma. This applies across all three of the main disciplines of field response: firefighters (Henderson & Van Hasselt, 2016; Jahnke, Poston, Haddock, & Murphy, 2016; Kim et al., 2018), police officers (Chopko, Palmieri, & Adams, 2015; Hem, Berg, & Ekberg, 2001; Price, 2017), and emergency medical services (EMS) responders (Berger et al., 2007; Donnelly, 2012). Many of the causes of the stress, PTSD, drug and alcohol abuse, suicidality, and other mental health issues experienced by field personnel are common to emergency dispatching as well, including shift work (Ma et al., 2013; Markus, Hartman, Brand, Holsboer-Trachsler, & Puhse, 2010), repeated exposure to trauma (Milligan-Saville et al., 2018; Rallings, 2000), and a professional culture that often downplays the mental health effects of the work or expressions of those effects (Brown & Campbell, 1990; Tuckey, Winwood, & Dollard, 2012), among many others.

However, while the events emergency dispatchers manage are identical to those handled by field responders, the working conditions of emergency dispatchers are very different—so much so that they experience unique risks as a result. Several studies have shown that the level of stress, burnout, and other mental health issues is as high among emergency dispatchers as among field responders (Lilly & Pierce, 2013; Meischke et al., 2015; Pierce & Lilly, 2012; Trachik et al., 2015), but few have identified the different causes of those outcomes among dispatchers. This chapter will review the work of emergency dispatchers in comparison to field responders and outline the unique risk factors faced by dispatchers, who by the nature of their work handle emergencies over the phone, rather than in person.

THE EMERGENCY DISPATCHER'S ROLE

The emergency dispatcher (sometimes referred to as an emergency calltaker) plays an unusual but critical role in public safety and emergency services. The first point of contact for anyone calling for emergency medical, fire, or police services, the emergency dispatcher is part information gatherer, part system manager, and part care provider (Clawson, Dernocoeur, & Murray, 2015).

As an information gatherer, the emergency dispatcher interfaces with the person calling for help—sometimes the patient, often someone else—to gather the relevant patient, situation/event, scene, and safety information, as well as information about persons like victims or suspects. Often, the emergency dispatcher works in all three of the disciplines of emergency services, taking police, medical, and fire calls as they come in and thus needing to gather different information for each type of situation. The outcome of this phase of the emergency dispatcher's job is the assignment of a dispatch code, the result of a complex triage system that determines the nature, severity, and complicating circumstances involved in an event. For example, if a caller reports that her father is experiencing chest pain, the emergency dispatcher would ask additional questions to identify the possible severity of his condition, such as questions about sweating and dizziness, the location and duration of the pain, and any medications he might have taken. All of this information would be combined to generate the dispatch code that best reflects the situation.

As a system manager, the emergency dispatcher manages all the public safety resources available in the service area, from assigning specific responders to incidents, to identifying and allocating the correct type and number of units, including everything from Basic Life Support ambulances to extrication equipment and police units. In this role, the emergency dispatcher applies his or her knowledge of the available resources to the dispatch code arrived at via information gathering, to determine exactly where to place resources. In the case of the caller reporting her father's chest pain, this would likely be a quick response involving medical crews; for a caller reporting a stolen bicycle, the response would involve police and would likely be either less urgent or involve just connecting the caller to an online or telephone incident reporting service. In some cases, emergency dispatchers may even connect callers to a wide range of resources, from poison control to nurse advice lines. Making an appropriate resource determination does not only affect the public safety system directly; it also has powerful effects on the safety of communities, by potentially reducing both emergency vehicle collisions and so-called "wake effect" collisions, as well as by ensuring that the highest-priority situations receive the highest-priority, and most appropriate, response.

Finally, as a care provider, the emergency dispatcher provides direct care over the phone, broadly known as pre-arrival instructions (PAIs). These can include everything from instructions for bystander cardiopulmonary resuscitation (CPR) or childbirth instructions to evacuation or lockdown protocols in active assailant situations or egress instructions for persons trapped in structure fires. Although the emergency dispatcher never lays a hand on a patient, lifts a hose, or arrests a suspect, he or she does provide direct care to the patient or caller during the critical minutes in which the field responders are on their way. One common way that emergency dispatchers provide care is by instructing callers to provide first aid to patients, such as instructing a mother to apply pressure to her child's cut to stop the bleeding.

And although they never treat patients or interact with victims directly, it is important to remember that emergency dispatchers' work is just as complex and professional as that of field responders. Emergency dispatchers have been shown to correctly identify high-acuity, high-severity conditions such as stroke (Clawson et al., 2016; Gardett, Olola, Scott, Broadbent, & Clawson, 2017; Jones et al., 2012; Mould-Millman et al., 2017; Ramanujam et al., 2008) and heart attack (Clawson et al., 2017; Scott et al., 2017) at least as well as field responders evaluating patients on scene, to accurately differentiate between high-and low-acuity conditions (Clawson et al., 2014; Scott et al., 2016), to provide high-quality CPR and other life-saving interventions (Bowbrow et al., 2014), and to effectively and quickly gather information that makes responders' jobs safer and more effective (Broadbent et al., 2018a; Broadbent et al., 2018b).

UNIQUE RISK FACTORS: VICARIOUS TRAUMA

The most obvious difference between the emergency dispatcher's work and that of field responders is distance. Unlike field responders, emergency dispatchers interact with callers, gather information, and provide help remotely. This remote work environment subjects emergency dispatchers to what has been termed "vicarious trauma." Contrary to common belief, vicarious trauma—experiencing the trauma of other people—is just as detrimental to mental health, and in some cases more so, than experiencing trauma directly (Cohen & Collens, 2013). One study found that peritraumatic stress, the distress experienced during and immediately after an event, was very high in emergency dispatchers, occurring in response to as many as 32% of the call types they handle (Pierce & Lilly, 2012). The same study found a relationship between this peritraumatic stress and PTSD.

McCann and Pearlman (1990) also refer to vicarious trauma, noting that the distance of the person from the trauma does not necessarily determine the amount of trauma experienced; and the *Diagnostic and Statistical Manual of Mental Disorders* (5th edition; American Psychiatric Association [APA], 2013) includes traumatic events occurring to others as one of the possible criteria for PTSD. For emergency dispatchers, the vicarious trauma experienced on the job is shaped by the role's unique characteristics. These characteristics can heighten exposure to, reduce ability to recover from, and increase the long-term effects of trauma.

"Relentless" Exposure

One of the most commonly-cited differentiators between the work of emergency dispatchers and that of field responders is the sheer volume and speed of incoming calls, which has been referred to as "relentless exposure" (Adams, Shakespeare-Finch, & Armstrong, 2015). While a paramedic, for example, may spend anywhere between 15 minutes and several hours handling a single incident, an emergency dispatcher is expected to identify the caller's problem and determine the appropriate response to send within 60 to 90 seconds. Even including additional time spent gathering address and other information, providing safety or life support instructions, and calming or supporting callers, emergency dispatchers often move from one call to another in a matter of a few minutes. Often, these calls occur immediately back-to-back.

A constant flood of such incidents is stressful in itself. But this deluge also significantly increases both the immediate and long-term effects of trauma because the dispatcher has no opportunity to process one event before moving to the next (Coxon et al., 2016), an issue that is compounded by the time pressure caused by required call-processing time standards (Tracy & Tracy, 1998). Moreover, in addition to dealing with large call volume, emergency dispatchers generally handle a wider variety of calls, and execute a greater variety of types of tasks, than field responders (Golding et al., 2017). An emergency dispatcher may very quickly switch from a medical call involving a non-breathing patient, to a low-urgency police call about a barking dog, to an informational call reporting a stolen bicycle, to a call involving a possible house fire. This variety, combined with the time pressure, adds to the sense of "relentlessness."

Vigilance

Another compounding factor for dispatchers' vicarious trauma is the unusual combination of a high percentage of mundane, even ridiculous or unimportant events with a very low percentage of critically important and even life-threatening events, which must be immediately identified from the "noise" of low-importance calls. Essentially, emergency dispatching is a full-time vigilance task.

A vigilance task is one in which the actor is "required to maintain their focus of attention and detect infrequent and unpredictable targets over extended periods of time" (Dillard et al., 2019). Perhaps the most common example of a life-critical vigilance task is air traffic control, in which controllers must constantly monitor many predictable and orderly events in order to catch the very rare, but incredibly dangerous, potential crashes. Emergency dispatchers' work is similar in that, contrary to popular understanding, most of the calls they handle are low-acuity, routine events, not true emergencies, such as minor car accidents, patients with minor illnesses, or reports of loud parties or barking dogs. Yet within this litany of lower-acuity calls lurk the true emergency calls, ranging from cardiac arrests to mass casualty incidents. Because any individual call could be one of these high-acuity incidents, emergency dispatchers must be constantly vigilant, maintaining attention to the signs of more serious problems while routinely (and courteously) handling the less-critical ones. Although field responders may be sent on some calls they perceive as low-importance or a waste of time, it is dispatchers who filter out and manage the vast majority of calls in which no immediate or critical assistance is needed. What is concerning for dispatcher mental health is the fact that vigilance tasks have been shown to correlate strongly with stress, particularly when the rare events have high consequences (Thackray, 1981). One recent study has found that, unlike almost every other type of work task, vigilance tasks are not perceived as less stressful when time is perceived as moving more quickly, i.e., when "time flies" (Dillard et al., 2019). In other words, even the highly-rewarding and fast-paced nature of emergency dispatching is not necessarily a buffer against the constant stress of vigilance.

Moreover, some evidence suggests that the vigilance-related stress of emergency dispatching may be increasing. Several studies have found that one of the most stressful elements of emergency call handling is the requirement to deal with "fake" or inappropriate calls—such as drunk or "pocket" dials— or calls for services not appropriate to emergency services (such as a person asking the emergency dispatcher to call their office because they are going to be late) (Tracy & Tracy, 1998; Forslund, Kihlgren, & Kihlgren, 2004). Given the ubiquity of cell phones, both types of "nuisance" calls are increasing, adding to the anger and frustration felt by emergency dispatchers when callers are seen as abusing the system, but also adding to the vigilance nature of the task by increasing the ratio of noncritical to true emergency calls. Not only does this increase the sense of having to maintain vigilance over long periods of low relevance; it also increases the dispatchers' sense that they may miss the important calls in the noise.

Powerlessness and Moral Injury

The combined elements of the emergency dispatcher's role as remote care provider add up to a sense of lack of control. Unlike field responders, who can immediately take action to mitigate a traumatic situation, no matter how tragic or terrifying, emergency dispatchers must "work through the caller," gathering information and providing advice and instructions through the person on the scene. That barriers to providing direct assistance are perceived as stressful has been demonstrated repeatedly (Adams, Shakespeare-Finch, & Armstrong, 2015; Forslund, Kihlgren, & Kihlgren, 2004; Golding et al., 2017;

Tracy & Tracy, 1998). Because of their very high sense of responsibility for the outcomes of the event (Burke, 1995; Carleton et al., 2018a), dispatchers experience extreme stress when they are unable to convince the caller to perform the necessary assistance for the patient, or when they hear events taking place (such as an assault) that they are powerless to change. This greater sense of powerlessness or helplessness in the face of trauma contributes directly to their experience of both immediate and long-term traumatic stress (Carleton et al., 2018b; Forslund, Kihlgren, & Kihlgren, 2004; Golding et al., 2017).

The cognitive activation theory of stress, as described by Ursin and Eriksen (2004), helps explain the extreme post-traumatic stress reaction emergency dispatchers feel when faced with their own powerlessness over a traumatic event. According to this theory, stress reactions occur when the desired state does not match the actual or achieved state, so stress is substantially increased when the individual perceives an inability to impact the final outcome—when he or she has no power to make the desired state occur. In their unique role in the system, emergency dispatchers may even feel greater powerlessness than untrained callers or bystanders on scene because they can compare their own role with that of the active responders they are dispatching to the scene; they know the responders will arrive to help but often feel powerless in the meantime. Such experiences are especially common among the many emergency dispatchers who have previously worked in the field, since they are well aware of what actions could be taken to help the patient or victim that they cannot provide (Palmer, 2014).

The perceived disconnect between what the emergency dispatcher wants to achieve, or knows should be done, and what is actually done by the caller or others on scene may also contribute to a condition known as "moral injury" (Shay, 2012). While PTSD generally applies to those who are threatened directly or are witnesses to a traumatic event, moral injury specifically applies to those whose role could be perceived as affecting the outcome—even the perpetrator. A moral injury, in brief, occurs when a person acts in a way that "violates deeply held moral values" (Shay, 2012). In some cases, moral injury can result directly from acting appropriately within a system that constrains the actor's behaviors; for example, it has been suggested that doctors experience moral injury when insurance systems or hospital rules require them to spend less time with patients or provide less-appropriate care than they feel their Hippocratic Oath requires (Bendix, 2019). Emergency dispatchers, who face similar time and system constraints, combined with the limitations of the remote care environment, likely experience similar feelings of disconnect between the care they know should be provided and what they are able to do.

Lack of Closure

Finally, the vicarious trauma experienced by emergency dispatchers is increased substantially by the lack of closure inherent in their remote position. Dispatchers regularly report that they rarely know the outcomes of the calls they handle and that this lack of closure increases their sense of powerlessness because they never know whether their actions were effective in providing help or not (Golding et al., 2017; Tracy & Tracy, 1998). This lack of closure has been associated with continuing hypervigilance, which is one of the arousal criteria associated with PTSD (APA, 2013). Emergency dispatchers described the state they experience as "just waiting" for another similar incident to occur because of heightened arousal from the previous event that never achieved closure (Adams, Shakespeare-Finch, & Armstrong, 2015).

UNIQUE RISK FACTORS: SYSTEMIC ALIENATION

In addition to their constant vicarious exposure to traumatic events over which they often feel powerless, emergency dispatchers also experience another unique set of stressors related to their unusual position as conduits between the public and the social support system. In his work on "street-level bureaucrats" (those who interact directly with the public as the "face" of a governmental organization), Michael Lipsky (2010) identifies four elements of what he terms the "alienation" of such workers: working only on individual "segments" of a problem, lacking control over work input, lacking control over work output, and lacking control over work pace (p.76-78). Both field responders and emergency dispatchers could be seen as experiencing all four of these conditions to some extent; however, as the intersection point among the public, responders, and the public health and public safety systems, emergency dispatchers are particularly at risk.

Lack of Control

More so even than field responders, emergency dispatchers lack control over their workflow (the input of their work) and its impact (the outcome). As was discussed above, dispatchers often feel that they have little power over the events they handle and that working through others—whether providing instructions to callers or sending responders to the scene—means that they don't have the impact on the outcome that they would like to have. Their powerlessness over outcome is somewhat mitigated, at least, because they are able to provide advice and instructions, gather relevant information to pass to responders, and provide access to help for patients and victims. In terms of input and work pace, they have no control at all. As Lipsky (2009) defines it, lack of control over input means lack of control over the client's circumstances when they enter the system. For emergency dispatchers, lack of control over input is reflected in the fact that callers often don't contact emergency services until it is too late to help, as in the case of a woman reporting the hanging suicide of her husband, who is clearly already dead (Tracy & Tracy, 1989). In the same way, a caller may report a chronic condition that has already been badly managed long before the call was made, or may be already engaged in an event or trapped in a situation, such as domestic violence, that it is not within the emergency dispatcher's ability to handle and that already existed before the dispatcher had any chance to intervene.

Emergency dispatchers cannot, in other words, determine when, whether, or why citizens will decide to call their emergency number; they can only attempt to apply the available solutions to the situations presented to them. Although this is true to some extent of field responders as well, their level of control over the input into their work is substantially higher—largely because of emergency dispatchers. When a dispatcher answers the phone, the situation could be almost anything; his or her job is to prioritize, to weed out the hang-ups and drunk dials, to assign low response priorities to non-urgent calls, and to send responders out, with as much information as possible, on the emergencies. As a result, field responders start out to any incident with significant information already in hand, and with the knowledge that a huge subset of non-urgent, accidental, and other types of calls have already been handled.

Lack of Recognition

One of the most distressing aspects of their location between the public and responders is that despite their powerlessness to change the situation, emergency dispatchers are often the ones blamed—from both sides. Callers often call back to the dispatcher over and over if responders do not arrive quickly, blaming the dispatcher for the delay even though he or she has no control over the activities of the responders (Tracy & Tracy, 1998); those in the calltaker position (rather than working on the radio) are most likely to be subject to this blame despite having the least control, since they do not even directly dispatch the units. On the other side, emergency dispatchers are often blamed by the field responders as well, often for gathering what field crews see as incomplete or inaccurate information (when they can only gather what the caller can or will provide); some even report receiving "abuse" from responders (Sprigg, Armitage, & Hollis, 2007).

Just as "powerlessness" is the key to understanding the level of vicarious trauma experienced by emergency dispatchers in handling emergency calls, the sense of being invisible to or separated from the rest of the public safety team is the key to understanding the work stress they experience in their position between the public and the responders. Dispatchers regularly report that both the public and responders lack an understanding of what dispatchers actually do and its complexity (Coxon et al., 2016; Golding et al., 2017) and that this lack of understanding leads them to feel invisible and undervalued. Many also report that they feel "divided" from the rest of the team and describe being excluded from debriefings, training, and other support and recognition opportunities (Adams, Shakespeare-Finch, & Armstrong, 2015; Burke, 1995). This divide separates them from the benefits that often otherwise goes along with high-stress work, such as a sense of camaraderie and a feedback loop to find out what happened following an event.

Oversight

Finally, emergency dispatchers report constant oversight as one of the systemic stressors of their position (Adams, Shakespeare-Finch, & Armstrong, 2014; Golding et al., 2017). Every single emergency call handled by an emergency dispatcher is recorded and can be recovered later for quality assurance, review, or questioning, creating the sense that any mistake made under time pressure may be reviewed and criticized later. Compared to this level of scrutiny, the work of field responders—who spend significant time in self-organized crews managing scene activities—has a high level of freedom of action and freedom from direct oversight. Such a difference contributes to the feeling among emergency dispatchers that they are not full, or fully-trusted, professionals with standing equal to other emergency service team members.

The Paradox of Powerlessness

In defining the cognitive activation theory of stress, Ursin and Eriksen (2004) note that "individuals working in a job where they have high demands, low control, and low social support carry the highest risk of illness and disease" (p. 579-580). Emergency dispatching could be described as fitting every one of these conditions at the highest level. Yet emergency dispatchers—like others in high-stress, life-critical, time-pressured fields—often report high levels of job satisfaction (Ujevic et al., 2018). As Mastracci, Guy, and Newman (2012) put it in their discussion of emotional labor, despite the fact that jobs involving high levels of emotional labor can be stressful and cause long-term emotional deficits for those who work in them, nonetheless "the more that emotional labor is performed, the higher is the worker's level of job satisfaction" (p. 36). Or as Golding et al. (2017) note, some dispatchers reported "gaining 'emotional competence'" as one of the benefits arising from the difficulties of their job or "appeared to enjoy the fast-paced and sometimes exciting environment" in which they worked. The difference, or the defining factor in achieving an overall sense of satisfaction despite the high level of unique traumatic and stressful exposure, appears to be a combination of self-efficacy (Golding et al., 2017) and inclusion (Adams, Shakespeare-Finch, & Armstrong, 2015).

Emergency dispatchers appear to feel far more control and far less trauma about events when they are given the opportunity—or, even better, the requirement and the tools—to provide immediate advice and instructions to help the caller or others on the scene. One study called this the "trump card" held by emergency dispatchers (Tracy & Tracy, 1998), the one way they could provide direct help to callers, patients, and victims in distress that was unique to their position as the first point of contact. Similarly, the sense that they were able to correctly determine and assign the priority level for the call gave them both a feeling of power over the situation and a sense of their own professional status within the system (Tracy & Tracy, 1998).

Similarly, inclusion in debriefing events "was found to assist emergency medical dispatchers with processing highly traumatic events by providing them with an avenue to discuss their concerns and with psychological closure and value" (Adams, Shakespeare-Finch, & Armstrong, 2015). The simple step of including emergency dispatchers in the training, closure, and celebration events common to emergency responder services could thus powerfully reduce their sense of hypervigilance and increase their perceived self-worth within the emergency response team.

Although relatively little research so far exists on the specific effects of their work on emergency dispatchers' mental health, it is clear that their jobs, far from being just another form of emergency response, are actually characterized by unique elements that would reward further study. And as more and more work of all kinds is done remotely, emergency dispatchers might provide valuable insight into the potential mental health effects of an increasingly mobile world characterized by interactions that are remote, time-pressured, critical, and yet absolutely reliant on effective interpersonal communications—a world increasingly like the one in which emergency dispatchers already live.

REFERENCES

Adams, K., Shakespeare-Finch, J., & Armstrong, D. (2015). An interpretative phenomenological analysis of stress and well-being in emergency medical dispatchers. *Journal of Loss and Trauma*, *20*(5), 430–448. doi:10.1080/15325024.2014.949141

American Psychiatric Association. (2013). *Diagnostic and statistical manual of mental disorders* (5th ed.). Arlington, VA: Author.

Bendix, J. (2019). The real reason docs burn out. *Medical Economics*, *96*(2), 14–25.

Berger, W., Coutinho, E. S., Figueira, I., Marques-Portella, C., Luz, M. P., Neylan, T. C., ... Mendlowicz, M. V. (2012). Rescuers at risk, a systematic literature review and meta-regression analysis of the worldwide current prevalence and correlates of PTSD in rescue workers. *Social Psychiatry and Psychiatric Epidemiology*, *47*(6), 1001–1011. doi:10.100700127-011-0408-2 PMID:21681455

Berger, W., Figueira, I., Maurat, A. M., Bucassio, E. P., Vieira, I., Jardim, S. R., ... Mendlowicz, M. V. (2007). Partial and full PTSD in Brazilian ambulance workers: Prevalence and impact on health and on quality of life. *Journal of Traumatic Stress*, *20*(4), 637–642. doi:10.1002/jts.20242 PMID:17721969

Boland, L. L., Kinzy, T. G., Myers, R. N., Fernstrom, K. M., Kamrud, J. W., Mink, P. J., & Stevens, A. C. (2018). Burnout and exposure to critical incidents in a cohort of emergency medical services workers from Minnesota. *The Western Journal of Emergency Medicine*, *19*(6), 987–995. doi:10.5811/westjem.8.39034 PMID:30429931

Bowbrow, B., Panczyk, M., Stolz, U., Sotelo, M., Vadeboncoeur, T., Sutter, J., ... Spaite, D. (2014). Statewide implementation of a standardized prearrival telephone CPR program is associated with increased bystander CPR and survival from out-of-hospital cardiac arrest. *Circulation*, *130*(22), A1.

Broadbent, M., Gardett, I., Knight, C., Scott, G., Clawson, J. J., & Olola, C. (2018b). Persons description reported to emergency police dispatch. *Annals of Emergency Dispatch & Response*, *6*(3), 21–27.

Broadbent, M., Knight, C., Warner, D., Williams, N., Scott, G., Clawson, J. J., ... Olola, C. (2018a). Weapons reported on-scene by callers to emergency police dispatch. *Annals of Emergency Dispatch & Response*, *6*(1), 19–25.

Brown, J., & Campbell, E. A. (1990). Sources of occupational stress in the police. *Work and Stress*, *4*(4), 305–318. doi:10.1080/02678379008256993

Burke, T. W. (1995). Dispatcher stress. *FBI Law Enforcement Bulletin*, *64*(10), 1–6.

Carleton, R. N., Afifi, T. O., Taillieu, T., Turner, S., El-Gabalawy, R., Sareen, J., & Asmundson, G. J. G. (2018a). Anxiety-related psychopathology and chronic pain comorbidity among public safety personnel. *Journal of Anxiety Disorders*, *55*, 48–55. PMID:29566981

Carleton, R. N., Afifi, T. O., Turner, S., Taillieu, T., LeBouthillier, D. M., Duranceau, S., ... Asmundson, G. J. G. (2018b). Suicidal ideation, plans, and attempts among public safety personnel in Canada. *Canadian Psychology*, *59*(3), 220–231. doi:10.1037/cap0000136

Carlier, I. V., Lamberts, R. D., & Gersons, B. P. (1997). Risk factors for posttraumatic stress symptomology in police officers: A prospective analysis. *The Journal of Nervous and Mental Disease*, *195*(8), 498–506. doi:10.1097/00005053-199708000-00004 PMID:9284863

Chopko, B. A., Palmieri, P. A., & Adams, R. E. (2015). Correlates of career traumatization and symptomology among active duty police officers. *Criminal Justice Studies*, *25*(1), 83–95. doi:10.1080/1478601X.2012.657905

Clawson, J., Scott, G., Gardett, I., Patterson, B., Barron, T., & Olola, C. (2014). Ability of a diabetic problems protocol to predict patient severity indicators determined by on-scene EMS crews. *Resuscitation*, *85*(s1), S111.

Clawson, J. J., Dernocoeur, K. B., & Murray, C. (2015). *Principles of Emergency Medical Dispatch*. Salt Lake City, UT: Priority Press.

Clawson, J. J., Gardett, I., Scott, G., Fivaz, C., Barron, T., Broadbent, M., & Olola, C. (2018, February). Hospital-confirmed acute myocardial infarction: Prehospital identification using the Medical Priority Dispatch System. *Prehospital and Disaster Medicine*, *33*(1), 29–35. doi:10.1017/S1049023X1700704X PMID:29223194

Clawson, J. J., Scott, G., Gardett, I., Youngquist, S., Taillac, P., Fivaz, C., & Olola, C. (2016). Predictive ability of an emergency medical dispatch stroke diagnostic tool in identifying hospital-confirmed strokes. *Journal of Stroke and Cerebrovascular Diseases*, *25*(8), 2031–2042. doi:10.1016/j.jstrokecerebrovasdis.2016.04.021 PMID:27256173

Cohen, K., & Collens, P. (2013). The impact of trauma work on trauma workers: A metasynthesis on vicarious trauma and vicarious posttraumatic growth. *Psychological Trauma: Theory, Research, Practice, and Policy*, *5*(6), 570–580. doi:10.1037/a0030388

Coxon, A., Cropley, M., Schofield, P., Start, K., Horsfield, C., & Quinn, T. (2016). "You're never just making one decision": Exploring the lived experiences of ambulance Emergency Operations Centre personnel. *Emergency Medicine Journal*, *33*(9), 645–651. PMID:27002162

Dillard, M. B., Warm, J. S., Funke, G. J., Nelson, T., Finomore, V. S., McClernon, C. K., ... Funke, M. E. (2019). Vigilance tasks: Unpleasant, mentally demanding, and stressful even when time flies. *Human Factors*, *61*(2), 225–242. doi:10.1177/0018720818796015 PMID:30216088

Donnelly, E. (2012). Work-related stress and posttraumatic stress in emergency medical services. *Prehospital Emergency Care*, *16*(1), 76–85. PMID:22128908

Forslund, K., Kihlgren, A., & Kihlgren, M. (2004). Operators' experiences of emergency calls. *Journal of Telemedicine and Telecare*, *10*, 290–297. PMID:15494088

Fullerton, C. S., Ursano, R. J., & Wang, L. (2004). Acute stress disorder, posttraumatic stress disorder, and depression in disaster or rescue workers. *The American Journal of Psychiatry*, *161*(8), 1370–1376. PMID:15285961

Gardett, I., Olola, C., Scott, G., Broadbent, M., & Clawson, J. J. (2017). Comparison of emergency medical dispatcher stroke identification and paramedic on-scene stroke assessment. *Annals of Emergency Dispatch & Response*, *5*(1), 6–10.

Golding, S. E., Horsfield, C., Davies, A., Egan, B., Jones, M., Raleigh, M., ... Cropley, M. (2017). Exploring the psychological health of emergency dispatch centre operatives: A systematic review and narrative synthesis. *PeerJ*, *5*, e3735. doi:10.7717/peerj.3735 PMID:29062596

Haugen, P. T., Evces, M., & Weiss, D. (2012). Treating posttraumatic stress disorder in first responders: A systematic review. *Clinical Psychology Review*, *32*(5), 370–380. doi:10.1016/j.cpr.2012.04.001 PMID:22561967

Hem, E., Berg, A. M., & Ekberg, O. (2001). Suicide in police – a critical review. *Suicide & Life-Threatening Behavior*, *31*(2), 224–233. doi:10.1521uli.31.2.224.21513 PMID:11459255

Henderson, S. N., Van Hasselt, V. B., LeDuc, T. J., & Couwels, J. (2016). Firefighter suicide: Understanding cultural challenges for mental health professionals. *Professional Psychology, Research and Practice*, *47*(3), 224–230. doi:10.1037/pro0000072

Jahnke, S. A., Poston, W. S. C., Haddock, C. K., & Murphy, B. (2016). Firefighting and mental health: Experiences of repeated exposure to trauma. *Work (Reading, Mass.)*, *53*(4), 737–744. doi:10.3233/WOR-162255 PMID:26890595

Jones, S. P., Carter, B., Ford, G. A., Gibson, J. M. E., Leathley, M. J., McAdam, J. J., ... Watkins, C. L. (2012). The identification of acute stroke: An analysis of emergency calls. *International Journal of Stroke*, *8*(6), 408–412. doi:10.1111/j.1747-4949.2011.00749.x PMID:22335960

Khatiban, M., Hosseini, S., Bikmoradi, A., Roshanaei, G., & Karampourian, A. (2015). Occupational burnout and its determinants among personnel of emergency medical services in Iran. *Acta Medica Iranica*, *53*(11), 711–716. PMID:26786993

Kim, J. E., Dager, S. R., Jeong, H. S., Ma, J., Park, S., Kim, J., ... Lyoo, I. K. (2018). Firefighters, posttraumatic stress disorder, and barriers to treatment: Results from a nationwide total population survey. *PLoS One*, *13*(1), e0190630. doi:10.1371/journal.pone.0190630 PMID:29304155

Lilly, M. M., & Pierce, H. (2013). PTSD and depressive symptoms in 911 telecommunicators: The role of peritraumatic distress and world assumptions in predicting risk. *Psychological Trauma: Theory, Research, Practice, and Policy*, *5*(2), 135–141. doi:10.1037/a0026850

Lipsky, M. (2010). *Street-level bureaucracy: dilemmas of the individual in public services*. New York, NY: Russell Sage Foundation.

Ma, C. C., Burchfiel, C. M., Andrew, M. E., Fekedulegn, T. A., Hartley, J. K., Gu, J. K., ... Charles, L. E. (2013). Shift work and work stress among police officers. *Annals of Epidemiology*, *23*(9), 596. doi:10.1016/j.annepidem.2013.06.080

Markus, G., Hartmann, T., Brand, S., Holsboer-Trachsler, E., & Puhse, U. (2010). The relationship between shift work, perceived stress, sleep and health in Swiss police officers. *Journal of Criminal Justice*, *38*(6), 1167–1175. doi:10.1016/j.jcrimjus.2010.09.005

Mastracci, S. H., Guy, M. E., & Newman, M. A. (2012). *Emotional labor and crisis response: working on the razor's edge*. Armonk, NY: M. E. Sharpe.

McCann, L., & Pearlman, L. A. (1990). *Psychological trauma and the adult survivor* (Vol. 21). New York, NY: Brunner/Mazel.

McQuerry Tuttle, B., Giano, Z., & Merten, M. J. (2018). Stress spillover and negative relationship functioning for law enforcement marriages. *The Family Journal (Alexandria, Va.)*, *26*(2), 246–252. doi:10.1177/1066480718775739

Meischke, H., Painter, I., Lilly, M., Beaton, R., Revere, D., Calhoun, B., ... Baseman, J. (2015). An exploration of sources, symptoms and buffers of occupational stress in 9-1-1 emergency call centers. *Annals of Emergency Dispatch & Response*, *3*(2), 28–35.

Milligan-Saville, J., Choi, I., Deady, M., Scott, P., Tan, L., Calvo, R. A., ... Harvey, S. B. (2018). The impact of trauma exposure on the development of PTSD and psychological distress in a volunteer fire service. *Psychiatry Research*, *270*, 1110–1115. doi:10.1016/j.psychres.2018.06.058 PMID:30190167

Mitani, S., Masatoshi, F., Keiji, N., & Shirakawa, T. (2006, July). Impact of post-traumatic stress disorder and job-related stress on burnout: A study of fire service workers. *The Journal of Emergency Medicine*, *31*(1), 7–11. doi:10.1016/j.jemermed.2005.08.008 PMID:16798146

Mould-Millman, N.-K., Meese, H., Alattas, I., Ido, M., Yi, I., Oyewumi, T., ... Yancey, A. (2018).. . *Prehospital Emergency Care*, *22*(6), 734–742. PMID:29596006

Palmer, C. G. (2014). Stress and coping in wildland firefighting dispatchers. *Journal of Emergency Management (Weston, Mass.)*, *12*(4), 303–314. PMID:25069024

Pierce, H., & Lilly, M. M. (2012). Duty-related trauma exposure in 911 telecommunicators: Considering the risk for posttraumatic stress. *Journal of Traumatic Stress*, *25*(2), 211–215. PMID:22467384

Price, M. (2017). Psychiatric disability in law enforcement officers. *Behavioral Sciences & the Law*, *35*(2), 113–123. doi:10.1002/bsl.2278 PMID:28303590

Rallings, M. (2000). *Police and trauma: A prospective examination of the psychological effects of occupational exposure to traumatic events* (Doctoral dissertation). Retrieved from WorldCat.

Ramanujam, P., Guluma, K. Z., Castillo, E. M., Chacon, M., Jensen, M. B., Patel, E., ... Dunford, J. V. (2008). Accuracy of stroke recognition by emergency medical dispatchers and paramedics—San Diego experience. *Prehospital Emergency Care*, *12*(3), 307–313. doi:10.1080/10903120802099526 PMID:18584497

Scott, G., Clawson, J., Fivaz, M. C., McQueen, J., Gardett, M. I., Schultz, B., ... Olola, C. (2016, February). Using on-scene EMS responders' assessment and electronic patient care records to evaluate the suitability of EMD-triaged, low-acuity calls for secondary nurse triage in 911 centers. *Prehospital and Disaster Medicine*, *31*(1), 46–57. doi:10.1017/S1049023X15005567 PMID:26758527

Scott, G., Clawson, J. J., Gardett, I., Broadbent, M., Williams, N., Fivaz, C., ... Olola, C. (2017). 9-1-1 triage of non-traumatic chest pain: Association with hospital diagnosis. *Prehospital Emergency Care*, *21*(4), 525–534. doi:10.1080/10903127.2017.1302530 PMID:28409655

Shay, J. (2012). Moral injury. *Intertexts*, *16*(1), 57–66.

Sprigg, C. A., Armitage, C. J., & Hollis, K. (2007). Verbal abuse in the National Health Service: Impressions of the prevalence, perceived reasons for and relationships with staff psychological well-being. *Emergency Medicine Journal*, *24*(4), 281–282. PMID:17384383

Thackray, R. I. (1981). The stress of boredom and monotony: A consideration of the evidence. *Psychosomatic Medicine*, *43*(2), 165–176. PMID:7267937

Trachik, B., Marks, M. R., Bowers, C., Scott, G., Olola, C., & Gardett, I. (2015). Is dispatching a traffic accident as stressful as being in one? Acute stress disorder, secondary traumatic stress, and occupational burnout in 911 emergency dispatchers. *Annals of Emergency Dispatch & Response*, *3*(1), 27–38.

Tracy, S. J., & Tracey, K. (1998). Emotion labor at 911: A case study and theoretical critique. *Journal of Applied Communication Research*, *26*(4), 390–411. doi:10.1080/00909889809365516

Tuckey, M. R., Winwood, P. C., & Dollard, M. F. (2012). Psychosocial culture and pathways to psychological injury within policing. *Police Practice and Research*, *13*(3), 224–240.

Ujevic, R. M., Prizmic, J., Barisin, A. B., Maras, M., & Luetic, L. (2018). Is there a difference in job satisfaction at emergency medicine service (EMS) team and EMS dispatchers? *Resuscitation*, *130S*, e140.

Ursin, H., & Eriksen, H. (2004). The cognitive activation theory of stress. *Psychoneuroendocrinology*, *29*(5), 567–592. doi:10.1016/S0306-4530(03)00091-X PMID:15041082

Chapter 5
The First, First Responder:
The Neglected Needs and Unique Challenges of Work as a 9-1-1 Telecommunicator

Michelle M. Lilly
Northern Illinois University, USA & 9-1-1 Recovers, LLC, USA

Zena Dadouch
https://orcid.org/0000-0002-3372-8028
Northern Illinois University, USA

Diana A. Robinson
Northern Illinois University, USA

ABSTRACT

Research on the health and wellness of emergency responders has continued to grow over the past two decades, demonstrating the profound impact of duty-related exposure to stress and trauma on responders' physical and mental health. The majority of this important literature has been conducted with field responders, including police officers and firefighters. As the first, first responder, the health and wellness of 9-1-1 telecommunicators has been largely neglected, despite the high levels of recurrent exposure to duty-related traumatic events among this population. This chapter reviews the current empirical literature on mental and physical health in 9-1-1 telecommunicators, followed by discussion on factors within the 9-1-1 work environment that may be responsible for elevated rates of mental and physical health problems. Prevention and intervention efforts for 9-1-1 telecommunicators are then discussed, followed by research showing the potentially profound impact of poor mental health on 9-1-1 telecommunicator performance.

DOI: 10.4018/978-1-5225-9803-9.ch005

INTRODUCTION

The health and safety of the general public depends largely on the efficiency and proficiency of emergency responders. From securing a dangerous scene, to delivering a baby, to saving a life while an injured person is rushed to the emergency department, the performance of emergency responders can make the difference between life and death. What is often obscured in the emergency response chain is the vital role played by 9-1-1 telecommunicators (TCs). As the first, first responder, 9-1-1 TCs answer calls placed by individuals who are often in extreme distress or in significant peril. The caller may be hysterical or may be suffering from an injury that makes it difficult to provide critical information to the 9-1-1 TC, such as location or nature of their injuries. The 9-1-1 TC must calm distressed callers while simultaneously securing the information needed to dispatch field responders. Field responders are provided crucial information about the caller and scene so that they can be prepared upon arrival. In some instances, the 9-1-1 TC may hear a caller's final breaths while they wait for field responders to arrive.

While many calls of an erroneous nature are made to 9-1-1 (e.g., asking what the time is), a 9-1-1 TC may handle multiple calls across a single shift in which there is a major medical emergency, including emergencies that involve children or possibly their own family members or friends. Over the course of a year, a 9-1-1 TC may be exposed to thousands of calls in which they are confronted with trauma and the suffering of others. The cumulative effects of such recurrent exposure to duty-related trauma enhances risk for a host of adverse psychological outcomes, including posttraumatic stress disorder (PTSD), depression, alcohol or substance abuse, and anxiety. In addition, the recurrent exposure may wear down the physical health of 9-1-1 TCs over time, leading to physical health complaints, obesity, and disease. Though limited, research on the psychological and physical health of 9-1-1 TCs will be reviewed in the next section.

While recurrent exposure to duty-related trauma enhances risk for a host of adverse outcomes, additional factors associated with the 9-1-1 work environment also enhance risk for stress-based pathology. Greater detail regarding the stressors associated with the 9-1-1 work environment are covered in this chapter. Briefly, 9-1-1 TCs are masters of multi-tasking, often having to integrate information from multiple screens in order to dispatch appropriate personnel while also receiving and recording information from callers. As a 24/7 industry, 9-1-1 TCs often encounter mandatory overtime if the call center is understaffed (which is a common occurrence in the industry) or if a colleague calls in sick. Shifts are often long and may be on a swing schedule. All of these factors can lead to exhaustion and difficulty achieving balance between the duties of work and home. Misconceptions among the general public regarding the work of 9-1-1 TCs and encountering the abuses of the 9-1-1 system by phony callers add to the stress and frustrations of work in the 9-1-1 industry.

In addition to these environmental factors, the nature of 9-1-1 calls amplifies the stress burden. Across many contexts, research suggests that the following four factors are among the strongest predictors of stress: novelty, lack of control, lack of predictability, and social evaluation. That is, events that present with novel features not previously encountered, events over which a person has limited control, events that are unpredictable, and events in which a person might be negatively evaluated or judged by others are often associated with the highest levels of stress. For 9-1-1 TCs, these factors are essentially a job description. This is especially true following the Freedom of Information Act (FOIA) in which a recording of a 9-1-1 call can be requested by anyone in the general public at any time. To ensure adequate performance, 9-1-1 centers emphasize the importance of quality assurance, which may be beneficial to the general public, but results in TCs being under the constant scrutiny of call center managers.

As the first, first responder, the accuracy and efficiency of the tasks performed by 9-1-1 TCs cannot be overstated. Small errors that delay the emergency response sequence could be fatal for a caller. Despite the integral role played by 9-1-1 TCs, research examining the health and wellness of this population has lagged significantly behind data collected on field responders. Further, the unique challenges associated with work as a 9-1-1 TC, and implications for intervention, are only now being recognized and addressed. This chapter begins with an overview of the empirical research on psychological and physical health in 9-1-1 TCs. This is followed by a description of aspects of work within the 9-1-1 industry that differentiates it from field responders, and how this enhances risk for adverse outcomes and presents challenges for intervention. Current efforts to develop and validate interventions targeting 9-1-1 will then be discussed, along with recommended approaches to treating stress- and trauma-based disorders. Finally, we include a brief discussion on the impact of psychopathology (i.e., PTSD and depression) on the cognitive functions necessary for optimal performance in the 9-1-1 industry.

HEALTH AND WELLNESS IN 9-1-1 TELECOMMUNICATORS

The long hours of sedentary, high mental demand computer work, coupled with the duty-related stressors of 9-1-1 TCs can have deleterious effects on the physical and mental health of these individuals. In addition to being the first contact for individuals summoning aid for potentially life-threatening crises, 9-1-1 TCs must maintain cognitive and emotional composure while simultaneously assimilating information from five to six computer screens. This includes making precise and rapid decisions that impact the caller and the emergency personnel to be dispatched. Furthermore, not being in direct contact with the event can lead TCs to experience feelings of helplessness and diminished self-efficacy (Adams, Shakespeare-Finch, & Armstrong, 2015; Shakespeare-Finch, Rees, & Armstrong, 2015).

Historically, research on occupational stress has focused on how police, firefighters, and emergency medical responders are impacted by duty-related stress, but has not included investigation of these factors among 9-1-1 TCs (Skogstad et al., 2013). Research examining the work-related stress of non-public safety call center employees has identified symptoms related to poor physical and mental health, reduced productivity, and technostress (i.e., emotional and physical stress related to technology and the fast-paced introduction of new technologies; Rameshbabu, Reddy, & Fleming, 2013). The sparse research that has examined the impact of duty-related stress on 9-1-1 TCs has identified similar stress symptomatology to that found among non-public safety call center employees. For instance, Meischke et al. (2015) examined a large sample of 9-1-1 TCs from the Pacific Northwest of the United States and determined that duty-related stress contributed to heightened reports of anger, excessive rumination, muscle tension, and sleep difficulties (i.e., trouble falling asleep and trouble staying asleep).

The psychological burden of being the first, first responder is illustrated in the prevalence of psychopathology reported by 9-1-1 TCs. Average levels of reported PTSD symptoms among 9-1-1 TCs have ranged from sub-clinical levels (Lilly & Pierce, 2012) to meeting criteria for probable PTSD (Lilly & Allen, 2015). The prevalence of PTSD among 9-1-1 TCs has ranged from 3.5% in an initial convenience sample of TCs (Pierce & Lilly, 2012) to 24.4% in a larger sample of TCs from across the United States (Lilly & Allen, 2015).

Although the literature addressing the physical and mental health needs of 9-1-1 TCs is in its infancy, a small amount of research has been generated regarding the predictors of psychopathology among this population. Research has demonstrated commonalities regarding predictors of psychopathology among 9-1-

1 TCs and other trauma-exposed populations (i.e., peritraumatic distress, coping strategies). Peritraumatic distress (i.e., distressing emotions present at the time of trauma) has been cited as a strong predictor of PTSD symptoms among various trauma-exposed populations, including sexual assault survivors, combat-exposed military personnel, and police officers (e.g., Brunet et al., 2001; Ozer, Best, Lipsey, & Weiss, 2003). Although they are not typically directly exposed to traumatic events, 9-1-1 TCs are not immune to experiencing peritraumatic distress. Among a sample of 9-1-1 TCs in the United States, measures of work-related events, peritraumatic distress, self-worth, and benevolence of the world were assessed in relation to measures of PTSD and depression symptoms (Lilly & Pierce, 2012). Findings from this study indicated that peritraumatic distress was significantly positively associated with PTSD and depression symptoms. Moreover, world assumptions, specifically self-worth and beliefs in the benevolence of the world, moderated the relationship between peritraumatic distress and psychopathology. When individuals endorsed low self-worth and beliefs that the world is not a benevolent place, heightened levels of distress were predictive of greater levels of PTSD and depression (Lilly & Pierce, 2012).

Coping strategies utilized in the aftermath of trauma exposure have also been cited as a strong predictor of PTSD symptoms (e.g., Schnider, Elhai, & Gray, 2007). Among 9-1-1 TCs, coping strategies have been examined as potential mediating factors in the relationship between childhood trauma exposure and PTSD symptoms (Allen, Mercer, & Lilly, 2016). Specifically, emotion-focused coping strategies (i.e., distancing, self-controlling, escape-avoidance, positive reappraisal) and problem-focused coping strategies (i.e., confrontive coping, seeking support, accepting responsibility, planful problem solving) were examined among a large sample of 9-1-1 TCs. Results indicated that three of four emotion-focused coping strategies (i.e., escape-avoidance, self-controlling, and positive reappraisal) were significant mediators in the relationship between childhood trauma exposure and PTSD symptoms, whereas no problem-focused coping strategies significantly mediated this relationship (Allen et al., 2016).

In addition to PTSD, depression is prevalent among 9-1-1 TCs, with rates of probable major depression reaching nearly 25% (Lilly & Allen, 2015). Numerous variables were examined in relation to psychopathology (i.e., depression, PTSD) in TCs including number of years of experience in the field, lifetime trauma exposure, levels of emotion regulation difficulties, event-related distress (i.e., peritraumatic distress and dissociation), anger, and neuroticism. Utilizing structural equation modeling (SEM), results indicated that levels of anger, neuroticism, and event-related distress were significant predictors of depression in TCs. Moreover, psychological inflexibility was the strongest predictor of psychopathology, indicating a potential intervention focus to reduce the negative impacts of duty-related trauma exposure (Lilly & Allen, 2015). The psychological inflexibility construct is now popularly referred to as experiential avoidance (Hayes, 2016), and is a target of cognitive-behavioral treatment, particularly Acceptance and Commitment Therapy (ACT; Hayes, Strosahl, & Wilson, 1999).

Additional factors have been shown to impact health outcomes among 9-1-1 TCs. In a large sample of 9-1-1 TCs in California, path analysis was used to explore the direct and indirect effects of work-related factors (e.g., burnout, work conditions, and work-life balance) on perceived stress, satisfaction with life, depression/anxiety, and physical health (Turner, Lilly, Gamez, & Kressler, 2019). Results revealed that burnout and work-life balance had a strong significant impact on outcomes. Burnout, for instance, was strongly associated with greater perceived stress, depression/anxiety, and physical health complaints, as well as lower satisfaction with life. Better work-life balance was associated with lower perceived stress and higher satisfaction with life. Notably, burnout had a significant indirect effect on each of the outcomes through stress. Said differently, greater burnout led to greater perceived stress, which in turn led to worse outcomes (i.e., higher depression/anxiety, lower physical health and satisfaction with life).

Although much of the first responder literature focuses on the negative trajectory of recovery for trauma-exposed individuals, there is research supporting positive psychological changes following trauma exposure. Although typically examined as a predictor of PTSD, the utilization of specific coping strategies has also been linked to posttraumatic growth (PTG). Posttraumatic growth is defined as perceived positive outcomes reported by individuals who have experienced trauma. Posttraumatic growth can occur in the domains of increased strengths, spiritual change, new life possibilities, and appreciation of life (Tedeschi & Calhoun, 1996). In an evaluation of 9-1-1 TCs, London, Mercer, and Lilly (2017) examined the potential for PTG (i.e., changes in domains of personal strength, new possibilities, relating to others, appreciation of life, and spiritual change) following childhood trauma exposure. Separate models were used to examine the effects of active coping (i.e., seeking support, problem solving, and positive reappraisal) and avoidant coping (i.e., escape avoidance, distancing, self-controlling) strategies on the relationship between childhood trauma exposure and PTG. Results indicated that childhood trauma had an indirect effect on PTG through active coping strategies, such that those with greater early trauma exposure developed adaptive coping habits that positively influenced perceptions of growth. Regarding avoidant coping strategies, results indicated an indirect effect of childhood trauma exposure on psychopathology and PTG, suggesting avoidant coping increases risk for psychopathology, but may also encourage perceptions of growth (London et al., 2017).

The negative outcomes associated with working as a 9-1-1 TC may be buffered by certain resilience factors. Among a sample of emergency medical dispatchers, Shakespeare-Finch et al. (2015) determined that social support and self-efficacy were important positive predictors of psychological well-being and significant negative predictors of PTSD. In their examination of a sample of 9-1-1 TCs in the Pacific Northwest, Meischke et al. (2015) demonstrated that mindfulness (i.e., an ability to pay attention to, recognize, and process one's experiences and emotions without judgement and in the moment) was associated with fewer symptoms of stress. Compassion satisfaction, which includes positive feelings derived from helping others, contributing to the greater good, and working with suffering individuals, has also been proposed as a potential buffer to the negative outcomes associated with working as a 9-1-1 TC (e.g., Figley, 2013; Meischke et al., 2015).

In addition to duty-related stress and negative impacts on mental health, 9-1-1 TCs are susceptible to duty-related physical health concerns. Being a 9-1-1 TC involves working long hours (often with mandatory overtime) and nonstandard schedules in rapid paced, high stress environments. All these factors, coupled with the sedentary nature of the position, can have adverse effects on one's physical health. Among a large sample of 9-1-1 TCs, Lilly, London, and Mercer (2016) examined the rates of obesity and physical health complaints. Regarding rates of obesity, more than half of the sample reported a body mass index (BMI) in the obese range, and nearly 30% of the sample met cutoff criteria for being overweight. In total, 83% of the sample reported height and weight that placed them in the overweight or obese category. Further, the sample endorsed experiencing headaches, back pains, sleeping difficulties/insomnia, muscle tension, and itchy eyes or skin, all of which can be attributed to the work environment. Notably, participants reported an average of 17 physical health complaints in the previous month alone (Lilly et al., 2016).

FACTORS UNIQUE TO 9-1-1 TELECOMMUNICATORS

As discussed in previous sections, the prevalence of psychological and physical health concerns detected in 9-1-1 TCs is troubling. Different job-related aspects unique to TCs distinguish them from field responders. This section discusses distinctive job characteristics of the 9-1-1 industry that increase the likelihood for this group to experience psychological and physical health difficulties.

Lack of Visual Information

The medium of exposure to traumatic content for TCs (i.e., audio) likely plays a major role in the aftereffects of such calls. Although there are assumptions that lack of direct exposure to the scene is protective for 9-1-1 TCs, it is argued that traumatic exposure in the form of audio can have severe emotional and cognitive impact. For instance, a recent study examined how listening to a story, in comparison to watching videos of scenes from famous literary works (e.g., Pride and Prejudice, A Game of Thrones), impact people's physiological reactions (Richardson et al., 2018). The researchers found that participants showed higher engagement with audiobooks than videos. Specifically, they displayed higher average heart rates while listening to audiobooks compared to watching videos. Additionally, they showed higher body temperatures; changes in body temperature indicate fluctuations in blood flow, a process regulated by the autonomic nervous system (ANS). Finally, listeners also showed higher ectodermal activity, which is a measure of emotional arousal (Critchley, 2002; Sequeira, Hot, Silvert, & Delplanque, 2009). Overall, the findings suggest greater emotional and cognitive activation while listening to audio files versus watching video clips.

Such findings extend directly to 9-1-1 TCs; listening to phone calls likely leads to an increase in telecommunicators' cognitive and emotional engagement. As noted above, it has been found that emotional and cognitive distress during traumatic exposure directly links to PTSD and depression in TCs (Lilly & Pierce, 2012). Compared to the Richardson et al. (2018) study, during which participants listened to audio files for an average of six minutes, TCs' jobs entail answering phone calls, day in and day out. On a typical 12-hour shift, a TC spends an estimated 10.5 hours answering between 40 to 120 phone calls separated by a six-second resting-period (Dicks, 2014; Wiegand, 2013); many of the phone calls are likely to be stressful or distressing. This intense and prolonged stimulation stemming from duty-related traumatic audio might lead to wear-and-tear to the ANS, increasing the risk of developing stress-related disorders (e.g., PTSD; Cacioppo et al., 1998; 2000) and weaker immune systems (Maier & Watkins, 1998), resulting in greater physiological concerns. Indeed, a recent dissertation project found that when exposing participants to either a 9-1-1 phone call or a news segment, those listening to the 9-1-1 calls had stronger physiological stress reactions (i.e., increased heart rate, breathing) compared to those who listened to the news segment (Hammelman, 2012).

Relatedly, Chow and colleagues (2014) used functional magnetic resonance imaging (fMRI) to assess brain activity of participants listening to one of three types of stories: action-packed, visually-vivid, or emotionally-charged. All three story types activated temporal lobes and Broca's area, a brain region linked to speech production. Of special interest were differences in activated areas between the story types. Specifically, action-based stories led to activation of areas within the premotor cortex. Visually-vivid stories led to activation of two regions linked with visuo-spatial processing. Finally, emotionally-charged stories led to activation in areas of the limbic system associated with emotional reactions. This suggests that beyond engaging essential "language areas", listening to stories leads to activation in perception-, action-, and emotion-related neurological systems (e.g., amygdala). Hence, it is possible that TCs listening to a large number of action-packed, visually-vivid, and/or emotionally-charged calls on a daily basis likely experience highly activated neurological systems (e.g., amygdala), which may partially explain the increased risk of psychopathology (Shin, Rauch, & Pitman, 2006).

Unknown Call Outcomes

In comparison to on-the-scene first responders who often learn the outcome or resolution of the emergency (e.g., domestically abused woman was taken to the emergency room and her abuser was taken into police custody), due to the fact that 9-1-1 TCs are physically removed from the scene, they often do not learn this information (Shakespeare-Finch et al., 2015). This lack of knowledge regarding call outcome might itself contribute to worse mental health for a variety of reasons. First, due to the nature of some calls, the caller might not be able to provide "the whole picture" or clear descriptions of the situation. This may leave the TC unable to provide the best assistance, which might lead to feelings of inadequacy and incompetence (Forslund, Kihlgren & Kihlgren, 2004). Further, "relay syndrome", when information goes from the person in distress to another and then eventually to the TC, has been found to lead to feelings of powerlessness, confusion, and stress (Forslund et al., 2004). To complicate matters further, even if TCs are able to gain a good understanding of the emergency, they may not learn the outcomes of the calls or receive "closure" and validation that their assistance made a difference (Shakespeare-Finch et al., 2015). Self-efficacy plays a protctive role in emergency workers (Cicognani, Pietrantoni, Palestini, & Prati, 2009) and 9-1-1 TCs (Shakespeare-Finch et al., 2015); however, the restricted ability to provide hands-on assistance and reduced likelihood of learning the outcomes of their assistance could negatively impact 9-1-1 TCs' self-efficacy and sense of competency. Over time, this is likely to increase baseline levels of stress and may lead to psychological exhaustion, anxiety, or depression.

Inability to Predict Calls

Telecommunicators are the first point of entry for most medical emergencies. They collect and decode as much information as possible and disseminate it in a timely and organized fashion to the next point of contact (e.g., fire personnel, police), who receive this information and continue to provide the necessary aid. Unlike field responders, 9-1-1 TCs rarely (if ever) have information regarding the details of the emergency prior to the incoming call (Burke, 1995; Burke, 2005). For instance, a dispatcher could receive a calm call regarding an abandoned car immediately followed by an incredibly distraught call about an unresponsive newborn baby. The inability to predict call content, and the instability in the nature of the calls, is an additional source of distress for TCs. Unpredictability is a core construct across fear and anxiety disorders (Mineka & Oehlberg, 2008), and studies have supported an increased risk for PTSD resulting from unpredictable aversive events in animal (Foa, Zinbarg, & Rothbaum, 1992) and human studies (Başoğlu, & Mineka, 1992; Grillon et al., 2009; Tobin, 1997).

Further, it is established that feeling in control helps diminish the effects of stressful events (Brennan & Riccio, 1975; Mineka Cook, & Miller, 1984), supporting the hypothesis that the uncontrollable nature of the calls would intensify distress levels in dispatchers. Individuals with PTSD seem to be oversensitive to unpredictability (Grillon et al., 2009), proposing that dispatchers living with posttraumatic stress symptoms (PTSS) likely experience added daily job-related distress. Research with this group strongly corroborates such conclusions, citing the difficulties they experience with lack of control, helplessness, unforeseeable events, powerlessness, uncertainty, and unknown outcomes (Adams et al., 2015; Forslund et al., 2004; Gurevich, Halpern, Brazeau, Defina, & Schwartz, 2009; Meischke et al., 2015; Tracy & Tracy, 1998; Wiegand, 2013). Relatedly, dispatchers struggling with traumatic stress are likely to get re-exposed to many of the same emergencies that triggered the posttraumatic reactions, causing a reactivation of earlier trauma memories and PTSD symptoms. Based on emotional processing theory (Foa & Kozak, 1986), a traumatic/feared experience or stimuli could form distorted fear networks made up of interconnected memories, behaviors, thoughts, and feelings. Any of the nodes in the network, including new traumas or the recurrence of the feared stimulus itself (e.g., another call regarding a suspected case of child sexual assault), would lead to the activation of the fear structure. Imaging studies further imply that creating a mental scene of a described situation could lead to a reactivation of a previous personal experience (i.e., prior traumatic call; Chow et al., 2014). Dispatchers are unable to identify the type of the emergency of the incoming call and are likely to be re-exposed to the type of emergency they have been adversely affected by, leading to an activation of the fear structure and consequently posttrauma reactions (e.g., distress, hyperarousal, withdrawal).

Trauma Load

Research has consistently supported a dose-response relationship between psychopathology and trauma exposure in general populations (Kira et al., 2008; van der Kolk, McFarlane, & Weisaeth, 1996) and in first responders such as police officers (Violanti et al., 2011), paramedics (Sofianopoulos, Williams, Archer, & Thompson, 2011), firefighters (Carey, Al-Zaiti, Dean, Sessanna, & Finnell, 2011), and 9-1-1 TCs (Adams et al. 2015; Pierce & Lilly, 2012; Trachik et al., 2015). That is, the greater amount of exposure over time, the greater the risk for symptoms of clinical conditions. TCs receive a large number of phone calls during each shift (Dicks, 2014); unsurprisingly, the number of traumatic calls has been found to significantly correlate with perceived lack of control and feelings of helplessness (Adams et al., 2015). In addition, experienced distress during the time of the stressful calls (i.e., peritraumatic distress) has predicted compassion fatigue (Troxell, 2008) and PTSD symptomatology (Pierce & Lilly, 2012) among 9-1-1 TCs. Further, the type of emergencies and the extent to which the calls are distressing (e.g., suicides, involving children, uncooperative callers) predicted higher PTSS levels in a sample of 9-1-1 TCs (Pierce & Lilly, 2012; Trachik et al., 2015). The traumatic work load has also been shown to predict feelings of burnout and compassion fatigue (Troxell, 2008), and 9-1-1 TCs experiencing PTSS endorse higher burnout (Trachik et al., 2015). Burnout is the result of severe stress and high ideals experienced by people working in "helping" professions (Freudenberger, 1980). Burnout has been shown to adversely impact performance and decrease job efficacy, particularly in high-risk environments (Bakker, Demerouti, & Euwema, 2005). On the other hand, dispatchers reported feeling guilt and blame for not being able to assist severely distressed callers due to being overworked or overwhelmed (Tracey & Tracey, 1998). Further, job stress has been shown to predict poor job satisfaction, which in turn increases risk of job turnover (Liu, 2005). Dispatchers endorse high job stress and intense demands, and a significant positive association between job demands and stress, anxiety, and depression has been detected (Wiegand, 2013). Finally, in addition to high levels of stress, dispatchers endorsed receiving low compensation for their job and lack of job security, which was also associated with increased daily stress (Wiegand, 2013).

Inability to Take Breaks

Considering the frequency of calls to dispatch centers, and the significantly lower number of 9-1-1 TCs compared to other emergency personnel (e.g., 108 dispatchers vs. 1000 paramedics in one urban center; Gurevich et al., 2009), 9-1-1 TCs are exposed to a higher number of potentially stressful incidents within each shift. For instance, it has been reported that in one 12-hour shift, a 9-1-1 TC answers emergency phone calls for approximately 10.5 hours (Dicks, 2014). Inadequate break time (Burke, 1995; Dicks, 2014; Driscoll, Tubbs, Habes, 2007; Gurevich et al., 2009; Ramey et al., 2017; Wiegand, 2013), a lack of a quiet space in which to take a break, recuperate, and regain composure (Burke, 1995; Forslund et al., 2004; Gurevich et al., 2009), and poor air quality, inadequate lighting, and ergonomics (Driscoll et al., 2007; Wiegand, 2013) have all been cited as amplifying work-related distress. Others have cited the guilt dispatchers feel when they need to take a break or when they want to take a day off (Dicks, 2014), and feeling extremely cautious before taking an unscheduled break out of fear that they might seem weak or unable to handle the job (Gurevich et al., 2009). Interestingly, 9-1-1 TCs with rotational shift-work (i.e., outside of the normal 9 a.m. to 5 p.m. schedule) and less break time are more likely to meet criteria for acute stress disorder (ASD) and PTSD compared to those who work a stable shift schedule (Shakespeare-Finch et al., 2015; Trachik et al., 2015).

Inadequate break time could lead to worsened well-being. An experienced threat produces a stress response that involves both psychological and physiological reactions operating outside of regular homeostasis, the state at which the body is maintained at optimal levels (Solomon & Heide, 2005). Once the threat, or in this case, the distressing phone call, dissipates, the body undergoes adaptive responses that return it to regular homeostatic functioning. However, there is a breakdown in the process of returning to this normal state of functioning in individuals with PTSD (Solomon & Heide, 2005). Hence, on-duty dispatchers with PTSS might need more time to return to homeostasis compared to those without PTSS. Without the recovery period, 9-1-1 TCs with elevated PTSS may experience increased distress and more difficulties in efficiently making decisions and performing duties (Gurevich et al., 2006). To complicate matters further, dispatchers are expected to display a calm and collected demeanor with the callers and to mask their own emotional reactions (Tracey & Tracey, 1998), which might be incredibly difficult during a strong fight-or-flight response, or during times when a 9-1-1 TC must answer a call before physiologically recovering from the previous call.

Pressures of Quality Assurance

Research has consistently shown that negative social evaluation is linked with higher stress and cortisol release (Dickerson & Kemeny, 2004). Cortisol is an important hormone with psychological and physiological impacts. A meta-analysis of over 200 laboratory studies concluded that rates of cortisol responses increased in situations when performance could be judged negatively by others. Further, when such social evaluations were uncontrollable, the changes in cortisol and adrenocorticotropic hormone were the largest, and recovery times were the longest (Dickerson & Kemeny, 2004). Extending such findings to 9-1-1 TCs, who are under constant monitoring and quality assurance checks, complicates issues further. If a 9-1-1 TC is unable to assist a caller, he or she may be blamed for failing to help, even if it was not in their control. In fact, 9-1-1 TCs report experiencing higher distress during phone calls due to concerns about negative evaluations if they are unable to perform their jobs well (Tracy & Tracey, 1998). Further, 9-1-1 TCs whose work was monitored and checked more often by superiors endorsed worse overall well-being (Charbotel et al., 2007). Those who felt unsupported by their managers while facing work-related difficulties (e.g., felt their managers were not willing to listen to problems, felt they could not talk to their managers) reported more anxiety and depression symptoms, and used more sick days than those who did not feel unsupported (Driscoll et al., 2007). Additionally, a general lack of recognition, appreciation, or support has been cited as a significant source of stress for this population (Behr, 2000; Charbotel et al., 2007; Forslund et al., 2004; Gurevich et al., 2009; Trachik et al., 2015; Troxell, 2008). On the other hand, having a supportive and concerned supervisor was found to be negatively associated with taking sick days (Martin, 2016), which supports the literature suggesting managerial styles can strongly impact wellbeing. Finally, as supervisors scrutinize different calls, dispatchers could constantly become re-exposed to highly distressing calls, which may trigger symptoms of PTSD.

Sedentary Nature

Due to the sedentary nature of the job, as hours are spent sitting down in front of computer monitors, 9-1-1 TCs often leave their shifts feeling physically exhausted (Wiegand, 2013). Of the most frequently endorsed physical complaints are headaches, attributed to looking at monitors for a prolonged period of time, and musculoskeletal pains (e.g., shoulder, back, and wrist pain) attributed to prolonged sitting and use of keyboards (Charbotel et al., 2007; Driscoll et al., 2007; Wiegand, 2013). Musculoskeletal pains have been positively linked with anxiety, depression, low job satisfaction, and low supervisory support in a sample of 9-1-1 TCs (Driscoll et al., 2007). Unsurprisingly, time spent in the field and in call centers has been positively linked with negative health complaints and outcomes (Lilly et al., 2016; Rameshbabu et al., 2013). Further, it was found that even those less than two years on the job reported high gastrointestinal difficulties and body pains (Rameshbabu et al., 2013). As noted earlier, elevated rates of obesity (i.e., 53.4%) have been detected in a large sample of TCs, and less than one in five TCs fell in the normal weight range (Lilly et al., 2016). In addition, inadequate sleep has been linked with worsened health in this group (Rameshbabu et al., 2013). Finally, high rates of absenteeism have been largely explained by acute illness and chronic diseases (Driscoll et al., 2007). These findings are unsurprising, as it is known that prolonged stress impacts the immune system, leading to higher release of glucocorticoids (i.e., stress hormones; Carlson, 2013). This directly suppresses the immune system's activity and possibly leads to higher incidences of disease. Feeling out of control and overwhelmed and living a sedentary life have been associated with weaker immune systems (Cohen, Tyrrell, & Smith, 1991; Knapp et al., 1992; Simpson & Guy, 2010). It is therefore unsurprising that physiological concerns are commonly reported by 9-1-1 TCs working in highly stressful settings.

PREVENTION AND INTERVENTION WITH 9-1-1 TELECOMMUNICATORS

This chapter has focused on the myriad pathways and factors that enhance risk for poor physical and mental health outcomes among 9-1-1 TCs. The good news is that effective interventions exist to reduce workplace stress and psychological conditions such as PTSD and depression. These will be described briefly in the upcoming pages. However, mental health practitioners cannot treat empty chairs. That is, the largest challenge in treating emergency responding populations, including 9-1-1 TCs, is the stigma associated with needing and seeking help. Like their field responding peers, center culture is marked by a privileging of stoicism, an emphasis on handling calls effectively while remaining emotionally untouched. To be affected by the emergency responding work is considered a sign of weakness or failure. This is further complicated by the avoidance that is part of the clinical picture of PTSD. That is, one of the symptoms of PTSD is strong avoidance of reminders of the traumatic event, including thoughts, memories, people, places, or things associated with the trauma. As many trauma-focused interventions require engaging with the traumatic memory, it can be difficult for 9-1-1 TCs to enter and remain in therapy through to completion. Further, the lack of energy and hopelessness common in disorders such as depression prevent individuals from finding the motivation to seek out and complete treatment. Unfortunately, conditions such as PTSD may persist for years without proper treatment, with a recent study showing that 39% of individuals will suffer a chronic course of PTSD without treatment (Santiago et al., 2013). These numbers are likely higher among individuals chronically re-exposed to emotionally-taxing or triggering experiences, such as what occurs for a 9-1-1 TC who continues to work in the industry. Several interventions for stress and psychological conditions are in development or are suggested as methods to better reach this critical population.

Stress Intervention for 9-1-1

Across the country, a number of work groups and training institutes have begun to conceptualize and develop interventions for the 9-1-1 industry. The majority of these interventions are focused on providing education regarding stress, distress, and coping, with the belief that knowledge breeds insight and behavioral change. There is also increased emphasis on training 9-1-1 professionals in the area of peer support with the confidence that creating healthier work environments in which TCs feel supported by, and can lean into, the relationships at work will provide systematic relief to a stressed industry. Though, to the authors' knowledge, a carefully designed and executed study evaluating the efficacy of a formalized peer support program has yet to be published, an emphasis on peer support is promising given the evidence showing the strong salutary impact of social support for stress, PTSD, and depression (Ozer et al., 2003; Gariepy, Honkaniemi, & Quesnel-Vallee, 2016), and the positive impact of social support in enhancing well-being among 9-1-1 TCs in particular (Shakespeare-Finch et al., 2015).

Another promising approach to stress reduction is mindfulness-based intervention (MBI). Mindfulness is an ancient concept, and its definition may change slightly depending on one's source of information. However, most recently, mindfulness has been defined as awareness that arises through paying attention, on purpose, in the present moment, non-judgmentally (Kabat-Zinn, Lipworth, & Burney, 1985). That is, individuals who are more mindful have a heightened ability to attend to one's physical, mental, and emotional experiences as they unfold in the moment, and do so with intent. Mindfulness includes intentionally attending to one's experience in the moment with a stance of openness and curiosity, as opposed to judgment and scrutiny. As an example, if you have ever reminded yourself while getting in the car that you need to drop something in the mailbox on your way to work, only to get to work and look over at the envelope in the passenger seat, you are likely in a state characterized by low mindfulness. Said differently, when operating on auto-pilot, you are likely in a state of mind<u>less</u>ness. It is perhaps unsurprising that low levels of mindfulness have been connected with greater reports of stress and distress, as well as poor mental health outcomes (Bergin & Pakenham, 2016; Brisbon & Lachman, 2017; Dixon & Overall, 2016), including in police officer recruits (Williams, Ciarrochi, & Deane, 2010) and 9-1-1 TCs (Meischke et al., 2015).

Mindfulness-based interventions focus on decreasing time spent on auto-pilot and increasing the frequency of time spent attending to and observing moment-to-moment experiences. When time is allocated to paying attention to one's lived experiences, the door is opened to choosing one's reactions rather than mindlessly engaging in unintended or misplaced behavior, or behavior that may make things worse (e.g., getting angry with loved ones after a hard day at work, overeating while engaging in a mindless task). A recent meta-analysis of studies ($N = 29$) that used MBI among individuals who were considered healthy (i.e., limited psychopathology) found MBI to have a large effect in reducing stress, as well as moderate effect sizes in terms of reducing anxiety, depression, and distress, and enhancing quality of life (Khoury, Sharma, Rush, & Fournier, 2015). In another meta-analysis of studies instituting MBIs to reduce psychological stress in the workplace ($N = 19$), Virgili (2015) found medium-to-large effect sizes from pre- to post-MBI, as well as medium-to-large effect sizes when comparing MBI to inactive control groups. One study found MBI to be associated with significant improvements in resilience, perceived stress, burnout, global mental health, global physical health, fatigue, sleep disturbance, and emotional functioning (Christopher et al., 2015). However, the study was limited by the small sample size ($N = 43$) and lack of a control group. Bergman, Christopher, and Bowen (2016) found decreases in organizational stress, operational stress, and anger as a function of MBI in another study of police officers.

Meischke and colleagues (2018) developed an online MBI tailored to 9-1-1 TCs with the assumption that learning to be mindful between calls or during breaks can decrease time spent on the auto pilot. The intervention aims to help 9-1-1 TCs notice when their heartrates increase, when their thoughts continue to race after a call is complete, or when they are perseverating on a call or work-related incident. This includes developing the ability to thwart self-judgment or self-beratement in case a call does not end well.

Over the course of the last five years, Dr. Meischke's team and the lead author collaborated on the development of an online mindfulness-based intervention for 9-1-1 TCs. An online approach was chosen because in-person approaches, particularly in-person group approaches, present a significant logistic challenge for the 9-1-1 industry. The resulting seven-week intervention is described in greater detail in an open access article (Meischke et al., 2018). Each week, individuals complete an online module of approximately 20-30 minutes in length, which includes a short video introducing the weekly theme, text describing the theme and activities, an audio-guided meditation exercise, suggestions for mindfulness activities for home and work, and a moderated discussion board. Audio-guided exercises are largely meditation-based, or are exercises designed to enhance mindfulness during daily activities (i.e., mindful movement).

To evaluate the efficacy of the intervention, the research team conducted a randomized control trial in which approximately half of the 323 participants were assigned to complete the intervention while the other half were placed in a waitlist condition (Lilly et al., under review). Participants completed measures of stress and mindfulness before participating in the intervention, upon completion of the intervention, and three-months after completing the intervention. Individuals who engaged in the intervention had a significantly greater drop in their stress scores when compared to participants who were on the intervention waitlist (Lilly et al., under review). The reduction in stress scores remained significant at three-month follow-up. The effect size of the intervention was in the moderate range, though it should be noted that the authors took a conservative approach to data analysis. That is, the research team included participants in the analysis who were assigned to the intervention but never actually completed a module. For those who more consistently engaged in the intervention, the impact was much greater. The intervention is now free and accessible to any and all 9-1-1 TCs interested in participating (www.nwcphp.org/training/opportunities/online-courses/stress-reduction-training-for-9-1-1-telecommunicators).

The development of empirically-supported stress interventions for emergency responders that can accommodate the scheduling needs of the population(s) is a great first start. However, results need to be replicated, and studies that incorporate rigorous methodology to examine the efficacy of approaches such as peer support and/or psychoeducational trainings are needed.

Psychological Intervention for 9-1-1 Telecommunicators

For 9-1-1 TCs who seek psychological treatment, options exist that have been empirically shown to reduce psychopathology. Predominantly, the most effective interventions for PTSD, depression, and substance use are cognitive-behavioral in nature. Cognitive behavioral interventions are typically time-limited and structured (i.e., consistent therapeutic targets are addressed with clients across sessions in a systematic way). These approaches attempt to help clients identify how their thinking affects their behaviors and mood, and conversely, provide guided input on behavioral changes that can enhance mood and thinking.

For PTSD in particular, there is a growing and robust literature identifying three treatment options that are most effective and supported by the Veteran's Administration and the National Center for PTSD (www.ptsd.va.gov). The three approaches include Cognitive Processing Therapy (CPT; Resick, Monson, & Chard, 2016), Prolonged Exposure (PE; Foa, Hembree, & Rothbaum, 2007), and Eye Movement Desensitization and Reprocessing (EMDR; Shapiro, 2017). CPT involves identifying and challenging negative cognitions that developed following, or were amplified by, a traumatic event. Self-statements such as "I should have known better" or "People are simply evil" are explored and challenged. PE is based on the principle that, because of avoidance, a traumatic memory has failed to be emotionally processed and integrated into a person's life narrative. Avoidance of the memory and trauma triggers leads to a failure to naturally habituate to the anxiety produced by the memory. Finally, EMDR involves thinking about an upsetting event while engaging in some form of bilateral stimulation, such as moving one's eyes back and forth or using hand tappers in each hand. While it is unclear how the bilateral stimulation aids in the improvements, there is a strong literature supporting EMDR as an empirically-supported treatment for PTSD.

Though rigorous evidence in support of these approaches specifically for 9-1-1 TCs cannot be found, there is no reason to believe that these approaches will not be effective for 9-1-1 TCs. However, the approaches do come at some cost. Traditional psychotherapeutic approaches are financially costly and require time and effort from clients, including preparing for sessions and transporting to and from sessions. Drop-out and lack of response to the interventions described above is higher than is ideal, ranging from 18% to 46% (Bradley, Russ, Dutra, & Westen, 2005; Foa et al., 2005; Hoge et al., 2014; Imel, Laska, Jakupcak, & Simpson, 2013; Resick et al., 2002; Schottenbauer, Glass, Arnkoff, Tendick, & Gray, 2008; Steenkamp, Litz, Hoge, & Marmar, 2015). To successfully complete CPT and PE, clients are encouraged to complete homework assignments out of session to help identify problematic thinking patterns and behaviors, and to practice new cognitions and behaviors. This can be intensive and may be experienced as time-consuming. Further, completing these interventions may be a challenge for 9-1-1 TCs who work long shifts, work non-standard hours, have a shift work schedule, or are required to stay for overtime unpredictably.

Two promising directions may relieve some of the burden for 9-1-1 TCs seeking treatment for PTSD or other conditions. The past five years have seen an explosion in the integration of telebehavioral health approaches. Using videoconferencing software, clients may be served remotely by trauma-trained experts, enhancing a sense of confidentiality in their call center or local community, reducing burden included in travel time to appointments, and assisting in scheduling at hours that may be less standard practice for mental health professionals working in a physical office. Though not consistent across providers, the convenience of seeing clients from one's home or local office may increase the provider's flexibility in scheduling and/or reduce burden on the provider when a client unexpectedly has to cancel due to mandatory overtime.

Another promising approach is Written Exposure Therapy (WET; Sloan, Marx, Bovin, Feinstein, & Gallagher, 2012). WET is a five-session intervention that includes writing about previous upsetting events and then engaging in limited processing of those written narratives with a trained practitioner. Research on the efficacy of WET, particularly WET compared to other empirically-supported treatments for PTSD, remains limited (Sloan, Marx, Lee, & Resick, 2018), but is growing. It may be a less invasive, less time-consuming approach that is experienced as more tolerable or portable than the other approaches. However, additional research is needed, particularly research that demonstrates that the effects of completing the WET protocol do not diminish substantially over time.

IMPLICATIONS OF POOR 9-1-1 HEALTH FOR PUBLIC HEALTH AND SAFETY

Prolonged exposure to stress has a wearing effect that can lead to psychological disorders and physical disease among emergency responders, including 9-1-1 TCs. Recurrent exposure to duty-related trauma also enhances risk for PTSD, as described earlier. As noted earlier, suffering from clinical disorders is associated with many concerning workplace outcomes that can affect center functioning, including absenteeism and job turnover (Driscoll et al., 2007; Kessler & Frank, 1997; Liu, 2005; Munce, Stansfeld, Blackmore, & Stewart, 2007; Wells et al., 2014), the financial costs of which are difficult to estimate and yet to be fully investigated.

Equally concerning is the impact of psychopathology on domains of cognitive functioning that are vital to competent performance among 9-1-1 TCs. Work within the 9-1-1 field requires strong to advanced cognitive skillsets and resources. To perform well, a 9-1-1 TC must have strong attentional capacity, concentration, and decision-making ability. Without these fundamental capacities, the likelihood of making an error or engaging in slow or poor decision making could mean the difference between life and death for a caller. Yet, difficulty with attention and concentration are common symptoms of PTSD (American Psychiatric Association [APA], 2013). Further, difficulty with concentration and decision-making are symptoms of depression (APA, 2013). This is to say that core symptoms of disorders that may be more likely to develop among 9-1-1 TCs have a direct impact on job performance through impaired attention, concentration, and decision-making ability.

Additional neurocognitive abilities integral to the performance of 9-1-1 TCs are also impacted by disorders such as PTSD, depression, and substance abuse. Working memory may be one example. Working memory is comparable to a mental workspace wherein an individual can hold brief pieces of verbal or visual information and manipulate those pieces of information as needed. For example, if a caller provides an address that does not seem correct, a 9-1-1 TC with good working memory can hold the address in memory and perhaps recognize that the caller is transposing numbers or words and make the correction. Processing speed is another neurocognitive domain that may be especially important in 9-1-1 performance. Simply, speed of processing is how quickly an individual can process incoming verbal or visual information. For a 9-1-1 TC, greater processing speed may directly impact how quickly the TC can take in and record verbal information, or dispatch appropriate personnel based on visually scanning a map. Job performance among 9-1-1 TCs may also be affected by verbal learning (i.e., acquiring, retaining, and recalling verbal information), verbal memory (i.e., memory of words and spoken language), spatial processing (i.e., seeing and then organizing and remembering visual input), and inhibitory control (i.e., ability to inhibit an impulse or inhibit a habitual, dominant response to stimuli). Many of these neurocognitive domains are core features of executive functioning (i.e., processes that regulate, control, and manage other cognitive processes, such as planning, working memory, attention, problem solving, verbal reasoning, inhibition, mental flexibility, and task switching).

A growing body of research has demonstrated connections between psychological health and neurocognitive performance. Meta-analyses, which consolidate data across empirical studies, have estimated the strength of these associations. In regard to PTSD, Scott and colleagues (2015) found that the largest associations between neurocognitive ability and PTSD were in the domains of verbal learning, processing speed, working memory, and verbal memory. Further, Polak and colleagues (2012) provided a systematic review and meta-analysis that demonstrated a statistically significant association between higher levels of PTSD and poorer executive functioning. A meta-analysis focusing on depression found similar links between depression and executive function, attention, and memory with effect sizes similar to those found for PTSD (Rock, Roiser, Riedel, & Blackwell, 2014). In regard to substance use, meta-analyses have shown deficits in short-term memory, sustained attention, and psychomotor speed among individuals who drank heavily the day before (Gunn, Mackus, Griffin, Munafo, & Adams, 2018). Further, Stephan and colleagues' (2017) meta-analysis of studies comparing individuals with and without alcohol use disorder demonstrated that alcohol use disorder is associated with greater deficits in planning, problem solving, and response inhibition, reflecting skills that translate directly to the work of a 9-1-1 TC.

In sum, the personal, financial, and social burden of poor health among 9-1-1 telecommunicators can be neither estimated nor ignored. Disorders shown to be prevalent in emergency responders, including within the 9-1-1 industry, have direct implications for duty-related performance, with potentially dire consequences to the general public. Prevention and intervention efforts must be prioritized to preserve the health and wellness of this invaluable population.

CONCLUSION

Though still limited in comparison to research on field responders, the early evidence suggests that 9-1-1 TCs are at risk for a host of mental and physical health outcomes that may directly impair performance. The cost associated with poor health among 9-1-1 TCs would be difficult to estimate, particularly when the cost may include loss of life for callers. With Next Generation 9-1-1 (NG911) on the horizon, which will make live video from callers a possibility, and thereby increase visual exposure and create larger multi-tasking demands for 9-1-1 TCs, the importance of enhancing 9-1-1 health cannot be overstated.

REFERENCES

Adams, K., Shakespeare-Finch, J., & Armstrong, D. (2015). An interpretative phenomenological analysis of stress and well-being in emergency medical dispatchers. *Journal of Loss and Trauma*, *20*(5), 430–448. doi:10.1080/15325024.2014.949141

Allen, C. E., Mercer, M. C., & Lilly, M. M. (2016). Duty-related posttraumatic stress symptoms in 911 telecommunicators: The roles of childhood trauma exposure and emotion-focused coping. *Journal of Aggression, Maltreatment & Trauma*, *25*(7), 686–701. doi:10.1080/10926771.2016.1175534

American Psychiatric Association. (2013). *Diagnostic and statistical manual of mental disorders* (5th ed.). Washington, DC: Author.

Bakker, A. B., Demerouti, E., & Euwema, M. C. (2005). Job resources buffer the impact of job demands on burnout. *Journal of Occupational Health Psychology*, *10*(2), 170–180. doi:10.1037/1076-8998.10.2.170 PMID:15826226

Başoğlu, M., & Mineka, S. (1992). The role of uncontrollable and unpredictable stress in post-traumatic stress responses in torture survivors. In M. Başoğlu (Ed.), *Torture and Its Consequences: Current Treatment Approaches* (pp. 182–225). New York, NY: Cambridge University Press.

Beaton, R. D., & Murphy, S. A. (1995). Working with people in crisis: Research implications. In C. R. Figly (Ed.), *Compassion fatigue: Coping with secondary traumatic stress disorder in those who treat the traumatized* (pp. 51–81). Philadelphia, PA: Brunner/Mazel.

Behr, R. (2000). *Under the headset: Surviving dispatcher stress*. Wildomar, CA: Staggs.

Bergin, A. J., & Pakenham, K. I. (2016). The stress-buffering role of mindfulness in the relationship between perceived stress and psychological adjustment. *Mindfulness*, *7*(4), 928–939. doi:10.100712671-016-0532-x

Bergman, A. L., Christopher, M. S., & Bowen, S. (2016). Changes in facets of mindfulness predict stress and anger outcomes for police officers. *Mindfulness*, *7*(4), 851–858. doi:10.100712671-016-0522-z

Bradley, R., Greene, J., Russ, E., Dutra, L., & Westen, D. (2005). A multidimensional meta-analysis of psychotherapy for PTSD. *The American Journal of Psychiatry*, *162*(2), 214–227. doi:10.1176/appi.ajp.162.2.214 PMID:15677582

Brisbon, N. M., & Lachman, M. E. (2017). Dispositional mindfulness and memory problems: The role of perceived stress and sleep quality. *Mindfulness*, *8*(2), 379–386. doi:10.100712671-016-0607-8 PMID:28344682

Brunet, A., Weiss, D. S., Metzler, T. J., Best, S. R., Neylan, T. C., Rogers, C., ... Marmar, C. R. (2001). The Peritraumatic Distress Inventory: A proposed measure of PTSD criterion A2. *The American Journal of Psychiatry*, *158*(9), 1480–1485. doi:10.1176/appi.ajp.158.9.1480 PMID:11532735

Burke, T. W. (1995). Dispatcher stress. *FBI Law Enforcement Bulletin*, *64*(10), 1–6.

Burke, T. W. (2005). Dispatch. In L. E. Sullivan & M. Simonetti (Eds.), *Encyclopedia of law enforcement* (Vol. 1, pp. 137–139). California: Sage.

Cacioppo, J. T., Berntson, G. G., Malarkey, W. B., Kiecolt-Glaser, J. K., Sheridan, J. F., Poehlmann, K. M., ... Glaser, R. (1998). Autonomic, neuroendocrine, and immune responses to psychological stress: The reactivity hypothesisa. *Annals of the New York Academy of Sciences*, *840*(1), 664–673. doi:10.1111/j.1749-6632.1998.tb09605.x PMID:9629293

Cacioppo, J. T., Burleson, M. H., Poehlmann, K. M., Malarkey, W. B., Kiecolt-Glaser, J. K., Berntson, G. G., ... Glaser, R. (2000). Autonomic and neuroendocrine responses to mild psychological stressors: Effects of chronic stress on older women. *Annals of Behavioral Medicine*, *22*(2), 140–148. doi:10.1007/BF02895778 PMID:10962707

Carey, M. G., Al-Zaiti, S. S., Dean, G. E., Sessanna, L., & Finnell, D. S. (2011). Sleep problems, depression, substance use, social bonding, and quality of life in professional firefighters. *Journal of Occupational and Environmental Medicine*, *53*(8), 928–933. doi:10.1097/JOM.0b013e318225898f PMID:21785370

Carlson Neil, R. (2013). *Physiology of behavior*. Boston: Pearson.

Charbotel, B., Croidieu, S., Vohito, M., Guerin, A. C., Renaud, L., Jaussaud, J., ... Bergeret, A. (2009). Working conditions in call-centers, the impact on employee health: A transversal study. Part II. *International Archives of Occupational and Environmental Health*, *82*(6), 747–756. doi:10.100700420-008-0351-z PMID:18704480

Chow, H. M., Mar, R. A., Xu, Y., Liu, S., Wagage, S., & Braun, A. R. (2014). Embodied comprehension of stories: Interactions between language regions and modality-specific neural systems. *Journal of Cognitive Neuroscience*, *26*(2), 279–295. doi:10.1162/jocn_a_00487 PMID:24047383

Christopher, M. S., Goerling, R. J., Rogers, B. S., Hunsinger, M., Baron, G., Bergman, A. L., & Zava, D. T. (2015). A pilot study evaluating the effectiveness of a mindfulness-based intervention on cortisol awakening response and health outcomes among law enforcement officers. *Journal of Police and Criminal Psychology*, *31*(1), 15–28. doi:10.100711896-015-9161-x

Cicognani, E., Pietrantoni, L., Palestini, L., & Prati, G. (2009). Emergency workers' quality of life: The protective role of sense of community, efficacy beliefs and coping strategies. *Social Indicators Research*, *94*(3), 449–463. doi:10.100711205-009-9441-x

Cohen, S., Tyrrell, D. A., & Smith, A. P. (1991). Psychological stress and susceptibility to the common cold. *The New England Journal of Medicine*, *325*(9), 606–612. doi:10.1056/NEJM199108293250903 PMID:1713648

Critchley, H. D. (2002). Electrodermal responses: What happens in the brain. *The Neuroscientist*, *8*(2), 132–142. doi:10.1177/107385840200800209 PMID:11954558

Dickerson, S. S., & Kemeny, M. E. (2004). Acute stressors and cortisol responses: A theoretical integration and synthesis of laboratory research. *Psychological Bulletin*, *130*(3), 355–391. doi:10.1037/0033-2909.130.3.355 PMID:15122924

Dicks, R. L. H. (2014). *Prevalence of PTSD Symptoms in Canadian 911 Operators* (Unpublished master's thesis). University of the Fraser Valley, Canada.

Dixon, H. C., & Overall, N. C. (2016). Dispositional mindfulness attenuates the link between daily stress and depressed mood. *Journal of Social and Clinical Psychology*, *35*(3), 255–268. doi:10.1521/jscp.2016.35.3.255

Driscoll, R. J., Tubbs, R. L., & Habes, D. J. (2007). *NIOSH health hazard evaluation report*. Retrieved from: https://www. cdc.gov/niosh/hhe/reports/pdfs/1997-0137-3026.pdf

Figley, C. R. (2013). Measuring compassion satisfaction as well as fatigue: Developmental history of the compassion satisfaction and fatigue test. In *Treating Compassion Fatigue* (pp. 115–128). New York, NY: Routledge.

Foa, E. B., Hembree, E. A., Cahill, S. P., Rauch, S. A. M., Riggs, D. S., Feeny, N. C., & Yadin, E. (2005). Randomized trial of prolonged exposure for posttraumatic stress disorder with and without cognitive restructuring: Outcome at academic and community clinics. *Journal of Consulting and Clinical Psychology*, *73*(5), 953–964. doi:10.1037/0022-006X.73.5.953 PMID:16287395

Foa, E. B., Hembree, E. A., & Rothbaum, B. O. (2007). *Prolonged exposure therapy for PTSD: Emotional processing of traumatic experiences*. Cambridge, UK: Oxford University Press.

Foa, E. B., & Kozak, M. J. (1986). Emotional processing of fear: Exposure to corrective information. *Psychological Bulletin*, *99*(1), 20–35. doi:10.1037/0033-2909.99.1.20 PMID:2871574

Foa, E. B., Zinbarg, R., & Rothbaum, B. O. (1992). Uncontrollability and unpredictability in posttraumatic stress disorder: An animal model. *Psychological Bulletin*, *112*(2), 218–238. doi:10.1037/0033-2909.112.2.218 PMID:1454893

Forslund, K., Kihlgren, A., & Kihlgren, M. (2004). Operators' experiences of emergency calls. *Journal of Telemedicine and Telecare*, *10*(5), 290–297. doi:10.1258/1357633042026323 PMID:15494088

Freudenberger, H. J. (1980). *Burnout: The high cost of high achievement*. Garden City, NY: Anchor Press.

Gariepy, G., Honkaniemi, H., & Quesnel-Vallee, A. (2016). Social support and protection from depression: Systematic review of current findings in Western countries. *The British Journal of Psychiatry*, *209*(4), 284–293. doi:10.1192/bjp.bp.115.169094 PMID:27445355

Griffiths, K. L., Mackey, M. G., & Adamson, B. J. (2007). The impact of a computerized work environment on professional occupational groups and behavioural and physiological risk factors for musculoskeletal symptoms: A literature review. *Journal of Occupational Rehabilitation*, *17*(4), 743–765. doi:10.100710926-007-9108-x PMID:17987369

Grillon, C., Pine, D. S., Lissek, S., Rabin, S., Bonne, O., & Vythilingam, M. (2009). Increased anxiety during anticipation of unpredictable aversive stimuli in posttraumatic stress disorder but not in generalized anxiety disorder. *Biological Psychiatry*, *66*(1), 47–53. doi:10.1016/j.biopsych.2008.12.028 PMID:19217076

Gunn, C., Mackus, M., Griffin, C., Munafo, M. R., & Adams, S. (2018). A systematic review of the next-day effects of heavy alcohol consumption on cognitive performance. *Addiction (Abingdon, England)*, *113*(12), 2181–2193. doi:10.1111/add.14404 PMID:30144191

Gurevich, M., Halpern, J., Brazeau, P., Defina, P. S., & Schwartz, B. (2009). Frontline stress behind the scenes: Emergency medical dispatchers. *Ryerson University, Do Psychology.*

Hammelman, J. (2013). *Physiological and psychological responses to 911 emergency tapes* (Doctoral dissertation). Retrieved from ProQuest dissertations and theses database. (Order No. 10138220)

Hartley, T. A., Violanti, J. M., Fekedulegn, D., Andrew, M. E., & Burchfiel, C. M. (2007). Associations between major life events, traumatic incidents, and depression among Buffalo police officers. *International Journal of Emergency Mental Health, 9*, 25–35. Retrieved from http:// www.ncbi.nlm.nih.gov/pubmed/11227748

Hayes, S. C. (2016). *Acceptance & Action Questionnaire (AAQ) and variations*. Jenison, MI: Association for Contextual Behavioral Science. Retrieved from https://contextualscience.org/acceptance_action_questionnaire_aaq_and_variations

Hayes, S. C., Strosahl, K. D., & Wilson, K. G. (1999). *Acceptance and commitment therapy: An experiential approach to behavior change*. New York, NY: Guilford Press.

Hoge, C. W., Grossman, S. H., Auchterlonie, J. L., Riviere, L. A., Milliken, C. S., & Wilk, J. E. (2014). PTSD treatment for soldiers after combat deployment: Low utilization of mental health care and reasons for dropout. *Psychiatric Services (Washington, D.C.)*, *65*(8), 997–1004. doi:10.1176/appi.ps.201300307 PMID:24788253

Imel, Z. E., Laska, K., Jakupcak, M., & Simpson, T. L. (2013). Meta-analysis of dropout in treatments for posttraumatic stress disorder. *Journal of Consulting and Clinical Psychology*, *81*(3), 394–404. doi:10.1037/a0031474 PMID:23339535

Kabat-Zinn, J., Lipworth, L., & Burney, R. (1985). The clinical use of mindfulness meditation for the self-regulation of chronic pain. *Journal of Behavioral Medicine*, *8*(2), 163–190. doi:10.1007/BF00845519 PMID:3897551

Kessler, R. C., & Frank, R. G. (1997). The impact of psychiatric disorders on work loss days. *Psychological Medicine*, *27*(4), 861–873. doi:10.1017/S0033291797004807 PMID:9234464

Khoury, B., Sharma, M., Rush, S. E., & Fournier, C. (2015). Mindfulness-based stress reduction for healthy individuals: A meta-analysis. *Journal of Psychosomatic Research*, *78*(6), 519–528. doi:10.1016/j.jpsychores.2015.03.009 PMID:25818837

Kira, I., Lewandowski, L., Templin, R., Ramaswamy, V., Ozkan, B., & Mohanesh, J. (2008). Measuring cumulative trauma dose, types and profiles using a development-based taxonomy of trauma. *Traumatology*, *14*(2), 62–87. doi:10.1177/1534765608319324

Kirmeyer, S. L., & Dougherty, T. W. (1988). Work load, tension, and coping: Moderating effects of supervisor support. *Personnel Psychology*, *41*(1), 125–139. doi:10.1111/j.1744-6570.1988.tb00635.x

Knapp, P. H., Levy, E. M., Giorgi, R. G., Black, P. H., Fox, B. H., & Heeren, T. C. (1992). Short-term immunological effects of induced emotion. *Psychosomatic Medicine*, *54*(2), 133–148. doi:10.1097/00006842-199203000-00002 PMID:1565752

Lilly, M. M., & Allen, C. E. (2015). Psychological inflexibility and psychopathology in 9-1-1 telecommunicators. *Journal of Traumatic Stress*, *28*(3), 262–266. doi:10.1002/jts.22004 PMID:25964163

Lilly, M.M., Calhoun, R., Painter, I., & Meischke, H. (under review). Destress 9-1-1: A randomized control trial of an online mindfulness-based intervention in reducing stress among emergency medical dispatchers.

Lilly, M. M., London, M. J., & Mercer, M. C. (2016). Predictors of obesity and physical health complaints among 911 telecommunicators. *Safety and Health at Work*, *7*(1), 55–62. doi:10.1016/j.shaw.2015.09.003 PMID:27014492

Lilly, M. M., & Pierce, H. (2013). PTSD and depressive symptoms in 911 telecommunicators: The role of peritraumatic distress and world assumptions in predicting risk. *Psychological Trauma: Theory, Research, Practice, and Policy*, *5*(2), 135–141. doi:10.1037/a0026850

London, M. J., Mercer, M. C., & Lilly, M. M. (2017). Considering the impact of early trauma on coping and pathology to predict posttraumatic growth among 9-1-1 telecommunicators. *Journal of Interpersonal Violence*, *00*(0), 1–23. doi:10.1177/0886260517716942 PMID:29294814

Maier, S. F., & Watkins, L. R. (1998). Cytokines for psychologists: Implications of bidirectional immune-to-brain communication for understanding behavior, mood, and cognition. *Psychological Review*, *105*(1), 83–107. doi:10.1037/0033-295X.105.1.83 PMID:9450372

Meischke, H., Lilly, M., Beaton, R., Calhoun, R., Tu, A., Stangenes, S., ... Baseman, J. (2018). Protocol: A multi-level intervention program to reduce stress in 9-1-1 telecommunicators. *BMC Public Health*, *18*(1), 570. doi:10.118612889-018-5471-0 PMID:29716576

Meischke, H., Painter, I., Lilly, M., Beaton, R., Revere, D., Calhoun, B., ... Baseman, J. (2015). An exploration of sources, symptoms, and buffers of occupational stress in 9-1-1 emergency call centers. *Annals of Emergency Dispatch & Response*, *3*(2), 28–35.

Mineka, S., Cook, M., & Miller, S. (1984). Fear conditioned with escapable and inescapable shock: Effects of a feedback stimulus. *Journal of Experimental Psychology. Animal Behavior Processes*, *10*(3), 307–323. doi:10.1037/0097-7403.10.3.307

Mineka, S., & Oehlberg, K. (2008). The relevance of recent developments in classical conditioning to understanding the etiology and maintenance of anxiety disorders. *Acta Psychologica*, *127*(3), 567–580. doi:10.1016/j.actpsy.2007.11.007 PMID:18226795

Munce, S. E., Stansfeld, S. A., Blackmore, E. R., & Stewart, D. E. (2007). The role of depression and chronic pain conditions in absenteeism: Results from a national epidemiologic survey. *Journal of Occupational and Environmental Medicine*, *49*(11), 1206–1211. doi:10.1097/JOM.0b013e318157f0ba PMID:17993924

Ozer, E. J., Best, S. R., Lipsey, T. L., & Weiss, D. S. (2003). Predictors of posttraumatic stress disorder and symptoms in adults: A meta-analysis. *Psychological Bulletin*, *129*(1), 52–73. doi:10.1037/0033-2909.129.1.52 PMID:12555794

Pierce, H., & Lilly, M. M. (2012). Duty-related trauma exposure in 911 telecommunicators: Considering the risk for posttraumatic stress. *Journal of Traumatic Stress*, *25*(2), 211–215. doi:10.1002/jts.21687 PMID:22467384

Polak, A. R., Witteveen, A. B., Reitsma, J. B., & Olff, M. (2012). The role of executive function in PTSD: A systematic review. *Journal of Affective Disorders*, *141*(1), 11–21. doi:10.1016/j.jad.2012.01.001 PMID:22310036

Rameshbabu, A., Reddy, D. M., & Fleming, R. (2013). Correlates of negative physical health in call center shift workers. *Applied Ergonomics*, *44*(3), 350–354. doi:10.1016/j.apergo.2012.09.002 PMID:23040668

Ramey, S. L., Perkhounkova, Y., Hein, M., Chung, S. J., & Anderson, A. A. (2017). Evaluation of stress experienced by emergency telecommunications personnel employed in a large metropolitan police department. *Workplace Health & Safety*, *65*(7), 287–294. doi:10.1177/2165079916667736 PMID:27941089

Resick, P. A., Monson, C. M., & Chard, K. M. (2016). *Cognitive processing therapy for PTSD: A comprehensive manual*. Boston: Guilford Press.

Richardson, D. C., Griffin, N. K., Zaki, L., Stephenson, A., Yan, J., Curry, T., & Devlin, J. T. (2018). Measuring narrative engagement: The heart tells the story. *bioRxiv*, 35–48. doi:10.1101/351148

Rock, P. L., Roiser, J. P., Riedel, W. J., & Blackwell, A. D. (2014). Cognitive impairment in depression: A systematic review and meta-analysis. *Psychological Medicine*, *44*(10), 2029–2040. doi:10.1017/S0033291713002535 PMID:24168753

Santiago, P. N., Ursano, R. J., Gray, C. L., ... Fullerton, C. S. (2013). A systematic review of PTSD prevalence and trajectories of DSM-5 defined trauma exposed populations: Intentional and non-intentional traumatic events. *PLoS One*, *8*(4), e59236. doi:10.1371/journal.pone.0059236 PMID:23593134

Schnider, K. R., Elhai, J. D., & Gray, M. J. (2007). Coping style use predicts posttraumatic stress and complicated grief symptom severity among college students reporting a traumatic loss. *Journal of Counseling Psychology*, *54*(3), 344–350. doi:10.1037/0022-0167.54.3.344

Scott, J. C., Matt, G. E., Wrocklage, K. M., Crnich, C., Jordan, J., Southwick, S. M., & ... . (2015). A quantitative meta-analysis of neurocognitive functioning in PTSD. *Psychological Bulletin*, *141*(1), 105–140. doi:10.1037/a0038039 PMID:25365762

Sequeira, H., Hot, P., Silvert, L., & Delplanque, S. (2009). Electrical autonomic correlates of emotion. *International Journal of Psychophysiology*, *71*(1), 50–56. doi:10.1016/j.ijpsycho.2008.07.009 PMID:18723054

Shakespeare-Finch, J., Rees, A., & Armstrong, D. (2015). Social support, self-efficacy, trauma and well-being in emergency medical dispatchers. *Social Indicators Research*, *123*(2), 549–565. doi:10.100711205-014-0749-9

Shapiro, F. (2017). *Eye movement desensitization and processing (EMDR) therapy*. Boston, MA: Guilford Press.

Shin, L. M., Rauch, S. L., & Pitman, R. K. (2006). Amygdala, medial prefrontal cortex, and hippocampal function in PTSD. *Annals of the New York Academy of Sciences*, *1071*(1), 67–79. doi:10.1196/annals.1364.007 PMID:16891563

Simpson, R. J., & Guy, K. (2010). Coupling aging immunity with a sedentary lifestyle: Has the damage already been done? A mini-review. *Gerontology*, *56*(5), 449–458. doi:10.1159/000270905 PMID:20029165

Skogstad, M., Skorstad, M., Lie, A., Conradi, H. S., Heir, T., & Weisæth, L. (2013). Work-related post-traumatic stress disorder. *Occupational Medicine*, *63*(3), 175–182. doi:10.1093/occmed/kqt003 PMID:23564090

Sloan, D. M., Marx, B. P., Bovin, M. J., Feinstein, B. A., & Gallagher, M. W. (2012). Written exposure as an intervention for PTSD: A randomized clinical trial with motor vehicle accident survivors. *Behaviour Research and Therapy*, *50*(10), 627–635. doi:10.1016/j.brat.2012.07.001 PMID:22863540

Sloan, D. M., Marx, B. P., Lee, D. J., & Resick, P. A. (2018). A brief exposure-based treatment vs cognitive processing therapy for posttraumatic stress disorder: A randomized noninferiority clinical trial. *JAMA Psychiatry*, *75*(3), 233–239. doi:10.1001/jamapsychiatry.2017.4249 PMID:29344631

Sofianopoulos, S., Williams, B., Archer, F., & Thompson, B. (2011). The exploration of physical fatigue, sleep and depression in paramedics: A pilot study. *Australasian Journal of Paramedicine*, *9*(1). doi:10.33151/ajp.9.1.37

Solomon, E. P., & Heide, K. M. (2005). The biology of trauma: Implications for treatment. *Journal of Interpersonal Violence*, *20*(1), 51–60. doi:10.1177/0886260504268119 PMID:15618561

Steenkamp, M. M., Litz, B. T., Hoge, C. W., & Marmar, C. R. (2015). Psychotherapy for military-related PTSD: A review of randomized clinical trials. *JAMA Psychiatry*, *314*(5), 489–500. doi:10.1001/jama.2015.8370 PMID:26241600

Stephan, R. A., Alhassoon, O. M., Allen, K. E., Wollman, S. C., Hall, M., Thomas, W. J., ... Grant, I. (2017). Meta-analyses of clinical neuropsychological tests of executive dysfunction and impulsivity in alcohol use disorder. *The American Journal of Drug and Alcohol Abuse*, *43*(1), 24–43. doi:10.1080/00952990.2016.1206113 PMID:27712350

Tedeschi, R. G., & Calhoun, L. G. (1996). The posttraumatic growth inventory: Measuring the positive legacy of trauma. *Journal of Traumatic Stress*, *9*, 455–471. doi:10.1002/jts.2490090305 PMID:8827649

Tobin, M. I. (1997). *Perceptions of uncontrollability, unpredictability, and life-threat, in the development of crime-related PTSD symptomology* (Doctoral dissertation). Retrieved from ProQuest dissertations and theses database. (Order No. AAM9639151)

Trachik, B., Marks, M., Bowers, C., Scott, G., Olola, C., & Gardett, I. (2015). Is dispatching to a traffic accident as stressful as being in one? Acute stress disorder, secondary traumatic stress, and occupational burnout in 911 emergency dispatchers. *Annals of Emergency Dispatch and Response*, *3*(1), 27–38.

Tracy, S. J., & Tracy, K. (1998). Emotion labor at 911: A case study and theoretical critique. *Journal of Applied Communication Research*, *26*(4), 390–411. doi:10.1080/00909889809365516

Troxell, R. M. (2008). *Indirect exposure to the trauma of others: The experiences of 911 telecommunicators* (Doctoral dissertation). Retrieved from ProQuest dissertations and theses database. (UMI number: 3335425)

Turner, K. D., Lilly, M. M., Gamez, A. M., & Kressler, K. (2019). Impact of work-related factors on stress and health among 9-1-1 call-takers and dispatchers in California. *Journal of Emergency Dispatch;* Advanced online publication.

van der Kolk, B., McFarlane, A., & Weisaeth, L. (1996). *Traumatic stress*. New York, NY: Guildford Press.

Violanti, J. M., Slaven, J. E., Charles, L. E., Burchfiel, C. M., Andrew, M. E., & Homish, G. G. (2011). Police and alcohol use: A descriptive analysis and associations with stress outcomes. *American Journal of Criminal Justice*, *36*(4), 344–356. doi:10.100712103-011-9121-7

Virgili, M. (2015). Mindfulness-based interventions reduce psychological distress in working adults: A meta-analysis of intervention studies. *Mindfulness*, *6*(2), 326–337. doi:10.100712671-013-0264-0

Wells, T. S., Bagnell, M. E., Miller, S. C., Smith, T. C., Gackstetter, G. D., & Boyko, E. J. (2014). U.S. Naval and Marine Corps occupations, posttraumatic stress disorder, depression risk, and absenteeism. *Journal of Workplace Behavioral Health*, *29*(2), 91–112. doi:10.1080/15555240.2014.899187

Wiegand, D. M. (2013). *Evaluation of job stress and work-related health concerns of a telephone call center*. Retrieved from: http://www.cdc.gov/niosh/hhe/reports/pdfs/2012-0211-3197. pdf

Williams, V., Ciarrochi, J., & Deane, F. P. (2010). On being mindful, emotionally aware, and more resilient: Longitudinal pilot study of police recruits. *Australian Psychologist*, *45*(4), 274–282. doi:10.1080/00050060903573197

KEY TERMS AND DEFINITIONS

9-1-1: The telephone number most people in the U.S. and several other countries dial in order to get help in the event of a fire, medical emergency, assault, or other accident.

Depression: A psychological disorder characterized by low mood, lack of positive emotion, and loss of interest or pleasure in typically-enjoyed activities, leading to impairment in daily functioning.

Dispatcher: A person whose job entails coordinating the actions of first responders in reaction to an emergency, providing those individuals with relevant details of the emergency to enhance responder performance.

Duty-Related Trauma: Emotional and/or psychological distress related to events encountered, or activities performed, on the job.

Emergency Responder: A person with specialized training who is the first to arrive and provide assistance at the scene of an emergency or natural disaster (e.g., paramedics, police officers, firefighters).

Posttraumatic Stress Disorder: A psychological disorder that can develop after experiencing or witnessing a life-threatening or highly stressful experience.

Telecommunicator: A person whose job is to coordinate communications between police officers, emergency personnel, and the public.

Chapter 6
Occupational Risk Factors and the Mental Health of Women Firefighters

Brittany Sara Hollerbach
National Development and Research Institutes, Inc., USA

ABSTRACT

Firefighting is an inherently dangerous occupation, yet little is known about the mental health of firefighters, and even less is known about women firefighters specifically. The purpose of this chapter is to examine relevant literature pertaining to firefighters and mental health with a specific focus on behavioral health aspects that may impact the mental health of women firefighters. There are key issues women in the fire service face that are likely related to their mental health including bullying and harassment, substance use, job satisfaction, fitness, protective gear, and injury. By identifying issues related to the mental health of women firefighters, the authors provide direction for future research and guidance for policy guidelines for the fire service.

INTRODUCTION

Firefighting is an inherently dangerous occupation, yet little is known about the mental health of firefighters, and even less is known about female firefighters. The objective of this chapter is to examine relevant literature pertaining to firefighters and mental health with a specific focus on behavioral health issues that may impact the mental health of women firefighters.

BACKGROUND

Firefighting is a dangerous and highly stressful occupation with high rates of injuries and line of duty deaths (Fahy, LeBlanc, & Molis, 2018; Evarts & Molis, 2018; Poplin, Harris, Pollack, Peate, & Burgess, 2011). The National Fire Protection Association (NFPA) estimated 58,835 firefighter injuries and 60

DOI: 10.4018/978-1-5225-9803-9.ch006

firefighter fatalities occurred in the line of duty in 2017 (Evarts & Molis, 2018). Additionally, there were 7,345 documented exposures to infectious diseases and 44,530 exposures to hazardous conditions (Evarts & Molis, 2018). Despite public perception of the sexy, muscular firefighter, firefighters also struggle with poor physical health (Jahnke, Poston, Haddock, & Jitnarin, 2013; Soteriades et al., 2005), high rates of being overweight and obesity (Soteriades et al., 2005; Kales, Polyhronopoulos, Aldrich, Leitao, & Christiani, 1999; Poston et al., 2011) and low fitness levels (Poston et al., 2011; Tsismenakis et al., 2009). On average, firefighters experience significant weight gain over the course of their career, and may put on 29-85 additional pounds (i.e., 1.15-3.4 lbs/year) (Tsismenakis et al., 2009). As a firefighter's weight increases, their cardiorespiratory fitness plummets and their risk of cardiovascular disease (CVD) increases (Durand et al., 2011). Other diseases related to being overweight and obesity include heart disease, stroke, type 2 diabetes, and certain types of cancers which are highly prevalent among the firefighter population (Poston et al., 2011; CDC, 2015). In 2017, 29 firefighters died while on duty due to cardiovascular events (Fahy et al., 2018). While there is a wealth of research that examines firefighters' physical health, there is limited data concerning the psychological health of these important tactical athletes.

Recent studies demonstrate that first responders suffer from elevated rates of depression, post-traumatic stress disorder (PTSD; Heyman, Dill, & Douglas, 2018). According to the Firefighter Behavioral Health Alliance (FBHA), 79 firefighters and 19 emergency medical technicians (EMTs) and paramedics died as the result of suicide in 2018 which is a rate higher than on-duty deaths (Firefighter Behavioral Health Alliance, 2018). Large metro departments have seen a spike in clustered firefighter suicides in recent years (Gist, Taylor, & Raak, 2011). With a rise in behavioral health issues amongst firefighters, the fire service is trying to address these issues through national standards, behavioral health programs, peer support, and research focused on these issues. Yet, often, academic research in the field of firefighter health and safety is not translated into fire service training nor reflected in policies and procedures. Although NFPA 1500: Standard on Fire Department Occupational Safety and Health Programs requires access to a behavioral health program that proposes assessment, counseling and treatment for such issues as stress, anxiety, and depression (National Fire Protection Association, 2018), many departments lack the resources to adequately implement such programs. Additionally, little is known about the physical or mental health impacts of firefighting for women (Jahnke et al., 2012; Stanley, Hom, Spencer-Thomas, & Joiner, 2017).

Women represent an incredibly small proportion of the fire service, even lower than the U.S. Marine Corps, where all members are expected to be combat ready (Women in Military Service for America Memorial Foundation, Inc. 2010). Despite representing a small percentage, over 85,100 women are on the front lines protecting communities across the U.S. (Haynes & Stein, 2017). According to the NFPA, women represent approximately 8.9% of volunteer and 3.7% of career firefighters (Haynes & Stein, 2017). Due to the fact that women represent a small percentage of the fire service, they often are overlooked in studies and excluded from statistical analysis due to their small sample size (Jahnke et al., 2012; Hollerbach et al., 2017). While all firefighters face environmental and occupational stressors, women in the fire service face additional barriers adversely affecting their health and wellness. The goal of this chapter is to explore what is known regarding the mental health of women in the fire service and to identify important gaps in that knowledge. Guidance for changing policies and procedures to better protect and diversify the fire service as a whole also will be addressed.

MAIN FOCUS OF THE CHAPTER

Recruitment and Retention

According to iWomen, the largest organization of women firefighters in the U.S., the low proportion of women in the fire service results from a combination of limited recruitment and low retention rates (Hulett, Bendick, Thomas, & Moccio, 2008; Horvath, 2013). Despite statements from national fire service organizations, including the International Association of Firefighters (IAFF; Fox, Hornick, & Hardin, 2006) and the International Association of Fire Chiefs (IAFC, 2018), promoting gender diversity within the fire service, rates of women firefighters remain extremely low (Jahnke et al., 2012; Haynes & Stein, 2017). There are many possible explanations for such low numbers of women in the fire service, including the psychological and physical strains of firefighting. Additionally, the culture of the fire service has been traditionally unaccepting of women (Hollerbach et al., 2017; Hulett et al., 2008; Horvath, 2013).

The Person-Environment Fit (PE-FIT) Model suggests that as the burdens and demands of one's occupation begin to exceed the ability of an employee to deal with them, this "lack of fit" contributes to overload, burden, role ambiguity, and conflicting role demands (Quick & Tetrick, 2003, p. 187). The resulting physical and psychological stress can lead to adverse behavioral consequences such as reduced productivity, increased absenteeism, turnover, employee burnout, and health-related issues (Quick & Tetrick, 2003). Research has found that women often are often given 'feminized' job tasks that restrict and challenge their success in non-traditional occupations. The same employment practices that favor men effectively lessen women's opportunities for promotion and lowers their chances of being seen as authoritative in their role (Reskin & Bielby, 2005). There is still a certain air of masculinity associated with the fire service, limiting the entry of women into the occupation (Perrott, 2016).

The collective intelligence of a diverse organization allows for differing points of view and strengths in working together to achieve the department's mission. Just as a government and its elected officials and leadership should reflect the demographics of the community they serve, so too should government agencies, such as the fire service, be representative of the citizens they protect (McNeil, 2008). Further diversifying the fire service begins with an examination of mental health issues affecting women, a growing minority group within the fire service.

Bullying and Harassment

The effects of workplace harassment on mental health are well-defined in the literature (Kessler, Mickelson, & Williams, 1999; Todorova, Falcon, Lincoln, & Price, 2010). Rosell et al. (1995) analyzed the difference in behavioral health outcomes of women firefighters that reported being sexually harassed and those that did not. They found that sexually harassed women firefighters reported higher job stress, sexual stereotyping, and acts of violence. Participants feared coming to work and used more sick leave than their non-harassed peers (Rosell, Miller, & Barber, 1995). Research has found more than 80% of women firefighters reported experiencing differential treatment based on gender, although only a small proportion of men felt that way (14%; Hulett et al., 2008; Griffith, Roberts, & Wakeham, 2016). This differential treatment included high levels of shunning/isolation (50.8%), verbal harassment (42.9%), sexual advances (30.2%), and assault (6.3%; Hulett et al., 2008).

Over 40% of women firefighters in current research reported that they frequently felt they had to work twice as hard to get the same treatment or evaluation and that they were watched more closely than other workers (Jahnke et al., under review). Of the specific types of gender-based harassment, women firefighters reported experiencing verbal (37.5%) and written harassment (12.9%), hazing (16.9%), sexual advances (37.4%), and assaults (5.1%) because of their gender while in the fire service (Jahnke et al., under review).

Research consistently finds an association between discrimination and harassment and a variety of mental (e.g., anxiety, depression, PTSD, self-rated health) and physical health outcomes (e.g., blood pressure, cardiovascular disease, diabetes, overall stress response, and a number of other medical conditions; Hulett et al., 2008; Kessler et al., 1999; Todorova et al., 2010; Rosell et al., 1995; Hom, Stanley, Spencer-Thomas, & Joiner, 2017; Krieger, 1999; Okechukqu, Souza, Davis, & de Castro, 2014; Pascoe & Smart Richman, 2009; Williams, Neighbors, & Jackson, 2003). Current research indicated that female firefighters who experienced a high severity of bullying and harassment were 300% more likely to report significant depressive symptoms (Jahnke et al., under review). Women firefighters who experienced moderate and severe discrimination and harassment also had negative mental health outcomes including higher prevalence of depressive symptoms, anxiety, and symptoms of PTSD. Additionally, women who experienced severe discrimination and harassment reported over 40% more poor health days in the last 30 days (Jahnke et al., under review). Hom and et al. (2017) found that a history of sexual harassment, discrimination, and other threats/harassment were significantly associated with a history of career suicidal ideation, in addition to other severe psychiatric symptoms including heightened anxiety, depression, more severe PTSD, and insomnia. Discrimination and harassment have significant impacts on physical and mental health outcomes on women in the fire service. Prevention efforts, training, and peer-support programs focused on this issue should be further explored.

Depression and Anxiety

Although firefighters are incredibly resilient, research suggests that many suffer negative psychological consequences from their experiences in the fire service. Studies have found high rates of acute stress disorder (26.5%) and elevated rates of those currently in the range of concern for depression (10.8-16.4%) among men in the fire service (Carey, Al-Zaiti, Dean, Sessanna, & Finnell, 2011; Fullerton, Ursano, & Wang, 2004). This is extreme when compared to the national average for civilians; in 2016, only 6.7% of all U.S. adults had at least one major depressive episode (National Institutes of Mental Health, 2019). Additionally, studies have found that firefighters in the depressed range reported significantly more poor mental health days than those not in the depressed range (Pyle et al., 2009). Depressed firefighters are more likely to be sleep deprived and to display hazardous drinking behaviors as well (Carey et al., 2011). While only about 4% of respondents reported low levels of social bonding among firefighters, those with poor mental wellbeing were more likely to report poor social bonding (Carey et al., 2011) which is an important mechanism for firefighter coping.

Firefighters often experience increased stress due to repeated exposures to trauma and they seem to know their jobs put them at risk. A study by Jahnke et al. (2012) found that firefighters across the country actually expressed a belief that their career would shorten their lives. Firefighters are plagued by psychological stress resulting from repeated exposure to trauma, sleep disruptions, injuries, and the risk for infectious disease (Jahnke et al., 2012). There is an emotional toll from repeated exposure to trauma that can lead to adverse mental health consequences (Jahnke et al., 2012). However, firefighters have consistently reported that talking with other firefighters was the most useful way of managing the emotional toll of their experiences, highlighting the importance of a supportive organization and access to peer support.

Jahnke et al. (2012) examined the health of women firefighters and found that, similar to their male colleagues, nearly a quarter of female firefighters were at risk for depression. Approximately 30% reported feeling nervous and stressed fairly or very often and 22% reported feeling angered because things were often outside of their control (Jahnke et al., 2012). To make matters worse, female firefighters with a history of discrimination or harassment on the job had significantly higher levels of anxiety and depression (Hom et al., 2017). Overall, female firefighters tend to have similar prevalence of mental health issues when compared to male firefighters. The problem arises when they are subject to adverse and pervasive differential treatment which has been shown to impact their health.

Posttraumatic Stress Disorder

Firefighters respond to incredibly dangerous and traumatic emergency incidents putting them at heightened risk of Posttraumatic Stress Disorder (PTSD). Depression and PTSD symptomatology (i.e., 'posttraumatic stress') often occur together (Martin et al., 2017) and, considering the high rates of depression found among firefighters, they are undoubtedly at risk for PTSD as well. Recent studies have, in fact, found between 14.0-31.8% of firefighters suffer from PTSD (Martin et al., 2017; Boffa et al., 2017; del Ben, Scotti, Chen, & Fortson, 2006) compared to only about 7-8% of the general population (US Department of Veterans Affairs, 2018). In addition, Boffa et al. (2017) found that 15.6% of firefighters in their study reported at least one suicide attempt during their firefighting career. PTSD has been shown to amplify the risk of suicide among firefighters (Boffa et al., 2017).

In addition to being linked to increased suicide risk, PTSD significantly impacts quality of life (QOL) and greater sleep disturbance (Chen et al., 2007). Jahnke et al. (2016) examined experiences of repeated exposure to trauma (RET) in a national sample of firefighters and found that RET resulted in a number of negative outcomes for firefighters including desensitization, irritability and cynicism, and intrusive flashbacks (Jahnke, Poston, Haddock, & Murphy, 2016). While some firefighters had a specific incident that they identified as negatively affecting them, most discussed the impact of repeatedly being exposed to traumatic events and the psychological toll that resulted from such experiences (Jahnke et al., 2016).

While research has examined PTSD among firefighters, published PTSD prevalence rates are not currently available for female firefighters. However, there have been numerous studies that show that differential treatment such as bullying, harassment, sexual assault, and other threats increase rates and severity of PTSD among women firefighters (Jahnke et al., under review; Hom et al., 2017). It is extremely important that more research be conducted to identify the prevalence of PTSD among firefighters, especially women. Additionally, interventions and treatment options should be explored to help firefighters manage PTSD symptoms.

Suicide

Elevated rates of depression and PTSD symptoms may be associated with increased suicide risk among firefighters (Stanley et al., 2019). Firefighters report high rates of suicidal ideation, plans, and attempts (46.8%, 19.2%, and 15.5%, respectively) when compared to both general (5.6–14.3%, 3.9%, and 1.9–8.7%, respectively) and military (3.8–13.9%, 5.3%, and 0.4–2.4%, respectively) populations (Nock et al., 2008;

Nock et al., 2014; Stanley, Horn, Hagan, & Joiner, 2015). The Firefighter Behavioral Health Alliance (FBHA) reported 98 firefighters died by suicide in 2017 (Firefighter Behavioral Health Alliance, 2019), which is more than the 86 total line of duty deaths that occurred in the fire service that year (US Fire Administration, 2019). The number of emergency responders who lose their lives to suicide may be even higher as the FBHA suggests that only approximately 40% of firefighter suicides are reported as such. Large metro departments have seen a spike in clustered firefighter suicides in recent years (Gist et al., 2011). Boffa et al. (2017) found 15.6% of the firefighters in their study reported at least one suicide attempt during their firefighting career.

So, what do we know about suicide and women firefighters? A recent CDC report on suicide rates by occupational group revealed that, among women workers, the highest rate of death by suicide was among protective service workers—a group that includes firefighters (Stanley et al., 2017; McIntosh, 2016). In 2017, Stanley et al. (2017) examined 313 women firefighters and found they reported elevated rates of suicidal thoughts and behaviors. For example, percentages of women firefighters reporting suicidal ideation, plans, and attempts were 37.7%, 10.9%, 3.5%, respectively (Stanley et al., 2017). While these rates may be higher than the general population, they appear lower than rates for men firefighters seen in the current literature. Further research is necessary to understand suicide risk among women firefighters. Further, research should explore firefighters' access to employee assistance including behavioral health programs tailored specifically to the fire service.

Substance Use

Substance use is common among first responders and includes problematic use of alcohol, tobacco, and prescription drug use, though little is known regarding the latter. According to the Dietary Guidelines for Americans 2015-2020 and the U.S. Department of Health and Human Services, moderate alcohol consumption is defined as up to one drink per day for women and up to two drinks per day for men. The National Institute on Alcohol Abuse and Alcoholism (NIAAA) defines "binge drinking" as a pattern of drinking that brings blood alcohol concentration (BAC) levels to 0.08 g/dL. This typically occurs after four drinks for women and five drinks for men, over a time span of two hours. Heavy alcohol use is defined as binge drinking on five or more days in the past month (National Institutes of Health, 2019). In similar populations (e.g. military), heavy drinking patterns can be as high as 67% among men and 9% among women, with binge drinking patterns occurring in 48% of men and 31% of women, higher than the general population (Fear et al., 2007).

Research has shown that firefighters "believed alcohol played an important role in the fire service, that high consumption was common, and the social norms supported alcohol consumption" (Jahnke, Poston, & Haddock, 2014). In a large study of male firefighters, Haddock et al. (2015) found that 85% of firefighters reported drinking alcohol, nearly half reported excessive drinking, and approximately one third reported binge drinking when off duty.

As with male firefighters, heavy and problem drinking are prevalent among women firefighters and are associated with negative occupational outcomes (Haddock, Poston, Jahnke, & Jitnarin, 2017). Haddock et al. (2017) examined over 1,000 women firefighters and found that more than 60% of the women in their study averaged two or more drinks (moderate to heavy drinking) on days when they consumed alcohol. Chief officers were more likely to consume two drinks per day compared to firefighters; otherwise, rank did not predict average consumption or binge drinking (Haddock et al., 2017). Problem drinking also was associated with negative health outcomes. For example, problem drinkers were more than 2.5

times more likely to have been diagnosed with depression or PTSD. Problem drinkers were nearly 40% more likely to have sustained an injury on the job in the past year and were less likely to recommend a career in the fire service to other women (Haddock et al., 2017). Recent research found that women experiencing moderate to high levels of workplace discrimination were also significantly more likely to be in the range of concern for alcohol misuse (Jahnke et al., under review).

Among 947 male firefighters, 21% were tobacco users. Of those who smoked, 34.5% used cigarettes, over half (53.2%) used smokeless tobacco (SLT), and 12.2% used both cigarettes and SLT (Jitnarin, Poston, Haddock, Jahnke, & Day, 2015). Tobacco users were significantly younger, had served fewer years in the fire service, were significantly more likely to engage in heavy and binge drinking, and were more likely to show signs of depressive symptoms compared to non-tobacco users (Jitnarin et al., 2015). Tobacco use rates were generally higher among women firefighters than their male colleagues and rates among women firefighters were similar to the rates of women in the military (Jahnke et al., 2012). Resources for substance use/misuse specific to firefighters should be identified and examined for validity in this population.

Job Satisfaction

Job satisfaction is an indicator of overall wellbeing and is related to individual health outcomes (Antecol & Cobb-Clark, 2006). Reported levels of job satisfaction are, however, difficult to accurately assess and may differ among different groups. For example, women and African Americans in the general population tend to report higher levels of job satisfaction even though on many objective measures their jobs are worse, which could stem from these groups having lower expectations (Antecol & Cobb-Clark, 2006; Bartel, 1981, & Clark, 1997). Most studies report that men firefighters have a high level of job satisfaction (Traut, Larsen, & Feimer, 2000; Wagner & O'Neill, 2012). Despite the barriers and differential treatment some women in the fire service face, those who stay in the profession tend to report higher levels of job satisfaction. In fact, 78% of the female firefighters in recent research reported they are satisfied with their job in the fire department (Jahnke et al., under review).

There are benefits of a collective and supportive fire service culture. The concept of "brotherhood" is deeply rooted in the American fire service (Crosby, 2007). The social bonds and connections among firefighters and within the firehouse are important factors in attenuating adverse mental health outcomes (Carey et al., 2011). It is important to feel a sense of belonging as a part of a group, as well as feeling supported by others. However, the adverse treatment many women in the fire service face can impact their job satisfaction, which research has shown impacts their health and their ability to do their jobs (Jahnke et al., under review).

Fitness

According to the Centers for Disease Control and Prevention (CDC; 2018), physical activity (PA) can be one of the best ways to improve both physical and mental health. However, male firefighters struggle with poor health and low levels of fitness. Overweight and obesity are highly prevalent, and in some cases >80% (Poston et al., 2011; Tsismenakis et al., 2009; Soteriades et al., 2008). Cardiac-related events consistently account for the majority of firefighter fatalities. In 2017, 29 line of duty deaths were related to sudden cardiac events (Fahy et al., 2018).

Female firefighters, on the other hand, seem to maintain a high level of fitness throughout their careers. For example, Jahnke et al. (2012) found that compared to male firefighters, women had more favorable body composition among both career and volunteers. Based on body mass index (BMI), the majority (66.7%) of female firefighters were classified in the normal weight category (range, 18.5–24.9 kg/m2), while only 16.7% were overweight and 16.7% were obese (Jahnke et al., 2012). Kirlin et al. (2017) found that, on average, female firefighters of all age groups met or exceeded the 12-MET professional standard for cardiorespiratory endurance; however, cardiovascular fitness declined with age (Kirlin, Nichols, Rusk, Parker, & Rauh, 2017; NFPA 1582; International Association of Firefighters, 2008). Current research found that 78% of female firefighters were regular exercisers according to the Self-Report Physical Activity Questionnaire (SRPA; Jahnke et al., under review). PA improves mental health and prevents weight gain (CDC, 2018). Fitness may be a key to improving the overall mental and physical health of firefighters. Research should examine women-specific fitness training for its efficacy in the fire service.

Gear

Most firefighters probably do not give the fit of their personal protective equipment (PPE) a second thought, but women often report ill-fitting PPE hinders their ability to do their job safely and effectively. According to iWomen in 2008, nearly 80% of the female firefighters surveyed reported ill-fitting protective gear. In addition, 14% reported ill-fitting self-contained breathing apparatus (SCBA) face pieces, a critical line of defense in a fire (Hulett et al., 2008). Nearly a decade later, a majority of the participants in a recent study still noted ill-fitting gear as a major threat to safety (Hollerbach et al., 2017). Women reported that bunker gear in their respective departments was made for men and they often had difficulty getting a good seal with an SCBA facepiece (Hollerbach et al., 2017). One participant said her department had to go through a lawsuit before they offered female-specific PPE (Hollerbach et al., 2017). Additionally, a number of chronic injuries may be due to inappropriately fitting gear. Feeling out of place or not having the necessary resources to do one's job has physical and psychological consequences such as lower productivity, absenteeism, turnover, burnout, and health-related issues (Quick & Tetrick, 2003). How can women be expected to survive in the fire service if they can't even get properly fitting PPE?

Injury

For years, the majority of fire service research has focused on male firefighters. The NFPA released its first report specific to the patterns of injury among women firefighters in 2017 (Campbell, 2017); however, unlike the NFPA annual injury report, this women-specific report only examined injuries that occurred on the fireground and likely underestimates the prevalence of injury among women firefighters. Despite its limitations, the report found that women firefighters experience similar injury causes (the majority overexertion/strain) on the fireground as their male counterparts (Evarts & Molis, 2018; Campbell, 2017). The NFPA report on women examined a five-year period and estimates that women firefighters sustained an average of 1260 injuries each year in the five-year period (from 2010-2014; Campbell, 2017).

Though they may experience the same types of injury, Liao et al. (2001) found that women firefighters experienced injuries more frequently than their male peers, with women firefighters reporting 33% more injuries than men. This relationship persisted even after controlling for factors such as age, race, tenure, personality, and secular trends (Liao, Arvey, Butler, & Nutting, 2001). Current research has shown that women often note a need to "prove" themselves in the firehouse and on the fireground, leading to taking on more than they are physically able or not asking for help, which puts them at increased risk of injury (Hollerbach et al., 2017). Further research should examine the types of injuries women firefighters sustain and policies and training programs should be explored to lessen the burden of injury in the fire service.

Reproductive Health

Limited research has examined reproductive health outcomes among firefighters. There is some data from the 1980's and '90s (Evanoff & Rosenstock, 1986) that reviewed the potential risks women firefighters face, but in general this area remains relatively unexplored. Reproductive risks for women include fireground and other hazardous response exposures (McDiarmid, Lees, Agnew, Midzenski, & Duffy, 1991), as well as the impact of shift work and sleep disturbances, high ambient temperatures, loud noises, and the physical and psychological strain of firefighting (Agnew, McDiarmid, Lees, & Duffy, 1991; Amani & Gill, 2013; Mahoney, 2010; Nurminen, 1998; Puttonen, Harma, & Hublin, 2010).

A recent study found an increased risk of male-factor infertility (46%) among Danish firefighters (Petersen, Hansen, Ebbehoej, & Bonde, 2018). It appears that the number of years serving as a firefighter attenuates the relationship with infertility, with those serving as a firefighter longer having a higher risk for infertility (Petersen et al., 2018). Firefighting hazards associated with increased risk of infertility include hyperthermia, loud noise, chemical and biological exposures, emotional trauma, and stress (Petersen et al., 2018). These hazards can reduce testosterone, weaken libido, and ultimately cause impotence (Agnew et al., 1991).

While there is some concern and limited research examining infertility in male firefighters, there is significant concern among women in the fire service who might want to have children (Jahnke, Poston, Jitnarin, & Haddock, 2018). Recent research suggests the uncertainty regarding the effects of firefighting on reproductive health may affect recruitment and retention of women in the fire service (Kehler et al., 2018). A study by Jahnke and colleagues found that only about a third of women firefighters reported a pregnancy during their career as a firefighter (Jahnke et al., 2018). It is unclear whether women firefighters choose to give birth before entering the fire service or if there are specific factors related to firefighting that discourage childbearing (Jahnke et al., 2018). Data suggests that, when women work in occupations in which formal limitations are high for reproduction (e.g. low benefit levels, gender segregated policies), women tend to delay or limit childbearing (Chesnais, 1996; Mills, Rindfuss, McDonald, & Te Velde, 2011; Neyer & Andersson, 2008). It is also possible given high rates of discrimination and harassment women face in the fire service (Hulett et al., 2008) that they decide against becoming pregnant because childbearing would limit their ability to fully participate in firefighting activities (Jahnke et al., 2018).

Additionally, for women in the fire service who do choose to get pregnant, few departments that have official policies in place to help them and their supervisors make decisions about when to restrict duties or disclose pregnancies to the department. Jahnke et al. (2018) found that, on average, women firefighters were at the end of their first trimester before they reported their pregnancy to their department, and most did not restrict their duties until the second or third trimester, while approximately 10% of women did not restrict their duties at all throughout their pregnancy (Jahnke et al., 2018). More research however is necessary to examine how long it is safe for women to remain on full active duty while pregnant.

There also is very little guidance for women firefighters regarding breastfeeding and how long after battling a fire it is safe to save breast milk. The only guidance currently available is pilot data from Burgess et al. (2015), which suggests that in order to limit potential exposure of toxins to their breastfeeding infants, women firefighters should pump and discard their breastmilk following a structural fire for 72 hours, and supplement using an alternative source. Further research is necessary to identify links between firefighting and infertility, as well as mechanisms to protect firefighters and their offspring. Further, practitioners need guidance specific to firefighters to give appropriate advice for new and expecting mothers.

SOLUTIONS AND RECOMMENDATIONS

There are initiatives, such as the IAFC Bullying, Harassment, and Workplace Violence Prevention Task Group, The First Twenty Tactical High Performance Program (TF20), and the Front Line Behavioral Health Intervention, targeted at improving the health and wellness of firefighters. The overall goal of these initiatives is to create a culture of dignity and respect in the fire service and improve the physical and mental health of firefighters. The fire service should continue to collaborate and combine efforts such as those mentioned above to enhance firefighter safety and promote diversity within its ranks.

FUTURE RESEARCH DIRECTIONS

Further research should examine policies and training in other occupations that may transfer to the fire service culture. Additionally, resources for assessing and treating mental health issues among firefighters are warranted. Future research is necessary to better connect firefighters to behavioral health providers and physicians and better train the providers specially trained to work with this unique population.

CONCLUSION

In a properly supported department, these numbers look much better. It is not just the fire service that is dangerous, it is what goes on behind the scenes where there is a real impact of bullying, harassment, and sexual assault. Research has found high rates of mental health concerns among firefighters, but some speculate that elevated rates among women means they cannot do the job. When one evaluates mental health in supportive environments, women perform nearly the same as men. A lot of these issues related to women firefighters and mental health are the product of being in an unsupportive and potentially toxic job environment. Current research is limited for female firefighters, especially regarding mental health outcomes. The data that exists suggest that there are limited trainings or resources specific for female firefighters and that women are still experiencing significant differential treatment in the fire service (Jahnke et al., 2012; Hollerbach et al., 2017; Hulett et al., 2008; Horvath, 2013; Fox et al., 2006; IAFC, 2016; Griffith et al., 2016; Jahnke et al., under review; Sinden et al., 2013). The barriers female firefighters face (e.g., harassment, inadequate training, ill-fitting gear, and a lack of resources) may lead to poor coping mechanisms including substance use and abuse, poor mental health, and an increased risk of injury. These barriers and the associated poor health outcomes may contribute to the low rates of recruitment and retention of women in the fire service.

ACKNOWLEDGMENT

Thank you to the researchers at the Institute for Biobehavioral Health Research for their dedication to this effort. Thank you to my fire service mentors, Bill Benjamin and Richard Lehmann, for their continued support and direction.

This research was supported by the Federal Emergency Management Agency [grant numbers EMW-2007-FP-02571 and EMW-2009-FP-01971]; the National Heart, Lung and Blood Institute at the National Institutes of Health [grant number R21HL119024]; and the American Heart Association [grant number 0830390N].

REFERENCES

Agnew, J., McDiarmid, M. A., Lees, P. S. J., & Duffy, R. (1991). Reproductive hazards of firefighting. I. Non-chemical hazards. *American Journal of Industrial Medicine*, *19*(4), 433–445. doi:10.1002/ajim.4700190403 PMID:2035545

Amani, R., & Gill, T. (2013). Shift working, nutrition and obesity: Implications for workforce health- a systematic review. *Asia Pacific Journal of Clinical Nutrition*, *22*(4), 505–515. PMID:24231009

Antecol, H., & Cobb-Clark, D. (2006). The sexual harassment of female active-duty personnel: Effects on job satisfaction and intentions to remain in the military. *Journal of Economic Behavior & Organization*, *61*(1), 55–80. doi:10.1016/j.jebo.2004.11.006

Bartel, A. P. (1981). Race differences in job satisfaction: A reappraisal. *The Journal of Human Resources*, *16*(2), 294–303. doi:10.2307/145514

Boffa, J. W., Stanley, I. H., Hom, M. A., Norr, A. M., Joiner, T. E., & Schmidt, N. B. (2017). PTSD symptoms and suicidal thoughts and behaviors among firefighters. *Journal of Psychiatric Research*, *84*, 277–283. doi:10.1016/j.jpsychires.2016.10.014 PMID:27810667

Burgess, D. (2015). *Firefighter breastmilk pilot study summary*. Report to the Arizona Fire Department.

Campbell, R. (2017). *Patterns of female firefighter injuries on the fireground*. Quincy, MA: National Fire Protection Association.

Carey, M. G., Al-Zaiti, S. S., Dean, G. E., Sessanna, L., & Finnell, D. S. (2011). Sleep problems, depression, substance use, social bonding, and quality of life in professional firefighters. *Journal of Occupational and Environmental Medicine/American College of Occupational and Environmental Medicine*, *53*(8), 928.

Centers for Disease Control and Prevention (CDC). (2015). *Adult obesity facts*. Retrieved from http://www.cdc.gov/obesity/data/adult.html

Centers for Disease Control and Prevention (CDC). (2018). *Physical Activity: Why it matters.* Retrieved from https://www.cdc.gov/physicalactivity/about-physical-activity/why-it-matters.html

Chen, Y. S., Chen, M. C., Chou, F. H. C., Sun, F. C., Chen, P. C., Tsai, K. Y., & Chao, S. S. (2007). The relationship between quality of life and posttraumatic stress disorder or major depression for firefighters in Kaohsiung, Taiwan. *Quality of Life Research: An International Journal of Quality of Life Aspects of Treatment, Care and Rehabilitation, 16*(8), 1289–1297. doi:10.100711136-007-9248-7 PMID:17668289

Chesnais, J. (1996). Fertility, family, and social policy in contemporary Western Europe. *Population and Development Review, 22*(4), 729. doi:10.2307/2137807

Clark, A. E. (1997). Job satisfaction and gender: Why are women so happy at work? *Labour Economics, 4*(4), 314–372. doi:10.1016/S0927-5371(97)00010-9

Crosby, F. (2007). *The Real Meaning of Brotherhood. Fire Engineering.* Retrieved from http://www.fireengineering.com/index/articles

del Ben, K. S., Scotti, J. R., Chen, Y. C., & Fortson, B. L. (2006). Prevalence of posttraumatic stress disorder symptoms in firefighters. *Work and Stress, 20*(1), 37–48.

Durand, G., Tsismenakis, A. J., Jahnke, S. A., Baur, D. M., Christophi, C. A., & Kales, S. A. (2011). Firefighters physical activity: Relation to fitness and cardiovascular disease risk. *Medicine and Science in Sports and Exercise, 43*(9), 1752–1759. doi:10.1249/MSS.0b013e318215cf25 PMID:21364484

Evanoff, B., & Rosenstock, L. (1986). Reproductive hazards in the workplace: A case study of women firefighters. *American Journal of Industrial Medicine, 9*(6), 503–515. doi:10.1002/ajim.4700090602 PMID:3740071

Evarts, B., & Molis, J. L. (2018). *United States Firefighter Injuries 2017.* Quincy, MA: National Fire Protection Association.

Fahy, R. F., LeBlanc, P. R., & Molis, J. L. (2018). *Firefighter Fatalities in the United States - 2017.* Quincy, MA: National Fire Protection Association.

Fear, N. T., Iversen, A., Meltzer, H., Workman, L., Hull, L., Greenberg, N., & Jones, M. (2007). Patterns of drinking in the UK Armed Forces. *Addiction (Abingdon, England), 102*(11), 1749–1759. doi:10.1111/j.1360-0443.2007.01978.x PMID:17935583

Firefighter Behavioral Health Alliance FF & EMS Suicide Deaths by Year and Type. (n.d.). Retrieved from http://www.ffbha.org/ff-ems-suicide-deaths-by-year-type/

Fox, K. A., Hornick, C. W., & Hardin, E. (2006). *International Association of Firefighters Diversity Initiative: Achieving and Retaining a Diverse Fire Service Workforce.* Washington, DC: IAFF.

Fullerton, C. S., Ursano, R. J., & Wang, L. (2004). Acute Stress Disorder, Posttraumatic Stress Disorder, and Depression in Disaster or Rescue Workers. *The American Journal of Psychiatry, 161*(8), 1370–1376. doi:10.1176/appi.ajp.161.8.1370 PMID:15285961

Gist, R., Taylor, V. H., & Raak, S. (2011). *Suicide surveillance, prevention, and intervention measures for the US Fire Service: Findings and recommendations for the suicide and depression summit.* Baltimore, MD: National Fallen Firefighters Foundation.

Griffith, J. C., Roberts, D. L., & Wakeham, R. T. (2016). Bullying at the Fire Station? Perceptions Based on Gender, Race and Sexual Orientation. *American International Journal of Social Sciences*, *5*, 34–44.

Haddock, C. K., Day, R. S., Poston, W. S., Jahnke, S. A., & Jitnarin, N. (2015). Alcohol use and caloric intake from alcohol in a national cohort of U.S. career firefighters. *Journal of Studies on Alcohol and Drugs*, *76*(3), 360–366. doi:10.15288/jsad.2015.76.360 PMID:25978821

Haddock, C. K., Poston, W. S., Jahnke, S. A., & Jitnarin, N. (2017). Alcohol Use and Problem Drinking among Women Firefighters. *Women's Health Issues*, *27*(6), 632–638. doi:10.1016/j.whi.2017.07.003 PMID:28822615

Haynes, H. J., & Stein, G. P. (2017). *US Fire Department Profile 2015.* Quincy, MA: National Fire Protection Association.

Heyman, M., Dill, J., & Douglas, R. (2018). *The Ruderman White Paper on Mental Health and Suicide of First Responders.* Boston, MA: Ruderman Foundation.

Hollerbach, B. S., Heinrich, K. M., Poston, W. S., Haddock, C. K., Kehler, A. K., & Jahnke, S. A. (2017). Current Female Firefighters' Perceptions, Attitudes, and Experiences with Injury. *International Fire Service Journal of Leadership & Management*, (11).

Hom, M. A., Stanley, I. H., Spencer-Thomas, S., & Joiner, T. E. (2017). Women firefighters and workplace harassment: Associated suicidality and mental health sequelae. *The Journal of Nervous and Mental Disease*, *205*(12), 910–917. doi:10.1097/NMD.0000000000000759 PMID:29088006

Horvath, C. (2013). Same old story: The biggest issues facing women firefighters today. *FireRescue1.* Retrieved from https://www.firerescue1.com/cod-company-officer-development/articles/1453190-Same-old-story-The-biggest-issues-facing-women-firefighters-today/

Hulett, D. M., Bendick, M., Thomas, S. Y., & Moccio, F. (2008). *A national report card on women in firefighting.* Madison, WI: International Association of Women in Fire and Emergency Services. Retrieved from https://www.i-women.org/wp-content/uploads/2014/07/35827WSP.pdf

IAFC President's Letter: Time to Lead on Diversity and Inclusion. (2016). Retrieved from https://www.iafc.org/on-scene/on-scene-article/president-s-letter-time-to-lead-on-diversity-and-inclusion

International Association of Firefighters. (2008). *The Fire Service Joint Labor Management Wellness-Fitness Initiative* (3rd ed.). Washington, DC: International Association of Firefighters.

Jahnke, S., Poston, W., Haddock, C., Jitnarin, N., Hyder, M., & Horvath, C. (2012). The health of women in the US fire service. *BMC Women's Health*, *12*(1), 39. doi:10.1186/1472-6874-12-39 PMID:23114186

Jahnke, S. A., Haddock, C. K., Jitnarin, N., Kaipust, C., Hollerbach, B. S., & Poston, W. S. C. (Manuscript submitted for publication). The prevalence and health impacts of frequent work discrimination and harassment among women firefighters in the US fire service. *BioMed Research International.* PMID:31016195

Jahnke, S.A., Poston, W.C., & Haddock, C.K. (2014). Perceptions of Alcohol use among US Firefighters. *Journal of Substance Abuse and Alcoholism*, *2*(2).

Jahnke, S. A., Poston, W. S., Jitnarin, N., & Haddock, C. K. (2018). Maternal and Child Health Among Female Firefighters in the US. *Maternal and Child Health Journal*, *22*(6), 922–931. PMID:29423588

Jahnke, S. A., Poston, W. S. C., Haddock, C. K., & Jitnarin, N. (2013). Obesity and incident injury among career firefighters in the central United States. *Obesity (Silver Spring, Md.)*, *21*(8), 1505–1508. PMID:23512940

Jahnke, S. A., Poston, W. S. C., Haddock, C. K., & Murphy, B. (2016). Firefighting and mental health: Experiences of repeated exposure to trauma. *Work (Reading, Mass.)*, *53*(4), 737–744. PMID:26890595

Jitnarin, N., Poston, W. S., Haddock, C. K., Jahnke, S. A., & Day, R. S. (2015). Tobacco use pattern among a national firefighter cohort. *Nicotine & Tobacco Research*, *17*(1), 66–73. doi:10.1093/ntr/ntu131 PMID:25145378

Kales, S. N., Polyhronopoulos, G. N., Aldrich, J. M., Leitao, E. O., & Christiani, D. C. (1999). Correlates of body mass index in hazardous materials firefighters. *Journal of Occupational and Environmental Medicine*, *41*(7), 589–595. PMID:10412100

Kehler, A., Jahnke, S.A., Haddock, C.K., Poston, W.S., Jitnarin, N., & Heinrich, K.M. (2018). Reproductive Health Concerns Among Female Firefighters. *International Fire Service Journal of Leadership and Management,* 12.

Kessler, R. C., Mickelson, K. D., & Williams, D. R. (1999). The prevalence, distribution, and mental health correlates of perceived discrimination in the United States. *Journal of Health and Social Behavior*, *40*(3), 208–230. PMID:10513145

Kirlin, L., Nichols, J., Rusk, K., Parker, R., & Rauh, M. (2017). The effect of age on fitness among female firefighters. *Occupational Medicine*, *67*(7), 528–533. doi:10.1093/occmed/kqx123 PMID:29016908

Krieger, N. (1999). Embodying inequality: A review of concepts, measures, and methods for studying health consequences of discrimination. *International Journal of Health Services: Planning Administration and Evaluation*, *29*(2), 295–352. PMID:10379455

Liao, H., Arvey, R., Butler, R., & Nutting, S. (2001). Correlates of work injury frequency and duration among firefighters. *Journal of Occupational Health Psychology*, *6*(3), 229–242. PMID:11482634

Mahoney, M. (2010). Shift Work, Jet Lag, and Female Reproduction. *International Journal of Endocrinology*. PMID:20224815

Martin, V., & Paulus, B. (2017). Alcohol use and suicidality in firefighters: Associations with depressive symptoms and posttraumatic stress. *Comprehensive Psychiatry*, *74*, 44–52. doi:10.1016/j.comppsych.2017.01.002 PMID:28092775

McDiarmid, M., Lees, P., Agnew, J., Midzenski, M., & Duffy, R. (1991). Reproductive hazards of firefighting II. Chemical hazards. *American Journal of Industrial Medicine*, *19*(4), 447–472. doi:10.1002/ajim.4700190404 PMID:2035546

McIntosh, W. L. (2016). Suicide rates by occupational group – 17 states, 2012. *Morbidity and mortality weekly report*, 65. PMID:27359167

McNeil, J. (2008). Diversity in the fire service: A problem or a solution? *Fire Engineering*, *161*(10), 129.

Mills, M. R., Rindfuss, R., McDonald, P., & Te Velde, E. (2011). Why do people postpone parenthood? Reasons and social policy incentives. *Human Reproduction Update*, *17*(6), 848–860. doi:10.1093/humupd/dmr026 PMID:21652599

National Fire Protection Association. (2013). NFPA 1582: Standard on Comprehensive Occupational Medical Program for All Fire Departments. Quincy, MA: NFPA, 98.

National Fire Protection Association. (2018). NFPA 1500: Standard on Fire Department Occupational Safety and Health Program. Quincy, MA: NFPA, 37.

National Institutes of Health. (n.d.). *Drinking Levels Defined*. Retrieved from https://www.niaaa.nih.gov/alcohol-health/overview-alcohol-consumption/moderate-binge-drinking

National Institutes of Mental Health. (n.d.). *Mental Health Information*. Retrieved from https://www.nimh.nih.gov/health/statistics/major-depression.shtml

Neyer, G., & Andersson, G. (2008). *Consequences of Family Policies on Childbearing Behavior: Effects or Artifacts?* (Vol. 34). Oxford, UK: Blackwell Publishing.

Nock, M. K., Borges, G., Bromet, E. J., Alonso, J., Angermeyer, M., Beautrais, A., ... Williams, D. (2008). Cross-national prevalence and risk factors for suicidal ideation, plans and attempts. *Journal of Psychiatry*, *192*(2), 98–105. doi:10.1192/bjp.bp.107.040113 PMID:18245022

Nock, M. K., Stein, M. B., Heeringa, S. G., Ursano, R. J., Colpe, L. J., Fullerton, C. S., ... Kessler, R. C. (2014). Prevalence and correlates of suicidal behavior among soldiers. *JAMA Psychiatry*, *71*(5), 514–522. doi:10.1001/jamapsychiatry.2014.30 PMID:24590178

Nurminen, T. (1998). Shift work and reproductive health. *Scandinavian Journal of Work, Environment & Health*, *24*, 28–34. PMID:9916814

Okechukwu, C. A., Souza, K., Davis, K. D., & de Castro, A. B. (2014). Discrimination, harassment, abuse, and bullying in the workplace: Contribution of workplace injustice to occupational health disparities. *American Journal of Industrial Medicine*, *57*(5), 573–586. doi:10.1002/ajim.22221 PMID:23813664

Pascoe, E. A., & Smart Richman, L. (2009). Perceived discrimination and health: A meta-analytic review. *Psychological Bulletin*, *135*(4), 531–554. doi:10.1037/a0016059 PMID:19586161

Perrott, T. (2016). Beyond 'Token' Firefighters: Exploring Women's Experiences of Gender and Identity at Work. *Sociological Research Online*, *21*(1), 1–14. doi:10.5153ro.3832

Petersen, K. U., Hansen, J., Ebbehoej, N. E., & Bonde, J. P. (2018, November). Infertility in a Cohort of Male Danish Firefighters: A Register-Based Study. *American Journal of Epidemiology*, 19. PMID:30452532

Poplin, G. S., Harris, R. B., Pollack, K. M., Peate, W. F., & Burgess, J. L. (2011). Beyond the fireground: Injuries in the fire service. *Injury Prevention*, *18*(4), 228–233. doi:10.1136/injuryprev-2011-040149 PMID:22117024

Puttonen, S., Harma, M., & Hublin, C. (2010). Shift work and cardiovascular disease - pathways from circadian stress to morbidity. *Scandinavian Journal of Work, Environment & Health, 36*(2), 96–108. doi:10.5271jweh.2894 PMID:20087536

Pyle, S., Graham, R., Suminski, R., Poston, W. S. C., Haddock, C. K., & Glaros, A. (2009). Depressive symptoms, self-rated mental health, daily functioning and job satisfaction among firefighters. *International Fire Service Journal of Leadership and Management, 3*(1), 19–24.

Quick, J., & Tetrick, L. E. (2003). *Handbook of occupational health psychology*. Washington, DC: American Psychological Association.

Reskin, B. F., & Bielby, D. D. (2005). A sociological perspective on gender and career outcomes.(wages, working hours). *The Journal of Economic Perspectives, 19*(1), 71–86.

Rosell, E., Miller, K., & Barber, K. (1995). Firefighting Women and Sexual Harassment. *Public Personnel Management, 24*(3), 339–350.

Sinden, K., Macdermid, J., Buckman, S., Davis, B., Matthews, T., & Viola, C. (2013). A qualitative study on the experiences of female firefighters. *Work (Reading, Mass.), 45*(1), 97–105. PMID:23241712

Soteriades, E. S., Hauser, R., Kawachi, I., Christiani, D. C., & Kales, S. N. (2008). Obesity and risk of job disability in male firefighters. *Occupational Medicine, 58*(4), 245–250. doi:10.1093/occmed/kqm153 PMID:18204003

Soteriades, E. S., Hauser, R., Kawachi, I., Liarokapis, D., Christiani, D. C., & Kales, S. N. (2005). Obesity and cardiovascular disease risk factors in firefighters: A prospective cohort study. *Obesity Research, 13*(10), 1756–1763. doi:10.1038/oby.2005.214 PMID:16286523

Stanley, I. H., Boffa, J. W., Tran, J. K., Schmidt, N. B., Joiner, T. E., & Vujanovic, A. A. (2019). Posttraumatic stress disorder symptoms and mindfulness facets in relation to suicide risk among firefighters. *Journal of Clinical Psychology*, 1–14. PMID:30672591

Stanley, I. H., Hom, M. A., Spencer-Thomas, S., & Joiner, T. E. (2017). Suicidal thoughts and behaviors among women firefighters: An examination of associated features and comparison of pre-career and career prevalence rates. *Journal of Affective Disorders, 221*, 107–114. doi:10.1016/j.jad.2017.06.016 PMID:28641147

Stanley, I. H., Horn, M. A., Hagan, C. R., & Joiner, T. E. (2015). Career prevalence and correlates of suicidal thoughts and behaviors among firefighters. *Journal of Affective Disorders, 187*, 163–171. doi:10.1016/j.jad.2015.08.007 PMID:26339926

Todorova, I. L. G., Falcón, L., Lincoln, A. K., & Price, L. L. (2010). Perceived discrimination, psychological distress and health. *Sociology of Health & Illness, 32*(6), 843–861. doi:10.1111/j.1467-9566.2010.01257.x PMID:20649891

Traut, C. A., Larsen, R., & Feimer, S. H. (2009). Hanging on or fading out? Job satisfaction and the long-term worker. *Public Personnel Management, 29*(3), 343–351. doi:10.1177/009102600002900304

Tsismenakis, A. J., Christophi, C. A., Burress, J. W., Kinney, A. M., Kim, M., & Kales, S. N. (2009). The obesity epidemic and future emergency responders. *Obesity (Silver Spring, Md.)*, *17*(8), 1648–1649. doi:10.1038/oby.2009.63 PMID:19300435

US Department of Veterans Affairs. (2018). *PTSD: National Center for PTSD*. Retrieved from https://www.ptsd.va.gov/understand/common/common_adults.asp

US Fire Administration. (n.d.). *Firefighter Fatality Search Results*. Retrieved from https://apps.usfa.fema.gov/firefighter-fatalities/fatalityData/list?deathYear=2018&offset=0&max=10

Wagner, S., & O'Neill, M. (2012). Job, Life, and Relationship Satisfaction for Paid-Professional Firefighters. *Journal of Loss and Trauma*, *17*(5), 423–438. doi:10.1080/15325024.2011.650129

Williams, D. R., Neighbors, H. W., & Jackson, J. S. (2003). Racial/Ethnic discrimination and health: Findings from community studies. *American Journal of Public Health*, *93*(2), 200–208. doi:10.2105/AJPH.93.2.200 PMID:12554570

Women in Military Service for America Memorial Foundation, Inc. (2010). *Statistics on Women in the Military*. Washington, DC: Women in Military Service for America Memorial Foundation.

KEY TERMS AND DEFINITIONS

Behavioral Health: The study of one's behavior and its influence on their health (both mental and physical).

Differential Treatment: Negative and pervasive inappropriate behavior directed at an induvial or individuals including bullying, harassment, assault, sexual assault, and threats.

Mental Health: The state of health (lack of disease or impairment) specific to one's mental status including an examination of stress, depression, anxiety, sleep status, and PSTD.

National Fire Protection Association: U.S. national governing body responsible for development and standardization of standard operating procedures and guidelines for the U.S. fire service.

Occupational Risk Factors: Refers to health risk factors associated with one's occupation.

PTSD: Posttraumatic stress disorder as defined in the literature; referring to a clinical stressful reaction to a traumatic event.

Tactical Athlete: Referring to a worker in a physically demanding and often dangerous occupation usually including military, police, and firefighters.

Women Firefighters: Referring to females in the occupation of firefighting including firefighters as well as leaders such as captains and chief officers.

Chapter 7
Critical Incident Stress Management:
A Comprehensive, Intergrative, Systematic, and Multi-Component Program for Supporting First Responder Psychological Health

Jeffrey T. Mitchell
University of Maryland, Baltimore County, USA

ABSTRACT

This chapter provides a clear overview of a peer support program for first responders. The field of Critical Incident Stress Management (CISM) was specifically developed to prepare emergency services personnel to psychologically manage significant traumatic events and to recover from the impact of psychological trauma. CISM services are based in the theoretical foundations of crisis intervention and CISM uses the lessons learned from the 150-year history of worldwide crisis intervention services. This chapter presents a history of crisis intervention that helps the reader to understand the core principles of crisis support. It then focuses on the numerous techniques that are incorporated into the Critical Incident Stress Management field. It summarizes key peer support procedures and practices. The chapter also describes the resiliency and the "AS IF" models that aid in the application of crisis intervention services. The chapter concludes with a summary of the evidence that supports CISM services.

INTRODUCTION

As the name implies, First Responders are people who get to emergencies first. They get involved when situations are chaotic and dangerous. Lives are frequently in jeopardy. Failure to take action quickly and act effectively can have dire consequences. Included in the First Responder category are law enforcement personnel, firefighters, EMS personnel, communications officers, federal agents, Search and Rescue

DOI: 10.4018/978-1-5225-9803-9.ch007

personnel, emergency and critical care nurses, disaster response personnel, medical doctors, especially in high risk environments like emergency and critical care centers and many members of the armed forces.

There are three terms that should come to mind when we think of First Responders:

- High Intensity
- High Reliability
- High Risk

High Intensity

High intensity work is fast-paced with one emergent situation often following closely on another. Sometimes multiple demanding situations are occurring simultaneously. On occasion, First Responders may work a scene of a major disaster. First Responders find that the stakes in their work are often very high. Mistakes and accidents are costly from many points of view. Mistakes in a field operation can delay final actions. The situation may spiral out of control. People can be seriously injured or they may die. The pressures for consistent maximum performance are great (Forstenzer, 1980; Hassling, 2000).

High Reliability

The term 'High Reliability' means that people in trouble can count on First Responders for help. They respond regardless of the weather or the circumstances or the threats. People who work in High reliability organizations cannot pick and choose which critical incidents they will handle. High Reliability organizations and the personnel who work for them have special training, specialized equipment, procedures or protocols. Substandard performance is unacceptable and dangerous. They are expected to function consistently and safely for the good of others.

High-Risk

Professions that are listed as high-risk are those whose members or employees experience considerable physical and psychological threats in their work. The word 'members' is used along with employees in the previous sentence because many people work as volunteers for high-risk organizations. Volunteer fire department personnel or volunteers who work at disaster sites for the Red Cross are examples of volunteer first responders who are exposed to some of the same physical and emotional threats as career employees. Rather than repeat, throughout this chapter, the fact that volunteers are involved in high-risk work, the words 'personnel,' 'members,' 'first responders,' 'emergency services' or 'employees' will be used somewhat interchangeably with the implication that both volunteers and career staff work as first responders.

This chapter is based on the premise that *high-risk organizations* are those in which the personnel face potential exposures to extreme stress or significant threats to their physical and emotional wellbeing. Highly stressful or threatening circumstances are viewed as a probable hazard associated with employment in these professions. Military and emergency services personnel such as law enforcement officers, fire fighters, search and rescue personnel, disaster workers, nurses, doctors and other medical staff are among the most well known psychologically high risk professions. They are not, however, the only professions in which there are considerable physical and emotional risks. The physical and psychological risks that are associated with mining, logging, ground transportation, aviation, and commercial fishing operations are well documented (Staff, Air Safety Week, 2001); Parker, 2006; US Department of Labor, 2008, a, b; 2009; Inglish, 2010).

Being on a list of high-risk professions should not be a badge of honor for any organization, agency or department. Risks must be managed and reduced wherever possible. The aim should always be high reliability, not maintaining the status quo of high-risk. These organizations must function reliably, consistently, effectively, and, above all else, safely.

As this chapter points out, one way to reduce and manage the psychological risk in First Responders is to develop peer support teams based on the principles of Critical Incident Stress Management.

CRITICAL INCIDENTS

Critical incidents are events that are so unusual or powerful that they can overwhelm the coping capacity of those who are exposed to them. A critical incident generates a strong, sometimes tumultuous, emotional reaction that is called a *crisis* or, occasionally, a *crisis reaction.* High-risk organizations like first response departments and agencies are justified in their concern about crisis reactions. They are typically accompanied by cognitive, emotional, physical, spiritual, and behavioral manifestations of stress. When people reach a state of intense emotional disturbance, their thinking may become disorganized and unclear. Exaggerated feelings can dominate one's reactions. When stress levels are high, mistakes may occur more frequently, and accident rates and personal injuries tend to climb. Psychological disequilibrium may appear, that is, a person's thinking ability is suppressed and one's feelings intensify to a point of being nearly out of control. In those circumstances, crisis intervention may be required to rebalance the person and assist him or her in resolving the situation. *Crisis intervention is the active, supportive, and temporary assistance given by family members, friends, colleagues and trained peer support personnel to others who are experiencing a period of acute distress* (Neil et al., 1974; Slaikeu, 1984).

Acts of violence, serious injuries to operations personnel, baby deaths, injured or ill children, deaths of adults, hostage takings, mistakes causing injury or deaths to others, and serious equipment failures that jeopardize mission effectiveness are just some of the critical incidents that may impact the emotional lives of people within the first responder organizations. Such stressful events are a relatively common occurrence. The ultimate critical incident would, of course, be a major disaster, but, thankfully, such horrific events are infrequent. Although they are high reliability organizations, first response agencies remain *high-risk organizations* for their employees. Crisis support programs like the Critical Incident Stress Management program have been designed to enhance the resiliency of employees in high-risk organizations.

Common Critical Incidents in First Responder Groups

- Work related deaths of colleagues (line of duty deaths)
- Serious work-related injuries to a colleague
- Suicide of a colleague
- Accidental killing or wounding of any innocent person in the performance of one's duties
- Events involving a high degree of personnel threat
- "Close calls" in which someone narrowly escaped being injured or killed

- Shooting incidents
- Seriously ill or injured children
- Major medical emergencies that occur while working on a patient
- Entrapped victims in a fire
- Handling the remains of the dead
- Threatening individuals interacting with first responders
- Violence from any source while performing one's job
- Damaged equipment that jeopardizes saving of a life.
- Serious accidents involving emergency response vehicles.
- Hazardous materials leaks that threaten operations personnel
- Acts of terrorism
- Disasters
- Murder scenes (especially if children are the victims)
- Fetal demise
- Medical errors causing injury or deaths to patients
- Baby deaths during delivery
- Listening to someone die on the phone while emergency units are being dispatched
- Other distressing experiences

CRITICAL INCIDENT STRESS

Critical incidents are seen as "turning point" events that can stimulate psychological growth or cause significant psychological damage. Critical incidents are typically considered horrible, terrible, awful, grotesque, overwhelming, frightening, threatening, or disgusting by those who experience them. They can generate a wide range of physical and psychological symptoms. Most people do recover reasonably rapidly after an exposure to a critical incident and do not require formal psychological intervention. If not managed carefully, however, it is possible that a critical incident can become the source of long-lasting conditions such as substance abuse, phobic reactions, depression, panic disorders or Posttraumatic Stress Disorder (PTSD). Critical incidents are, therefore, the starting point for Critical Incident Stress.

The term, *Critical Incident Stress*, was developed in the mid 1970's to describe an expected and typical response of normal, psychologically healthy people after an exposure to an extraordinary traumatic event (the critical incident). It originated from a need to have non-clinical terminology that could be easily understood by and appropriately applied to emergency services, military, and disaster response personnel. Critical Incident Stress is a term that is routinely used to describe the cognitive, physical, emotional, behavioral, and spiritual reactions of people who experience psychologically disturbing events frequently, but not always, as a result of their jobs. The key factor in Critical Incident Stress is the exposure to the critical incident. Without exposure to the traumatic event, the Critical Incident Stress reaction would not be possible. Some mental health professionals use the phrase Critical Incident Stress as a synonym for terms like "post traumatic stress," "traumatic stress," and "post trauma syndrome." Those terms, however, are generally viewed as being more rooted in clinical psychology and, thus, are less acceptable to hardy people, such as military and emergency services personnel, who periodically encounter severe psychological threats, unusually distressing circumstances, gory sights and sounds, and other unsettling critical incidents (Mitchell, 1982,1983, 2001, 2006).

Formulation of the Concept

The primary concept that underlies the term Critical Incident Stress is that healthy, well-functioning people can undergo enormously stressful circumstances and have powerful reactions to those experiences, but not be inherently weak, or psychologically impaired prior to the traumatic event. In fact, because they are typically hardy or resilient people, they can usually resist the ill effects of stress, bounce back from the shock and disruption associated with the experience, recover from critical incident stress, and resume normal life functions within a relatively short time of their exposure to the traumatic event.

In the majority of cases, early support lessens the duration of the symptoms. This is especially so when early psychological support is provided by peer support teams. Family, friends and colleagues are also important in providing support. The signs and symptoms of Critical Incident Stress can lessen within a few days of the critical incident. Symptoms lasting beyond three weeks, however, indicate a need for intensified supportive intervention and possibly professional care. Support provided by people who are specially trained in crisis intervention and who use a combination of supportive processes generally has a greater positive impact on the speed and efficiency of recovery for people suffering through Critical Incident Stress. The works of Gerald Caplan, Robert Jay Lifton, Richard S. Lazarus, and Suzanne C. Kobassa are the most succinct if one wishes to delve more deeply into theoretical underpinnings of Critical Incident Stress (Caplan, 1961,1964,1969; Lifton, 1970, 1973, 1993;Lazarus, 1966, 1969; Kobassa, 1979, 1982).

Although they had been used in verbal presentations to emergency personnel for several years during the 1970's, the words "critical incident," when utilized to indicate an event that generates the critical incident stress reaction, first appeared in the literature in 1982 and the term "critical incident stress" appeared in the following year. Since then, many hundreds of articles using those terms have been written both in peer-reviewed journals and in popular publications. Numerous books have also been published on the topic of Critical Incident Stress (Mitchell, 1982, 1983, 2007; Everly and Mitchell, 2008).

Signs and Symptoms of Critical Incident Stress

Most people, who are in a state of crisis and go through Critical Incident Stress, describe the following five characteristics of the condition:

1. They perceive that the critical incident was threatening, powerful, or overwhelming.
2. They are unable to manage the disruptive impact of the critical incident with their usual coping skills.
3. They experience increased fear, tension, and mental confusion.
4. They experience considerable subjective discomfort.
5. In a short time, they can proceed to an intense state of emotional crisis that is accompanied by the signs and symptoms of Critical Incident Stress.

Critical Incident Stress manifests itself differently in each person. The volume and intensity of stress signs and symptoms may vary considerably. Subjective perceptions of the traumatic event may contribute substantially to how disruptive the experience is for individuals and thus may lessen or intensify the person's Critical Incident Stress reaction. There are, however, relatively common patterns of stress reactions after critical incidents. People typically react with a combination of the following:

- Mental confusion and disorganization
- Difficulties in decision making and problem solving
- Intense anxiety, shock, denial and disbelief
- Anger, agitation and rage
- Helplessness
- Lowered self esteem
- Loss of self confidence
- Fear
- Feeling emotionally subdued or depressed
- Feelings of intense grief
- Emotional numbness
- Apathy
- Withdrawal from others
- Increase use of alcohol or other substances
- Periods of excessive activity to avoid thinking of the traumatic experience
- Loss of faith
- Cessation of the practice of religion
- Physical reactions such as nausea, shakes, headaches, intestinal disturbance, chest pain or difficulty breathing (Everly, 1989).

Caution: *Always rule out medical conditions first. It would be a mistake to assume that people's reactions are caused solely by psychological trauma. Medical staff should evaluate chest pain, difficulty breathing or any other severe physical conditions as soon as possible. Mental health professionals should evaluate severe psychological symptoms as soon as possible after medical conditions have been ruled out or stabilized.*

The above list is, by no means, exhaustive. Since so many diverse symptoms can be associated, directly or indirectly, with Critical Incident Stress, a complete list of symptoms would not be feasible or useful here. Any cognitive, physical, emotional, behavioral, or spiritual symptom can be caused by or made worse by stress.

When people reach a state of intense emotional disturbance, their thinking becomes disorganized and unclear. Exaggerated feelings dominate one's reactions. If a person's thinking ability is suppressed and one's feelings explode out of control, outside "crisis intervention" or "Critical Incident Stress Management" may be required to rebalance the person, assist them in resolving the situation, and in facilitating a return to adaptive functions.

CRISIS AND CRISIS INTERVENTION

In the section on "Critical Incidents" above, it was stated that critical incidents may generate a strong emotional reaction called a *crisis* or a *crisis reaction.* We will now look a little more closely at the concepts associated with the term crisis. Peer support and Critical Incident Stress Management Programs were developed specifically to assist people through crises.

Crisis: An acute emotional, cognitive and physical ***reaction*** to a powerful, horrible, awful, terrifying, threatening, or grotesque stimulus or to an overwhelming demand or circumstance.

Types of Crises

There are two types of crises. There are *maturational crises* and there are *situational crises.* Maturational crises occur as a result of common life's stages such as being a teenager, moving away from home, marriage, divorce, aging, retirement, and issues surrounding the end of life.

Characteristics of Crises

1. Disruption to one's general state of psychological balance
2. Usual coping mechanisms fail
3. Distress, impairment, or dysfunction (Caplan, 1964).

Crisis Intervention

The entire field of Critical Incident Stress Management (CISM) is actually an organized and structured program of crisis intervention. CISM is based on the history, theory, principles and practices of crisis intervention.

Crisis intervention is a ***temporary, active, and supportive*** entry into the life situation of an individual or of a group during a period of extreme distress. *Different intervention procedures are used for individuals than those that are used for groups* (Caplan, 1964; Mitchell, 1981).

A Brief History of Crisis Intervention

Knowing the history of the field of crisis intervention helps us to understand better the objectives and methods of crisis intervention that have been developed over time and which are now incorporated into the CISM field. There is a rich history of crisis intervention that dates back to the wars and disasters of the past century and a half (APA, 1964; Artiss, 1963; Caplan, 1961, 1964; Crocq et al, 1999; Crocq, 2007; 1981; Freeman, 1979; Lindemann, 1944; Roberts, 2005; Salmon, 1919; Stierlin, 1909). It was not until the French documented and applied the use of rudimentary crisis intervention techniques in the Franco-Prussian war in 1870-71 that the approach to helping people in a state of crisis became somewhat organized and structured. Medical personnel employed simple procedures such as removing distressed soldiers from the front lines, in other words, reducing war stimuli. They gathered together soldiers from the same units to take advantage of the bonds of friendship that were already well established. They also provided nutritious meals, fluids, rest, and an opportunity to talk to medical personnel. This was done near the front lines. Soldiers could still hear cannon fire in the distance, but were in no immediate danger. They were able to calm distressed soldiers and restore the majority of them to function on the battlefield. Those basic approaches to crisis intervention still have value today (Crocq et al, 1999; Crocq, 2007).

In 1906, Eduard Stierlin, a Swiss psychiatrist, provided psychological support to the victims and family members of miners after a great mining disaster killed 1100 miners in northern France near the border with Germany. Similar to the approach of the French in the Franco-Prussian war, providing information and guidance and placing people with their family members helped to calm highly distressed people who were awaiting word of their loved ones who were in the mine (Stierlin, 1909).

In World War I, The Americans, under the leadership of psychiatrist, Dr. Thomas Salmon, followed the French example and cared for American soldiers with psychological support services provided immediately behind the front lines. About 65% returned to combat in 3 or 4 days. Without crisis support only 40% returned to combat and that took 3 to 4 weeks. Salmon's study was one of the earliest studies of early psychological intervention and the result were very positive (Salmon, 1919).

Since the World War II, Crisis intervention has also been known as "psychological first aid," "Emotional first aid," and "early psychological intervention." The same history, theory base, and core principles apply regardless of name of the support program (Lindemann, 1944; Appel et al., 1946; American Psychiatric Association, 1954; Mitchell and Everly, 2001).

The use of the term, "Psychological First Aid" can be traced to before World War II. (Dewey, 1933) It appeared in civilian and military circles and meant a variety of support services. One WWII London rescuer, later wrote, "Every night, from dusk to dawn, the German bombs fell upon them. Woolton suggested that I might go down about six o'clock when the 'all clear' sounded and see what I could do to help. I found that, as they came out of the shelters, what comforted them was a kiss and a cup of tea." (Robert Boothby, 1978; Mitchell, 2017).

Other authors describe Psychological First Aid as a *debriefing tool* for soldiers or for the US Merchant Marine. (Blain, Hoch, & Ryan, 1945). One prominent British author states that Psychological First Aid was employed as group counseling sessions for soldiers following battle. (Terr, 1992).

In 1944, after the horrific Cocoanut Grove fire in Boston, Massachusetts, Erik Lindemann and Gerald Caplan established the principles and the core practices are still used today (Lindemann, 1944).

By the mid 1950's, at the beginning of the "Cold War," Psychological First Aid was commonly applied in disasters (American Psychiatric Association Committee on Civil Defense, 1954). In fact, at that time Psychological First Aid was seen as a very broad spectrum of support services to assist people in crisis. Consider, for a moment, the following quote from F.C. Thorn, editor of the *Journal of Clinical Psychology* in 1952:

Prophylactically, [from the prevention point of view], it is probable that many disorders could be nipped in the bud if prompt attention could be given...First aid treatment by its very nature should be very flexible and expedient, utilizing every possible method of achieving results... (Thorn, 1952).

By the 1960s Gerald Caplan had clearly demonstrated his knowledge and skill in crisis intervention and his writings stand out as benchmarks against which we can measure all other crisis intervention programs.

In the early 1970's, Jeffrey T. Mitchell, the author of this chapter, of the University of Maryland, Baltimore County began writing about the needs of emergency personnel for crisis support after traumatic events. He developed many of the crisis intervention procedures used around the world today. His work is the foundation of a broad-spectrum crisis intervention program known as Critical Incident Stress Management (CISM) (Mitchell, 1982, 1983, 2001; Mitchell and Mitchell, 2006).

The International Critical Incident Stress Foundation (ICISF) was co-founded by Dr. George S. Everly, Jr. and Dr. Jeffrey T. Mitchell in 1989. It provides crisis intervention and stress management training to many thousands of people each year. ICISF is known for its support services to emergency personnel and many other populations. It has a network of over 1500 Critical Incident Stress Management teams that operate in about one hundred countries.

Crisis Intervention support services have been utilized in thousands of disasters and uncountable numbers of smaller tragedies. Theses supportive interventions have made a difference in the lives of literally hundreds of thousands of people. Crisis Intervention services continue to be developed, expanded, and refined under the leadership of the International Critical Incident Stress Foundation, as well through the efforts of numerous Federal, State and private entities (Mitchell 2007, 2017)

Providers of Crisis Intervention

Some mental health professionals provide crisis intervention services. It is often used in the early stages of therapy to calm distressed clients and to gain an understanding of the circumstances that have caused the state of crisis. First responders, however, are the most frequent providers of crisis intervention services.

Dr. Gerald Caplan, in the early 1970's, said at large conference on crisis intervention in Baltimore, Maryland that "*…excellent help may be provided by friends, family and colleagues who do not have formal mental health training.*" It was his remarks that encouraged the development of peer support programs around the world.

Crisis intervention services should always serve as a link to formal mental health services when such services are necessary.

Goals of Crisis Intervention

1. Lower emotional tension, stabilize the person, mobilize a person's resources, and mitigate the impact of the traumatic event.
2. Normalize their reactions and facilitate normal recovery processes, in normal people who are experiencing normal reactions to abnormal events.
3. Restore individuals to adaptive functions and to enhance unit cohesion and unit performance in homogeneous groups.
4. Identification of individuals who may need professional care and to assure that those individuals have access to appropriate referrals.

Principles of Crisis Intervention

1. **Simplicity**: People respond to simple, not complex issues, during a crisis. Interventions should be simple.
2. **Brevity**: Short contacts from a few minutes up to about 1 hour. It is typical to have 3-5 contacts to complete crisis intervention work.
3. **Innovation**: Crisis Intervention providers must be creative to manage unique and emotionally painful situations. Thinking of novel solutions is often necessary.
4. **Pragmatism:** Suggestions must be practical if they are to work in resolving a crisis.
5. **Proximity:** Most effective crisis intervention contacts occur closer to the operational zone or in someone's comfort zone. In crisis intervention, we still make "house calls."
6. **Immediacy:** A crisis reaction demands rapid intervention. Delays cause more pain and complications.

7. **Expectancy**: When possible, the crisis intervener works to set up expectations of a reasonable positive outcome.

NOTE: Proximity, Immediacy, and Expectancy were the first recorded principles of crisis intervention. Dr. Thomas Salmon developed them in WWI. Battalion psychiatrists such as Dr. Artiss added Brevity and Simplicity as crisis intervention principles in WWII. Dr. Karl Slaikeu added Innovation and Pragmatism in 1984. These seven principles today are the core principles of crisis intervention (Artiss, 1963; Salmon, 1919; Slaikeu, 1984).

The principles of Crisis Intervention are used daily by CISM teams around the world. An expanded description of these principles is, therefore justified at this point in the chapter. It is important that members of a CISM team, sometimes referred to as a "Critical Incident Response Program" (CIRP), adhere closely to this basic set of seven operational principles when providing crisis intervention services of any type (ALPA, 1997; Bailey and Hightower, 1996; LiBassi, 1987).

Proximity is the first principle of crisis intervention. Crisis work is often provided in surroundings familiar to the people who need support. Many crisis intervention tactics are applied in the field or at worksites or in schools, churches and many other locations that do not in any way resemble offices of mental health professionals (Bohl, 1991,1995).

The second principle is *immediacy*. People in a crisis appreciate help as soon as possible after being exposed to a traumatic experience. The longer they wait, the less likely crisis intervention will be effective (Lindy, 1985).

The third principle is that of *expectancy*. Early in the intervention, the provider of crisis intervention should instill some hope that it is possible to manage and resolve the situation (Salmon, 1919; Kardiner and Spiegel, 1947; Solomon and Benbenishty, 1986; Robinson and Mitchell, 1993).

The fourth principle is *brevity*. The luxury of abundant time is usually absent in a crisis. Actions to assist people in crisis are generally brief (Parad & Parad, 1968).

The fifth principle is *simplicity*. People do not handle complexity very well in the midst of a crisis. Therefore, crisis support personnel should focus on selecting solutions that are easy for a distressed person to apply. Simple, well thought out interventions will be the most effective in the majority of cases (Vogt et al, 2007; Wee et al, 1999, Western Management Consultants, 1996).

It is usually helpful if crisis workers have some creativity when they are working in extraordinary and challenging circumstances. The ability to be *innovative* in the face of unusual, threatening, and disturbing situations is a key to good crisis intervention and the sixth major principle of crisis intervention. Appropriate helpful interventions may have to be developed on the spot.

Finally, the seventh principle is that whatever crisis interventions are chosen in a crisis should be *practical*. Impractical solutions are no solutions at all. People struggling through a painful experience may view those who make impractical suggestions as insensitive and uncaring.

Peer support team members are encouraged to *keep the seven primary principles of crisis intervention in mind*. Crisis intervention is helpful when it is applied in accordance with those principles. Crisis support personnel should avoid establishing outcome expectations that are far beyond its capabilities. In other words, crisis intervention cannot cure disease or significant mental disturbance. It is not a cure for Post Traumatic Stress Disorder, a condition that is among the most serious reactions to a critical incident. It can, however, reduce stress symptoms and it can function as a bridge to professional care for those who may need more than what crisis intervention can provide.

The "AS-IF" Approach to Crisis Intervention

The "A" stands for Assessment

There are two essential elements that are part of the assessment.

1. The incident Including:
    a. The *nature* of the incident (what happened?)
    b. The *magnitude* of the incident (how horrible or terrible is it?)
2. The *impact* on (reactions of) those involved in the incident

The "S" Stands for Strategy

The strategy is based upon the following five considerations:

1. **Theme**: The theme is the basic information regarding the incident. It includes the circumstances of the event, the threats associated with the event, and other concerns, considerations, problems or issues that are connected to the event. Themes influence CISM decision-making. Themes can change the priority order of the target populations. They may also influence the types of crisis interventions selected and the timing of those interventions. Themes can cause us to select different support providers to accommodate the needs of those in a state of crisis.
2. **Target**: Who needs crisis intervention? Who does not? Crisis support personnel need to know who was involved in the incident and to what extent were they involved.
3. **Types**: What types of interventions are most likely to be helpful? The right tools need to be selected to assist the people involved in the crisis.
4. **Timing**: The most appropriate timing is essential in intervening during a crisis. Certain interventions become less effective or useless if they delayed. Other interventions are more effective if they are held off for a relatively brief period of time until people are ready to receive those services and achieve the maximum benefits.
5. **Team**: It is important to send the right person or people from the CISM team to provide the crisis intervention services. Efforts should always be made to match the responding team member(s) to the people who need the assistance and to their specific needs in the situation.

The "I" Stands for Interventions

Note the plural in the word "interventions". Crisis Intervention is best when it is a blend of several crisis intervention techniques. Stand-alone interventions are never appropriate. At the very least, crisis intervention personnel always need to follow-up with the people they assist. No assumptions should be made that everything is okay simply because one crisis intervention service was provided.

There are many techniques or tools in the Critical Incident Stress Management toolbox. They include, but are not limited to, the following:

- Pre-incident planning, preparation
- Assessment
- Strategic planning
- Individual contacts (one-on-one)
- Informational group interventions (RITS and CMB)
- Interactive group interventions (defusing and CISD)
- Family support
- Follow-up services
- Organizational consultation
- Pastoral crisis intervention
- Referrals for additional care
- Post incident lessons learned and provide education to others about those lessons

The "F" Stands for Follow-Up

It is essential, in crisis intervention, to check on the welfare of those we have attempted to help. This can be accomplished by means of phone calls; personal contacts and visits to their work sites or homes, and also by referrals for additional care, if that were needed.

The steps to cover the "F" portion of this crisis intervention model are:

1. Inquire about the wellbeing of the individual
2. Determine the needs that must be addressed
3. Refer if necessary or complete the crisis intervention work

In crisis intervention, treat people "AS IF" they were your own and that you love them. (Mitchell, 2010)

CRITICAL INCIDENT STRESS MANAGEMENT

CISM: Definitions, Models, and Tools

The Resiliency Model in Crisis Work and Critical Incident Stress Management

CISM Background

From the very beginning, Critical Incident Stress Management (CISM) was, and continues to be, a crisis system based on a **resiliency model.** It aims at building *resistance* before exposure to traumatic events. It focuses on *rebounding* from stress. In those cases where people need additional care, the CISM program is uniquely positioned to assist individuals in finding appropriate professional care to help them *recover* from traumatic experience.

Resistance

Resistance is the ability of individuals, groups, organizations, and entire populations to resist distress, impairment, and dysfunction. One way to look at resistance is to think about it as if it were a certain degree of immunity. If we make ourselves resistant enough, we can ward off many of the harmful effects of traumatic incidents.

Resistance is the foundation of resilience. Resistance can be developed. Providing training and education, encouraging healthy living and exercise, and enhancing life style, behaviors and attitudes, long before the traumatic event strikes, are the best methods to develop resistance. If you build resistance you also enhance resilience. Resistance (and thus resilience) is built up by preparation for stressful experiences and the practice of stress management skills. In summary, resistance is the build-up of protective factors to make us stress-resistant.

Protective factors include self-esteem, optimism, improved nutrition, appropriate sleep habits, social support, family life, exercise, recreation and relaxation, avoidance of non-prescription drugs and tobacco, and limitation of alcohol use.

Resilience

Resilience is the ability of a person to rapidly rebound or recoil from distress, and to rise above adversity. Every person is born with some resilience, but the work done in building resistance improves our ability to be resilient over time and especially when faced with adversity.

Recovery

The resolution, repair, reconstruction, restoration, and rebuilding of the human spirit, mind, and body after sustaining the damages incurred by prolonged, extreme, or overwhelming distress.

- Recovery is about regaining control
- Recovery re-establishes resilience
- Recovery means we come to terms with the experiences that hurt us, shocked us and drained our resilience
- Recovery is reigniting the spark that lights the flame that makes life worth living
- Be prepared to seek help. Recovery is very difficult without a support system.
- Recovery frequently takes the support and guidance of professionals
- Family, Friends and Colleagues should also take a role in a person's recovery
- Recovery is part of resilience.
- Recovery means you have the resilience and the courage to reignite the spark.

CISM Definition

Critical Incident Stress Management (CISM) is a *comprehensive, integrated, systematic, and multi-component crisis intervention program.* It is interesting to note that the initials, CISM, can be used in two ways as it is in the previous sentence. First, CISM represents the title of the program, Critical Incident Stress Management. Second, the same initials, CISM, can be viewed as a description of the program – comprehensive, integrated, systematic and multi-component. CISM is versatile, practical, and effective. It is a common sense stress management system. It can do much to alleviate distress and to maintain healthy levels of function for first responders and many other populations.

C = Critical C = Comprehensive
I = Incident I = Integrated
S = Stress S = Systematic
M = Management M = Multi-tactic

Since its development in the 1970's, CISM has spread rapidly into many different types of agencies, organizations, and services in over fifteen hundred communities around the world. The United Nations developed its own internal CISM program to assist UN workers throughout its multi-national community (United Nations Department of Safety and Security, 2007 a, b, c).

Critical Incident Stress Management (CISM) is, first and foremost, a *subset* of the field of crisis intervention. A subset is defined as a collection of elements within a certain category that are clearly related to each other and which can be found within a larger "umbrella" category. All of the elements contained within a subset (CISM) can be found within the main category (crisis intervention). From its inception Critical Incident Stress Management (CISM) was deeply rooted in the field of crisis intervention. Therefore, the many elements of a CISM program are all crisis intervention elements and they share the same history, theoretical foundations, principles, goals, strategies, procedures, methods and techniques associated with crisis intervention. *CISM is neither psychotherapy nor a substitute for psychotherapy. It is a support service.*

CISM Interventions

CISM is best described as a "package" of crisis intervention tactics that are strategically woven together. The main objectives of a CISM program are to:

1. **Mitigate** the impact of a traumatic event;
2. **Facilitate** normal recovery processes in normal people, who are having normal reactions to traumatic events;
3. **Restore** individuals, groups and organizations to adaptive function;
4. **Identify** people within an organization or a community who would benefit from additional support services or a referral for further evaluation and, possibly, medical or psychological treatment.

A basic model of a CISM program has several key components. They include:

- Assessment of the magnitude or severity of a critical incident as well as its impact on the personnel.
- Planning, education, resiliency building, policy development, and peer support team preparation.
- Strategic planning so that the proper *targets* of an intervention are identified and the correct *types* of interventions are selected for application at the most advantageous *time*. In developing a strategic action plan, the *themes* that might influence decision- making must be considered. Finally, the most appropriate *team* must be selected to provide the best services.
- A flexible, multi-tactic approach utilizing specific models for individual or group interventions.
- Listening skills and individual crisis intervention
- Informational groups
- Interactive groups (must be homogeneous)
- Personal and community resilience

- Follow-up services including phone calls, visits to work sites or homes, and advice to supervisors or administration when necessary.
- Links to professional referrals when personnel would benefit from such contacts.

As noted above, a CISM program encompasses a package of many tactics or tools that may be necessary under different circumstances. The table below lists the types of interventions, the targets and timing of the interventions, as well as the potential goals of the interventions.

SUMMARY OF COMMONLY USED CRISIS INTERVENTION TACTICS

See Table 1.

CISM Teams

The management of the potential physical and psychological risks to first responders involves the establishment of well organized, appropriately trained, and efficient crisis support programs. The aim of such programs should be to build a *high resiliency organization* that can resist overwhelming stress, bounce back from a traumatic event and recover its personnel to healthy, functional levels. Fortunately, when it comes to support services for an organization's personnel, first responders are not facing an unchartered course. The age of pioneering efforts for crisis support is over. CISM services for first responders has a history that is now approaching five decades and these programs have taken on great importance as they have consistently demonstrated their value. Experience clearly indicates the positive effects when crisis intervention services are applied for first responders for common daily critical incidents as well as in major accidents (Vogt & Leonhardt, 2006; Tomkins et al., 1996; Everly, 2019).

PRACTICAL GUIDELINES FOR EFFECTIVE PEER SUPPORT PROGRAMS

1. Every successful crisis-oriented staff support program is ***comprehensive***. That is, it has elements in place before, during, and after traumatic events. Additionally, it is ***programmatic***. That is, it is endorsed by the administration and built into the fabric of the organization. Administration and union "buy-in" or acceptance of a support program is essential to the program's survival. Although they remain independent units, peer support programs must communicate, coordinate, and link their efforts with the organization's leaders and with human services, employee assistance and psychological resources within an organization.
2. A key to effective peer support programs is the presence of **dedicated, enthusiastic, leaders** who actively work toward enhancing the peer support team at every opportunity.
3. Well-developed first responder peer support programs are ***integrated***. That is, all of the elements of a program are interrelated and blended with one another. The combined effects of an integrated program are far more powerful than any single element.

Table 1.

Intervention / Tactic	Timing	Target Group	Potential Goals
Pre–event Planning/Preparation	Prior to exposures to traumatic events	Anticipated target or even victim populations	Resistance building. Enhance resiliency anticipatory guidance
Assessment	Pre-intervention	Those directly and indirectly exposed	Determine need for intervention
Strategic planning	Pre-event / early stages of event	Actual and anticipated exposed populations	Improve overall crisis response
Individual Crisis Intervention (includes "Psychological First Aid")	Whenever needed	Individuals as needed	Assessment, screening, education, reduction of acute distress, triage, referral
Informational groups: a) Rest Information Transition Services (RITS) {formerly known as "demobilization"} b) Crisis Management Briefings Large Group "psychological First Aid"	Operation shift disengagement Ongoing large scale events As needed During or after event.	Emergency operations personnel Any size group needing information, guidance, instructions. Large heterogeneous groups	Decompression, ease transition, screening, triage, guidance, meet basic needs Respite, refreshment preliminary support Information, rumor control, increase group cohesion, lower tension and anxiety in the group. Enhance appropriate behaviors
Informational session for small sized group crisis intervention (conversational somewhat similar to a CMB but with only a few people)	During and after the event May be repeated as needed May use the CMB format even though the group size is quite small	Community groups seeking information and resources. Usually non-emergency groups. Often heterogeneous 3-6 in attendance	Provide information, control rumors, reduce acute distress, increase cohesion, facilitate resilience, screening and triage
Interactive Groups: a) Defusing (group "psychological first aid") b) Critical Incident Stress Debriefing (CISD)	Up to 8 to 12 hours after the event Post event 24-72 hours – ideal sometimes 5 -10 days. Longer times after disaster (3-4 weeks)	Homogeneous groups only; usually small unit-sized groups; same exposure to the traumatic event Homogeneous groups only with equal trauma exposure (workgroups, teams)	Stabilization, ventilation, reduction of acute distress, screening, information, increase cohesion and facilitate resilience Restore unit cohesion and unit performance
Family crisis intervention	Pre-event preparation Post event support as needed	Families of victims as well as Emergency personnel	Wide range of interventions Preparation CMB, individual, other as needed
Organizational / community intervention, consultation	Pre event preparation Support post event as needed	Organizations, businesses, agencies impacted by trauma	Improve preparedness and response. Leadership guidance. Assist in recovery
Pastoral Crisis Intervention	Before, during, after as needed	Individual, RITS, defusing, CMB, faith based crisis intervention	Faith-Based support
Follow-up / Referral	Some follow-up is always necessary; Referrals as needed	Intervention recipients, other exposed individuals and groups	Assure continuity of care. Refer as necessary

Source: (Mitchell, 2017, Tables used with permission)

4. First responder personnel are best sustained by a ***systematic*** program or "support package" which has phases, segments, or logical steps. Peer support programs should, therefore, take a few simple steps such as, resting personnel and talking with them on an individual basis, before increasing the complexity, number, and duration of the available crisis interventions after a distressing event.
5. Effective peer support programs must be ***multi-tactic*** in approach. Many different types of support services must be available since every person will have a somewhat different response to a highly stressful event. Each person will have different needs after a traumatizing experience.
6. Although it is part of a **C**omprehensive, **I**ntegrated, **S**ystematic and **M**ulti-tactic (CISM) approach, ***linkages to a wide range of resources*** is an important enough element of a first responder crisis support program or peer support program to be repeated here. Additional assistance, beyond the capabilities of the peer support team, may be necessary.
7. Crisis support teams are most effective when they are run and staffed by ***peer support personnel*** and backed up by mental health professionals who are trained in Critical Incident Stress Management (CISM) (Mitchell, 2004).
8. **Properly trained.** The International Critical Incident Stress Foundation, a non profit organization, offers 46 different courses to prepare people to serve on a CISM team. ICISF can be reached at www.icisf.org.

EFFECTIVENESS OF CISM

The literature to date suggests that crisis intervention, in the form of a Critical Incident Stress Management program, has positive effects on the reduction of stress symptoms. When applied by properly trained personnel who adhere to the standards of practice, CISM programs may play a preventative role against the development of long-range psychological problems (Adler et al. 2008, 2009; Amir et al., 1998; Bohl, 1991, 1995;, Boscarino, 2005, 2011; Campfield and Hills, 2001; Castro and Adler 2011; Chemtob et al., 1997; Dealh et al., 2000; Dyregrov, 1998; Eid et al., 2001; Everly, Flannery & Mitchell, 2000; Everly et al. 2001; Flannery, 2005; Jenkins, 1996; NATCA, 2003;North et al, 2002; Nurmi, 1999; Regel, 2007, 2010; Richards, 2001; Roberts, 2005; Robinson and Mitchell, 1993; Vogt et al., 2004; Vogt et al, 2006; Vogt et al., 2007; Wee et al., 1999; Western Management Consultants, 1996; Everly, 2019).

In one particularly interesting series of studies directly related to the aviation industry, Vogt and his colleagues (2004, 2006, 2007) performed a cost-benefit analysis of the German Air Traffic Control Services' (Deutsche Flugsicherung, DFS) CISM program. The authors describe the applications of the CISM peer support program within air-traffic control systems after "loss of separation" incidents (when two radar blips merge into one on the screen). An unforeseen loss of separation between aircraft is a major threat to the professional self-image of an air traffic controller officer. Such incidents are generally distressing reminders to the controllers of the ever present risk of life-threatening aviation accidents. Prior to the development of a CISM support program, German Air Traffic Control Officers lost an average of three days from work per incident because of distress. About 30 of these lost of separation events occur per month in the crowded skies above Europe (Vogt et al, 2004, 2006, 2007).

An analysis by Vogt and his colleagues (2004, 2006, 2007) indicates that, since the introduction of the CISM peer support program in 1997, no air traffic controller reported a single lost day for stress related to a loss of separation critical incident. The estimated fiscal benefits associated with the prevention of absenteeism or reported stress-related illness while at work actually exceeded the program's costs by several times. The study concludes that a combination of factors assures the effectiveness of peer provided crisis intervention. They include a *clear model, well-trained providers and adherence to the standards and protocols of good practice* (Vogt et a, 2004, 2006, 2007).

Dr. George S. Everly, Jr., recently published a review of over 100 studies on crisis intervention and Critical Incident Stress Management that indicate positive effects of CISM. CISM is therefore in the realm of evidence-based interventions. Several of the studies are Randomized Controlled Trials (RCT) which are considered the "gold standard" of research designs (Adler et al., 2008; Campfield and Hills, 2001; Deahl et al, 2000; Everly, 2019; Richards, 2001;Tuckey and Scott, 2014).

THE ROLE OF THE CRITICAL INCIDENT STRESS DEBRIEFING IN A CISM PROGRAM

Critical Incident Stress Debriefing

The author of this chapter, Dr. Jeffrey T. Mitchell of the University of Maryland, Baltimore County, developed the interactive group process called Critical Incident Stress Debriefing (CISD) in 1974. The first publication on CISD appeared in 1983 in the *Journal of Emergency Medical Services.* Even in that first article, many types of interventions were presented as part of a broad, systematic approach to managing distress in emergency personnel now known as Critical Incident Stress Management (CISM) (Mitchell 2007 Mitchell and Everly, 2001; Mitchell, 2017).

The Critical Incident Stress Debriefing was developed solely as a *support service* for *homogeneous groups* who had experienced a traumatic event. The word "support" means: *to help keep a person or a group stable. Support also means to care for people, to sustain them, or to reinforce the individual or the group*. Other meanings for the word support are: *to give active help and encouragement; to help in a crisis; to provide active assistance; to provide comfort; or to bear some of the weight.* The word support best describes what CISM teams do when they provide a CISD. As stated earlier, a CISD is neither psychotherapy nor is it a substitute for psychotherapy. It was never intended to be a therapy process or to be used as a cure for any physical or mental problem or disorder. It is really about unit cohesion and unit performance.

The CISD should never be used in isolation from other interventions. Stress management education, for instance, is desirable long before personnel are traumatized by a specific incident. At the very least, follow-up is always required whenever a CISD is provided. For a number of reasons, the CISD process has received a great deal of unnecessary attention during the last decade. Some of that undue attention may have generated misinformation and faulty applications of the model. The material in this chapter provides accurate information on the CISD process.

A Critical Incident Stress Debriefing (CISD) is an interactive *group support process* designed specifically for application with homogeneous (primary) groups that have experienced roughly the same level of exposure to the same traumatic event. It is a group crisis intervention procedure. Although it has been used successfully with a wide range of homogeneous populations, such as school children, businesses and industries, it should be kept in mind that it was originally developed for operational groups such as first responders who know each other and who share both a common history and positive relationships with one another. *It is inappropriate to use the CISD group crisis intervention process with groups that are heterogeneous. Likewise, it is inappropriate to use the CISD model with individuals.*

The CISD process was never designed for individual primary victims such as those who are ill, injured, medicated, psychotic, or who are hospital patients, victims of violence, people with suicidal ideation, or people currently undergoing grave personal threat. It is an *egregious (outrageous or flagrant) violation* of the standard principles and practices of CISD to apply this group crisis intervention process to individual women who had difficult pregnancies, complicated deliveries, miscarriages, or stillborn babies. It is also an *egregious violation* of the standards of practice to apply the CISD interactive group crisis intervention process to individual auto accident victims, sexual assault victims, burn victims and dog bite victims. These misguided and horribly flawed applications of the CISD group crisis intervention model are unequivocally condemned. CISD should *only* be used with appropriate *homogeneous* groups.

Homogeneous Groups

Three conditions are necessary for a group to be a homogeneous group.

1. There must be ***existing relationships among the group members*** before the traumatic event occurred.
2. There must be a ***shared history***. That shared history includes the fact that the group members experienced the same traumatic experience.
3. Sufficient ***time together*** should have elapsed so that the ***group members are thought of as if one***.

Goals of CISD

The main goals of a CISD are to support the *primary group* after a shared traumatic experience and to restore the unit's cohesion and performance. **The CISD is a not a treatment or a cure for any form of mental disorder, including Posttraumatic Stress Disorder (PTSD).** *Any possible preventative value against PTSD would be of a secondary nature, not primary*. The prevention of PTSD is *not* listed as one of the primary goals of the CISD process. The actual goals of the CISD process are:

1. Mitigation of the crisis response,
2. Assist in the *restoration of the group's ability to function* and
3. *Identification of individuals within the small homogeneous group who might need additional support or a referral* for professional care.

The CISD interactive crisis intervention group process plays an important role in screening and referral.

CISD Is Not a Stand-Alone Process

Although it is an important process for stressed homogeneous groups, the *CISD is not a stand-alone process*. It should always be used as only one component of a comprehensive program that includes at least assessment, individual support, and follow-up services. The CISD interactive group crisis support process is only one element of the larger, comprehensive, integrative, systematic and multi-component CISM program (Mitchell, 2017).

Benefits of CISD

There are many benefits of the interactive group CISD process. It provides:

1. Practical information that serves as a useful guide for the group members' recovery from a traumatic experience.
2. A CISD may also help the group members understand that they are not alone in the trauma experience.
3. Help is available if they want it. It is generally reassuring to the members of the group to know that they are not unique and that others may be experiencing the same physical and emotional effects.
4. The CISD aims at normalizing the reactions that the group members are experiencing after the critical incident.

NOTE: The benefits of the CISD can only be realized when the interactive group process is conducted by trained personnel. Reading this book without practical training is insufficient to achieve a proper level of skill to provide the CISD process.

Stages of the CISD Process

There are seven steps or stages in the small group CISD process. They are presented here to round out this brief discussion on CISD as a component of a larger, more comprehensive, CISM program. **Proper training in CISM is a necessity before one attempts to utilize the CISD process.**

1. *Brief introduction* by the crisis team members
2. Facts phase or a *brief situation review*
3. Thought phase or f*irst impressions* of the traumatic event
4. Aspects of the event that produced the *greatest personnel impact* on the group members
5. *Signals of distress*
6. Teaching phase or s*tress information and guidelines for recovery*
7. Re-entry phase or *Summary*

The preponderance of the studies cited in the literature on CISD indicate a positive effect if two conditions are in place. The first is that people who conduct the small group CISD process are properly trained to do so. The second condition is that the providers of the service must adhere to the standard of practice for the CISD primary group support process that have been established and promulgated since 1983 (Mitchell and Everly 2017; Everly 2019).

CONCLUSION

This chapter began with a discussion of high intensity / high-risk organizations in which the employees are subjected to extremely elevated levels of stress and circumstances that threaten their physical and mental health. It then noted that high-risk organizations should also be High Reliability Organizations. Consistency in performance, efficiency, and a safety consciousness are the hallmarks of High Reliability Organizations.

The author reviewed evidence that when well-designed Critical Incident Stress Management programs are in place and the CISM personnel are *properly trained and adhere to the standards of CISM practice,* that a new meaning for "high reliability organizations" may be applicable. That is, first responder personnel will function effectively within *"High Resiliency Organizations"* that can resist stress, manage it when it arises, and restore personnel to maximal levels of performance and unit cohesion.

Peer support programs using the principles of CISM have proven Gerald Caplan's words that *excellent help in a crisis could come from paraprofessionals or family members or from friends helping friends.* Whether it is a situation involving personal grief, a family crisis, or an air disaster, first responder CISM team members respond with skill, care and concern. Crisis support personnel have demonstrated the enormous value of crisis intervention teams. It is likely that the number of peer support programs will expand in the coming years. Peer support personnel in the emergency services have clearly made a difference in the lives of their fellow responders throughout the nearly fifty-year history of their important work.

REFERENCES

Adler, A., Bliese, P. D., McGurk, D., Hoge, C. W., & Castro, C. A. (2009). Battlemind debriefing and battlemind training as early interventions with soldiers returning from Iraq: Randomization by platoon. *Journal of Consulting and Clinical Psychology*, *77*(5), 928–940. doi:10.1037/a0016877 PMID:19803572

Adler, A., Litz, B., Castro, C. A., Suvak, M., Thomas, J. L., Burrell, L., ... Bliese, P. D. (2008). A group randomized trial of critical incident stress debriefing provided to U.S. peacekeepers. *Journal of Traumatic Stress*, *21*(3), 253–263. doi:10.1002/jts.20342 PMID:18553407

Air Line Pilots Association (ALPA). (1997). *Critical Incident Response Program Guide*. Herndon, VA: ALPA.

American Psychiatric Association. (1954). *First Aid for Psychological Reactions in Disasters*. Washington, DC: American Psychiatric Association.

Amir, M., Weil, G., Kaplan, Z., Tocker, T., & Witzum, E. (1998). Debriefing with group psychotherapy in a homogenous group of non-injured victims of a terrorist attack: A prospective study. *Acta Psychiatrica Scandinavica*, *98*(3), 237–242. doi:10.1111/j.1600-0447.1998.tb10074.x PMID:9761413

Appel, J. W., Beebe, G. W., & Hilgardner, D. W. (1946). Comparative incidence of neuropsychiatric casualties in World War I and World War II. *The American Journal of Psychiatry*, *102*(2), 196–199. doi:10.1176/ajp.103.2.196 PMID:21001991

Artiss, K. (1963). Human behavior under stress: From combat to social psychiatry. *Military Medicine*, *128*(10), 1011–1015. doi:10.1093/milmed/128.10.1011 PMID:14055063

Bailey, W., & Hightower, S. (1996). *Critical Incident Response Program*. Dallas, TX: Southwest Airlines Pilots' Association, Transport Workers Union.

Bohl, N. (1991). The effectiveness of brief psychological interventions in police officers after critical incidents. In J. T. Reese, J. Horn, & C. Dunning (Eds.), *Critical Incidents in Policing, Revised* (pp. 31–38). Washington, DC: Department of Justice.

Bohl, N. (1995). Measuring the effectiveness of CISD. *Fire Engineering,* 125-126.

Boscarino, J. A., Adams, R. E., & Figley, C. R. (2005). A Prospective Cohort Study of the Effectiveness of Employer-Sponsored Crisis Interventions after a Major Disaster. *International Journal of Emergency Mental Health*, *7*(1), 31–44. PMID:15869077

Boscarino, J. A., Adams, R. E., & Figley, C. R. (2011). Mental health service use after the world trade center disaster: Utilization trends and comparative effectiveness. *The Journal of Nervous and Mental Disease*, *199*(2), 91–99. doi:10.1097/NMD.0b013e3182043b39 PMID:21278537

Campfield, K., & Hills, A. (2001). Effect of timing of critical Incident Stress Debriefing (CISD) on posttraumatic symptoms. *Journal of Traumatic Stress*, *14*(2), 327–340. doi:10.1023/A:1011117018705 PMID:11469160

Caplan, G. (1961). *An approach to Community Mental Health*. New York: Grune and Stratton.

Caplan, G. (1964). *Principles of Preventive Psychiatry*. New York: Basic Books.

Caplan, G. (1969). Opportunities for school psychologists in the primary prevention of mental health disorders in children. In A. Bindman & A. Spiegel (Eds.), *Perspectives in Community Mental Health* (pp. 420–436). Chicago: Aldine.

Castro, C. A., & Adler, A. B. (2011). Re-conceptualizing combat-related posttraumatic stress disorder as an occupational hazard. In A. B. Adler, P. B. Bliese, & C. A. Castro (Eds.), *Deployment Psychology: Evidence-Based Strategies to Promote Mental Health in the Military* (pp. 217–242). Washington, DC: American Psychological Association. doi:10.1037/12300-009

Chemtob, C., Tomas, S., Law, W., & Cremniter, D. (1997). Post disaster psychosocial intervention. *The American Journal of Psychiatry*, *134*, 415–417. PMID:9054792

Crocq, L. (1999). *Les Traumatismes psychiques de guerre*. Paris, France: Odile Jacob.

Crocq, L., Dalligand, L., Villerbu, L., Tarquinio, C., Duchet, C., Coq, J. M., ... Vitry, M. (2007). *Traumatismes psychiques: Prise en charge psychologique des victims*. Paris, France: Elsevier-Masson.

Deahl, M., Srinivasan, M., Jones, N., Thomas, J., Neblett, C., & Jolly, A. (2000). Preventing psychological trauma in soldiers. The role of operational stress training and psychological debriefing. *The British Journal of Medical Psychology*, *73*(1), 77–85. doi:10.1348/000711200160318 PMID:10759052

Dyregrov, A. (1998). Psychological debriefing: An effective method? *TRAUMATOLOGYe*, *4*(2), Article 1.

Eid, J., Johnsen, B. H., & Weisaeth, L. (2001). The effects of group psychological debriefing on acute stress reactions following a traffic accident: A quasi-experimental approach. *International Journal of Emergency Mental Health*, *3*, 145–154. PMID:11642192

Everly, G. (1989). *A clinical guide to the treatment of the human stress response*. New York, NY: Plenum Press. doi:10.1007/978-1-4613-0741-9

Everly, G. (2019). *Critical Incident Stress Management (CISM) and Psychological Crisis Intervention: a Practical Review of Research*. Severna Park, MD: Resiliency Science Institutes International.

Everly, G. S. Jr, Flannery, R. B. Jr, Eyler, V., & Mitchell, J. T. (2001). Sufficiency analysis of an integrated multi-component approach to crisis intervention: Critical Incident Stress Management. *Advances in Mind-Body Medicine*, *17*, 174–183. PMID:11572844

Everly, G. S. Jr, Flannery, R. B. Jr, & Mitchell, J. T. (2000). Critical Incident Stress Management (CISM): A review of the literature. *Aggression and Violent Behavior*, *5*(1), 23–40. doi:10.1016/S1359-1789(98)00026-3

Everly, G. S. Jr, & Mitchell, J. T. (2008). *Integrative Crisis Intervention and Disaster Mental Health*. Ellicott City, MD: Chevron Publishing Corporation.

Flannery, R. B. (2005). *Assaulted Staff Action Program (ASAP): Fifteen years of Empirical Findings*. Paper presented at the 8th World Congress on Stress Trauma and Coping: Crisis Intervention: Best Practices in Prevention, Preparedness and Response, Baltimore, MD.

Forstenzer, A. (1980, July). Stress, the psychological scarring of air crash rescue personnel. *Firehouse*, 50-52.

Frederick, C. J. (Ed.). (1981). *Aircraft Accidents: Emergency Mental Health Problems*. Washington, DC: National Institute of Mental Health, U.S. Department of Health and Human Services.

Freeman, K. (1979). CMHC responses to the Chicago and San Diego airplane disasters. *Technical Assistance Center Report*, *2*(1), 10–12.

Hassling, P. (2000). Disaster management and the Gothenburg fire of 1998: When first responders are blamed. *International Journal of Emergency Mental Health*, *2*(2), 267–273. PMID:11217158

Inglish, P. (2010). *Top 10 Most Dangerous Jobs 2007-2010 Hub Pages Elite Jobs*. Retrieved from Hubpages.com/hub/Most_Dangerous_

Jenkins, S. R. (1996). Social support and debriefing efficacy among emergency medical workers after a mass shooting incident. *Journal of Social Behavior and Personality*, *11*, 447–492.

Kardiner, A., & Spiegel, H. (1947). *War, Stress, and Neurotic Illness*. New York: Hoeber.

Kobassa, S. C. (1979). Stressful life events, personality, and health: An inquiry into hardiness. *Journal of Personality and Social Psychology*, *37*, 1–11. PMID:458548

Kobassa, S. C., Maddi, S. R., & Kahn, S. (1982). Hardiness and Health: A prospective study. *Journal of Personality and Social Psychology*, *42*(1), 168–177. doi:10.1037/0022-3514.42.1.168 PMID:7057354

Lazarus, R. S. (1966). *Psychological Stress And The Coping Process*. New York: McGraw-Hill.

Lazarus, R. S. (1969). *Patterns of Adjustment and Human Effectiveness*. New York: McGraw-Hill.

Leonhardt, J. (2006). Critical Incident Stress Management (CISM) in Air Traffic Control (ATC). In J. Leonhardt & J. Vogt (Eds.), *Critical Incident Stress Management CISM in Aviation* (pp. 81–91). Aldershot, UK: Ashgate Publishing Company.

LiBassi, M.D. (1987). Employee Trauma Recovery Program. In Personnel Resources, Local Procedures Manual. Dallas, TX: American Airlines.

Lifton, R. J. (1970). *History and Human Survival: Essays on the Young and the Old, Survivors and the Dead, Peace and War, and on Contemporary Psychohistory*. New York: Random House.

Lifton, R. J. (1973). *Home from the War: Vietnam Veterans—Neither Victims nor Executioners*. New York: Simon & Schuster.

Lifton, R. J. (1993). *The Protean Self: Human Resilience in an Age of Fragmentation*. New York: Basic Books.

Lindemann, E. (1944). Symptomatology and management of acute grief. *The American Journal of Psychiatry*, *101*(2), 141–148. doi:10.1176/ajp.101.2.141 PMID:8192191

Lindy, J. (1985). The trauma membrane and other clinical concepts derived from psychotherapeutic work with survivors of natural disasters. *Psychiatric Annals*, *15*(3), 153–160. doi:10.3928/0048-5713-19850301-06

Mitchell, J. T. (1982). The psychological impact of the Air Florida 90 Disaster on fire-rescue, paramedic and police officer personnel. In Mass Casualties: a lessons learned approach, accidents, civil disorders, natural disaster, terrorism. Washington, DC: Department of Transportation. (DOT HS 806302)

Mitchell, J.T. (1982, Fall). Recovery from rescue. *Response, the Magazine of Emergency Management*, 7-10.

Mitchell, J. T. (1983). When disaster strikes … The critical incident stress Debriefing process. *Journal of Emergency Medical Services*, *13*(11), 49–52. PMID:10258348

Mitchell, J. T. (2004). Characteristics of Successful Early Intervention Programs. *International Journal of Emergency Mental Health*, *6*(4), 175–184. PMID:15635898

Mitchell, J. T. (2006). A brief history of Crisis Intervention in Aviation. In J. Vogt & J. Leonhardt (Eds.), *Critical Incident Stress Management in Aviation*. Hampshire, UK: Ashgate Publishing Limited.

Mitchell, J. T. (2007). *Group Crisis Support: Why it works, When and How to Provide It*. Ellicott City, MD: Chevron Publishing.

Mitchell, J. T. (2017). *Critical Incident Stress Management: Group Crisis Intervention* (5th ed.). Ellicott City, MD: International Critical Incident Stress Foundation.

Mitchell, J. T., & Everly, G. S. Jr. (2001). *Critical Incident Stress Debriefing: An operations manual for CISD, Defusing and other group crisis intervention services* (3rd ed.). Ellicott City, MD: Chevron.

Mitchell, S. G., & Mitchell, J. T. (2006). Caplan, Community and Critical Incident Stress Management. *International Journal of Emergency Mental Health*, *8*(1), 1–10. PMID:16573247

NATCA/FAA. (2003). *You are Not Alone: Critical Incident Stress Management Program*. Washington, DC: NATCA / FAA.

Neil, T., Oney, J., DiFonso, L., Thacker, B., & Reichart, W. (1974). *Emotional First Aid*. Louisville: Kemper-Behavioral Science Associates.

North, C., Tivis, C., McMillen, J., Pfefferbaum, B., Cox, J., Spitznagel, E., ... Smith, E. (2002). Coping, functioning, and adjustment of Rescue workers after the Oklahoma City bombing. *Journal of Traumatic Stress*, *15*, 171–175. PMID:12092908

Nurmi, L. (1999). The sinking of the Estonia: The effects of Critical Incident Stress Debriefing on Rescuers. *International Journal of Emergency Mental Health*, *1*, 23–32. PMID:11227750

Parad, L., & Parad, H. (1968). A study of crisis oriented planned short –term treatment: Part II. *Social Casework*, *49*(7), 418–426. doi:10.1177/104438946804900705

Parker, J.G. (2006, April). Watching the Clock. Safety and Health, 44-47.

Regel, S. (2007). Post-trauma support in the workplace: The current status and practice of critical incident stress management (CISM) and psychological debriefing (PD) within organizations in the UK. *Occupational Medicine*, *57*(6), 411–416. doi:10.1093/occmed/kqm071 PMID:17728314

Regel, S. (2010). Does psychological debriefing work? *Healthcare Counseling and Psychotherapy Journal.*, *10*(2), 14–18.

Richards, D. (2001). A field study of critical incident stress debriefing versus critical incident stress management. *Journal of Mental Health (Abingdon, England)*, *10*(3), 351–362. doi:10.1080/09638230124190

Roberts, A. (2005). Bridging the Past and Present to the Future of Crisis Intervention and Crisis Management. In A. Roberts (Ed.), *Crisis Intervention Handbook: Assessment, Treatment and Research* (3rd ed.). New York: Oxford University Press.

Robinson, R., & Mitchell, J. (1993). Evaluation of psychological debriefings. *Journal of Traumatic Stress*, *6*, 367–382.

Salmon, T. S. (1919). War neuroses and their lesson. *New York Medical Journal*, *108*, 993–994.

Slaikeu, K. A. (1984). *Crisis intervention: A handbook for practice and research.* Boston, MA: Allyn and Bacon, Inc.

Solomon, Z., & Benbenishty, R. (1986). The role of proximity, immediacy, and expectancy in frontline treatment of combat stress reaction among Israelis in the Lebanon War. *The American Journal of Psychiatry*, *143*(5), 613–617. doi:10.1176/ajp.143.5.613 PMID:3963249

Staff. (2001, May 21). Aviation Workplace Safety Lags Other Industries. *Air Safety Week.*

Stierlin, E. (1909). *Psycho-neuropathology as a result of a Mining Disaster March 10, 1906*. Zurich: University of Zurich.

Tompkins, M., Morin, W., Campbell, A., Hudson, D., Sumwalt, R., Johnson, J., ... Bracken, J. (1996). *Air Line Pilots Association: Critical Incident Response Program Manual*. Herndon, VA: ALPA.

Tuckey, M. R. (2007). Issues in the debriefing debate for the emergency services. *Clinical Psychology: Science and Practice*, *14*(2), 106–116. doi:10.1111/j.1468-2850.2007.00069.x

Tuckey, M. R., & Scott, J. E. (2013). Group critical incident stress Debriefing with emergency services personnel: A randomized controlled trial. *Anxiety, Stress, and Coping*, *27*(1), 38–54. PMID:23799773

United Nations Department of Safety and Security CISMU Staff. (2007a). *UNDSS CISMU Certification Training For Counselors. DSS Newsletter*. New York: United Nations Secretariat, Department of Safety and Security.

United Nations Department of Safety and Security CISMU Staff. (2007b). *New crisis and stress management training program launched. I Seek (May 2, 2007)*. New York: United Nations Secretariat.

United Nations Department of Safety and Security CISMU Staff. (2007c). *Certification training in Crisis and Stress Management. New York: UN Department of Safety and Security, Consultative Working Group on Stress in Collaboration with the International Critical Incident Stress Foundation, the American Academy of Experts in Traumatic Stress and the Comite National de L'urgence Medico-Psychologigue*. New York: United Nations, Department of Safety and Security.

United States Department of Labor, Bureau of Labor Statistics. (2008a). *Fatal Occupational Injuries Resulting from Transportation incidents and Homicides, All United States*. Washington, DC: US Department of Labor.

United States Department of Labor, Bureau of Labor Statistics. (2008b). *Fatal Occupational injuries by event or exposure, 2007-2008*. Washington, DC: US Department of Labor.

United States Department of Labor, Bureau of Labor Statistics. (2009). National Census of Fatal Occupational Injuries in 2008. Bureau of Labor Statistics News.

Vogt, J., & Leonhardt, J. (Eds.). (2006). *Critical Incident Stress Management in Aviation*. Hampshire, UK: Ashgate Publishing Limited.

Vogt, J., Leonhardt, J., Koper, B., & Pennig, S. (2004). Economic Evaluation of CISM – A Pilot Study. *International Journal of Emergency Mental Health*, *6*(4), 185–196. PMID:15635899

Vogt, J., Pennig, S., & Leonhardt, J. (2007). Critical Incident Stress Management in air traffic control and its benefits. *Air Traffic Control Quarterly*, *15*(2), 127–156. doi:10.2514/atcq.15.2.127

Wee, D. F., Mills, D. M., & Koelher, G. (1999). The effects of Critical Incident Stress Debriefing on emergency medical services personnel following the Los Angeles civil disturbance. *International Journal of Emergency Mental Health*, *1*, 33–38. PMID:11227752

Western Management Consultants. (1996). *The Medical Services Branch CISM Evaluation Report*. Edmonton, Canada: WMC.

Chapter 8
Application and Integration of Psychological First Aid in First Responder Organizations

Emily F. Brucia
San Francisco VA Health Care System, USA

Matthew J. Cordova
Palo Alto University, USA

Angelique Finestone
Palo Alto University, USA

Josef I. Ruzek
Palo Alto University, USA & Stanford University, USA

ABSTRACT

First responders are exposed to many potentially traumatic events throughout their careers. Given the risk of adverse mental and physical health outcomes secondary to frequent trauma exposure, access to culturally-sensitive, evidence-informed early intervention is paramount. Critical Incident Stress Management (CISM) and components therein (e.g., Critical Incident Stress Debriefing, peer support) represent the most commonly utilized early interventions within first responder organizations. Limited research has evaluated these models, and evaluation of early interventions presents many challenges due to characteristics of first responder cultures and organizational demands and constraints. Psychological First Aid (PFA) is a widely endorsed and promising evidence-informed early intervention model grounded in research on trauma recovery and resilience. This chapter examines the theoretical underpinnings and core actions of PFA and describes the potentially diverse applications of PFA within first responder organizations and concludes by discussing recommendations and future directions.

DOI: 10.4018/978-1-5225-9803-9.ch008

INTRODUCTION

First responders are exposed to many critical incidents (e.g., Carlier, Voerman, & Gersons, 2000; Malcolm, Seaton, Perera, Sheehan, & Van Hasselt, 2005) or potentially traumatic events that "may cause a given individual's emotional resources to become over-taxed, resulting in a spectrum of reactions from exhaustion to increased and unrelenting mental health symptomology" (Maguen et al., 2009, p. 754). For example, research suggests police officers are exposed to an average of 166 – 188 critical incidents during their careers (Chopko, Palmieri, & Adams, 2015; Weiss et al., 2010). Not surprisingly, first responders are at elevated risk for PTSD, depression, and alcohol use disorders (Berger et al., 2012; Kleim & Westphal, 2011).

Given the potential for adverse mental health outcomes secondary to frequent trauma exposure, access to culturally-sensitive, evidence-informed early intervention is paramount. While definitions of early intervention vary, it has been viewed as secondary prevention efforts occurring in the immediate (0-48 hours) or acute (a few weeks later) phases following a potentially traumatic event (Litz, 2008). Current early interventions within first responder organizations often include elements of the multi-component Critical Incident Stress Management (CISM) model (Everly, Flannery, & Mitchell, 2000; Mitchell & Everly, 2001). However, CISM has not been rigorously evaluated, has not specifically been studied with first responders, and includes components (e.g., Critical Incident Stress Debriefing) that have been called into question (Bisson, McFarlane, Rose, Ruzek, Watson, 2009; Brucia, Cordova, & Ruzek, 2017; Bryant, 2007; Fox et al., 2012; Rose, Bisson, Churchill, & Wessely, 2002; Ruzek et al., 2007; Tuckey, 2007; Van Emmerik, Kamphuis, Hulsbosch, & Emmelkamp, 2002). Thus, evidence-based early interventions for first responders have not been established and there are realistic challenges to implementing standardized approaches in first responder organizations.

Psychological First Aid (PFA, Forbes et al., 2011) is a specified set of early post-trauma helping behaviors derived from research-based principles (Hobfoll et al., 2007). While multiple models exist, this chapter will focus on a PFA approach collaboratively developed by the Child Stress Traumatic Network and National Center for PTSD (Brymer et al., 2006). Although this model has great potential, it has yet to be empirically validated for use in first responder populations.

This chapter will initially discuss critical incident exposure and mental health sequelae in first responders and highlight first responder cultures as an important context in which support programs must be designed. Current critical incident and early intervention models will then be reviewed, followed by examination of the theoretical underpinnings and actions of PFA (Forbes et al., 2011) and descriptions of the potential diverse applications with first responders. The chapter will conclude by identifying methodological and organizational challenges in the development, implementation, and evaluation of PFA, and discuss future directions. While first responders (e.g., emergency medical services, fire, dispatch, law enforcement) at large will be considered there will be an emphasis on law enforcement personnel and organizations given the state of the literature.

TRAUMA EXPOSURE AND MENTAL HEALTH OUTCOMES

In the United States (U.S.), civilians' lifetime risk of trauma exposure ranges from 37-92% and the prevalence rate of PTSD is 6.8% (Kearns, Ressler, Zatzick, & Rothbaum, 2012; Litz, Gray, Bryant, & Adler, 2002). While psychological distress following trauma exposure will resolve naturally for most individuals, those who continue to experience symptoms beyond 3 months are at increased risk for chronic conditions (Kessler, Sonnega, Bromet, Hughes, & Nelson, 1995; Litz et al., 2002). Identified risk factors for PTSD include perceived life threat during the traumatic event, peri-traumatic responses, previous trauma exposure, self and family psychiatric history, insecure attachment style, and limited social support (e.g., DiGangi et al., 2013; Kearns et al., 2012; Ogle, Rubin, & Siegler, 2015; Renaud, 2008; Woodhouse, Ayers, & Field, 2015). Female gender, younger age, and certain personality traits (e.g., neuroticism, hostility, trait anger, anxiety, and dissociation) are also associated with increased risk of PTSD (e.g., Brewin, Andrew, & Valentine, 2000; DiGangi et al., 2013; Litz et al., 2002; Maguen et al., 2009).

First responders are significantly more likely than the general public to be exposed to critical incidents. For example, research suggests the average 30-year police officer is exposed to between 166 – 188 critical incidents (Chopko et al., 2015; Weiss et al., 2010), and Marin (2012) posited that number may be as high as 250 critical incidents. Berger and colleagues' (2012) meta-analysis suggested that 10% of emergency service workers (e.g., police officers, firefighters, paramedics) worldwide have PTSD, with approximately 400,000 cases in the U.S. alone (Haugen et al., 2012). Prevalence rates of PTSD in police officers range from 4.7% to 19%, suggesting approximately 135,000 U.S. police officers have the condition; many more may experience subthreshold PTSD (Berger et al., 2012; Carlier, Lamberts, & Gersons, 1997; Komarovskaya et al., 2011; Marin, 2012; O'Hara, 2012). Risk factors for PTSD in first responders include cumulative trauma exposure, environmental and work stress, avoidant coping and difficulties problem solving, and poor social support (Beaton & Murphy, 1993; Brondolo, Wellington, Brady, Libby, & Brondolo, 2008; Evans, Pistrang, & Billings, 2013; Haugen et al., 2012; Kleim & Westphal, 2011; Maguen et al., 2009; Marchand, Nadeau, Beaulieu-Prevost, Boyer, & Martin, 2015; Marmar et al., 2006; Meyer, Zimering, Daly, Knight, Kamholz, & Gulliver, 2012; Phillips, LeardMann, Gumbs, & Smith, 2010; Royle, Keenan, & Farrell, 2009).

Beyond PTSD, the most commonly diagnosed psychiatric conditions in first responders are Alcohol Use Disorders and Major Depressive Disorder (MDD) (Kleim & Westphal, 2011). Sterud, Hem, Ekeberg, and Lau (2007) found that 17.7% of male and 9.1% of female Norwegian police officers (N = 2,372) endorsed hazardous alcohol use. Compared to the general American population (5.2%), rates of depressive symptoms are higher in female (12.5%) and male (6.1%) police officers (Violanti & Drylie, 2008). Stanley, Hom, and Joiner's (2016) systematic review of 63 studies on suicide in police, firefighters, and EMTs/paramedics identified elevated risk of suicidal thoughts and behaviors. Between 2008 – 2012, police officers were twice as likely to die by suicide than be killed in the line of duty (Marin, 2012).

FIRST RESPONDER CULTURES

While there are many first responder sub-cultures, police, fire, and emergency medical services personnel share common characteristics including unique indoctrination procedures, a strong sense of duty, discipline and compliance with rules and authority, and strong allegiance to their organizations, which have hierarchical command structures and long-standing traditions (Brauer, 2016; Cassan, 2010; Liedenbaum, 2011). Norms include working unusual schedules, exposure to inordinate amounts of danger, special privileges (e.g., arrest power), and the ability of superiors to cancel leave due to work demands (Brauer, 2016). Further cross-cutting first responder values and behaviors include communalism, separateness from civilians ("the thin blue line") and isolation from society, keeping work-related concerns in-house, caring for others before self ("mission-first," self-sacrifice), exhibition of physical and emotional strength, and compartmentalization and suppression of emotion (Kirschman, 2007).

Importantly, first responder cultures and beliefs about self, other, and the world may pose real and perceived barriers to seeking informal support and/or formal mental health treatment. Mental health issues are often stigmatized, particularly given that many community calls involve responding to mental health crises, and disclosure of emotional distress or mental health concerns may be viewed as weakness. (Kirschman, Kamena, & Fay, 2014). While these attitudes and coping strategies may be viewed as resilient and foster effective first responder work in the short-term, they may inhibit expression, detection, and treatment of mental health problems in this population (Haugen, McCrillis, Smid, & Nijdam, 2017; Kirschman et al., 2014; Wester, Arndt, Sedivy, & Arndt, 2010).

COMMON INTERVENTIONS FOR FIRST RESPONDERS

Given characteristics of first responder cultures and organizational demands and constraints, the development, implementation, and evaluation of critical incident interventions presents many challenges. In the 1990s, Mitchell and Everly (2001; Everly et al., 2000a) developed the multi-component Critical Incident Stress Management (CISM) model. CISM is a comprehensive stress management model utilized by some first responder organizations, with the primary aim to provide various types of mental health support to first responders, their families, and their organizations at various time points before and after a critical incident (Everly & Mitchell, 1999; Everly et al., 2000a; Everly, Lating, & Mitchell, 2000b). CISM includes pre-critical incident psychoeducation about stress reactions and stress management, and assessment of the needs of first responders during or immediately following a critical incident. The model further calls for a group defusing intervention to assess current needs within 12-hours post-critical incident, followed by a Critical Incident Stress Debriefing (CISD) in the subsequent days or weeks. CISM also includes peer support and chaplaincy services, consultation with organization and community administrators to tailor the model as appropriate for the setting, referrals for ongoing psychological distress, and debrief-the-debriefer sessions (Sheehan, Everly, & Langlieb, 2004).

Some meta-analytic studies have reviewed the effectiveness of CISM interventions. Everly, Flannery, and Eyler (2002) conducted a meta-analysis investigating the effectiveness of eight CISM interventions on outcomes, including PTSD symptoms. Results demonstrated large mean effect sizes, suggesting delivery of CISM interventions may mitigate adverse psychological outcomes of trauma. However, these naturalistic studies were not conducted with first responders, and contained many methodological limitations that limited generalizability and the ability to draw definite conclusions.

Within many first responder organizations, isolated CISM components are utilized as stand-alone interventions that are not embedded within the multi-component stress management model. Psychological debriefings are the longest-standing and most common critical incident intervention for first responders, though debriefing structures and content can vary dramatically between organizations and there is confusion in the literature about the definition of debriefings (Bisson et al., 2009; Brucia et al., 2017; Litz et al., 2002; Tuckey, 2007). First developed in the early 1980s, Critical Incident Stress Debriefing (CISD) is the most frequently utilized group critical incident intervention for first responders and is comprised of seven phases: Introduction, Fact, Thought, Reaction, Symptom, Teaching, and Re-entry (Malcolm et al., 2005; Mitchell, 1983). While very limited research has evaluated CISD delivered to first responders (e.g., Bohl, 1995; Carlier, Lamberts, Van Uchelen, & Gersons, 1998; Carlier et al., 2000), multiple meta-analytic studies concluded that both CISD and non-CISD stand-alone group psychological debriefings do not reduce psychological distress or prevent PTSD and may even exacerbate symptoms (Bisson, Jenkins, Alexander, & Bannister, 1997; Bisson et al., 2009; Brucia et al., 2017; Bryant, 2007; Carlier et al., 1998; Carlier et al., 2000; Fox et al., 2012; NIMH, 2002; Gene-Cos, 2006; Rose et al., 2002; Ruzek et al., 2007; Tuckey, 2007; Van Emmerik et al., 2002). Notably, the CISM manual explicitly states that CISD is not intended to be delivered as a stand-alone intervention.

In the U.S., Canada, and globally, there is a proliferation of peer support programs in emergency medical services, fire, and law enforcement organizations (Papazoglou & Tuttle, 2018). Although informal peer support has been an integrated part of police culture for decades, some police departments offer formal peer support programs as a way to support the psychological health of officers (Benner, 1982; Graf, 1986; Kamena, Gentz, Hays, Bohl-Penrod, & Greene, 2011; Waters & Ussery, 2007). To this end, the International Association of Chiefs of Police (IACP, 2016) developed Peer Support Guidelines, which provide guidance and flexible recommendations for creating and maintaining a formal peer support program within an organization. Peer support members are specially trained co-workers who serve to normalize and validate the range of decisions (e.g., tactical, emotional) made by officers (IACP, 2016; Kirschman et al., 2014). Peer support members may be particularly well-suited to identify officers in increased distress, and because of the peer relationship, distressed officers may be more amenable to sharing (M. Bloesch, 2018, personal communication; Kirschman et al., 2014). Peer support programs have numerous intended effects, including providing emotional, social, and practical support to those in distress due to personal and work-related issues, and helping officers navigate the challenges of policing (IACP, 2016). Peer support programs may protect against the adverse outcomes of trauma exposure, may reduce feelings of shame, embarrassment, abandonment, and rejection, and may increase help seeking behavior (Graf, 1986; Flannery, 2015; Kirschman et al., 2014).

Limited research has evaluated the effectiveness of peer support programs in reducing psychiatric morbidity (Brucia et al., 2017; Grauwiler, Barocas, & Mills, 2008). Berg, Hem, Lau, Haseth, and Ekeberg (2005) found greater work injuries and perceived job pressures in a nationwide sample of Norwegian police ($N = 3272$) who worked in districts lacking peer support programs and whose populations were greater than 50,000 people. These findings highlight the importance of peer involvement in early intervention programs.

Several support structures for first responders have emerged outside of the workplace. National peer-to-peer organizations have developed (e.g., The Badge of Life, 2018; Concerns of Police Survivors (C.O.P.S.), 2018; COPLINE) in an effort to increase awareness of mental health, support bereaved survivors of duty-related deaths, and prevent suicide (Samuels, 2018). Other innovative models of care include residential treatment programs (e.g., First Responder Support Network) for first responders with posttraumatic stress reactions (e.g., Brucia, 2018; Dunnigan, 2012; Fay, Kamena, Benner, & Buscho, 2006).

In some fashion, CISM model, CISD, and peer support all incorporate information about coping and fostering social connectedness in the immediate aftermath of a traumatic event. However, these interventions have limited empirical support, particularly with first responders. Given the complex organizational demands, diverse roles, and multiple critical incident exposures of first responders, flexible, empirically-informed, principle-based approaches to early intervention are needed.

CORE PRINCIPLES AND ACTIONS OF PSYCHOLOGICAL FIRST AID

Developed to be utilized in the immediate aftermath of a traumatic event and delivered by mental health and/or disaster response workers, Psychological First Aid (PFA) (Forbes et al., 2011) is an early intervention with primary goals of reducing acute distress and facilitating individual and community short- and long-term resilience, adaptive coping, and functioning (Brymer et al., 2006). The basic standards of PFA are consistent with research on trauma-related risk and resilience, practical for field settings (e.g., emergency departments, staging areas, feeding locations), appropriate for use in individuals across the developmental lifespan (e.g., children, adolescents, adults), and designed to be delivered in flexible and culturally sensitive ways (Forbes et al., 2011). PFA has multiple basic objectives identified as eight core actions: 1) contact and engagement, 2) safety and comfort, 3) stabilization, 4) information gathering regarding current needs and concerns, 5) practical assistance, 6) connection with social support, 7) information on coping, and 8) connection with appropriate services (Brymer et al., 2006; Ruzek et al., 2007; Uhernik & Husson, 2009). Importantly, PFA acknowledges that trauma survivors will experience a range of reactions, that not all survivors will experience chronic symptoms, and that natural recovery is common.

PFA emerged from five core theory-based principles that are rooted in empirical support and that highlight mechanisms of trauma recovery (Hobfoll et al., 2007). The five central intervention principles are promotion of safety, calming, self- and collective efficacy, connectedness, and hope. These principles can guide organizational responses to work-related trauma exposures at the individual, group, organizational, and community levels, including workforce education, peer support, specialist counseling, media communications, and organizational ceremonies and practices (Hobfoll et al., 2007). Further, the underlying principles of PFA are generative tenets that can be creatively applied in culturally appropriate, flexible ways. The following text will describe the five core theory-based principles underlying PFA and the core actions of PFA that map onto these principles; it will also discuss the particular relevance and application of these principles and actions for first responders. These broad principles and core actions are potentially applicable at multiple levels; mental health providers may provide PFA to first responders, and first responders may deliver PFA to each other and to those in the public they serve. Given that many PFA components are nested within multiple underlying principles and core actions, those most salient to each will be discussed.

Safety

Traumatic events threaten self and other physical and psychological safety. In the face of real or perceived on-going danger, the human body is hardwired to make biological and survival driven behavioral and cognitive adaptations (van der Kolk & Saporta, 1993). Bryant and colleagues (2007) posited that promotion of safety in both humans and animals is associated with regulating biological responses, such as the fight-flight-freeze response, that maintain anxiety and fear. Traumatic events also impact safety-related cognitions and threat appraisal such that the ability to realistically appraise threats can be compromised, increasing the likelihood that ambiguous and neutral stimuli will be experienced as real threats (Ehlers & Clark, 2000; Foa & Rothbaum, 1998). As such, beliefs about self- and other- safety and the dangerousness of community environments have important implications for trauma-related mental health sequelae.

Self and other safety concerns map onto two core actions of PFA. Contact and engagement, PFA's first core action, encourages those in response roles to develop non-intrusive and compassionate human connections with trauma survivors (Forbes et al., 2011). Specifically, PFA recommends introducing oneself, explaining one's role, and inquiring about immediate needs while respecting confidentiality and upholding relevant ethical and legal standards. The second core action of PFA is focused on the promotion of immediate and ongoing physical and psychological safety and comfort (Forbes et al., 2011; Hobfoll et al., 2007). Re-establishing safety at multiple levels (i.e., individual, group, organization, and community) is emphasized, and ensuring immediate and ongoing physical safety is paramount. Depending on environmental circumstances and personal needs, this may include basic actions like removing sharp objects (e.g., broken glass), asking about the need for medications, eyeglasses, wheelchairs, or other mobility devices, or provision of blankets. It is also critical to assess for ongoing threats to self or others and to identify individuals who may be in shock and in need of immediate medical and/or psychiatric attention.

Given unique cultural factors and the significant risk of work-related trauma exposure in first responder populations, re-establishing physical and emotional safety in the immediate aftermath of a traumatic event may be challenging. Re-establishing physical and emotional safety is likely best delivered via bottom-up and top-down approaches. Immediate bottom-up approaches may include providing first responders with information about tactical response activities and available services, giving them the opportunity to ask questions about what may happen next, and providing support for acute stress and/or grief reactions. Top-down approaches may include dissemination of accurate, organized, and timely information by first responder administrators and other leaders (Shalev & Freedman, 2005). To create a more comfortable physical environment and promote social interactions with colleagues who are coping adequately, organizational leaders may designate a separate staging/recovery area in a safe area for respite, attention to practical needs (e.g., hunger, thirst), and social connection.

Safety-related beliefs are particularly salient for first responders and may present unique challenges to immediate and ongoing post-trauma interventions. First responder training and experiences may alter and/or reinforce prior beliefs and contribute to the development of new self, other, and world safety-related beliefs (Brucia, 2018; Kirschman, 2007; Kirschman et al., 2014; Terpstra & Schapp, 2013). Beginning in the academy, police officers are trained to be suspicious and skeptical of others and to view civilians as "suspects" and potential sources of danger. Research examining risk factors of PTSD in male firefighter cadets ($N = 82$) found that those with fewer negative and catastrophic beliefs prior to work-related trauma exposure were at decreased risk of PTSD one year later (Bryant & Guthrie, 2005). Later in their careers, self and other safety concerns may generalize to broader distrust of non-police individuals, politicians, command staff, and administrators, who may be perceived as unable to understand policing demands, experiences, and culture (Terpstra & Schapp, 2013). Many negative safety-related beliefs held by first responders may prove functionally adaptive in some aspects of the job, but may contribute to psychological distress and dysfunction in other work and non-work contexts. Providing psychoeducation (see below) about trauma reactions and coping on an ongoing basis, including at the onset of first responders' careers as well as in the immediate aftermath of traumatic events, may be one particularly useful way to protect against development of problematic beliefs about personal and community safety.

In the immediate aftermath of a traumatic event, individuals delivering PFA to first responders may encounter individuals whose self and other safety and trust-related beliefs inhibit engagement with mental health providers, and this may be compounded by self- and other-stigma as well as label avoidance (Corrigan, Watson, & Barr, 2006; Goldstein, 2005). Importantly, practical (e.g., duty-related responsibilities) and systemic barriers (e.g., organizational policies that prohibit interactions with others prior to evidence collection and formal statements) may further impede contact and engagement with first responders in need, and compound safety-related beliefs and stigma that contribute to reluctance to utilize social support and mental health services. A clear understanding of organizational policies and procedures as well as depth and breadth of knowledge of first responder culture is critical for otherwise well-intentioned mental health providers.

Calming

The second underlying principle of PFA is promotion of calming (Hobfoll et al., 2007). Increased emotionality, anxiety, and hypervigilance and/or affective detachment and numbing are common responses to traumatic events. However, if these symptoms are maintained over time they can interfere with basic needs, such as eating, sleeping, or hydration, and contribute to impairment in concentration, completion of routine tasks, and social connectedness (Goenjian, Karayan, Pynoos, Minassian, Najarian, Steinberg, et al., 1997; Goenjian, Walling, Steinberg, Karavan, Najarian, & Pynoos, 2005; Hobfoll et al., 2007). There is also a well-demonstrated relationship between stress and trauma and adverse physical health outcomes (e.g., cardiovascular, autoimmune disease, chronic pain, GI conditions), as well as increased utilization of healthcare services (Engelhard, van den Hout, Weerts, Hox, & van Doormen, 2009; Hoge, Terhakopian, Castro, Messer, & Engel 2007). Physical and emotional calming may be promoted via psychoeducation that identifies and normalizes early trauma responses, formal relaxation training methods (e.g., breathing, mindfulness, meditation), and relaxing activities that enable teams and individuals to find calm across their daily routines. Indeed, most evidence-based psychosocial post-trauma interventions include promotion of calming as a critical component (e.g., Bryant, Harvey, Dang, Sackville, & Basten, 1998; Foa & Rothbaum, 1998; Foa, Hembree, & Rothbaum, 2007), and an indicator of successful treatment completion is attainment of mastery and calming over the traumatic memory (Forbes et al., 2011).

Promotion of calming relates to the third and fourth core actions of PFA. Stabilization, the third core action, aims to calm and orient overwhelmed survivors who may be numb, unresponsive, confused, or incapacitated by anxiety and worry by engaging individuals in calming strategies. The fourth core action of PFA focuses on identification of current needs and concerns and gathering additional information (Forbes et al., 2011). While multiple factors in the field may limit what and how much information is gathered, PFA suggests asking questions in an effort to clarify the following: nature and severity of experiences during that trauma, death of and/or separation from colleagues and if relevant, family and loved ones, concerns about immediate or ongoing danger, history of exposure to trauma, physical illness and psychiatric conditions and need for medications, losses (e.g., home, neighborhood, property, business), strong feelings of guilt or shame, suicidality and homicidality, access to social support, and/or historical or current substance use. PFA also recommends enlisting nearby family members or friends to comfort the individual, engaging the individual in conversation about their current concerns, remaining calm and quiet, and providing orienting information (e.g., next steps) (Forbes et al., 2011).

Promotion of calming in first responders is vital given research demonstrating first responders are more frequently diagnosed with stress-related physical illnesses than the general population, though it may be challenging (Alkus & Padesky, 1983; Centre for Occupational and Environmental Health, 2000; Marin, 2012). Their training to suppress outward signs of physical and emotional stress enables effective action in response to victims but may reduce awareness and self-regulation of heightened internal states. That said, helping first responders learn to recognize their own distress and arousal and re-establish calm may be accomplished through a variety of strategies. Psychoeducation specific to common psychological, emotional, and physiological reactions during the stabilization phase may also serve to normalize and validate first responders' reactions and challenge negative safety-, doubt-, and stigma-related beliefs (e.g., "I'm losing it; I'm not safe because my reactions") and emotional distress, which may in turn foster increased coping self-efficacy. Referrals for professional mental health services may likely utilize cognitive-behavioral and exposure strategies to increase self-awareness of antecedents of anxious distress, gently challenge beliefs, and increase coping self-efficacy (see below). For example, in the immediate aftermath of a traumatic event, anxiety management techniques might include physical, mental, emotional, and self-soothing grounding strategies, such as diaphragmatic breathing and progressive muscle relaxation, which have been found to reduce anxiety and counter intense emotionality (Foa & Rothbaum, 1998; Somer et al., 2005).

Calming interventions for first responders are being implemented. Some police departments in the U.S. and Canada are creating "quiet" rooms for rest, relaxation, or meditation, furnished with comfortable recliners and televisions (McHugh, 2019; PoliceOne, 2017). Christopher and colleagues (2015) evaluated an 8-week Mindfulness-Based Resilience Training (MBRT) program for police officers ($N = 43$) and found significant improvements in self-reported mindfulness, physical and emotional health, perceived stress, burnout, emotion regulation (e.g., anger), resilience, sleep difficulties, and fatigue. These approaches reflect proactive, early organizational-level interventions that may foster calming coping strategies and restoration of homeostasis following critical incidents. In contrast, interventions such as CISD, which involve emotional processing and ventilation, may exacerbate disequilibrium at precisely the time when recently traumatized individuals are attempting to restore calmness (Bisson et al., 2009).

Gathering information about current concerns may guide tailored responses to first responders. For example, emotionally flooded first responders may benefit from immediate and ongoing use of grounding and calming strategies. Alternatively, individuals expressing intense negative self, other, and/or worldviews may benefit from immediate and ongoing use of cognitive interventions (e.g., reframing, gentle thought challenging, crafting more realistic/flexible beliefs). First responders may also present with culturally-unique concerns. For example, specific types of critical incidents (e.g., officer involved shootings) may initiate organizational policies that require an officer's duty weapon be removed from their possession. Approaching the function of firearms from a self-psychology perspective, Feldmann and Johnson (1992) suggested that weapons serve to combat feelings of powerlessness and vulnerability and maintain self-cohesion. As such, police officers who have their duty weapon removed from their possession following a critical incident may feel particularly uneasy and unsafe. To ease such concerns some departments ensure that a replacement weapon is available and provided to officers as appropriate (M. Bloesch, 2019, personal communication).

Self and Collective Efficacy

Promotion of self- and collective efficacy is the third principle underpinning PFA. Trauma can overwhelm one's coping resources and contribute to feelings of powerlessness and helplessness (Hobfoll et al., 2007). The concept of self-efficacy emerged from social cognitive theory (Bandura, 1997) and may be defined as beliefs that one can successfully implement a particular behavior and that one's "actions are likely to lead to generally positive outcomes, principally through self-regulation of thoughts, emotions, and behavior" (Hobfoll et al., 2007, p. 293). Most individuals draw from a broad array of learned adaptive and maladaptive coping strategies in an effort to self-regulate following trauma exposure. Research suggests that the development of trauma-specific adaptive coping self-efficacy is particularly beneficial for trauma recovery and resilience (Benight & Harper, 2002), and that those with greater coping self-efficacy may naturally select more adaptive, action-oriented strategies compared to those with lower self-efficacy (Luszczynska, Benight, & Cieslak, 2009).

Bandura (1997, p. 477) defined collective efficacy as "a group's shared belief in its conjoint capability to organize and execute the course of action required to produce given levels of attainment." Given the action-oriented nature of first responder careers, the development and maintenance of collective efficacy vital as it promotes action (Cicognani, Pietrantoni, Palestini, & Prati, 2009). Importantly, self-efficacy and collective efficacy are often interwoven; solving large-scale problems requires the collaboration of multiple people and systems.

Self- and collective efficacy are associated with the fifth core action of PFA, which consists of offering practical assistance, identifying and clarifying the most pertinent need(s), and discussing the action plan (Forbes et al., 2011). Accessing and retaining resources is associated with post-trauma recovery and may foster self- and collective efficacy (Forbes et al., 2011). For first responders, practical assistance may include organizational and peer support, religious activities, briefings, meetings, mourning rituals, and dissemination of information and resources (Benight, 2004; Cicognani et al., 2009; de Jong, 2002; Sampson, Raudenbush, & Earls, 1997). Providing and helping first responders maintain access to these resources may improve self-efficacy, contribute to restoration of dignity and empowerment, buffer against a loss of hope, and promote optimism, a sense of predictability, positive beliefs, and for some religious faith.

To cope with their complex job duties, responsibilities, and exposures, first responders need to be familiar with and confident in their ability to use a broad range of strategies. Learning and rehearsing strategies for problem-focused coping, sleep hygiene, managing media exposure, relaxation, and engagement in pleasurable activities that foster positive emotions such as joy, curiosity, humor, and love, may result in more effective coping (Hobfoll et al., 1991, 2007).

Some cultural norms underlie maladaptive coping. For example, first responder culture condones drinking as a coping strategy. High rates of problematic alcohol use in police officers have been documented and may have the unintended long-term effect of decreasing self-efficacy (Kirschman, 2007; Larson, Eyerman, Foster, & Grfoerer, 2007; Richmond, Wodak, Kehoe, & Heather, 1998).

Given the collaborative and interdependent nature of their work in high risk, stressful situations, first responders are likely to develop collective efficacy beliefs about situations they can master as a group (Cicognani et al., 2009). However, discrepancies may exist between their beliefs about the abilities of their frontline colleagues versus the abilities of command staff and organizational leadership. Further, positive outcome expectations may depend on a just world view (i.e., good things happen to good people, bad things happen to bad people). First responders may be at risk of lower collective efficacy due to past work-related stressors and trauma, organizational demands, childhood and civilian trauma exposure, and minority stress/trauma. Formal assessment and education about the impact of past learning experiences on individual and group beliefs, and training to identify and evaluate maladaptive beliefs and formulate more helpful thoughts may foster greater self- and collective efficacy.

Connectedness

The fourth principle of PFA is connectedness. Trauma can be isolating and alienating, and social support is one of the strongest post-trauma protective factors against PTSD and suicide (Bernert, Kim, Iwata, & Perlis, 2015; DiGangi et al., 2013; Ozer, Best, Lipsey, & Weiss, 2008; Vallieres, Azaiez, Moreau,

LeBlanc, & Morin, 2014; Van Orden et al., 2010). Survivors often yearn for immediate connection to those with whom they have a strong relationship (e.g., family, close friends, clergy, colleagues), and social support immediately after a traumatic event serves multiple functions, including normalization and validation of emotional reactions and facilitation of problem-solving (Hobfoll et al., 2007). Talking with supportive others can help individuals process emotions and develop a coherent and realistic understanding of traumatic experiences (Lepore, 2001). In contrast, social constraints related to talking about trauma, whether objectively imposed by others' behavior or subjectively experienced due to one's expectations or perceptions, can inhibit trauma processing and pose obstacles to natural recovery (Lepore & Revenson, 2007; Belsher, Ruzek, Bongar & Cordova, 2012).

Establishing and connecting survivors with social support is the sixth core action of PFA. Social support may include emotional support, physical and material assistance, social connection, feeling valued and needed, reassurance of self-worth and that others are reliable, and advice and information. PFA advocates guiding those who are reluctant to seek social support to consider what type of support might be helpful and who they may feel comfortable approaching.

Social support is associated with reduced distress in a range of first responder populations. Specifically, among police officers, social support has been found to protect against mental health disorders, hopelessness, and suicide, and to increase recovery rates from PTSD, even in the absence of a formal treatment intervention (De Terte, Stephens, & Huddleston, 2014; Klimley, Van Hasselt, & Stripling, 2018; Marchand et al., 2015; Violanti et al., 2016). Stanley et al. (2018) found that among firefighters social support received from coworkers, supervisors, family, and friends buffered against the development of PTSD. Dispatchers displayed higher rates of burnout, stress, and anxiety when they perceived a lack of social support (Klimley et al., 2018; Burke, 1995; Kirmeyer & Dougherty, 1988). Regehr, Goldberg, Glancy, and Knott (2002) found that current social support was associated with paramedics' tendency to use mental health stress leave.

While families are often the primary source of support following a traumatic event, it is common for first responders, particularly police officers, to experience a decrease in social support from non-law enforcement family and friends as they progress through their careers (Gilmartin, 2002; Violanti & Drylie, 2008). This decline in support may be influenced by beliefs that "others can't understand me and my job," a desire to not burden family and friends with the stress of first responder work, substance use, emotional numbing and distancing, and feelings of isolation.

First responder peer support programs provide social support in a variety of situations and can be designed to integrate PFA principles and core actions. Although some organizational peer support programs incorporate chaplains as part of the CISM model, these programs tend to emphasize collegial peer support (Gillespie, 2017). In addition to work-related peer and spiritual support, encouraging connection with multiple sources of social support, including connecting first responders with their family members, non-first responder friends, and other community-based social, religious/spiritual, and recreational groups, is especially important. Further, departmental peer support programs may also implement programming specific to first responders' significant others, partners, children, and extended family.

Hope

Instilling hope is of central importance following a traumatic event. Trauma can shatter world-views and contribute to feelings of despair and hopelessness (Janoff-Bulman, 1992). Hope is commonly defined as a "positive, action-oriented expectation that a positive future goal or outcome is possible" (Haase,

Britt, Coward, & Leidy, 1992). Hobfoll, Briggs- Phillips, and Stines (2003) note that this view of hope may be more consistent with Western, upper-class, and white majority culture, and based on a notion of "rugged individualism" that overlooks realities of those who experience racism, poverty, and/or mass trauma. More inclusively, hope may be viewed as a sense of strength and optimism for recovery. Maintenance of hope is a resilience factor; optimism following a traumatic event is associated with a favorable outcome (Hobfoll et al., 2007).

The seventh core action consists of providing psychoeducation about common stress reactions and coping strategies, which may foster hopefulness about trauma recovery and resilience. As previously discussed, trauma survivors may be alarmed by their stress reactions and their baseline coping tools may be ineffective following trauma exposure. Providing reassurance about trauma responses and teaching a range of adaptive coping strategies may enhance a sense of self-efficacy and foster goal-oriented coping. These coping strategies may include seeking social support, accessing information and resources, engaging in distracting, enjoyable activities and physical exercise, maintaining a normal schedule to the extent possible, utilizing relaxation methods such as calming self-talk, journaling, and grounding. PFA also recommends identifying and modifying maladaptive coping strategies (e.g., substance use, overworking, excessive self/other blame, lack of self-care).

Referring survivors to additional services is the eighth core action of PFA. Providing information about professional support services may instill hope, contribute to calming, and foster a plan for action. Recommended referrals might include mental health care, medical treatment, social support services, and drug and alcohol support groups. When possible, PFA recommends warm hand-offs (i.e., provider-to-provider communication about survivors), which can ease the transition for survivors, increase sense of being cared for, and decrease the burden survivors may feel to "re-tell" their story to multiple providers.

Psychoeducation and referrals for first responders should be couched in terms that are consistent with first responder culture. Ideally, this would include education, during training/academy and then on an ongoing basis, about common trauma responses, the trajectory of and obstacles to natural recovery, the strengths and potential liabilities of first responder culture with regard to emotional and physical well-being (e.g., "it is not a sign of weakness to experience distress, even when it persists"), and adaptive and maladaptive coping. Education should also be provided regarding formal empirically-supported treatment options for post-trauma distress and their efficacy. Organizations should maintain a network of mental health professionals that have the cultural competence and evidence-based training to work effectively with first responders and should take steps to reduce stigma and barriers to initiating treatment (e.g., confidentiality of referrals, warm hand-offs when feasible, assurance that seeking treatment will not negatively influence job status or promotion).

In sum, promotion of safety, calming, connectedness, self- and collective efficacy, and hope are the core evidence-informed elements that guided the design of PFA and are integral components of many evidence-based treatments (Hobfoll et al., 2007). The underlying principles of PFA are interrelated; feeling physically and psychologically safe and calm may increase one's sense of coping self-efficacy and hope for recovery, which may increase likeliness of social connectedness, and positive outcomes of social support likely enhance a sense of individual and collective efficacy (de Jong, 1995; Hobfoll et al., 2007).

METHODOLOGICAL AND ORGANIZATIONAL CHALLENGES

Significant methodological and organizational challenges to evaluating and implementing PFA in first responder organizations exist. In general, conducting evaluations of PFA is difficult. Most broadly, PFA is not a structured, one-size-fits-all approach. It is not surprising that there are no published RCTs of PFA given practical and ethical challenges of assessing pre-trauma functioning, randomizing trauma survivors to treatment modalities, delivering replicable interventions in the field, monitoring what is actually happening during those helping encounters (i.e., fidelity, replicability), retaining participants, and obtaining consistent follow-up data.

Evaluation of PFA will be especially challenging in first responder populations, particularly police officers. First, it is likely that PFA would be integrated as one of many components of a peer support program and would not exist as a stand-alone model. Second, although law enforcement peer support program guidelines exist (e.g., IACP, 2011), departments vary in their application of these guidelines. Third, the intended effects of peer support programs are conceptually unclear and may include outcomes both for those whom the first responder helps and interacts with and for first responder themselves. These might be as wide-ranging as detection of symptoms/impairment, prevention of chronic and impairing psychiatric conditions, receipt of professional support/treatment, maintenance of on-the-job functioning, prevention of adverse events, reduction of needed stress leave or workman's compensation cases, and improved employee retention. Fourth, it is ethically and functionally challenging to conduct RCTs, resulting in the self-selection of officers who choose and are selected to participate in peer-support programs. Fifth, it would be rare to obtain a true baseline level of functioning prior to a given critical incident and few psychological assessments have been normed and validated for police officers (Robinson & Mitchell, 1993; Malcolm et al., 2005). Thus, it is acknowledged that rigorous research evaluation of PFA outcomes faces complex obstacles.

Challenges in implementing PFA in first responder organizations are also anticipated. Strong leadership support is needed, and must be sustained across changes in personnel and organizational change. Effective training methods are required to ensure mastery of PFA skills and routine ongoing use in day-to-day practice. Optimal training in PFA would likely entail didactics, observed role-plays with feedback, and ongoing supervision and case consultation. Such continuing support is needed to help trainees continue to apply their skills and reach a level of familiarity and confidence that will lead to continued use. Should they be mastered, the new ways of helping included in PFA will need to negotiate cultural barriers, including previous ways of doing business and countervailing norms of behavior. It remains challenging to encourage openness and sharing of thoughts and feelings in organizations characterized by a commitment to placing others before self and norms of "emotional strength" (Kirschman, 2007). Finally, it may be necessary to alter staffing patterns, shift rotations, use of organizational space, and allocation of resources in order to make it possible for newly trained helpers to successfully deploy their skills. All these considerations mean that leaders intent on building effective PFA programs will need to think beyond simply adding training workshops to include planning for sustained use in the context of local factors and challenges of encouraging busy people to do things differently in busy organizations, where the focus on community service under emergency conditions may push to the side considerations of staff wellbeing. Additionally, ensuring the confidentiality of peer-to-peer supports and referrals for professional services is paramount given internalized stigma about mental health concerns among first responders.

RECOMMENDATIONS AND FUTURE DIRECTIONS

As demonstrated above, developing, implementing, and evaluating evidence-based or evidence-informed early interventions for first responders following trauma exposure poses many practical, methodological, and organizational challenges. There is an alarming paucity of research demonstrating that the historically implemented early intervention models (e.g., CISD/CISM, peer support programs) are effective at ameliorating acute psychological distress, preventing trauma- and stressor-related disorders, and promoting a natural recovery (Everly et al., 2000a; Everly et al., 2000b; Tuckey, 2007). Clearly, there is a need for innovative, integrative early intervention work-related stress management models that expand on the traditional CISM model or offer novel ideas; this would facilitate assessment of the centrality of critical incident exposure and its interaction with other stressors (e.g., poor relationship with supervisor, overall workplace functioning, family stressors). With high-stress, physically and emotionally taxing jobs, frequent exposure to potentially traumatic events, and higher rates of stress-related physical illnesses, depression, PTSD, alcohol use disorder, and suicide compared to the general population, there is an urgent need for flexible, adaptable, and evidence-based early interventions for first responders. PFA is a promising and widely endorsed evidence-informed model grounded in theories of trauma recovery and resilience. PFA may be particularly well-matched for first responders because it 1) expands on currently culturally accepted interventions (e.g., peer support programs), 2) can be delivered on both mental health provider to first responder and peer-to-peer bases, and 3) may enhance first responders' skill-sets when caring for those they serve. As such, PFA may be diversely utilized and integrated within first responder organizations for an array of purposes. More specifically, multi-component PFA interventions could include staff education and preparation for stressful aspects of the job, response to critical incidents, team-building/morale, peer response programs, specialized crisis counseling and/or treatment, and family programs.

Detailed below are several evidence-informed recommendations. First, the beginning of a first responder career should include comprehensive psychoeducation about common mental health issues, coping strategies, self-care, peer/social support, and resources, and this should be reinforced throughout their careers via continued training. Second, it is recommended that first responders be trained in PFA (Forbes et al., 2011), and that these interventions be utilized in the immediate aftermath of a critical incident and integrated into peer support programs. Such training would likely enhance first responders' knowledge and skill-set in supporting their colleagues and have the added benefit of enhancing their skill-sets when serving their constituents. For example, first responders are exposed to mass disaster and hostage situations, distressed survivors and family members, suicidal and homicidal suspects who may be armed and dangerous, and deaths of adults and children secondary to suicide, homicide, accidents, and natural causes (Golden, Jones, & Donlon, 2014; Kleim & Westphal, 2011). First responders additionally provide emergency medical care and engage in handling of human remains (Golden, Jones, & Donlon, 2014; Kleim & Westphal, 2011). As such, PFA training may facilitate their ability and self-efficacy to provide psychological and practical support to victims and may protect against the experience of a loss of coping ability. More specifically, PFA may provide a clear, organized mental template that first responders can use when tasked with providing psychological and practical support to trauma survivors in the immediate aftermath of a traumatic event. PFA also provides recommendations for death notifications and body identification, which may be particularly relevant for first responders tasked with this challenging role.

Third, it is recommended that first responder organizations develop peer support programs, particularly in light of research demonstrating social support as a primary protective factor of PTSD and related mental health sequelae. With regard to peer support, it is recommended that peer support programs follow the IACP Peer Support Guidelines (2016) and are confidential, provide ongoing monitoring and support as indicated, and utilize targeted and appropriate interventions for specific problems. For the field to advance, and to ensure that services are actually helping, there will be a need for conceptual clarity about the intended effects of peer support programs. Fourth, it is recommended that intentional efforts be undertaken to assimilate peer support programs as a culturally-normed component of first responder organizations.

Beyond PFA, there is also a need to develop evidence-based teaching interventions to train those who provide peer support, and to tailor these trainings to the variety of existing first responder subcultures. It is now well established that, by themselves, simple training workshops are unlikely to effectively add to staff skills and change routine practice. Instead, they need to be followed by a period of supervision and consultation as trainees try out the new skills and make them their own. A few preliminary yet promising interventions have emerged, including Marks and colleagues (2017) peer support training program titled Recognize, Evaluate, Advocate, Coordinate, and Track (REACT). This four-module training program was designed to promote psychological health and prevent stress injuries in first responders.

Internet and mobile technologies offer significant opportunities to innovation. Given recent technological advances and the potential value of integrating mobile-health into early intervention responses, PFA Mobile was developed and is available for download on iOS and Android operating systems. The mobile app is provides a broad and comprehensive overview of PFA, including the five evidence-informed principles and basic objectives, information about who should deliver PFA and where it should be used, PFA guidelines (e.g., how to engage survivors, recommended behaviors to avoid), and considerations for cultural/diversity factors and supporting at-risk populations. The mobile app contains sections about PFA in practice, the eight core actions, and common reactions across the lifespan (e.g., infants/toddlers, preschool-age, school-age, adolescents, adults). There is also a section within the app that allows for providers to create a survivor needs form as a quick and practical way to keep track of individuals with whom providers come into contact. Provider self-care is another component of the PFA mobile application, including a provider self-assessment and information about self-care before, during, and after relief work. Lastly, the PFA mobile app includes a resource section with direct links to SAMHSA's Disaster Distress Helpful, the National Suicide Prevention Hotline, FEMA, and National Center for PTSD and National Child Traumatic Stress Networks.

At present there is no published research evaluating PFA. While RCTs may not be tenable due to aforementioned methodological and organizational challenges, there is a need for program evaluation research of PFA that is generalizable to first responder cultures, although there are still many obstacles (e.g., funding, organizational support) to conducting this type of research. At present, little is known about whether programs (e.g., CISD/CISM) accomplish their intended objectives, so managers cannot adequately evaluate the cost-effectiveness of their initiatives and, most important, it remains unclear if these programs are effectively reducing individual distress. There is a need to evaluate PFA peer support programs on multiple outcomes such as PTSD, depression, substance/alcohol use, suicide, and social and occupational functioning, and quality of life (e.g., Wessely & Deahl, 2003), and to consider the role of stigma of mental health and broader organizational context in which peer support programs are developed, implemented, and evaluated.

Perhaps most importantly, in order for leadership to manage effectively and for peer support and other procedures to benefit staff members, it is important that organizations conduct periodic assessments of staff well-being and areas for concern. This information can be gathered anonymously, to evaluate PFA programs and inform their improvement and redesign. Further, first responder organizations are likely to benefit from collaboration with academic partners in order to evaluate current models of support and to develop and investigate innovative and potentially more effective proactive, preventative interventions as well as posttraumatic early intervention models for first responders, who fulfill vital and complex roles in society.

REFERENCES

Alkus, S., & Padesky, C. (1983). Special problems of police officers: Stress-related issues and interventions. *The Counseling Psychologist*, *11*(2), 55–64. doi:10.1177/0011000083112010

Badge of Life. (2018). *Psychological survival for police officers.* Retrieved from https://www.badgeoflife.org

Bandura, A. (1997). *Self-efficacy: The exercise of control.* New York: Freeman.

Beaton, R. D., & Murphy, S. A. (1993). Sources of occupational stress among firefighters/EMTs and firefighters/paramedics and correlations with job-related outcomes. *Prehospital and Disaster Medicine*, *8*(2), 140–150. doi:10.1017/S1049023X00040218 PMID:10155458

Belsher, B. E., Ruzek, J. I., Bongar, B., & Cordova, M. J. (2012). Social constraints, posttraumatic cognitions, and posttraumatic stress disorder in treatment-seeking trauma survivors: Evidence for a social-cognitive processing model. *Psychological Trauma: Theory, Research, Practice, and Policy*, *4*(4), 386–391. doi:10.1037/a0024362

Benight, C. C., & Harper, M. L. (2002). Coping self-efficacy perceptions as a mediator between acute stress response and long-term distress following natural disasters. *Journal of Traumatic Stress: Official Publication of The International Society for Traumatic Stress Studies*, *15*(3), 177–186. doi:10.1023/A:1015295025950 PMID:12092909

Benner, A. (1982, August). *Concerns cops have about shrinks.* Paper presented at the annual meeting of the American Psychological Association, San Francisco, CA.

Berg, A. M., Hem, E., Lau, B., Haseth, K., & Ekeberg, O. (2005). Stress in the Norwegian police service. *Occupational Medicine*, *55*(2), 113–120. doi:10.1093/occmed/kqi023 PMID:15757985

Berger, W., Coutinho, E. S. F., Figueira, I., Marques-Portella, C., Luz, M. P., Neylan, T. C., ... Mendlowicz, M. V. (2012). Rescuers at risk: A systematic review and meta-regression analysis of the worldwide current prevalence and correlates of PTSD in rescue workers. *Social Psychiatry and Psychiatric Epidemiology*, *47*(6), 1001–1011. doi:10.100700127-011-0408-2 PMID:21681455

Bernert, R. A., Kim, J. S., Iwata, N. G., & Perlis, M. L. (2015). Sleep disturbances as an evidence-based suicide risk factor. *Current Psychiatry Reports*, *17*(3), 15. doi:10.100711920-015-0554-4 PMID:25698339

Bisson, J. I., Jenkins, P. L., Alexander, J., & Bannister, C. (1997). Randomised controlled trial of psychological debriefing for victims of acute burn trauma. *The British Journal of Psychiatry*, *171*(1), 78–81. doi:10.1192/bjp.171.1.78 PMID:9328501

Bisson, J. I., McFarlane, A. C., Rose, S., Ruzek, J. I., & Watson, P. J. (2009). Psychological debriefing for adults. In E. B. Foa, T. M. Keane, M. J. Friedman, & J. A. Cohen (Eds.), *Effective treatments for ptsd (pp. 83 - 104)*. New York, NY: The Guilford Press.

Bohl, N. (1995). Measuring the effectiveness of CISD: A study. *Fire Engineering.*, *148*(8), 125–126.

Brauer, B. R. (2016). The fire and emergency services culture: Can it be changed? *Fire Engineering*. Retrieved from https://www.fireengineering.com/articles/print/volume-169/issue-8/features/the-fire-and-emergency-services-culture-can-it-be-changed.html

Brewin, C. R., Andrew, B., & Valentine, J. D. (2000). Meta-analysis of risk factors for posttraumatic stress disorder in trauma-exposed adults. *Journal of Consulting and Clinical Psychology*, *68*(5), 748–766. doi:10.1037/0022-006X.68.5.748 PMID:11068961

Brondolo, E., Wellington, R., Brady, N., Libby, D., & Brondolo, T. J. (2008). Mechanism and strategies for preventing post-traumatic stress disorder in forensic workers responding to mass fatality incidents. *Journal of Forensic and Legal Medicine*, *15*(2), 78–88. doi:10.1016/j.jflm.2007.04.007 PMID:18206823

Brucia, E. (2018). *The effects of residential treatment at the West Coast Post-trauma Retreat on police officers with PTSD* (Unpublished doctoral dissertation). Palo Alto University, Palo Alto, CA.

Brucia, E., Cordova, M. J., & Ruzek, J. I. (2017). Critical incident interventions: Crisis response and debriefings. In C. Mitchell & E. H. Dorian (Eds.), *Police psychology and its growing impact on modern law enforcement* (pp. 119–142). Hershey, PA: IGI Global. doi:10.4018/978-1-5225-0813-7.ch006

Bryant, R. A. (2007). Early intervention for post-traumatic stress disorder. *Early Intervention in Psychiatry*, *1*(1), 19–26. doi:10.1111/j.1751-7893.2007.00006.x PMID:21352105

Bryant, R. A., & Guthrie, R. M. (2005). Maladaptive appraisals as a risk factor for posttraumatic stress: A study of trainee firefighters. *Psychological Science*, *16*(10), 749–752. doi:10.1111/j.1467-9280.2005.01608.x PMID:16181434

Bryant, R. A., Harvey, A. G., Dang, S. T., Sackville, T., & Basten, C. (1998). Treatment of acute stress disorder: A comparison of cognitive-behavioral therapy and supportive counseling. *Journal of Consulting and Clinical Psychology*, *66*(5), 862–866. doi:10.1037/0022-006X.66.5.862 PMID:9803707

Brymer, M., Jacobs, A., Layne, C., Pynoos, R., Ruzek, J., Steinberg, A., & Watson, P. (2006). *Psychological First Aid: Field Operations Guide* (2nd ed.). National Child Traumatic Stress Network and National Center for PTSD.

Burke, T. W. (1995). Dispatcher stress. *FBI Law Enforcement Bulletin*, *64*(10), 1. Retrieved from https://paloaltou.idm.oclc.org/login?url=https://search.ebscohost.com/login.aspx?direct=true&db=a9h&AN=9510252868

Carlier, I. V. E., Lamberts, R. D., & Gersons, B. P. R. (1997). Risk factors for post-traumatic stress symptomatology in police officers: A prospective analysis. *The Journal of Nervous and Mental Disease*, *185*(8), 498–506. doi:10.1097/00005053-199708000-00004 PMID:9284863

Carlier, I. V. E., Lamberts, R. D., Van Uchelen, A. J., & Gersons, B. P. (1998). Disaster-related post-traumatic stress in police officers: A field study of the impact of debriefing. *Stress Medicine*, *14*(3), 143–148. doi:10.1002/(SICI)1099-1700(199807)14:3<143::AID-SMI770>3.0.CO;2-S

Carlier, I. V. E., Voerman, A. E., & Gersons, B. P. R. (2000). The influence of occupational debriefing on post-traumatic stress symptomatology in traumatized police officers. *The British Journal of Medical Psychology*, *73*(1), 87–98. doi:10.1348/000711200160327 PMID:10759053

Cassan, D. (2010). Police and socialisation in France and in England: How do they stand towards the community policing model? *Journal of Police Studies*, *3*(16), 243–260.

Centre for Occupational and Environmental Health. (2000). *Occupational Physicians Reporting Activity. Quarterly Report.* Manchester, UK: University of Manchester.

Chopko, B. A., Palmieri, P. A., & Adams, R. E. (2015). Critical incident history questionnaire replication: Frequency and severity of trauma exposure among officers from small and midsize police agencies. *Journal of Traumatic Stress*, *28*(2), 157–161. doi:10.1002/jts.21996 PMID:25808672

Christopher, M. S., Goerling, R. J., Rogers, B. S., Hunsinger, M., Baron, G., Bergman, A. L., & Zava, D. T. (2015). A pilot study evaluating the effectiveness of a mindfulness-based intervention on cortisol awakening response and health outcomes and law enforcement officers. *Journal of Police and Criminal Psychology*, *31*(1), 15–28. doi:10.100711896-015-9161-x

Cicognani, E., Pietrantoni, L., Palestini, L., & Prati, G. (2009). Emergency workers' quality of life: The protective role of sense of community, efficacy beliefs and coping strategies. *Social Indicators Research*, *94*(3), 449–463. doi:10.100711205-009-9441-x

C.O.P.S. (2018). *Concerns of police survivors.* Retrieved from https://www.concernsofpolicesurvivors.org

Corrigan, P. W., Watson, A. C., & Barr, L. (2006). The self-stigma of mental illness: Implications for self-esteem and self-efficacy. *Journal of Social and Clinical Psychology*, *25*(8), 875–884. doi:10.1521/jscp.2006.25.8.875

de Jong, J. T. V. M. (1995). Prevention of the consequences of man–made or natural disaster at the (inter)national, the community, the family and the individual level. In S. E. Hobfoll & M. W. de Vries (Eds.), *Extreme stress and communities: Impact and intervention* (pp. 207–229). Boston: Kluwer. doi:10.1007/978-94-015-8486-9_9

de Jong, J. T. V. M. (Ed.). (2002). *Trauma, war and violence: Public mental health in sociocultural context.* New York, NY: Plethnum-Kluwer. doi:10.1007/b109606

De Terte, I., Stephens, C., & Huddleston, L. (2014). The development of a three part model of psychological resilience. *Stress and Health*, *30*(5), 416–424. doi:10.1002mi.2625 PMID:25476966

Devilly, G. J., Gist, R., & Cotton, P. (2006). Ready! Fire! Aim! The status of psychological debriefing and therapeutic interventions: In the workplace and after disasters. *Review of General Psychology*, *10*(4), 318–345. doi:10.1037/1089-2680.10.4.318

DiGangi, J. A., Gomez, D., Mendoza, L., Jason, L. A., Keys, C. B., & Koenen, K. C. (2013). Pretrauma risk factors for posttraumatic stress disorder: A systematic review of the literature. *Clinical Psychology Review*, *33*(6), 728–744. doi:10.1016/j.cpr.2013.05.002 PMID:23792469

Dunnigan, R. (2012). *Emergency responders' trauma symptoms following the west coast post- trauma retreat recovery program* (Unpublished doctoral dissertation). Alliant International University, San Francisco, CA.

Ehlers, A., & Clark, D. M. (2000). A cognitive model of posttraumatic stress disorder. *Behaviour Research and Therapy*, *38*(4), 319–345. doi:10.1016/S0005-7967(99)00123-0 PMID:10761279

Engelhard, I. M., van den Hout, M. A., Weerts, J., Hox, J. J., & van Doornen, L. J. (2009). A prospective study of the relation between posttraumatic stress and physical health symptoms. *International Journal of Clinical and Health Psychology*, *9*(3).

Evans, R., Pistrang, N., & Billings, J. (2013). Police officers' experiences of supportive and unsupportive social interactions following traumatic incidents. *European Journal of Psychotraumatology*, *4*(1), 1–9. doi:10.3402/ejpt.v4i0.19696 PMID:23516046

Everly, G. S. Jr, Flannery, R. B. Jr, & Eyler, V. A. (2002). Critical incident stress management (CISM): A statistical review of the literature. *The Psychiatric Quarterly*, *73*(3), 171–182. doi:10.1023/A:1016068003615 PMID:12143079

Everly, G. S. Jr, Flannery, R. B. Jr, & Mitchell, J. T. (2000a). Critical incident stress management (CISM): A review of the literature. *Aggression and Violent Behavior*, *5*(1), 23–40. doi:10.1016/S1359-1789(98)00026-3

Everly, G. S., Lating, J. M., & Mitchell, J. T. (2000b). Innovations in group crisis intervention: Critical incident stress debriefing (CISD) and critical incident stress management (CISM). In A. Roberts (Ed.), *Crisis intervention handbook: Assessment, treatment, and research* (pp. 77–97). New York: Oxford University Press.

Everly, G. S., & Mitchell, J. T. (1999). *Critical Incident Stress Management (CISM): A New Era and Standard of Care in Crisis Intervention* (2nd ed.). Chevron Pub.

Fay, J., Kamena, M. D., Benner, A., & Buscho, A. (2006). A residential milieu treatment approach for first-responder trauma. *Traumatology*, *12*(3), 255–262. doi:10.1177/1534765606294991

Feldmann, T. B., & Johnson, P. W. (1992). The selfobject function of weapons: A self psychology examination. *The Journal of the American Academy of Psychoanalysis*, *20*(4), 561–576. doi:10.1521/jaap.1.1992.20.4.561 PMID:1291544

Flannery, R. B. (2015). Treating psychological trauma in first responders: A multi-modal paradigm. *The Psychiatric Quarterly*, *86*(2), 261–267. doi:10.100711126-014-9329-z PMID:25403791

Foa, E. B., Hembree, E. A., & Rothbaum, B. O. (2007). *Prolonged exposure therapy for ptsd: Emotional processing of traumatic experiences*. New York, NY: Oxford University Press.

Foa, E. B., & Rothbaum, B. O. (1998). *Treating the trauma of rape: Cognitive–behavioral therapy for PTSD*. New York: Guilford.

Forbes, D., Lewis, V., Varker, T., Phelps, A., Andrea, P., O'Donnell, M., ... Creamer, M. (2011). Psychological first aid following trauma: Implementation and evaluation framework for high-risk organizations. *Psychiatry, 74*(3), 224–239. doi:10.1521/psyc.2011.74.3.224 PMID:21916629

Fox, J. H., Burkle, F. M. Jr, Bass, J., Pia, F. A., Epstein, J. L., & Markenson, D. (2012). The effectiveness of psychological first aid as a disaster intervention tool: Research analysis of peer-reviewed literature from 1990 - 2010. *Disaster Medicine and Public Health Preparedness, 6*(3), 247–252. doi:10.1001/dmp.2012.39 PMID:23077267

Gene-Cos, N. (2006). Post-traumatic stress disorder: The management of PTSD in adults and children in primary and secondary care. *The Psychiatrist, 30*(9), 357–357.

Gillespie, E. (2017, May 14). *First responders' selfless service leaves them vulnerable to PTSD's toll: Programs aim to help those who face trauma daily.* Retrieved from https://www.columbian.com/news/2017/may/14/first-responders-selfless-service-leaves-them-vulnerable-to-ptsds-toll/

Gilmartin, K. (2002). *Emotional survival for law enforcement: A guide for officers and their families.* Tucson, AZ: E-S Press.

Goenjian, A. K., Karayan, I., Pynoos, R. S., Minassian, D., Najarian, L. M., Steinberg, A. M., & Fairbanks, L. A. (1997). Outcome of psychotherapy among early adolescents after trauma. *The American Journal of Psychiatry, 154*(4), 536–542. doi:10.1176/ajp.154.4.536 PMID:9090342

Goenjian, A. K., Walling, D., Steinberg, A. M., Karavan, I., Najarian, L. M., & Pynoos, R. (2005). A prospective study of posttraumatic stress and depressive reactions among treated and untreated adolescents 5 years after a catastrophic disaster. *The American Journal of Psychiatry, 162*(12), 2302–2308. doi:10.1176/appi.ajp.162.12.2302 PMID:16330594

Golden, L. L., Jones, R. T., & Donlon, K. (2014). Delayed treatment seeking following the April 16th shootings at Virginia Tech: Impact on a first responder. *Clinical Case Studies, 13*(5), 391–404. doi:10.1177/1534650113512174

Goldstein, D. B. (2005). A comparison of utilization of peer support services and perceived stigma within the Vermont State Police. *Forensic Examiner, 14*(3), 44–48.

Graf, F. A. (1986). The relationship between social support and occupational stress among police officers. *Journal of Police Science and Administration, 14*(3), 178–186.

Grauwiler, P., Barocas, B., & Mills, L. G. (2008). Police peer support programs: Current knowledge and practice. *International Journal of Emergency Mental Health, 10*(1), 27–38. PMID:18546757

Haase, J., Britt, T., Coward, D., Leidy, N., & Penn, P. E. (1992). Simultaneous concept analysis of spiritual perspective, hope, acceptance, and self-transcendence. *Image--the Journal of Nursing Scholarship, 24*(2), 141–147. doi:10.1111/j.1547-5069.1992.tb00239.x PMID:1601456

Haugen, P. T., Evces, M., & Weiss, D. S. (2012). Treating posttraumatic stress disorder in first responders: A systematic review. *Clinical Psychology Review*, *32*(5), 370–380. doi:10.1016/j.cpr.2012.04.001 PMID:22561967

Haugen, P. T., McCrillis, A. M., Smid, G. E., & Nijdam, M. J. (2017). Mental health stigma and barriers to mental health care for first responders: A systematic review and meta- analysis. *Journal of Psychiatric Research*, *94*, 218–229. doi:10.1016/j.jpsychires.2017.08.001 PMID:28800529

Hobfoll, S., Watson, P., Bell, C., Bryant, R., Brymer, M. J., Friedman, M. J., ... Ursano, R. J. (2007). Five essential elements of immediate and mid-term mass trauma intervention: Empirical evidence. *Psychiatry*, *70*(4), 283–315. doi:10.1521/psyc.2007.70.4.283 PMID:18181708

Hobfoll, S. E., Briggs-Phillips, M., & Stines, L. R. (2003). Fact or artifact: The relationship of hope to a caravan of resources. In R. Jacoby & G. Keinan (Eds.), *Between stress and hope: From a disease-centered to a health-centered perspective* (pp. 81–104). Westport, CT: Praeger.

Hobfoll, S. E., Spielberger, C. D., Breznitz, S., Figley, C., Folkman, S., Lepper-Green, B., ... van der Kolk, B. (1991). War-related stress: Addressing the stress of war and other traumatic events. *The American Psychologist*, *46*(8), 848–855. doi:10.1037/0003-066X.46.8.848 PMID:1928937

Hoge, C. W., Terhakopian, A., Castro, C. A., Messer, S. C., & Engel, C. C. (2007). Association of posttraumatic stress disorder with somatic symptoms, health care visits, and absenteeism among Iraq War veterans. *The American Journal of Psychiatry*, *164*(1), 150–153. doi:10.1176/ajp.2007.164.1.150 PMID:17202557

International Association of Chiefs of Police (IACP). (2016). *Peer support guidelines*. Retrieved from https://www.theiacp.org/sites/default/files/all/p-r/Psych-PeerSupportGuidelines.pdf

Janoff–Bulman, R. (1992). *Shattered assumptions: Toward a new psychology of trauma*. New York: Free Press.

Kamena, M. D., Gentz, D., Hays, V., Bohl-Penrod, N., & Greene, L. W. (2011). Peer support teams fill an emotional void in law enforcement agencies. *The Police Chief*, *78*(8), 80–84.

Kearns, M. C., Ressler, K. J., Zatzick, D., & Rothbaum, B. O. (2012). Early intervention for PTSD: A review. *Depression and Anxiety*, *29*(10), 833–842. doi:10.1002/da.21997 PMID:22941845

Kessler, R. C., Sonnega, A., Bromet, E., Hughes, M., & Nelson, C. B. (1995). Posttraumatic stress disorder in the national comorbidity survey. *Archives of General Psychiatry*, *52*(12), 1048–1060. doi:10.1001/archpsyc.1995.03950240066012 PMID:7492257

Kirmeyer, S. L., & Dougherty, T. W. (1988). Work load, tension, and coping: Moderating effects of supervisor support. *Personnel Psychology*, *41*(1), 125–139. doi:10.1111/j.1744-6570.1988.tb00635.x

Kirschman, E. (2007). *I love a cop: What police families need to know* (Rev. ed.). New York, NY: The Guilford Press.

Kirschman, E., Kamena, M. D., & Fay, J. (2014). *Counseling cops: What clinicians need to know*. New York, NY: The Guilford Press.

Kleim, B., & Westphal, M. (2011). Mental health in first responders: A review and recommendation for prevention and intervention strategies. *Traumatology*, *17*(4), 17–24. doi:10.1177/1534765611429079

Klimley, K. E., Van Hasselt, V. B., & Stripling, A. M. (2018). Posttraumatic stress disorder in police, firefighters, and emergency dispatchers. *Aggression and Violent Behavior*, *43*, 33–44. doi:10.1016/j.avb.2018.08.005

Komarovskaya, I., Maguen, S., McCaslin, S. E., Metzler, T. J., Madan, A., Brown, A. D., ... Marmar, C. R. (2011). The impact of killing and injuring others on mental health symptoms among police officers. *Journal of Psychiatric Research*, *45*(10), 1332–1336. doi:10.1016/j.jpsychires.2011.05.004 PMID:21658717

Larson, S. L., Eyerman, J., Foster, M. S., & Gfroerer, J. C. (2007). *Worker substance use and workplace policies and programs (DHHS Publication No. SMA 07 – 4273, Analytic Series A-29)*. Rockville, MD: Substance Abuse and Mental Health Services Administration, Office of Applied Studies.

Lepore, S., & Revenson, T. (2007). Social constraints on disclosure and adjustment to cancer. *Social and Personality Psychology Compass*, *1*(1), 313–333. doi:10.1111/j.1751-9004.2007.00013.x

Lepore, S. J. (2001). A social–cognitive processing model of emotional adjustment to cancer. In A. Baum & B. L. Andersen (Eds.), *Psychosocial interventions for cancer* (pp. 99–116). Washington, DC: American Psychological Association. doi:10.1037/10402-006

Liedenbaum, C. (2011). *Policing between task and implement: A comparative study of the basic police in the Netherlands and North Rhine-Wesphalia*. Nijmegen: WLP.

Litz, B. T. (2008). Early intervention for trauma: Where are we and where do we need to go? A commentary. *Journal of Traumatic Stress*, *21*(6), 503–506. doi:10.1002/jts.20373 PMID:19107726

Litz, B. T., Gray, M. J., Bryant, R. A., & Adler, A. B. (2002). Early intervention for trauma: Current status and future directions. *Clinical Psychology: Science and Practice*, *9*(2), 112–134. doi:10.1093/clipsy.9.2.112

Luszczynska, A., Benight, C. C., & Cieslak, R. (2009). Self-efficacy and health-related outcomes of collective trauma: A systematic review. *European Psychologist*, *14*(1), 51–62. doi:10.1027/1016-9040.14.1.51

Maguen, S., Metzler, T. J., McCaslin, S. E., Inslicht, S. S., Henn-Haase, C., Neylan, T. C., & Marmar, C. R. (2009). Routine work environment stress and PTSD symptoms in police officers. *The Journal of Nervous and Mental Disease*, *197*(10), 754–760. doi:10.1097/NMD.0b013e3181b975f8 PMID:19829204

Malcolm, A. S., Seaton, J., Perera, A., Sheehan, D. C., & Van Hasselt, V. B. (2005). Critical incident stress debriefing and law enforcement: An evaluative review. *Brief Treatment and Crisis Intervention*, *5*(3), 261–278. doi:10.1093/brief-treatment/mhi019

Marchand, A., Nadeau, C., Beaulieu-Prévost, D., Boyer, R., & Martin, M. (2015). Predictors of posttraumatic stress disorder among police officers: A prospective study. *Psychological Trauma: Theory, Research, Practice, and Policy*, *7*(3), 212–221. doi:10.1037/a0038780 PMID:25793514

Marin, A. (2012). *In the line of duty: Investigation into how the Ontario Provincial Police and the Ministry of Community Safety and Correctional Services have addressed operational stress injuries affecting police officers*. Ontario Ombudsman.

Marks, M. R., Bowers, C., DePesa, N. S., Trachik, B., Deavers, F. E., & James, N. T. (2017). REACT: A paraprofessional training program for first responders – A pilot study. *Bulletin of the Menninger Clinic*, *81*(2), 150–166. doi:10.1521/bumc.2017.81.2.150 PMID:28609149

Marmar, C. R., McCaslin, S. E., Metzler, T. J., Best, S., Weiss, D. S., Fagan, J., & Neylan, T. (2006). Predictors of posttraumatic stress in police and other first responders. *Annals of the New York Academy of Sciences*, *1071*(1), 1–18. doi:10.1196/annals.1364.001 PMID:16891557

McHugh, J. (2019). *Yoga mats in the squad room.* Retrieved from https://psmag.com/magazine/yoga-mats-in-the-squad-room

Meyer, E. C., Zimering, R., Daly, E., Knight, J., Kamholz, B. W., & Gulliver, S. B. (2012). Predictors of posttraumatic stress disorder and other psychological symptoms in trauma-exposed firefighters. *Psychological Services*, *9*(1), 1–15. doi:10.1037/a0026414 PMID:22449083

Mitchell, J. T. (1983). When disaster strikes: The critical incident stress debriefing process. *Journal of Emergency Medical Services*, *8*(1), 36–39. PMID:10258348

Mitchell, J. T., & Everly, G. S. (2001). *Critical Incident Stress Management: Basic Group Crisis Interventions*. Ellicott City, MD: International Critical Incident Stress Foundation.

National Institute of Mental Health (NIMH). (2002). *Mental health and mass violence: Evidence-based early psychological intervention for victims/survivors of mass violence. A workshop to reach consensus on best practices. (NIH Publication No. 02- 5138).* Washington, DC: U.S. Government Printing Office.

O'Hara, A. (2012, August). Badge of life: Police mental health. *Badge of Life Newsletter,* 1–3.

Ogle, C. M., Rubin, D. C., & Siegler, I. C. (2015). The relation between insecure attachment and posttraumatic stress: Early life versus adulthood traumas. *Psychological Trauma: Theory, Research, Practice, and Policy*, *7*(4), 324–332. doi:10.1037/tra0000015 PMID:26147517

Ozer, E. J., Best, S. R., Lipsey, T. L., & Weiss, D. S. (2008). Predictors of posttraumatic stress disorder and symptoms in adults: A meta-analysis. *Psychological Trauma: Theory, Research, Practice, and Policy*, *S*(1), 3–36. doi:10.1037/1942-9681.S.1.3

Papazoglou, K., & Tuttle, B. M. (2018). Fighting police trauma: Practical approaches to addressing psychological needs of officers. *SAGE Open*, *8*(3). doi:10.1177/2158244018794794

Phillips, C. J., LeardMann, C. A., Gumbs, G. R., & Smith, B. (2010). Risk factors for posttraumatic stress disorder among deployed US male marines. *BMC Psychiatry*, *10*(52), 1–11. PMID:20579379

PoliceOne. (2017, January 30). *VA cops decompress in "quiet rooms."* Retrieved from https://www.policeone.com/health-fitness/articles/284889006-Va-cops-decompress-in-quiet-rooms/

Regehr, C., Goldberg, G., Glancy, G. D., & Knott, T. (2002). Posttraumatic symptoms and disability in paramedics. *Canadian Journal of Psychiatry*, *47*(10), 953–958. doi:10.1177/070674370204701007 PMID:12553131

Renaud, E. F. (2008). The attachment characteristics of combat veterans with PTSD. *Traumatology*, *14*(3), 1–12. doi:10.1177/1534765608319085

Richmond, R. L., Wodak, A., Kehoe, L., & Heather, N. (1998). How healthy are the police? A survey of life-style factors. *Addiction (Abingdon, England)*, *93*(11), 1729–1737. doi:10.1046/j.1360-0443.1998.9311172910.x PMID:9926535

Robinson, R. C., & Mitchell, J. T. (1993). Evaluation of psychological debriefings. *Journal of Traumatic Stress*, *6*(3), 367–382. doi:10.1002/jts.2490060307

Rose, S. C., Bisson, J., Churchill, R., & Wessely, S. (2002). Psychological debriefing for preventing post traumatic stress disorder (PTSD). *Cochrane Database of Systematic Reviews*, (2): CD000560. doi:10.1002/14651858.CD000560 PMID:12076399

Royle, L., Keenan, P., & Farrell, D. (2009). Issues of stigma for first responders accessing support for post traumatic stress. *International Journal of Emergency Mental Health*, *11*(2), 79–86. PMID:19927494

Ruzek, J. I., Brymer, M. J., Jacobs, A. K., Layne, C. M., Vernberg, E. M., & Watson, P. J. (2007). Psychological first aid. *Journal of Mental Health Counseling*, *29*(1), 17–49. doi:10.17744/mehc.29.1.5racqxjueafabgwp

Sampson, R. J., Raudenbush, S. W., & Earls, F. (1997). Neighborhoods and violent crime: A multilevel study of collective efficacy. *Science*, *277*(5328), 918–924. doi:10.1126cience.277.5328.918 PMID:9252316

Samuels, S. (2018). *COPLINE: National law enforcement officers hotline.* Retrieved from http://www.copline.org

Sheehan, D. C., Everly, G. S., & Langlieb, A. (2004). Current best practices coping with major critical incidents. *FBI L. Enforcement Bulletin*, *73*(9), 1–13.

Stanley, I. H., Hom, M. A., Chu, C., Dougherty, S. P., Gallyer, A. J., Spencer-Thomas, S., ... Joiner, T. E. (2018). Perceptions of belongingness and social support attenuate PTSD symptom severity among firefighters: A multistudy investigation. *Psychological Services*. doi:10.1037er0000240 PMID:29595287

Stanley, I. H., Hom, M. A., & Joiner, T. E. (2016). A systematic review of suicidal thoughts and behaviors among police officers, firefighters, EMTs, and paramedics. *Clinical Psychology Review*, *44*, 25–44. doi:10.1016/j.cpr.2015.12.002 PMID:26719976

Sterud, T., Hem, E., Ekeberg, O., & Lau, B. (2007). Occupational stress and alcohol use: A study of two nationwide samples of operational police and ambulance personnel in Norway. *Journal of Studies on Alcohol and Drugs*, *68*(6), 896–904. doi:10.15288/jsad.2007.68.896 PMID:17960308

Terpstra, J., & Schaap, D. (2013). Police culture, stress conditions and working styles. *European Journal of Criminology*, *10*(1), 59–73. doi:10.1177/1477370812456343

Tuckey, M. R. (2007). Issues in the debriefing debate for the emergency services: Moving research outcomes forward. *Clinical Psychology: Science and Practice*, *14*(2), 106–116. doi:10.1111/j.1468-2850.2007.00069.x

Uhernik, J. A., & Husson, M. A. (2009). Psychological first aid: An evidence informed approach for acute disaster behavioral health response. *Compelling counseling interventions. VISTAS*, *200*(9), 271–280.

Vallieres, A., Azaiez, A., Moreau, V., LeBlanc, M., & Morin, C. M. (2014). Insomnia in shift work. *Sleep Medicine*, *15*(12), 1440–1448. doi:10.1016/j.sleep.2014.06.021 PMID:25277664

Van der Kolk, B. A., & Saporta, J. (1993). Biological response to psychic trauma. In J. P. Wilson & B. Raphael (Eds.), *International handbook of traumatic stress syndromes* (pp. 25–33). Boston, MA: Springer. doi:10.1007/978-1-4615-2820-3_2

Van Emmerik, A. A., Kamphuis, J. H., Hulsbosch, A. M., & Emmelkamp, P. M. (2002). Single session debriefing after psychological trauma: A meta-analysis. *Lancet*, *360*(9335), 766–771. doi:10.1016/S0140-6736(02)09897-5 PMID:12241834

Van Orden, K. A., Witte, T. K., Cukrowicz, K. C., Braithwaite, S. R., Selby, E. A., & Joiner, T. E. (2010). The interpersonal theory of suicide. *Psychological Review*, *117*(2), 575–600. doi:10.1037/a0018697 PMID:20438238

Violanti, J. M., Andrew, M. E., Mnatsakanova, A., Hartley, T. A., Fekedulegn, D., & Burchfiel, C. M. (2016). Correlates of hopelessness in the high suicide risk police occupation. *Police Practice and Research*, *17*(5), 408–419. doi:10.1080/15614263.2015.1015125 PMID:26752981

Violanti, J. M., & Drylie, J. J. (2008). *Copicide: Concepts, cases, and controversies of suicide by cop*. Springfield, IL: Charles C. Thomas Publisher, LTD.

Waters, J. A., & Ussery, W. (2007). Police stress: History, contributing factors, symptoms, and interventions. *Policing: An International Journal of Police Strategies & Management*, *30*(2), 169–188. doi:10.1108/13639510710753199

Weiss, D. S., Brunet, A., Best, S. R., Metzler, T. J., Liberman, A., Pole, N., & Marmar, C. R. (2010). Frequency and severity approaches to indexing exposure to trauma: The critical incident history questionnaire for police officers. *Journal of Traumatic Stress*, *23*(6), 734–743. doi:10.1002/jts.20576 PMID:21171134

Wessely, S., & Deahl, M. (2003). Psychological debriefing is a waste of time. *The British Journal of Psychiatry*, *183*(1), 12–14. doi:10.1192/bjp.183.1.12 PMID:12835237

Wester, S. R., Arndt, D., Sedivy, S. K., & Arndt, L. (2010). Male police officers and stigma associated with counseling: The role of anticipated risks, anticipated benefits and gender role conflict. *Psychology of Men & Masculinity*, *11*(4), 286–302. doi:10.1037/a0019108

Woodhouse, S., Ayers, S., & Field, A. P. (2015). The relationship between adult attachment style and post-traumatic stress symptoms: A meta-analysis. *Journal of Anxiety Disorders*, *35*, 103–117. doi:10.1016/j.janxdis.2015.07.002 PMID:26409250

Chapter 9
The HEROES Project:
Building Mental Resilience in First Responders

Alex R. Thornton
Indiana University, Kelley School of Business, USA

Daniel M. Blumberg
https://orcid.org/0000-0001-8925-8689
Alliant International University, USA

Konstantinos Papazoglou
Yale School of Medicine, USA

Luciano Giromini
https://orcid.org/0000-0002-9540-4803
University of Turin, Italy

ABSTRACT

The chapter introduces the HEROES Project, an online training resource that develops mental resilience. The goal is to provide the reader with insight into a resource that can be used as an adjunct to employee assistance programs, critical incident stress debriefing, and counseling. The HEROES Project is the first virtual training course that combines the therapeutic tools of clinical and organizational psychology and provides first responders access to a self-driven wellness program. This respects many first responders' preference for anonymous and private self-care, while the autonomous nature of the training reinforces for all first responders that they are ultimately responsible for maintaining their own wellness.

DOI: 10.4018/978-1-5225-9803-9.ch009

PROBLEM STATEMENT

In the course of their careers, first responders are routinely and repeatedly exposed to direct and vicarious traumatic events (Kleim & Westphal, 2011). The stress resulting from such repetitive exposure to trauma can cause a number of physical and emotional challenges, and if left unchecked, the symptoms can lead to changes in behavior. Many of these problems can be ameliorated through skills training, including techniques designed to boost resilience. Skills training, such as use of firearms, emergency vehicle operations, and defensive tactics, typically requiring updates and re-certifications at regular intervals, has long been a mandate for first responders (Gjefle & Vikari, 2012). However, training programs that treat mental resilience as a perishable skill, which requires intermittent training, are not afforded the same level of organizational commitment. The HEROES Project fills this void by helping first responders develop the skills to effectively withstand the negative implications of workplace stress and repetitive exposure to trauma. The intervening influence of mental resilience in the face of critical incidents provides first responders with coping strategies for handling routine and traumatic stressors.

First responders are often reluctant to seek help when experiencing reactions to work-related stressors (Hyland et al., 2015). Common objections to mental wellness initiatives include stigma, fear of receiving a diagnosis, and discomfort with traditional therapeutic approaches to managing the stressors of the job (Wester, Arndt, Sedivy, & Arndt, 2010). The HEROES Project takes a proactive, preventative perspective of critical incident stress management and provides first responders with resilience training through a series of independent online training sessions. Pulling from multiple psychological disciplines, the curriculum is based on the development of Positive Psychological Capital (PsyCap) and utilizes the tools of Cognitive Behavior Therapy (CBT).

The present chapter introduces the HEROES Project, an online training resource that develops mental resilience. The goal is to provide the reader with insight into a resource that can be used as an adjunct to employee assistance programs, critical incident stress debriefing, and counseling. The HEROES Project is the first virtual training course that combines the therapeutic tools of clinical and organizational psychology and provides first responders access to a self-driven wellness program. This respects many first responders' preference for anonymous and private self-care, while the autonomous nature of the training reinforces for all first responders that they are ultimately responsible for maintaining their own wellness.

POSITIVE PSYCHOLOGICAL CAPITAL

Successfully staffing a first-response organization, in a perfect world, means finding top performers who excel at building relationships in the community and who are proficient problem-solvers. Traditionally, meeting those expectations meant honing in on human capital, recognized widely as the level of education and experience an employee brings to the job (Seligman & Csikszentmihalyi, 2000). However, in high-stress and multifaceted positions where employees are expected to execute the mission autonomously and are likely to be exposed repeatedly to direct and vicarious trauma, proactive measures must be taken to ensure individual wellness. The creation of advanced learning content requires enhancing the mental characteristics that research has shown have the most powerful influence over the body's response to fear and uncertainty (Hetrick, Purcell, Garner, & Parslow, 2010).

An attitude of self-development is necessary to strengthen and maintain those skills; such a mindset looks beyond "who you are," and focuses instead on "who you are becoming" or ultimately who your "best self" is (Luthans, Youssef, & Avolio, 2006, p. 20). The development of PsyCap encourages this progressive perspective and is characterized by:

(1) having confidence (self-efficacy) to take on and put in the necessary effort to succeed at challenging tasks; (2) making a positive attribution (optimism) about succeeding now and in the future; (3) persevering toward goals and, when necessary, redirecting paths to goals (hope) in order to succeed; and (4) when beset by problems and adversity, sustaining and bouncing back and even beyond (resilience) to attain success (Luthans, Youssef, et al., 2006, p. 3).

Constructing PsyCap involves character-building techniques that shift the mindset away from doing what has always been done toward a consistent practice of self-improvement with an eye on what will be needed to meet future expectations. Anticipating needs requires the identification of strategic, actionable goals, expected and unexpected roadblocks to achievement of those goals, building relationships that will provide resources when challenges arise, and crafting contingency plans that ensure forward progress, even in small-win capacities. Through an objective personal evaluation process, areas for improvement are identified and, with the assistance of respected peers, weaknesses are fleshed out and turned into strengths.

The impact of PsyCap characteristics extends beyond confidence handling ambiguous situations into an attitude of flexible leadership in the midst of critical incidents. High levels of PsyCap have been connected to elevated emotional intelligence and organizational commitment, and a decrease in stress and anxiety for employees in obscure and ever-changing environments (Newman, Ucbasaran, Zhu, & Hirst, 2014). The influencing power of one person with high PsyCap levels reaches well beyond his or her immediate sphere of influence (Luthans, Avey, Avolio, & Peterson, 2010) and, over time, has been proven to positively impact the PsyCap levels of others.

COGNITIVE BEHAVIOR THERAPY

Consistently, CBT is viewed as the most efficacious traditional psychological treatment of depression and a host of anxiety disorders (Stirman et al., 2013). As such, it is a logical starting place for ensuring that the HEROES curriculum adheres to the therapeutic process and uses the tools that place self-improvement into the hands of the client. At its core, CBT is talk therapy. Therapists guide their patients through activities with the goal of identifying and replacing faulty thought patterns and feelings, which tend to negatively influence behavior and the meaning applied to various situations ("Beck Institute for Cognitive Behavior Therapy," 2015). Common tools used by CBT therapists include: 1) formulation, which is a map that provides visual current-state assessments and goals for the future; 2) journaling; 3) homework assignments; 4) self-help books; and 5) behavioral experiments whereby patients identify problems between thoughts, feelings, and behaviors. This approach has effectively treated numerous mental health disorders including PTSD, anxiety, substance abuse, and depression.

In the HEROES Project, the fundamentals of the CBT therapeutic process partner closely with those of PsyCap and are echoed in the curriculum. Each lesson includes a homework assignment requiring that the material be applied and practiced. Journaling, writing impact statements, and building a strategic goal map align with the homework component used in CBT to help clients personalize the lessons learned. By training first responders to develop the specific characteristics of hope, self-efficacy, resilience, optimism, empathy, and socialization, the best of PsyCap in organizational psychology and CBT in clinical psychology combine to provide wellness resources.

This interdisciplinary training program adheres to the wisdom of more than 40 years of psychology. The foundation that makes CBT successful was matched with the core characteristics built in PsyCap. Additionally, the active learning tools used within both disciplines were applied to the curriculum to allow first responders the ability to apply knowledge and to measure their own progress. As such the HEROES Project is a resource that, in its design, meets first responders where they are. The proactive, preventative nature of this training program makes it a solid choice for first responders who are just starting out in the profession, have recently experienced a traumatic event, or who are facing a major life change. That the course is completed remotely online sets it apart from every other type of proactive resilience training.

HEROES: TRAINING COMPONENTS

Each online lesson corresponds to one of the letters in the HEROES project: Hope, Efficacy, Resilience, Optimism, Empathy, and Socialization. Use of the word *project* was also deliberate. Participants start a project in lesson one and continue it throughout the training. They are then encouraged after conclusion of the training to regularly update it over the course of their careers. Each training activity adds an essential element to the project, challenging trainees to apply lessons to their own lives.

The training is self-paced. Trainees are able to take as much time as they want to critically evaluate and apply the learning outcomes. Each lesson includes a video lecture delivered by the project author with downloadable lecture notes focused on learning outcomes. Trainees are virtually introduced Mitch Kazjer, a police officer who survived being shot on the job, and are provided with short video clips throughout the training, wherein he details his journey to resilience. Additional resources such as podcasts, books, and articles that are particularly relevant to the development of resilience are made available to the trainees as adjuncts to the lesson materials. At the conclusion of the training program, first responders receive a certificate of achievement.

The HEROES Curriculum

Hope

The trigger point for seeking professional help in many CBT patients is experiencing hopelessness, feeling demoralized, or living with a sense of fog or confusion (Von Brachel, Teismann, Feider, & Margraf, 2019). From the therapist's perspective, the central goal is foster hope in patients. Developing hope requires distinguishing between wishful thinking and goals that can be acted upon (Niles, In, & Amundson, 2014). Snyder's (2002) hope theory, a foundation of traditional psychological treatment for hopeless patients, clearly specifies that hope cannot be based on fantasy but must instead specify goals with a plan for attainment.

Action-oriented hope in PsyCap is developed when a person goes beyond setting goals by tapping into personal motivation to achieve (Niles, Yoon, Balın, & Amundson, 2010). Snyder (2000, 2002) clarified that there are two types of hope: dispositional and state. Dispositional hope endures while state hope is emotionally based and focused on fleeting desires. The goal-setting exercise in the HEROES Project clarifies the difference between each and requires that trainees evaluate goals to determine whether they are emotional (state-like) or realistic (dispositional). People with high levels of hope focus on health-maintenance, cope well when faced with trauma and adversity, build relationships with people close to them, are less likely to use avoidance to deal with challenges, and experience less long-term anxiety and depression (Rand & Cheavens, 2009).

On a large wall or cork board, trainees create wellness quadrants from left to right, reading Mental, Emotional, Spiritual, Physical, Professional, and Financial. Once the foundation is crafted, then trainees consider what their potential is within each quadrant. In short, they are tasked with answering the question, "What achievement in this area of my life would make me feel like I am meeting my potential?" The answers are then translated into specific, measurable, attainable, realistic, and timely goals. The act of placing the goals on the board solidifies in the trainees' minds what to reach for and focus on as the training progresses.

Self-Efficacy

As early as the days of Albert Bandura's Social Cognitive Theory (1997, 2005), the construct with perhaps the most extensive research support is efficacy. In CBT, self-efficacy is defined as the degree of conviction a person has that s/he has the capacity to successfully execute the behavior needed to produce a specific outcome (Brown et al., 2014). A number of studies have shown the influence that self-efficacy has on performance (Sadri & Robertson, 1993; Stajkovic & Luthans, 1998). Stajkovic and Luthans define self-efficacy in PsyCap as "the individual's conviction or confidence about his or her abilities to mobilize the motivation, cognitive resources or courses of action needed to successfully execute a specific task within a given context" (Stajkovic & Luthans, 1998, p. 66).

Efficacy stands out from the other constructs in HEROES, due to the specific in-task focus. Low levels of efficacy indicate that a person believes that efforts to overcome challenges are futile, a belief which increases anxiety and stress (Bandura, 2007). Adversely, those with high levels of self-efficacy view challenges as surmountable, provided they have the ability, necessary resources, and are dedicated to putting forth the necessary effort to reach goals.

Developing self-efficacy is accomplished through the use of mastery experiences, behavior modeling, psychological/physiological arousal, and social persuasion (Bandura, 1997) Combining CBT and PsyCap perspectives, self-efficacy develops by returning to the project started in lesson one on hope. Trainees examine the goals they set and begin to develop in-role confidence by first identifying small wins along the journey to goal-attainment that, when met, will add to their motivation moving forward. Each of these goals adheres to at least one of Bandura's (1977) four developmental requirements of self-efficacy. To meet a mastery experience, for instance, the small win needs practice to perfect the behavior. To adhere to the social persuasion component, trainees receive external encouragement from someone who believes they can do anything to which they have set their minds. No matter to which of Bandura's developmental areas the small win adheres, they must stipulate which resources are most likely to help motivate them to stay the course.

Resilience

Resilience in CBT is defined as persistence in the face of roadblocks, accepting circumstances that cannot be changed, and adapting to challenges so that it is possible to bounce back from major stressors (Bonanno, 2004). The historic attitude taken in CBT about developing resilience was centered on the maintenance of treatment gains and the management of a potential for relapse (Hammond, 2000). Recent advances in the understanding of resilience have resulted in changes to the way resilience is viewed and the types of CBT treatments applied to develop it (Padesky, 2006). Resilience is now understood to be a preventative characteristic, providing a buffer protecting against the physical and psychological health consequences of distressing experiences (Yi, Vitaliano, Smith, Yi, & Weinger, 2008). Resilience comes naturally for some and requires learning and practice in others, but fluctuates throughout life depending on the effort put in to develop and maintain it (Kuyken, Padesky, & Dudley, 2009). The four-step process to develop resilience includes the acknowledgement of strengths, the creation of a personal model of resilience, application to life challenges, and practice (Padesky & Mooney, 2012).

Resilience in PsyCap is somewhat different than traditional definitions. It is defined as a person's ability to rebound from conflict, failure, increased responsibility, setbacks, progress, and positive events, into a stronger strategic place than before (Block & Kremen, 1996; Luthans, 2002; Masten & Garmezy, 1985). Because first responders are repeatedly exposed to incredible challenges, the PsyCap definition of resilience, which includes the use of past experiences to build character, provides an excellent framework. Identifying positive emotions associated with the successful negotiation of past experiences – whether they were positive or negative – increases resilience in the face of negativity (Tugade & Fredrickson, 2004). Considered the most valuable positive resource in stressful, turbulent workplace environments, resilience prepares people to transition smoothly, adjust, and rebound during times of organizational upheaval (Makawatsakul & Kleiner, 2003).

Within the HEROES Project, building resilience begins by identifying resilient beliefs (e.g., "I have overcome difficulty before") and constructs behaviors that build on those beliefs. In HEROES, resilience hinges on the ability to objectively evaluate past life experiences, pulling out the positive emotions felt as a result of overcoming challenges and creating a plan for how to respond if faced with a similar event in the future. To do this, trainees are tasked with engaging the help of respected peers to evaluate past experiences. The purpose of the evaluation is: 1) to objectively identify what was done well (personal strengths) and what could have been done differently to effect a more positive outcome (creating a personal model of resilience); 2) to decide how to apply the past to the future (application); and, 3) to participate as an active observer in future mastery exercises (practice).

Optimism

In CBT, optimism is planning process that, when acted upon, results in the kind of intentional grit that drives a person forward even in the face of challenging circumstances (Chaves, Lopez-Gomez, Hervas, & Vazquez, 2019). The distinctive difference between CBT's definition and the way optimism is viewed as a PsyCap resource is specific to the longevity of the perspective (Luthans, Avey, Avolio, Norman, & Combs, 2006). In PsyCap, optimism is built through the planning and execution of small wins. By focusing optimism on an incremental task, trainees are not being expected to develop an overarching positive view of the world. By removing the worldview component of optimism, HEROES training continues to promote achievement and confidence by task. This mentality furthers the value placed on small wins and reinforces the fact that building mental resilience is a journey.

Through the PsyCap lens, optimists approach problems and challenges and handle adversity differently than pessimists (Luthans et al., 2010). Instead of simply expecting the best, they put plans in place that require them to acknowledge what might cause failure and then gather resources to apply to a situation that would increase the likelihood of success. Learning optimism leads to the belief that more effort will change the outcome. This attitude reflects a tenacious problem solver who, when faced with failure, sees it as temporary and continues working until the goal is accomplished. When one strategy fails, seek wisdom to build a new one. If that strategy does not result in the intended outcome, determine why and begin again with the optimistic belief that a solution can be found.

Empathy

Many research studies have evaluated empathy, generally defined as a person's sensitivity and ability to understand the mental states of others, as a necessary characteristic in public service (Parra, 2013). Empathy allows a person to see the perspective of others (Chenault, Martin, & Matusiak, 2016). An underlying theme in the research has been whether empathy is a trait or a developable characteristic (Grant, 2014). Recent advances in psychology reveal that empathy develops early in some people, but requires time to mature to its full capacity (Singer, 2006). In others, empathy is cultivated through a variety of life experiences (Oxley, 2011).

In the HEROES project, trainees are exposed to the concept of tactical empathy through the use of research and a podcast interview with criminal justice expert, Dr. Michael Schlosser (Kosor, 2019). Mastering the art of tactical empathy requires the employment of empathy phrases like, "I understand where you're coming from. If I were in your situation, I'd probably be upset too." The learning activity in this section of the course personalizes the value of empathy through a written impact statement. Trainees are tasked with writing about an event in the past that caused them great distress, and then evaluating that event to uncover what they had control over, what was beyond their control, and what their emotional reactions entailed. The goal is to broaden self-awareness to a point where one can tap into past experiences in order to empathize with those going through difficulties.

Socialization

The psychological definition of socialization is found in the act of sharing, either in written format or verbally (Kazantzis & Dattilio, 2010). Sharing past traumatic experiences allowed trainees to promote a culture of awareness about the impact of trauma while building relationships that will help with coping strategies in the future. In the CBT context, the act of sharing often takes place with a counselor present or through a homework assignment given by the therapist to share with a loved one. The PsyCap approach allows for socialization to take place with anyone to whom (a) the learner is comfortable revealing personal information, and (b) the learner believes would benefit from a deeper understanding of what drives his/her decisions and behaviors. Accepting the feedback of others, particularly those with social influence, is proven to be a motivating factor for wellness (Bandura, 1977). To the socialization process, PsyCap adds the additional step of analyzing how trauma has influenced – positively and negatively – the way they approach personal and professional situations (Knaevelsrud & Maercker, 2007).

The tendency to isolate after a traumatic experience is particularly prevalent in the helping professions (Von Brachel et al., 2019). Socialization brings to the surface emotions that may have led to isolation. Sharing past traumas not only encourages first responders to seek feedback from someone about harboring faulty thinking, such as blaming themselves for an uncontrollable outcome, it also aids in the process of forgiveness and re-engagement into social activities. This creates the kind of environment where first responders can acknowledge the need for change in an effort to be well.

MENTAL RESILIENCE THROUGH HEROES

The progression from the development of hope through the socialization experience takes first responders on a journey of self-discovery. At the launch of the training, the goal-mapping activity establishes what they most desire to achieve with the understanding that actively pursuing their goals initiates their journey to wellness. The confidence-building process they undergo in the self-efficacy, resilience, and optimism portions of the course builds healthy anticipation for future success. Along the way, they learn to identify and strategically plan for roadblocks by collecting the resources that will make the journey easier. Empathy training reminds them of their responsibility to approach each situation with a fresh perspective as well as awareness that their attitude has an incredible impact on the outcome. Socializing their own experiences brings them face-to-face with buried tragedy and, through the assistance of people they respect, helps them build a healthy perspective. Continued application and practice of the lessons in HEROES results in mental resilience: the ability to withstand the negative influences of change, uncertainty, and fear with limited negative psychological impact.

Trainee Feedback

Hope

Homework in the Hope session requires trainees to build a strategic goal map, evaluating their potentials within six wellness areas: mental, physical, emotional, spiritual, financial, and professional. In reviewing trainees' work, hope for the future was clearly the theme. Trainee statements included, "I've always had a general idea of what I wanted to accomplish, but seeing it up on my wall made the goals more real somehow. I put my project up on the wall where I have to look at it every day and it's really helping me prioritize" and "For the first time, I've put a lot of thought into each of my goals. Now, every morning when I have my coffee I find myself really thinking about what I'm working to accomplish and throughout the day, I continue to go back to my goals and remind myself of what's important. It's a nice change of pace to be looking forward to something again."

Self-Efficacy

Trainees conduct a self-evaluation that requires focus on each goal with the identification of resources they either already have available or could obtain through education, practice, or asking for help from others. A theme that emerges centers on a renewed appreciation for personal skills and talents as well as a willingness to adjust their goals to reflect new priorities. For instance, trainees commented, "I used to play the guitar to blow off steam and, until now, I didn't realize that playing was a necessary resource for managing my stress. The other day I pulled it out of storage and played it again. I can't believe something so simple made me feel better than I have in a long time" and "After thinking about my professional goal to one day work with other cops in distress, I decided to adjust my mental goal so that I could focus on finishing my degree. I even enrolled in night school! I have a plan and am determined to make it happen."

Resilience

The homework in the section on resilience requires trainees to seek objective performance evaluations from peers they respect. To do so, they have to physically visit a member of their department and explain why they chose to seek an evaluation from that person. In doing so, trainees began the process of building a relationship based on mutual respect. Using a scenario from their own lives, they then ask the respected peer to objectively analyze performance with two questions in mind. (1) What was done well? (2) What was done poorly? After listening to the evaluation, they then apply the feedback in deciding what to do differently if faced with similar situations in the future.

The trainees convey two primary themes: the value of respected peers' feedback in planning for future difficulties and an appreciation of peer wisdom. Research into outcomes stemming from peer evaluation support greater creativity and the free flow of communication in the workplace (Shellenbarger, 2014). Trainee comments support this assertion and resulted in statements like, "Even though he's someone I respect, it was a challenge for me to ask him for feedback. I found that the courage it took me to acknowledge a need for help was just as valuable as the advice he gave me for doing better next time" and "I've been doing this job a long time and honestly, didn't think this old dog could learn new tricks. The young man I approached showed me a much easier way to do something I've been doing for decades. I should have swallowed my pride and asked sooner!"

Optimism

The homework assignment for developing optimism requires trainees to purposefully listen to their own self-talk, notating whether it was positive or negative and whether it was accurate or not. A primary theme based on these internal evaluations is unhealthy assumptions of future potential based on negative past experiences. For instance, a repetitive comment made by first responders is, "I never really listened to the voice inside my head and now I know why. It's very negative and most of the time, tells me why not to do something based on a bad choice I made in the past, as if since I messed up before, I'll probably mess up again so why try." As optimism is built by task, trainees are assigned the additional step of identifying behaviors associated with each strategic goal that would increase the likelihood that they will successfully achieve their potential. Comments stemming from that work included, "When I think about achievement, now I think about what I need to do to get it done" and "It takes effort, but I purposely correct the voice inside my head and replace the negative assumption with positive reality."

Empathy

Using past experiences to communicate empathy to others is a valuable skill for first responders. Trainees are tasked with writing an impact statement about something in the past that has influenced their wellness. In writing the statement, they identify what they could control and over what they had zero control. They also commented on their emotional states as the event unfolded and in the days and weeks that followed. Many trainees comment that this was the most difficult, yet most powerful part of the training. The primary theme communicated through this activity is acceptance. Trainee comments include, "If not for this training, I never would've worked through what happened that night" and "I didn't think I'd ever be able to get past what happened, but seeing it in writing and forcing myself to look at what I had control over helped me to see that there was nothing I could do to change the outcome."

Socialization

To support the basic human need for community, trainees learn how to recognize warning signs of isolation and are tasked with sharing their impact statements with someone who would benefit from deeper insight into their thought processes and behaviors, which stemmed from past trauma. To honor the importance of sharing something very personal as well as the value of being chosen to hear something so personal, the trainees are instructed to intentionally plan for a quiet place and sufficient time for the conversation.

Comments about this experience focus consistently on closure. Trainees express their thankfulness for the overwhelming sense of relief they feel after sharing their impact statement with someone. A number of trainees choose to meet with former work partners while others share with spouses or friends. "I chose to meet with my former partner. She was on scene with me the night he died. I read my impact statement to her and she sat there silently for a long time. Then, she started talking about how she'd been feeling the same way for years but hadn't ever been comfortable saying anything. We talked for hours and after, both of us promised to keep talking to each other about the job from then on."

The experiential feedback from first responders at the conclusion of the training clearly supports the need for intentionally focusing on wellness at both the individual and organizational levels. Trainees overwhelmingly express a fresh perspective of what wellness is and a renewed vigor for pursuing it through the continued use of the strategic map. A number of comments echo the statement that, "This project wasn't at all what I expected it to be, but in a good way. I've never had anyone tell me what wellness actually is, let along show me using my own goals and past experiences. Now that I've established my own wellness plan, I'm going to approach my department about using a similar tool in our performance evaluations. Everyone should be using something like this because it forces you to take ownership of your choices."

IMPLICATIONS FOR THE FIRST-RESPONSE CULTURE

In addition to the individual benefits experienced in the lives of the first responders who complete the HEROES Project, there are organizational benefits that are equally powerful. Public safety executives and first-responder agency administrators have the incredible responsibility of protecting the workforce that protects and serves the people. A reality of such leadership is handling civilian complaints, responding to serious allegations, and standing at the podium in front of a bank of media microphones answering questions. To do both impeccably requires a strategic approach to wellness. When organizations provide tools like the HEROES Project, the commitment to a culture of health and wellness is prioritized. For instance, Chief Jean-Michael Blais of the Halifax Police Department, used his own PTSD diagnosis to create a culture of mental-health awareness within his police department (Bresge, 2016).

The implications of the training are directly leveled at the culture of the first-responder profession. Leaders have made critical incident stress awareness a matter of importance. However, many stress management efforts either target a specific public safety population or are implemented only after exposure to a critical incident. With the HEROES project, executives within the first-responder community can provide all of their employees with psychological resilience training. The training can be given throughout first responders' careers to help establish wellness, to intervene when something threatens wellness, and to reinforce and maintain their individualized wellness plans.

The HEROES Project can benefit organizations by creating a culture of wellness and resilience. Implementing the HEROES Project delivers the message to personnel that the organization prioritizes health, wellness, and resilience, and cares for those in distress. When something malfunctions in an organization, a punitive, authoritarian, or autocratic way of processing issues will more likely lead to cynicism, absenteeism, low morale, and low performance, which increase the risk for health-related difficulties. On the other hand, principles at the center of the HEROES Project instill a sense of hope and caring within the organization.

The HEROES Project is effective across different stages of first responders' careers. The Program will benefit all first responders of an organization covering the newly hired to seasoned veterans. In an anonymous, self-paced way, first responders gain confidence that mental health challenges experienced in the line of duty are reversible and that positive change is possible.

CONCLUSION

Traditional approaches to wellness among first responders tend to be very reactionary. The unique nature of the HEROES Project is found in its proactive development of the psychological and behavioral skills necessary to form mental resilience. Additionally, it was intentionally crafted as a resource that conquers the stigma so frequently attached to mental health treatment. To overcome the most frequent objections raised about using wellness tools, the HEROES Project is accessible virtually, from the privacy of home, completed with anonymity, and progressed through at the pace most comfortable to the trainee. Solving for the reasons first responders are uncomfortable with wellness initiatives increases the likelihood that they will approach it as a valuable training tool and apply the lessons to their personal and professional lives.

Using the techniques learned in the HEROES Project, first responders develop strategies to cope with the mind-body's reactions during and after potentially traumatic situations. Additionally, by broadening the scope of mission-focused activities, they become driven to achieve more in the face of adversity, learn to allocate the necessary resources to overcome challenges, seek wisdom from well-respected colleagues, and approach each situation objectively. With every success, there is another ambitious goal waiting in the wings to be focused on and immediately followed by action. With every setback, another opportunity to learn. The results are well-rounded autonomous leaders who intentionally build mental resilience to trauma through the development of hope, efficacy, resilience, optimism, empathy, and socialization: HEROES.

REFERENCES

Bandura, A. (1977). Self-efficacy: Toward a unifying theory of behavioral change. *Psychological Review*, *84*(2), 191–215. doi:10.1037/0033-295X.84.2.191 PMID:847061

Bandura, A. (1997). *Self-efficacy: The exercise of Control*. New York, NY: W.H. Freeman and Company.

Bandura, A. (2005). The evolution of social cognitive theory. In K. G. Smith & M. A. Hitt (Eds.), *Great minds in management: The process of theory development* (pp. 9–35). New York, NY: Oxford University Press.

Bandura, A. (2007). An agentic perspective on positive psychology. In S. J. Lopez (Ed.), *Positive psychology: Expecting the best in people* (pp. 167–196). Westport, CT: Greenwood Publishing Company.

Beck Institute for Cognitive Behavior Therapy. (2015). Retrieved from https://beckinstitute.org/

Block, J., & Kremen, A. M. (1996). IQ and ego-resiliency: Conceptual and empirical connections and separateness. *Journal of Personality and Social Psychology*, *70*(2), 349–361. doi:10.1037/0022-3514.70.2.349 PMID:8636887

Bonanno, G. A. (2004). Loss, Trauma, and Human Resilience: Have We Underestimated the Human Capacity to Thrive After Extremely Aversive Events? *The American Psychologist*, *59*(1), 20–28. doi:10.1037/0003-066X.59.1.20 PMID:14736317

Bresge, A. (2016). *Halifax police chief making mental health, PTSD a priority*. Retrieved from https://www.ctvnews.ca/canada/halifax-police-chief-making-mental-health-ptsd-a-priority-1.2849866

Brown, L. A., Wiley, J. F., Wolitzky-Taylor, K., Roy-Byrne, P., Sherbourne, C., Stein, M. B., ... Craske, M. G. (2014). Changes in self-efficacy and outcome expectancy as predictors of anxiety outcomes from the calm study. *Depression and Anxiety*, *31*(8), 678–689. doi:10.1002/da.22256 PMID:24619599

Chaves, C., Lopez-Gomez, I., Hervas, G., & Vazquez, C. (2019). The Integrative Positive Psychological Intervention for Depression (IPPI-D). *Journal of Contemporary Psychotherapy*, 1–9. doi:10.100710879-018-9412-0

Chenault, S., Martin, J., & Matusiak, R. E. (2016). The Ripple Effect: Empathy Statements of Participants of an Impact of Crime on Victims Class. *Corrections: Policy, Practice and Research*, *1*(3), 196–214. doi:10.1080/23774657.2016.1210994

Gjefle, A., & Vikari, V. (2012). Training to the rescue: First responders power up skills while cutting costs. *Public Management*, *41*(3), 35–38.

Grant, L. (2014). Hearts and Minds: Aspects of Empathy and Wellbeing in Social Work Students. *Social Work Education*, *33*(3), 338–352. doi:10.1080/02615479.2013.805191

Hammond, D. C. (2000). Clinical Corner. *Journal of Neurotherapy*, *4*(3), 93–97. doi:10.1300/J184v04n03_07

Hetrick, S. E., Purcell, R., Garner, B., & Parslow, R. (2010). Combined pharmacotherapy and psychological therapies for post traumatic stress disorder (PTSD). *Cochrane Database of Systematic Reviews.* doi:10.1002/14651858.CD007316.pub2 PMID:20614457

Hyland, P., Boduszek, D., Dhingra, K., Shevlin, M., Maguire, R., & Morley, K. (2015). A test of the inventory of attitudes towards seeking mental health services. *British Journal of Guidance & Counselling, 43*(4), 397–412. doi:10.1080/03069885.2014.963510

Kazantzis, N., & Dattilio, F. M. (2010). Definitions of homework, types of homework, and ratings of the importance of homework among psychologists with cognitive behavior therapy and psychoanalytic theoretical orientations. *Journal of Clinical Psychology, 66*(7), 758–773. doi:10.1002/jclp.20699 PMID:20527055

Kleim, B., & Westphal, M. (2011). Mental health in first responders: A review and recommendation for prevention and intervention strategies. *Traumatology, 17*(4), 17–24. doi:10.1177/1534765611429079

Knaevelsrud, C., & Maercker, A. (2007). Internet-based treatment for PTSD reduces distress and facilitates the development of a strong therapeutic alliance: A randomized controlled clinical trial. *BMC Psychiatry, 7*(1), 13. doi:10.1186/1471-244X-7-13 PMID:17442125

Kosor, R. (2019, February 9). *The command post: If it feels good, don't say it.* [Audio Podcast].

Kuyken, W., Padesky, C. A., & Dudley, R. (2009). *Collaborative case conceptualization: Working effectively with patients in cognitive– behavioral therapy*. New York, NY: Guilford Press.

Luthans, F. (2002). The need for and meaning of positive organizational behavior. *Journal of Organizational Behavior, 23*(6), 695–706. doi:10.1002/job.165

Luthans, F., Avey, J. B., Avolio, B. J., Norman, S. M., & Combs, G. M. (2006). Psychological capital development: Toward a micro-intervention. *Journal of Organizational Behavior, 27*(3), 387–393. doi:10.1002/job.373

Luthans, F., Avey, J. B., Avolio, B. J., & Peterson, S. J. (2010). The development and resulting performance impact of positive psychological capital. *Human Resource Development Quarterly, 21*(1), 41–67. doi:10.1002/hrdq.20034

Luthans, F., Youssef, C. M., & Avolio, B. J. (2006). *Psychological Capital: Developing the Human Competitive Edge*. New York: Oxford University Press. doi:10.1093/acprof:oso/9780195187526.001.0001

Makawatsakul, N., & Kleiner, B. H. (2003). The effect of downsizing on morale and attrition. *Management Research News, 26*(2/3/4), 52–62. doi:10.1108/01409170310783998

Masten, A. S., & Garmezy, N. (1985). Risk, Vulnerability, and Protective Factors in Developmental Psychopathology. In B. Lahey & A. E. Kazdin (Eds.), *Advances in Clinical Child Psychology* (pp. 1–52). New York: Plenum. doi:10.1007/978-1-4613-9820-2_1

Newman, A., Ucbasaran, D., Zhu, F., & Hirst, G. (2014). Psychological capital: A review and synthesis. *Journal of Organizational Behavior, 35*(S1), S120–S138. doi:10.1002/job.1916

Niles, S. G., In, H., & Amundson, N. (2014). Using an Action Oriented Hope-Centered Model of Career Development. *Journal of Asia Pacific Counseling*, *4*(1), 1–13. doi:10.18401/2014.4.1.1

Niles, S. G., Yoon, H. J., Balın, E., & Amundson, N. E. (2010). Using A Hope-Centered Model Of Career Development in Challenging Times. *Turkish Psychological Counseling and Guidance Journal*, *4*. Retrieved from http://dergipark.gov.tr/download/article-file/200146

Oxley, J. C. (2011). The Moral Dimensions of Empathy: Limits and Applications in Ethical Theory. New York, NY: Palgrave Macmillan.

Padesky, C. A. (2006). *The next phase: Building positive qualities with cognitive therapy*. Invited address presented at the International Congress of Cognitive Psychotherapy, Göteborg, Sweden.

Padesky, C. A., & Mooney, K. A. (2012). Strengths-Based Cognitive-Behavioural Therapy: A Four-Step Model to Build Resilience. *Clinical Psychology & Psychotherapy*, *19*(4), 283–290. doi:10.1002/cpp.1795 PMID:22653834

Parra, A. (2013). Cognitive and Emotional Empathy in Relation to Five Paranormal/Anomalous Experiences. *North American Journal of Psychology*, *15*(3), 405–612.

Rand, K. L., & Cheavens, J. S. (2009). Hope Theory. In S. J. Lopez & C. R. Snyder (Eds.), *The Oxford Handbook of Positive Psychology* (2nd ed.; pp. 323–333). New York: Oxford University Press.

Sadri, G., & Robertson, I. T. (1993). Self-efficacy and Work-related Behaviour: A Review and Meta-analysis. *Applied Psychology*, *42*(2), 139–152. doi:10.1111/j.1464-0597.1993.tb00728.x

Seligman, M. E. P., & Csikszentmihalyi, M. (2000). Positive psychology: An introduction. *The American Psychologist*, *55*(1), 5–14. doi:10.1037/0003-066X.55.1.5 PMID:11392865

Shellenbarger, S. (2014, Jun 24). Work & family: Better responses to criticism at work - nobody likes negative feedback from the boss; taking it well requires humility and self-awareness. *Wall Street Journal*. Retrieved from https://libcatalog.atu.edu:443/login?url=https://search.proquest.com/docview/1539355996?accountid=8364

Singer, T. (2006). The neuronal basis and ontogeny of empathy and mind reading: Review of literature and implications for future research. *Neuroscience and Biobehavioral Reviews*, *30*(6), 855–863. doi:10.1016/j.neubiorev.2006.06.011 PMID:16904182

Snyder, C. R. (2000). *Handbook of hope: Theory, measures, and applications*. San Diego, CA: Academic Press.

Snyder, C. R. (2002). Hope Theory: Rainbows in the Mind. *Psychological Inquiry*, *13*(4), 249–275. doi:10.1207/S15327965PLI1304_01

Stajkovic, A. D., & Luthans, F. (1998). Social cognitive theory and self-efficacy: Goin beyond traditional motivational and behavioral approaches. *Organizational Dynamics*, *26*(4), 62–74. doi:10.1016/S0090-2616(98)90006-7

Stirman, S. W., Gutiérrez-Colina, A., Toder, K., Esposito, G., Barg, F., Castro, F., ... Crits-Christoph, P. (2013). Clinicians' Perspectives on Cognitive Therapy in Community Mental Health Settings: Implications for Training and Implementation. *Administration and Policy in Mental Health*, *40*(4), 274–285. doi:10.100710488-012-0418-8 PMID:22426739

Tugade, M. M., & Fredrickson, B. L. (2004). Resilient Individuals Use Positive Emotions to Bounce Back From Negative Emotional Experiences. *Journal of Personality and Social Psychology*, *86*(2), 320–333. doi:10.1037/0022-3514.86.2.320 PMID:14769087

Von Brachel, R., Teismann, T., Feider, L., & Margraf, J. (2019). Suicide ideation as a predictor of treatment outcomes in cognitive-behavioral therapy for unipolar mood disorders. *International Journal of Clinical and Health Psychology*, *19*(1), 80–84. doi:10.1016/j.ijchp.2018.09.002 PMID:30619501

Wester, S. R., Arndt, D., Sedivy, S. K., & Arndt, L. (2010). Male police officers and stigma associated with counseling: The role of anticipated risks, anticipated benefits and gender role conflict. *Psychology of Men & Masculinity*, *11*(4), 286–302. doi:10.1037/a0019108

Yi, J. P., Vitaliano, P. P., Smith, R. E., Yi, J. C., & Weinger, K. (2008). The role of resilience on psychological adjustment and physical health in patients with diabetes. *British Journal of Health Psychology*, *13*(2), 311–325. doi:10.1348/135910707X186994 PMID:17535497

Chapter 10
Disaster Responder Self-Care, Self-Compassion, and Protective Factors:
A Pilot Study on Responders' Resilience and Competence

Gargi Roysircar
Antioch University New England, USA

Allyssa M. Lanza
Psychological Solutions, USA

Marie F. Macedonia
Antioch University New England, USA

ABSTRACT

The study examined the relationships among resilience, self-care, self-compassion of first responders. In addition, the study assessed the contributions of protective and risk factors to responders' resilience and disaster response competencies. Five research hypotheses and three research questions were examined with Pearson r correlations, multiple regressions, one t-test, one MANOVA, and post hoc tests, showing significant and meaningful results. In addition, the internal consistency reliabilities of the DRCQ scales were investigated which were strong to very strong. It was hypothesized and shown that there were significant positive relationships among self-care, self-compassion, and resilience. A second hypothesis was retained that the two dimensions of self-care (i.e., self-care practices and physical safety) were predictors of self-compassion. Responders who consciously observed self-care practices fostered and strengthened self-compassion and vice versa.

DOI: 10.4018/978-1-5225-9803-9.ch010

INTRODUCTION

Natural and human-made disasters are a fact of life. Disaster responders serving their fellow human beings in the aftermath of disasters are exposed to great pressures in the line of humanitarian work. The very nature of their work is determined by unpredictable catastrophes that tear down emergency support infrastructure. Disaster responders leave behind the comforts of home and family to provide care and support to survivors of traumatic circumstances, often in the most precarious environments. They work and live in less-than-basic accommodations available to rescue workers. Disaster responders are at risk for emotional exhaustion, social isolation or loneliness, decreased job satisfaction, interpersonal relationship problems, and low self-concept (Shapiro, Brown, & Biegel, 2007). Studies have shown that the PTSD rate can reach 32% for individuals involved in rescue and recovery (Dass-Brailsford, 2010; Fullerton, Ursano, & Wang, 2004). This is compared to the rate of PTSD for the general public estimated at 3.5% for men and 9.7% for women. However, research has also shown that protective factors (e.g., training, adequate self-care) can enhance responders' resilience to vicarious traumatization (Brodeur, 2009; Howlett & Collins, 2014). The present study was undertaken because there is no assessment research on the positive mental health of disaster responders.

The study investigated the relationships of self-care, self-compassion, and disaster response competencies with the resilience of disaster responders. Furthermore, the study investigated the content validity and internal consistencies of the Disaster Response Competency Questionnaire (DRCQ) as an instrument appropriate for assessing good mental health of disaster responders. At the conclusion of the study, there is a discussion of the applications of self-care, psychological first-aid, and prevention training for disaster responders to help them sustain good mental health.

Disaster responders are at significant risk for mental health issues, and yet there is a gap in the literature on how to address their specific needs. The present study specifically addresses the well-being needs of first responders. The first responder literature is sometimes applied to disaster responders though the two populations have nuanced differences in roles and resources. First responders are described as people who respond professionally to crises. They are the police, firefighters, and emergency medical response teams. In some circumstances, additional people may act in first responder roles, such as medical personnel, the military, veterans, or lay people who are willing to help in the moment of an emergency. Disaster responders, on the other hand, are often defined as people working to rebuild and heal communities after a large-scale breakdown in infrastructure (Macedonia, 2018). While many first responders also serve in disaster response scenarios, not all first responders have disaster response experience or formal training in disaster response (Lanza, Roysircar, & Rodgers, 2018). Disaster responders may be formally trained professional responders (such as FEMA workers, the military national guard, or American Red Cross responders), or they may be people temporarily in disaster responder roles because of the needs of the situation (such as mental health workers, electrical line workers, road repair workers, or volunteers). The disaster responder population varies from the first responder population in the type of events to which they are vicariously exposed, the length of time to which they are exposed to the effects of devastation, and the effects of working without traditionally available resources (Lanza et al., 2018).

Disaster responders also have barriers to accessing mental health treatment. The care of volunteers is not a high priority for relief organizations that are already burdened by responding to the overwhelming effects of natural and/or human-made disasters (Ehrenreich & Elliott, 2004). Responders experiencing the impact of trauma work often do not reach out for help because of their culture of grit and stoicism. Research has shown that some first responders internalize stigma at the prospect of revealing to others their perceived vulnerability and feelings of inadequacy when they are negatively affected by their work (Boudreau, 2015; Lanza et al., 2018). The study saw a need for access to mental healthcare for disaster responders.

On the other hand, there have been attempts to integrate mental healthcare into disaster response. As conceptualized by Roysircar (Roysircar, 2008, 2009a, 2010; Roysircar, Podkova, & Pignatiello, 2013), it is psychosocial programming for sufferers of disasters to return to normal levels of functioning. Mental health professionals who serve as disaster responders initiate this recovery in disaster-affected communities by providing prevention, postvention, and treatment outreach, such as, trauma counseling and psychoeducation (Bowman & Roysircar, 2012; Lanza et al., 2018; Roysircar, 2013; Roysircar, Pignatiello, Lanza, & Irigoyen, 2015); as well as assessment of children's resilience, vulnerability, and trauma coping to improve disaster counseling services (Roysircar, Colvin, Afolayan, Thompson, & Robertson, 2017; Roysircar, Geisinger, & Thompson, 2019). Parenting skills in coping are also addressed through focus groups of parents, extended kin, and orphanage caregivers (Roysircar, Thompson, & Geisinger, in press).

Disaster responders who may suffer vicarious traumatization also need to be assessed for mental health issues and provided treatment. The well-being of disaster responders is important to the communities they serve. Multiple groups are affected when responders quit their work because of burnout and illness. Harrison and Westwood (2009) stated, "when individuals trained in the helping professions abandon the field, because of a perceived burden of caring and an insufficient ability to balance work with other aspects of life, this constitutes an enormous loss of resources and potentials" (p. 204). The cost of disaster responders suffering burnout, compassion fatigue, or vicarious traumatization is significant and translates into absenteeism, turnover, decreased job satisfaction, mental health disorders, and lower rates of productivity and effectiveness (Maslach, Schaufeli, & Leiter, 2001). There are also human costs (e.g., poor care to patients), structural costs (e.g., destabilization of team organization), and monetary costs (e.g., replacement of workers). Finally, this results in great costs to the disaster-affected community experiencing trauma and needing help with recovery. Thus, disaster responders need help to be healthy, so that they can help others. The study's theoretical orientation and variables of interest are defined next.

STRENGTHS-BASED APPROACH TO STUDY DISASTER RESPONDERS

The strength-based approach differs from traditional psychological models that have focused on deficits and pathology as a central focus and area of intervention (Seligman & Csikszentmihalyi, 2000). Rather, a strength-based approach encourages psychologists to understand and identify assets that promote well-being. With a strength-based approach, psychologists acknowledge challenges, while also identifying positive ways of adaptation to life experiences. Resilience is one aspect of a strength-based perspective and along with human strengths is central to positive psychology that emphasizes good mental health, adaptive functioning, hope, optimism, love, vocational development, perseverance, and courage (American Psychological Association [APA], 2017; Chang, Downey, Hirsch, & Lin, 2016). Michael Rutter's (1985) study on children provided one of the earliest definitions of resilience. Rutter conducted research on children whose parents suffered from mental disorders and found that not all children went on to develop psychopathology as adults. Rutter defined resilience as the absence of psychopathology, which, however, represents a deficit model. Currently, resilience is defined as sustained competence under stress, which is a strengths-based perspective (Masten, Best, & Garmezy, 1990).

Resilience

Though there is not one operational definition of resilience, the construct can be conceptualized as, "effective coping and adaptation in the face of major life stress" (Tedeschi & Kilmer, 2005, p.231). Resilience can be understood as the sum of experience and knowledge acquired over time through one's survivor experiences and from one's local community of sufferers; and that a combination of individual, family, and environmental factors leads to resilience outcomes (Agaibi & Wilson, 2005; Alvord & Grados, 2005; Glicken, 2006). Friborg et al. (2006), Masten and Narayan (2012), and Roysircar et al. (2017, 2019, in press) present two assumptions regarding resilience. First, it stems from people encountering challenging situations, and second, these situations require them to utilize resources that are internal (self-regulation, problem-solving skills, positive views of self, motivation to be effective) and external (familial, communal, religious coping) to achieve competence outcome through traumatic events and contexts.

Self-Care

Roysircar (2008, 2018) describes self-care as a multidimensional concept in which psychological and physical well-being aspects are interdependent and lead to enhanced quality of life and a sense of fulfillment. Furthermore, integrating self-care practices into the daily lives of disaster responders serves as a safeguard against vicarious traumatization (Roysircar, 2008). The use of self-care practices is expected to foster resilience in disaster responders. From the point of view of the helping professions, self-care is not only a beneficial practice to people involved in the care of others in order to remain physically and psychologically healthy, it is a necessity, an integral part of ethical practice (Norcross & Barnett, 2007), and a moral imperative (Carroll, Gilroy, & Murra, 1999). The APA Ethical Principles and Code of Conduct (2002, amended 2010 and 2017) state the necessity for providers to be self-aware of any personal problems that might impair their ability to work effectively with clients and to take active steps to receive assistance (see Standard 2.06, Personal Problems and Conflicts). The American Counseling Association Code of Ethics (2005) states clearly the importance of self-care, recommending counselors to "engage in self-care activities to maintain and promote their emotional, physical, mental, and spiritual well-being to best meet their professional responsibilities" (See Section C, introduction, p.8). Norcross and Barnett (2007) stated "self-care is not restricted to intervention after professional competence has been compromised; it is a continuous, proactive process throughout our careers)" (para 18).

Self-Compassion

Self-compassion is kindness and forgiveness directed toward oneself (Germer & Neff, 2013; Smith, 2015) and may counteract self-stigma (Roysircar et al., in press). Self-compassion is relevant to all people, but particularly to individuals in situations that might bring pervasive feelings of personal inadequacies, failures, and mistakes, and has been associated with lower pathology and depressive disorders (Barnard & Curry, 2011; MacBeth & Gumley, 2013). Self-compassion enhances resilience by lessening emotion dysregulation (Germer & Neff, 2013; Leary, Tate, Adams, Allen, & Hancock, 2007). In addition, Neff and Pommier (2012) associated self-compassion with positive attitudes towards others: altruism, greater empathy, perspective taking, and forgiveness. Smith (2015) suggests that there are three fundamental aspects to self-compassion: mindfulness, common humanity, and self-kindness. Mindfulness is "the ability to be present and aware of one's thoughts, feelings, and experiences in the moment" (Smith, 2015, p.17) and allows people to reach a balance in their perspective of their shortcomings and their successes. Common humanity enables people to view their shortcomings in the larger context of the greater world, which allows them to experience a sense of connection with others when facing challenges and avoiding isolation (Smith, 2015). Smith showed that self-kindness, which is soothing in challenging times, resulted in higher levels of happiness and resilience in older adults. Disaster responders who perform in overwhelming conditions may often challenge their sense of worth and ask themselves if they are making a difference in the task-at-hand. Some training models (cf. Roysircar, 2009b) teach volunteer responders to express self-compassion in their daily self-reflection notes, healing themselves first before healing others.

DISASTER RESPONSE COMPETENCIES

Disaster response competencies are a set of skills that are particular to individuals who serve in disaster settings. These skills encompass the ability to "calibrate wide-spread loss and tragedy and differentiate individual and group differences in trauma reactions, accompanied with individual and community-appropriate intervention responses" (Roysircar, 2012, p. 1). For more information, see the Measure section that describes different assessed competencies.

VICARIOUS TRAUMATIZATION

Vicarious traumatization refers to a transformation in trauma workers' inner experience resulting from empathic engagement with survivors' trauma material (Dass-Brailsford, 2010). These effects are cumulative and permanent, affecting both professional and personal lives. The effects of vicarious traumatization include significant disruptions in one's sense of meaning, connection, identity, and world view, as well as in one's affect tolerance and interpersonal relationships (Lanza et al., 2018).

PROTECTIVE FACTORS AND RISK FACTORS

Protective factors are micro systems in the environment, such as family, school, community, place of worship, group solidarity, organizational resources, and healthcare clinics, which act to reduce the likelihood of a negative outcome despite adversity (APA, 2017; Lightsey, Jr., 2006). Risk factors are macrosystemic and structural influences on a local community (e.g., poverty, marginalization of a minority group, disparities), which increase the likelihood of a negative outcome (APA, 2017; Lightsey, Jr., 2006).

RESEARCH HYPOTHESES AND QUESTIONS

The study's rationale and literature review led to six research hypotheses and three questions. Because this was a pilot study, the design was correlational and the analyses were kept simple.

Hypothesis 1. Resilience, Self-care, and Self-compassion have significant positive relationships with each other.

Hypothesis 2. Self-care dimensions have positive significant relationships with self-compassion.
Hypothesis 3. Self-care practices have significant negative relationships with vicarious traumatization.
Hypothesis 4. Select protective factors and risk factors are related to resilience.
Hypothesis 5. Disaster responders who received longer prevention training have higher scores on disaster response competencies, resilience, self-care, self-compassion, and protective factors than those who received a shorter period of training.
Hypothesis 6. DRCQ has acceptable content validity and internal consistency reliabilities.
Question 1. Is high self-compassion found in the majority of the responders?
Question 2. Is there a sex difference in the practice of self-care among responders?
Question 3. Are responder preparedness, organizational support from work place, age, and social status related disaster response competencies?

METHOD

Effect Size Estimation

To determine the necessary number of participants required for the study, the authors assumed to detect a small to medium effect size for an expected sample of $N = 75$-100 for the statistical analyses of Pearson r correlations, two tests of difference, and three simple linear multiple regressions. This would result in an estimated statistical power of .80 at $p < .05$ for the hypotheses tested. Seventy-seven participants were sought for the needed effect size. A few participants ($n = 10$) had a maximum of 20 missing responses out of 204 items of the DRCQ. These missing responses were taken care of by the use of mean replacement (i.e., the mean score of the entire sample for a particular item).

Participants

Among the participants, 71 (94.8%) self-identified as volunteer responders, while four (5.2%) reported being professional responders. All participants (100%) reported participating in response work within the past 5 years. Of the 77 participants, 44 (65.7%) were women and 23 (34.3%) were men. Their age ranged widely from 22 years of age to 74, with a mean of 40 years of age. Thirty-three (49.3%) participants self-identified as Black/African American/Black American, while 22 (32.8%) as White/White American.

Table 1. Participant racial and ethnic demographic data

Racial/Ethnic Identity	*n*	Percentage
Black/African American	33	49.3%
White/White American	22	32.8%
Arabic/Middle Eastern	8	11.9%
Asian/Asian American	1	1.5%
Latino/Hispanic/Latinx	1	1.5%
Multiracial	2	3%

Note. $n = 67$. Four participants did not report their race, ethnicity, or nationality.

Table 2. Participants' involvement in large scale disasters

Disaster	*n*	Percentage
Hurricanes	36	52.2%
Tsunamis	26	37.7%
Earthquakes	21	30.4%
Community Violence	20	29.0%
Pandemics	15	21.7%
Wild Fires	10	14.5%
Wars	6	8.7%

Note. $n = 69$.

Eight participants (11.9%) self-identified as Arabic/Middle Eastern, two (3.0%) as Multiracial, one as Asian (1.5%), and one as Latino/Hispanic/Latinx (1.5%). A majority (67.2%) consisted of racial, ethnic, and nationality minorities. Forty (59.7%) participants self-identified as blue collar/working middle class, 17 (25.4%) as middle class, while 10 (14.9%) as upper middle class. A large majority of the participants (85.1%) was middle class. See Table 1 for racial and ethnic demographic data.

Of the participants, 37 (55.2%) were married, 11 (16.4%) lived with a partner/significant other, and 12 (17.9%) were in a dating relationship. Five (7.5%) participants self-identified as single, one (1.5%) as divorced, and one as widowed (1.5%). A large majority (89.5%) reported being in relationships. Participants relied on different support systems when performing disaster relief work: partner/spousal support and family (66.7%), co-workers (73.9%), close friends (87%), and spiritual community members (37.7%). A large majority (89.6%) reported having social support systems.

All participants reported diverse experiences with disaster relief work. Their involvement in large-scale disasters varied, ranging from 1 to 10 with a mean of 3.1. See Table 2 for participants' involvement in various types of large-scale disasters.

Measure: The Disaster Response Competencies Questionnaire (DRCQ)

The purpose of the Disaster Response Competencies Questionnaire (DRCQ) (Roysircar, 2008, 2009a, 2010), first, is to screen and do ongoing assessment of disaster responders (pre, midway, post, follow-up). Second, the DRCQ fills a gap in the assessment of disaster responder services because no such instrument exists as of now. Third, the DRCQ uses a positive framework of community resilience as its theoretical basis (Roysircar, 2009b, 2012; Roysircar et al., 2013). Fourth, the DRCQ was submitted for a review by a panel of three experts who had responded to disasters as mental health practitioners as well as have conducted research on disaster responders (**Brodeur**, 2009; **Lanza** et al., 2018; Roysircar, Pignatiello, Lanza, & **Irigoyen**, 2015). The experts judged positively the face and content validity of the DRCQ, while providing some recommendations for fine-tuning some wording; expanding a few content areas; and reducing some other content areas. A complete report and the qualitative analyses of the experts' review of the DRCQ's content and face validity are provided by Macedonia (2018). The DRCQ, a copyrighted instrument, may be obtained from Gargi Roysircar (groysircar@antioch.edu). Copyright laws do not allow the display of copyrighted measures. However, examples of items are provided here.

The DRCQ in the present study had 204 items that covered Demographic Information and the topics of Resilience, Self-Care Practices, Self-Compassion, Disaster Response Competencies, Protective Factors, and Risk Factors. The DRCQ uses a Likert-type scale of 1 to 4, with 1 = *strongly disagree* and 4 = *strongly agree*, with higher scores indicating stronger positive attributes. However, lower scores on Risk Factors indicate participants are in less at-risk conditions and less at risk for vicarious traumatization. Fourteen items were reverse scored to control for participant response biases.

Demographic Items

There were 15 items that asked questions in a multiple-choice format on sex, age, race and ethnicity, social class, relational status, support people, types of disaster work done, number of large-scale disaster work done, populations served, cultural diversity of populations served, formal training in disaster work, training gained through experience, access to debriefing, and disaster organizations' support for responders. Among four open-ended questions, one was analyzed for the present study ("How many large-scale disaster situations have you been involved in helping?"). Open-ended answers to this question were coded quantitatively for analyses.

Resilience

Resilience was measured by 23 items. Items included dispositional characteristics: Optimism (e.g., "I love what I do"); flexibility (e.g., "I consider myself to be open-minded and flexible); self-efficacy for disaster work (e.g., "I was able to manage my emotions to respond to difficult situations"); using a resilience framework in disaster work (e.g., "I avoided pathologizing, instead emphasizing what were normal reactions to abnormal situations"); and sense of purpose and achievement (e.g., "My recovery work has provided me with a sense of making a difference in the world"). Items also include external support: social support (e.g., "I have at least one best friend and confidante"); family relationships (e.g., "I stay in contact with family through regular visits, e-mails, phone calls, text messages, and holiday meals"); spirituality and religiousness (e.g., "I see religion as a support for both the survivors of a disaster and those helping them"); group orientation (e.g., "I believe that our human nature brings us together to work for common goals").

Self-Care Practices

Self-care practices measured by 19 items included emotional self-care (e.g., "Rather than letting my emotions well up, I sought a mental healthcare provider upon my return home"), physical self-care (e.g., "I used many ways to deal with the stress associated with disaster work, like physical and mental relaxation"), social self-care (e.g., "In times of need, I always have someone to talk to"), familial/relational self-care (e.g., "I accept help from my family members"), and safety and security concerns (e.g., I frequently monitored my own safety while delivering disaster relief services").

Self-Compassion

There were 6 items that measured self-compassion (e.g., "I avoid negative people who do not share my best interest at heart"; "I recognized that my actions, while not typical to my own behavior, were normal for a person who had been in a disaster situation"; and "I was proud of myself for the challenges I faced and the ability to overcome many obstacles"). These items were scattered throughout the DRCQ and were identified by the present authors as representing self-compassion.

Disaster Response Competencies

Disaster response competencies were measured by 40 items on: social competence in disaster work (e.g., "In a disaster situation, I easily adapted to a new group"); integrative and flexible practices (e.g., "I relinquished prior roles, identities, and preconceived notions of what "should be" in any disaster work"); collaborative work (e.g., "I provided assistance in whatever way needed by the stakeholders"); psychosocial interventions (e.g., "The disaster has provided an opportunity to the community to work together"); listening to stories of loss and grief from large numbers of survivors (e.g., "I was willing to listen to people talk about their disaster experiences"); multicultural responsiveness in disaster work (e.g., "The history of the disaster community was unknown to me" [reverse scored]; and assessment of community culture of a disaster setting (e.g., "Prior to entering the area I knew the predominant religion of the people and the community's socioeconomic status"). Ethics were also included and its items measured the ethical challenges of disaster work (e.g., "I was familiar with my organization's code of ethics").

Protective Factors

Protective factors were measured by 5 items on: preparedness for disaster work (e.g., "I was mentally prepared to face ethical dilemmas, environmental stresses, and possible vicarious traumatization"). Responders' preparedness also included psychological first-aid training, reflective listening skills training, and knowledge of what challenges to expect.

Risk Factors

Risk factors were measured by 28 items on: low responder SES (e.g., "I find it hard to make ends meet"); low organizational support (e.g., "My organization was very supportive of staff that experienced work-related stress" [reverse scored]); low survivor SES (e.g., "unemployment in the disaster area I served was above the national average"); environmental stresses (e.g., "I worked in physically demanding and unpleasant conditions"); and vicarious traumatization (e.g., "I had repeated exposure to others' traumatization and tragedies").

Procedure

At the onset of the project, Dr. Roysircar obtained the approval of her university's Institutional Review Board. She obtained participants through snowball sampling. The announcement on the study was passed to other key informants believed to be interested in the topic. This technique was specifically employed in rural regions of New Hampshire (NH) and Mississippi (MS) since Roysircar, by virtue of working in NH and MS, had the opportunity to "spread the word" to colleagues. To recruit participants in MS, Dr. Roysircar invited responders who had attended her disaster resilience workshops (Roysircar, 2008) in Mississippi.

A recruitment message was sent to disaster relief organizations and disaster training sites: FEMA Disaster Training; American Red Cross Training; SAMSHA's Training; Disaster Training International; Northwest Center for Public Health Practice; and University of South Dakota-Disaster Mental Health Institute. These contacts were requested to forward the message to responders and trainees that they knew. A link to the informed consent document and the survey was included in the message. A diverse and adequate sample size was hoped, but recognizing, at the same timw, the limited population of disaster responders and trained volunteers. Participants were directed to the research website, psychdata.com, which provided a link to answer voluntarily and anonymously the DRCQ. Participants read an Informed Consent Form prior to answering. Participants were offered a participation incentive. They were given a choice between entering a drawing to win a $50 amazon gift card, having five dollars donated on their behalf to the American Red Cross by Dr. Roysircar, or not receiving anything. Surveys carried neither names nor codes nor IP addresses. The website that hosted the survey has the ability to have participants taken to a separate and unlinked webpage at the end of the study where email addresses could be entered for rewards.

Data Analyses

Data analyses included examining the DRCQ's internal consistency reliabilities. Pearson r correlation analyses for Self-Care, Self-Compassion, and Resilience were performed. A t-test, a MANOVA, and post hoc tests were conducted to examine differences in group scores. Simple linear multiple regression analyses investigated predictors.

DRCQ Internal Consistency Reliabilities

See Table 3 for Cronbach's alpha values for the DRCQ scales, which may be considered strong to very strong.

Table 3. Cronbach's alpha values for DRCQ scales

DRCQ Scales	Items	α
Disaster Response Competencies	40	.89
Resilience	23	.87
Self-Care Practice	19	.88
Self-Compassion	6	.70
Protective Factors	5	.80
Risk Factors	28	.80

Note. $N = 77$.

TESTS OF RESEARCH HYPOTHESES AND QUESTIONS

Hypothesis 1: *There are significant positive relationships among resilience, self-care, and self-compassion.*

Self-care and self-compassion were significantly correlated to a moderate degree ($r = .59$, $p = .000$), while showing themselves to be different constructs. Self-care and resilience were significantly correlated to a moderate degree ($r = .51$, $p= .000$), while also showing themselves to be different constructs. A very strong correlation was found for self-compassion and resilience ($r = .86$, $p = .000$), suggesting either possible multicollinearity in the measurement of the two constructs or convergent validity. The DRCQ, as developed by Roysircar (2008, 2009a, 2010), did not have a specific scale on self-compassion. The present authors selected items from within the DRCQ on the basis of their knowledge of the self-compassion literature, and they proposed that these items assessed self-compassion.

Hypothesis 2: *Self-care dimensions are related to self-compassion.*

A simple linear multiple regression analysis was conducted to test the hypothesis that self-care practices (broad coverage of self-care and physical safety self-care) are related to self-compassion, supporting the hypothesis, $R^2 = .409$, $F(2, 74) = 25.63$, $p < .001$, showing an overall moderate effect size. Individual predictors self-care contributed significant variance to self-compassion ($\beta = .381$, $p < .00$), as did physical safety and security ($\beta = .357$, $p < .001$). See Table 4 for the regression results.

Table 4. Summary of a simple linear multiple regression analysis of self-care and physical safety as predictor variables with self-compassion as the criterion variable

	B	*SEB*	**β**	*t*	*p*
(Constant)	1.475	.258		5.726	.000
Self-Care	.275	.074	.381	3.700	.000
Physical Safety	.302	.087	.357	3.465	.001

Note. n = 76. Criterion Variable = Self-Compassion.

Hypothesis 3: *Self-care (i.e., self-care practices and physical safety) has negative relationships with vicarious traumatization.*

A Pearson *r* correlational analysis showed a significant negative moderate correlation between self-care and vicarious traumatization ($r = -.38$, $p = .000$) and a modest significant negative correlation between physical safety and vicarious traumatization ($r = -.22$, $p = 00$). Given that self-care and physical safety had a significant moderate correlation with each other ($r =. 50$, $p = .00$), self-care practices that cover several areas of self-care may relate more strongly in the inverse direction with vicarious traumatization in disaster responders than physical safety. See Table 5 for the correlations.

Table 5. Pearson correlations among vicarious trauma, self-care, and physical safety

	Vicarious Trauma	Self-Care	Physical Safety
Vicarious Trauma	1.00		
Self-Care	-.380**	1.00	
Physical Safety	-.223**	.499**	1.00

Note. N = 77. ** Correlation is significant at the 0.01 level (One-tailed).

Hypothesis 4: *Protective factors and risk factors are related to resilience.*

A simple linear multiple regression analysis was conducted to determine if protective factors (an overall average score) and risk factors (an overall average score) were significant predictors of resilience in disaster responders, showing, $F(1, 76) = 30.703$, $p < .001$, with $R^{2}= .290$. Protective factors were strong predictors of resilience, $\beta = .539$, $p<.001$, $t\ (75) = 5.54$, while risk factors were not, $\beta = -.032$, p = ns. See Table 6 for the regression results. The t value for risk factors was negative, showing an appropriate inverse relationship between risk factors and resilience.

Table 6. Summary of a simple linear multiple regression analysis of protective factors and risk factors as predictor variables with resilience as the criterion variable

	B	*SEB*	β	*t*	*p*
(Constant)	2.451	.180		13.651	.000
Protective Factors	.303	.055	.539	5.541	.000
Risk Factors	*-.032*	*.122*	-.030	-.259	.797

Note. N = 77. Criterion Variable = Resilience.

Hypothesis 5: *Disaster responders who received longer prevention training have higher scores in disaster response competencies, resilience, self-care, self-compassion, and protective factors than responders who receive a shorter period of training.*

Responders who reported prevention training for more than 4 weeks (n = 24) and responders who reported prevention training for 1 day to 4 weeks (n = 53) were compared. A MANOVA showed a significant difference between the two prevention training groups, $F(4.00, 72.00) = 4.82$, $p < .002$, partial eta squared = .21, a small overall effect size. Significant between-subject effects were found on: Self-Care: $F(1,.998) = 13.58$, $p < .000$, partial eta squared = .15; Protective Factors: $F(1,.708) = 13.56$, $p < .000$, partial eta squared = .15; Disaster Response Competencies: $F(1, .708) = 12.89$, $p < .001$, partial eta squared = .15; Resilience: $F(1, .38) = 5.51$, $p < .02$, partial eta squared = .07; and Self-Compassion: $F(1, .573) = 7.59$, $p < .007$, partial eta squared = .092. Responders who had received training for a longer period had higher scores on self-care, protective factors, disaster response competencies, resilience, and self-compassion; however, the effect sizes were small. (Partial eta squared is a measure in which the effects of other independent variables and interactions are partialled out. Nowadays, partial eta squared is widely cited as a measure of effect size). See Table 7 for the means and standard deviations of the two training time groups.

Table 7. Descriptive statistics for the impact of training time on self-compassion, resilience, disaster competency, and protective factors

	Training Time	*n*	*M*	*SD*
Self-Care	1 day - 4 weeks	53	2.92	.237
	4 weeks and more	24	3.17	.334
Self-Compassion	1 day - 4 weeks	53	3.21	.257
	4 weeks and more	24	3.39	.310
Resilience	1 day - 4 weeks	53	3.38	.235
	4 weeks and more	24	3.54	.318
Disaster Competency	1 day - 4 weeks	53	3.02	.210
	4 weeks and more	24	3.22	.280
Protective Factors	1 day - 4 weeks	53	3.12	.451
	4 weeks and more	24	3.52	.436

Note. n =77.

Research Question 1

This question examined if a majority of responders practiced self-compassion. Participants endorsed items according to the following Likert scale: 1= Strongly Disagree, 2= Disagree, 3= Agree, 4= Strongly Agree. A cut-off score was identified. Answers of "agree" or lower indicated low self-compassion. Responders who endorsed an answer higher than "agree" on the self-compassion items indicated a high self-compassion score. A frequency count indicated that the majority of respondents (n = 56, 72.7%) reported high self-compassion scores.

Research Question 2

This question examined the possibility of a sex difference in the practice of self-care among disaster responders. A t-test was performed to examine the difference between women (n = 44) and men (n = 23) responders' self-care scores. Results indicated that women (M =3.28, SD = .31) and men (M = 3.27, SD = .30) did not differ on levels of self-care, $t(65)$ = -.1.00, p = .920, n.s.

Research Question 3

A simple linear multiple regression analysis was conducted to determine if age, low organizational support from place of work, low responder socioeconomic status, and protective factors predicted disaster response competencies. A significant regression equation was found, $F(4, 61) = 11.016, p <.001$, with $R^2 = .419$, an overall moderate effect size. Only Protective factors predicted disaster competencies β = .596, $t(61) = 6.07, p < .001$. Responder low socioeconomic status (a risk factor) contributing negative variance to disaster response competencies came close to significance. See Table 8 for regression results of Risk Factors and Protective Factors for Disaster Competencies.

Table 8. Summary of a simple linear multiple regression analysis of responder age, low organizational support, low socioeconomic status, and protective factors as predictor variables with disaster competency as the criterion variable

	B	*SEB*	β	*t*	*p*
(Constant)	2.002	.294		6.810	.000
Age	.001	.002	.060	.582	.563
LOS	.066	.057	.119	1.163	.249
LRSES	-.104	0.57	-.180	-1.835	.071
PF	.310	.051	.596	6.069	.000

Note. *n*=65. Criterion Variable = Disaster Competency; LOS = Low Organization Support; LRSES = Low Responder Socioeconomic Status; PF = Protective Factors.

DISCUSSION

The study examined the relationships among resilience, self-care, and self-compassion of disaster responders and assessed the contributions of protective factors to responders' resilience and disaster response competencies. Five research hypotheses and three research questions were examined with Pearson r correlations, multiple regressions, and tests of difference that showed significant results and were meaningful. In addition, the internal consistency reliabilities of the DRCQ that assessed disaster responder variables of interest to the study were strong to very strong.

Significant Findings

Self-Care, Self-Compassion, and Resilience

It was hypothesized and shown that there were significant positive relationships among self-care, self-compassion, and resilience. The correlation between self-compassion and resilience was very strong, potentially suggesting convergent validity. A second hypothesis was retained that the two dimensions of self-care (i.e., self-care practices and physical safety) were predictors of self-compassion. Responders who observed more self-care practices showed more self-compassion and vice versa. In fact, a strong majority of the participants ($n = 56$, 72.7%) reported high self-compassion scores, endorsing an answer higher than "agree" on the self-compassion question.

There was no sex difference in the practice of self-care. Awareness of the challenges of disaster work may positively change in both men and women's attitudes of stoicism, toughness, and heroism (Lanza et al., 2018; Roysircar et al., 2015). It is possible that both women and men were equally informed about the benefits of self-care practices perhaps due to prevention training in work-related stress (e.g., attending self-care workshops). For instance, the participants reported high social and familial support in the demographic items, suggesting that they were practicing relational and social self-care (Roysircar, 2018) and were not isolated, which can lead to depression.

Self-Care and Vicarious Traumatization

Self-care practices were negatively correlated with vicarious traumatization. This finding is significant because it suggests some actionable options for promoting resilience in disaster responders. Vicarious traumatization is insidious and develops over time in responders before symptoms become obvious and debilitating (Baird & Jenkins, 2003). Self-care practices might be used as a preventative tool to build resilience and reduce vicarious traumatization in disaster responders before their exposure in fieldwork. Training in self-care through prevention programing for disaster responders was provided by Roysircar (2008) for responders of Hurricane Katrina and Rita in Louisiana and Mississippi and for providers in a primary care clinic in a disaster-affected very poor urban community in Haiti (Roysircar et al., in press). The authors of the present study suggest that self-care training is something feasible to implement in all disaster response organizations.

Protective Factors, Resilience, and Disaster Response Competencies

Research has shown that disaster responders are exposed to various stressors and are vulnerable to vicarious traumatization (Daas-Brailsford, 2010; Lanza et al., 2018; Roysircar, 2008). The study showed that protective factors (i.e., responder preparedness including psychological first-aid training, reflective listening skills training, knowledge of ethical, environmental, and emotional challenges to expect) predicted resilience (see also Howlett & Collins, 2014). This finding implies a need to emphasize training and preparation of disaster responders to prevent stress, burnout, compassion fatigue, or even trauma. Prevention programming may not always be possible because disasters are unpredictable and the response force is often mostly composed of volunteers with little experience in disaster work. Building resilience in responders through prevention training in preparation for a specific mission may support their ability to work in the field longer, remain efficient care providers to survivors, be less prone to mental illnesses, and reduce human, structural, and financial costs to the disaster-affected community (Lanza et al., 2018).

One hypothesis guiding the study was to determine if (a) protective factors (defined in the previous paragraph), (b) organizational support from place of work, (c) age, and (d) social status predicted disaster response competencies. Only protective factors predicted responders' competencies. Along the same line of implications expressed in the previous paragraph, results for another hypothesis showed that participants who trained for a longer period of time had higher scores on disaster response competencies, resilience, self-care, self-compassion, and protective factors than those who trained for a briefer period of time. These findings place further emphasis on the timing and optimal length of training necessary to prepare less experienced disaster responders prior to sending them into the field.

A negative correlation came close to significance between responder low socioeconomic status (a risk factor) and disaster response competencies. The sample was composed of middle class and upper-class responders, which might have contributed to the negative correlation. A more varied sample with responders from modest economic backgrounds may have shown a different result. However, the implication may be that volunteering is a class privilege, which people of humble means cannot afford because they need to work daily for a living.

Strengths of the Study

It is to be noted that the sample was diverse with a majority of women and racial and ethnic minorities. The question that arises is whether women and racial and ethnic minorities are more responsive to societal suffering and large-scale human needs. There was no intentional recruitment or oversampling of these underrepresented populations. In addition, the age range covered a large lifespan (22 to 74 years old, with a mean of 40 years), indicating that the study was attractive to a diverse age group of responders, not just college students doing service learning for credit. The sample, in fact, had considerable experience in responding to large scale disasters ($n = 69$). The study was unique in the collection of data from populations that are often not represented or studied in significant numbers in general survey studies or experimental designs (APA, 2017; Arnett, 2008). Other strengths of the study were its insights into self-care practices, self-compassion, resilience, disaster response competencies, and protective factors that may benefit disaster responders, particularly from minority populations. The study may exemplify how mainstream psychological concepts, such as, trauma coping, competencies, protective factors may be adapted for and applied to multicultural service providers (APA, 2017). For instance, the findings might indicate that there are no generational differences in self-care practices and self-compassion among disaster responders and that these healthy behaviors are of interest to responders of all ages.

Limitations of the Study

One weakness of the study was its mostly quantitative design. Offering open-ended questions to participants would have enriched the study with personal, unique information on self-care practices that might not have been considered in the original design of the DRCQ. There, were, however, four open-ended questions, and the answers to only one question were coded for analyses. Another weakness of the study was the use of means imputation, which has some statistical limitations. While means imputation is still commonly used in research, it may be helpful for future research to replicate this study with other data replacement methodology. The correlation design of the pilot study was a weakness because causal effects were not presented.

Finally, there may be some limitations in generalizing the findings to professional disaster responders. The sample was primarily volunteer responders, and it may be assumed that there is a larger variance in their disaster competency training experiences than those of professional responders. Competency training may be more valuable for volunteer populations, who may have as little as no understanding of what to expect in a disaster scenario (Lanza et al., 2018); whereas training benefits may taper for professionals who have moderate to large amount of trainings and experiences.

Self-Compassion Scale

Originally, the DRCQ did not have items specifically based on the construct of self-compassion. Once the idea to explore self-compassion was considered by the authors, a scale was formed pulling together items that were the most closely related to the construct of self-compassion. This scale had good internal consistency reliability, suggesting that the construct was satisfactorily assessed. The items, however, could be strengthened by adding contents on common humanity, mindfulness, and self-kindness (Smith, 2015). Examples of suggested items are as follows: “When I think I did not help someone enough, I pause and come to believe that others feel the same as I do and I am not alone” (e.g., common humanity);

"When I feel useless or challenged, I reflect immediately on times when I felt useful and successful" (e.g., mindfulness); and "When I feel challenged or discouraged, I tell myself I work to the best of my ability and I do a good job" (e.g., self-kindness).

Suggestions for Future Research

Study's Replication in Other Professions

Future research might examine if the findings of the current study could be extended to professionals in health and social services fields. For example, a similar study could be conducted with providers who are exposed to stressful and often traumatic situations (e.g., social case managers, nurses), placing them at risk for vicarious traumatization or burnout. The DRCQ could be adapted to assess professional responders, such as active-duty military forces, fire fighters, the police, and emergency medical technicians. The results of diverse studies might reveal different results in self-care practices and self-compassion than shown in the present study, especially as these relate to societal, work, and cultural stigma about mental health disorders in providers who are labeled as heroes.

Use of the DRCQ

The present pilot study has shown the initial usefulness of the DRCQ as an assessment measure for disaster response competencies, resilience, and self-care practices, indicating strong internal consistency reliabilities and significant positive and negative correlations among variables, tests of difference, and multiple regression, providing meaningful conceptualizations and implications. This pilot study suggests possibilities of the DRCQ's usage and more research on the DRCQ like exploratory factor analyses to learn about the latent dimensionality of its scales. Regarding usage, the measure can be used for evaluating responders prior to their departure for a disaster site; as an on-going tool when disaster responders are in the field and help to identify their lack of self-care while exposed to duress; and finally used after responders have returned from disaster work to assess possible gains made or an area of self-care that might need attention. With some accommodations, the DRCQ can be used to assess personnel from any professions at risk for vicarious traumatization or burnout.

ACKNOWLEDGMENT

Gargi Roysircar, Professor Emerita of Psychology, Antioch University, has been awarded the American Psychological Association's (APA) 2019 International Humanitarian Award and APA's Div. 35 Psychology of Women's 2019 Psychotherapy with Women Research Award. Allyssa Lanza is a licensed clinical psychologist practicing in Maryland and Virginia with a focus on treating trauma disorders. Marie Macedonia is a postdoctoral fellow at Greater Nashua Mental Health Center, Nashua, NH, where she manages an integrated co-occurring treatment program and a team of case managers/therapists, and has a caseload of clients. This research was supported by the Foundation of the Mid-South in partnership with the America Red Cross and Antioch University's Faculty Mini-Grant. Roysircar thanks alumni/ae of Disaster Shakti of Antioch University New England for joining her in disaster mental health service and research nationally and internationally. They are Drs. Michael Brodeur, Allyssa Lanza, Abimbola

Afolayan, Ashland Thompson, Sarajane Rodgers, Josefina Irigoyen, Michiko Ishibashi, Brian Denietolis, Perrin Tellock, Thomas Hulslander, Katherine Russell, Kelsey Moran, Molly Conley, Kevin O'Leary, Megan Marsh, Elizabeth Briggs, Katie Reynolds, Sarah Hersey, Kristen Robinson, Linda Lee, Kate Airey, Alison Roy, Anders Goranson, Claire Dunnett, Daniel Greif, and Stephanie Miller.

REFERENCES

Agaibi, C. E., & Wilson, J. P. (2005). Trauma, PTSD, and resilience: A review of the literature. *Trauma, Violence & Abuse*, *6*(3), 195–216. doi:10.1177/1524838005277438 PMID:16237155

Alvord, M. K., & Grados, J. J. (2005). Enhancing resilience in children: A proactive approach. *Professional Psychology, Research and Practice*, *36*(3), 238–245. doi:10.1037/0735-7028.36.3.238

American Counseling Association. (2005). *ACA Code of Ethics*. Alexandria, VA: Author.

American Psychological Association. (2002). Ethical principles of psychologists and code of conduct. *American Psychologist*, *57*(12), 1060–1073. doi:10.1037/0003-066X.57.12.1060 PMID:12613157

American Psychological Association. (2017) *Multicultural Guidelines: An ecological approach to context, identity, and intersectionality*. Retrieved from http://www.apa.org/about/policy/multicultural-guidelines.aspx

Arnett, J. (2008). The neglected 95%: Why American psychology needs to become less American. *American Psychologist*, *63*(70), 602–614. doi:10.1037/0003-066X.63.7.602 PMID:18855491

Baird, S., & Jenkins, S. (2003). Vicarious traumatization, secondary traumatic stress, and burnout in sexual assault and domestic violence agency staff. *Violence and Victims*, *18*(1), 71–86. doi:10.1891/vivi.2003.18.1.71 PMID:12733620

Barnard, L. K., & Curry, J. F. (2011). Self-compassion as a mechanism of change in mindfulness and acceptance-based treatments. In R. A. Baer (Ed.), *Assessing mindfulness and acceptance processes in clients: Illuminating the theory and practice of change* (pp. 135–153). Oakland, CA: New Harbinger Publications.

Boudreau, M. (2015). Africentric Resilience Training: A prevention program for African American soldiers. *Dissertations & Theses*. 229. Retrieved from https://aura.antioch.edu/etds/229

Bowman, S., & Roysircar, G. (2011). Training and practice in trauma, catastrophes, and disaster counseling. *The Counseling Psychologist*, *39*(8), 1160–1181. doi:10.1177/0011000010397934

Brodeur, M. D. (2009). *Assessment of resilience and its protective factors in disaster volunteers* (Doctoral dissertation). Retrieved from ProQuest Dissertations and Theses database. (UMI No. 3385340)

Carroll, L., Gilroy, P. J., & Murra, J. (1999). The moral imperative: Self-care for women psychotherapists. *Women & Therapy*, *22*(2), 133–143. doi:10.1300/J015v22n02_10

Chang, E. C., Downey, C. A., Hirsch, J. K., & Lin, N. J. (Eds.). (2016). *Cultural, racial, and ethnic psychology book series. Positive psychology in racial and ethnic groups: Theory, research, and practice.* Washington, DC: American Psychological Association. doi:10.1037/14799-000

Daas-Brailsford, P. (2010). Secondary trauma among disaster responders. In P. Daas-Brailsford (Ed.), *Crisis and disaster counseling* (pp. 213–228). Thousand Oaks, CA: SAGE. doi:10.4135/9781452275093.n14

Ehrenreich, J. H., & Elliott, T. L. (2004). Managing stress in humanitarian aid workers. *Peace and Conflict, 10*(1), 53–66. doi:10.120715327949pac1001_4

Friborg, O., Hjemdal, O., Rosenvinge, J. H., Martinussen, M., Aslaksen, P. M., & Flaten, M. A. (2006). Resilience as a moderator of pain and stress. *Journal of Psychosomatic Research, 61*(2), 213–219. doi:10.1016/j.jpsychores.2005.12.007 PMID:16880024

Fullerton, C. S., Ursano, R. J., & Wang, L. (2004). Acute stress disorder, posttraumatic stress disorder, and depression in disaster or rescue workers. *The American Journal of Psychiatry, 161*(8), 1370–1376. doi:10.1176/appi.ajp.161.8.1370 PMID:15285961

Germer, C. K., & Neff, K. D. (2013). Self-compassion in clinical practice. *Journal of Clinical Psychology, 69*(8), 856–867. doi:10.1002/jclp.22021 PMID:23775511

Glicken, M. D. (2006). *Learning from resilient people: Lessons we can apply to counseling and psychotherapy*. Thousand Oaks, CA: Sage Publications.

Harrison, R. L., & Westwood, M. J. (2009). Preventing vicarious traumatization of mental health therapists: Identifying protective practices. *Psychotherapy (Chicago, Ill.), 46*(2), 203–219. doi:10.1037/a0016081 PMID:22122619

Howlett, S. L., & Collins, A. (2014). Vicarious traumatization: Risk and resilience among crisis support volunteers in a community organization. *South African Journal of Psychology. Suid-Afrikaanse Tydskrif vir Sielkunde, 44*(2), 180–190. doi:10.1177/0081246314524387

Lanza, A., Roysircar, G., & Rodgers, S. (2018). First responder mental healthcare. Evidence-based prevention, postvention, and treatment services. *Professional Psychology, Research and Practice, 49*(3), 193–204. doi:10.1037/pro0000192

Leary, M. R., Tate, E. B., Adams, C. E., Allen, A. B., & Hancock, J. (2007). Self-compassion and reactions to unpleasant self-relevant events: The implication of treating oneself kindly. *Journal of Personality and Social Psychology, 92*(5), 887–890. doi:10.1037/0022-3514.92.5.887 PMID:17484611

Lightsey, O. R. Jr. (2006). Resilience, meaning, and well-being. *The Counseling Psychologist, 34*(1), 96–107. doi:10.1177/0011000005282369

MacBeth, A., & Gumley, A. (2012). Exploring compassion: A meta-analysis of the association between self-compassion & psychopathology. *Clinical Psychology Review, 32*(6), 545–552. doi:10.1016/j.cpr.2012.06.003 PMID:22796446

Macedonia, M. (2018). *Self-Care and self-compassion of first responders: Predictors of resilience* (Doctoral Dissertation). Antioch University New England. https://aura.antioch.edu/etds/431/

Maslach, C., Schaufeli, W., & Leiter, M. (2001). Job burnout. *Annual Review of Psychology, 52*(1), 397–422. doi:10.1146/annurev.psych.52.1.397 PMID:11148311

Masten, A. S., Best, K. M., & Garmezy, N. (1990). Resilience and development: Contributions from the study of children who overcome adversity. *Development and Psychopathology, 2*(4), 425–444. doi:10.1017/S0954579400005812

Masten, A. S., & Narayan, A. J. (2012). Child development in the context of disaster, war, and terrorism: Pathways of risk and resilience. *Annual Review of Psychology, 63*(1), 227–257. doi:10.1146/annurev-psych-120710-100356 PMID:21943168

Neff, K. D., & Pommier, E. (2012). The relationship between self-compassion and other-focused concern among college undergraduates, community adults, and practicing mediators. *Self and Identity, 12*(2), 160–176. doi:10.1080/15298868.2011.649546

Norcross, J. C., & Barnett, J. E. (2007). Self-care as ethical imperative. *National Register of Health Service Psychologists*. Retrieved from https://www.nationalregister.org/pub/the-national-register-report-pub/the-register-report-spring-2008/self-care-as-ethical-imperative/

Roysircar, G. (2008). *Building community resilience in Mississippi: Self-care for disaster response workers and caregivers (Grantor: Foundation of the Mid-South in partnership with the America Red Cross)*. Keene, NH: Antioch University New England, Multicultural Center for Research and Practice.

Roysircar, G. (2009a, August). *Resilience and self-care of Katrina responders: Outcomes and evaluations*. Paper presented at the annual conference of the American Psychological Association, Toronto, Canada.

Roysircar, G. (2009b). The big picture of social justice advocacy: Counselor, heal society and thyself. *Journal of Counseling and Development, 87*(3), 288–295. doi:10.1002/j.1556-6678.2009.tb00109.x

Roysircar, G. (2010). *Development of the Disaster Response Competencies Questionnaire (DRCQ): A Pilot Study. (Faculty Mini Grant, Antioch University New England)*. Keene, NH: Antioch University New England, Multicultural Center for Research and Practice.

Roysircar, G. (2012). Development of the Disaster Response Competencies Questionnaire (DRCQ): A pilot study. Grant application to the National Science Foundation, Arlington, VA.

Roysircar, G. (2018). Chapter 2: Counselor role and functions, professional ethics, stress, and self-care. In E. Ginter, G. Roysircar, & L. Gerstein (Eds.), Theories and strategies of counseling and psychotherapy: Relevance across cultures and settings (pp. 22-47). Thousand Oaks, CA: SAGE.

Roysircar, G., Colvin, K. F., Afolayan, A. G., Thompson, A., & Robertson, T. W. (2017). Haitian children's resilience and vulnerability assessed with House-Tree-Person (HTP) drawings. *Traumatology, 23*(1), 68–81. doi:10.1037/trm0000090

Roysircar, G., Geisinger, K., & Thompson, A. (2019). Haitian children's disaster trauma: Validation of pictorial assessment of resilience and vulnerability. *The Journal of Black Psychology*. doi:10.1177/0095798419838126

Roysircar, G., Pignatiello, V., Lanza, A., & Irigoyen, J. (2015, August). *A qualitative study of a disaster counseling model*. Paper presented at the annual conference of the American Psychological Association, Montreal, Canada.

Roysircar, G., Podkova, M., & Pignatiello, V. (2013). Crisis intervention, social class, and counseling: Macrolevel disaster effects. In W. M. Liu (Ed.), *The Oxford Handbook of social class in counseling* (pp. 144–163). New York, NY: Oxford University Press. doi:10.1093/oxfordhb/9780195398250.013.0009

Roysircar, G., Thompson, A., & Geisinger, K. (in press). Mothers' and children's trauma coping among the poor in Haiti: Mixed methods study of community-level research. *American Psychologist.*

Rutter, M. (1985). Resilience in the face of adversity: Protective factors and resistance to psychiatric disorder. *The British Journal of Psychiatry*, *147*(6), 598–611. doi:10.1192/bjp.147.6.598 PMID:3830321

Seligman, M., & Csikszentmihalyi, M. (2000). Positive psychology: An introduction. *American Psychologist*, *55*(1), 5–14. doi:10.1037/0003-066X.55.1.5 PMID:11392865

Shapiro, S., Brown, K., & Biegel, G. (2007). Teaching self-care to caregivers: Effects of mindfulness-based stress reduction on the mental health of therapists in training. *Training and Education in Professional Psychology*, *1*(2), 105–115. doi:10.1037/1931-3918.1.2.105

Smith, J. L. (2015). Self-compassion and resilience in senior living residents. *Seniors Housing & Care Journal*, *23*(1), 17–31. doi:10.7748/ns.2017.e10671

Tedeschi, R. G., & Kilmer, R. P. (2005). Assessing strengths, resilience, and growth to guide clinical interventions. *Professional Psychology, Research and Practice*, *36*(3), 230–237. doi:10.1037/0735-7028.36.3.230

Chapter 11

Bridging the Gaps:
Toward Effective Collaboration Between Peer Supporters and Behavioral Health Professionals

Fatima Dobani
Baylor Scott & White Health, USA

Michelle L. Pennington
Baylor Scott & White Health, USA

Elizabeth Coe
Baylor Scott & White Health, USA

Patrick Morrison
International Association of Fire Fighters, USA

Suzy Bird Gulliver
Baylor Scott & White Health, USA

ABSTRACT

Peer support, as part of a recovery-oriented approach to treatment, is a valuable resource across various clinical and nonclinical populations. Specifically, in fire service, peer support may bridge the gap between firefighters' behavioral health needs and access to professional services. The current chapter summarizes the literature on peer support utility, presents data on barriers to treatment, and describes the roles clinicians can fill in partnering with fire service peer support to enhance the quality and reach of behavioral health services offered to fire service personnel. Finally, future research directions are outlined to continue the conversation about how to improve collaborations between peer supporters, clinicians, and others working to support the needs and strengths of firefighters.

DOI: 10.4018/978-1-5225-9803-9.ch011

INTRODUCTION

Firefighters are tasked with preventing fires and preserving life and property. As such, they are required to be on the frontline of emergencies including, but not limited to: fires, multiple casualty events, natural disasters, and community traumas such as shootings, terrorist acts, and explosions. Firefighters may also be exposed to line of duty deaths, critical injuries, and suicides of fellow fire service members. These events have the potential to be traumatic for firefighters, and research demonstrates that repeated exposure to potentially traumatic events (PTEs) may have serious repercussions on firefighters' behavioral and physical health (Byrne & Espnes, 2008; Corneil, Beaton, Murphy, Johnson, & Pike, 1999; Murphy, Beaton, Pike, & Johnson, 1999; Wu, Yin, Xu, & Zhao, 2011). Although many firefighters complete their employment without developing a behavioral or physical health disorder, prevalence rates of depression, PTSD, cancer, suicide and substance misuse are higher among firefighters compared to the general population (Carey, Al-Zaiti, Dean, Sessanna, & Finnell, 2011; Haddock, et al., 2012; Javidi & Yadollahie, 2012; NIMH, 2017; CDC, 2017; Dill & Loew, 2012).

Because of the pervasiveness of behavioral health issues within fire service, having access to resources such as Employee Assistance Programs (EAPs), Member Assistance Programs (MAPs), and professional behavioral health clinicians can be useful to firefighters. While many fire departments provide resources such as EAPs and MAPs, and some provide direct access to clinicians, various barriers may prevent firefighters from seeking treatment through these means (Halpern, Gurevich, Schwartz, & Brazeau, 2009). The overarching objective of this chapter is to highlight how peer supporters, in collaboration with behavioral health professionals, may help bridge the gaps between firefighters' behavioral health needs and access to professional services. Towards this end, this chapter summarizes the literature on peer support utility, presents information on barriers to treatment, describes ways clinicians can effectively partner with fire service peer support to enhance the quality and reach of firefighter-focused behavioral health services, and outlines future research directions to continue improving collaborations between peer supporters, clinicians, and others working to support the needs and strengths of firefighters.

BACKGROUND

Overview of Peer Support

Evidence for peer support dates back as early as the 18th century, when a physician in France employed recovered patients at his hospital (Davidson, Bellamy, Guy, & Miller, 2012). Today, peer support has evolved into a system of care with applications in nearly every field, including fire service. Peer supporters may be paid employees or unpaid volunteers. A peer supporter may be a professional in a related field (e.g., a retired firefighter with a counseling degree) or a paraprofessional (e.g., a firefighter with no formal counseling education, but 15 years of sobriety). Peer supporters may also be individuals who do not have lived experience with specific symptomology, yet are naturally drawn to that role (e.g., the "confidante" of the firehouse).

The concept of peer support entails those with similar backgrounds being able to relate to one another in a way that supports authentic empathy and validation, thereby fostering wellness (Mead & Macneil, 2006). By using their own lived experiences or successful recovery stories, peer supporters can provide guidance and support to individuals (Clossey, Solomon, Hu, Gillen, & Zimm, 2018). Peer supporters can offer a range of services including but not limited to: teaching individuals about their diagnosis, offering emotional support, connecting individuals to resources and other individuals in the community, and role modeling (Clossey, et al., 2018). Peer supporters can also support individuals in ways that may be considered beyond the scope of clinicians (Hoey, Ieropoli, White, & Jefford, 2008), such as through advocacy or social services.

In populations presenting with common behavioral health concerns, peer support has been shown to decrease substance use and depression; increase hopefulness, engagement with care, activation, self-care, and sense of well-being; and improve relationships with providers (Chinman, Shoai, & Cohen, 2010). In populations presenting with less common, serious mental illness, Fuhr and colleagues (2014) concluded that peer services may be superior to standard psychiatric care in increasing quality of life and hope, and equivalent to clinician-delivered services in terms of symptom reduction. Moreover, peer support is adaptable to alternative delivery methods, such as online (Melling & Houguet- Pincham, 2011).

Dorgo and colleagues (2009; 2013) conducted a study in which they examined the effectiveness of a peer support program among older adults. Results indicate that the peer support program significantly improved fitness of the older adults and the peer support program had high retention rates. Moreover, a meta-analysis by Pfeiffer and colleagues (Pfeiffer, Heisler, Piette, Rogers, & Valenstein, 2011) found that peer support was superior to usual care in reducing depressive symptoms, and peer support was as good as professionally delivered group cognitive-behavioral therapy (gCBT) in reducing symptoms of depression. Among a group of police officers, Donahue (1977) found that peer support led to improvements in communication and empathy skills.

In summary, peer supporters may serve as effective gatekeepers and facilitators of behavioral health treatment. In fire service, peer support may serve a particularly important function as a bridge across the gaps between firefighters' behavioral health concerns, which occur at a high rate (Byrne & Espnes, 2008), and access to services, which occurs at a lower-than-expected rate (Gulliver et al., 2018). The following section outlines some of these gaps and barriers in greater detail.

GAPS IN BEHAVIORAL HEALTH CARE FOR FIREFIGHTERS

Barriers to Treatment

Although resources such as EAPs are provided to address firefighters' behavioral and physical health concerns, firefighters report limited use of EAPs (McMahon, 2010). Gulliver and colleagues (2018) conducted an online survey in which they examined access, attitudes, and preferences of 2,156 firefighters towards behavioral health services. The results of this study revealed different barriers to treatment: concerns about confidentiality, self-stigma, a lack of culturally competent clinicians, and negative expectations of treatment. A literature search also indicated structural and logistic barriers endorsed by firefighters, preventing them from seeking services.

Fire culture emphasizes the importance of social support among colleagues (North et al., 2002). As such, the bonds made between firefighters are unlikely to be replicated by professionals. Firefighters may be hesitant to confide in professionals, as they believe private information may be leaked to the rest of fire service (Løvseth & Aasland, 2010). Concern about confidentiality is one reason firefighters may be resistant to using EAPs. Depending on the structure of a fire department, EAPs may have to report out to city management. This may result in termination for firefighters who disclose detrimental information. Gulliver and colleagues (2018) reported 51% of firefighters endorsed a fear of breach in confidentiality as a barrier to treatment.

Stigma is another barrier that prevents firefighters from seeking treatment. Fire culture often refers to "feelings" as an "F" word, wherein firefighters view feelings as a taboo discussion topic and may feel discomfort when faced with vulnerable emotions (Halpern, et al., 2009). Gulliver and colleagues (2018) reported that only 3% of firefighters would think less of other firefighters utilizing behavioral health services, but 43% of firefighters reported stigma-related barriers were preventing participation in behavioral health services, and 29% of firefighters believed using behavioral health services may damage their firefighter reputation, which suggest that firefighters feel self-stigma as opposed to perceived public-stigma to seeking help. Self-stigma is an individual's belief that their illness makes them weak (Watson, Corrigan, Larson, & Sells, 2007), leading to internalized devaluation and disempowerment (Corrigan, 2002). Hom and colleagues (Hom, Stanley, Ringer, & Joiner, 2016) also found that firefighters' concerns about embarrassment and harm to one's reputation were significantly associated with service non-use.

Eighty-eight percent of firefighters reported that having a clinician who understands their work culture is an important component of a behavioral health program and 53% of firefighters reported clinicians who were unaware of the work culture as a barrier to treatment (Gulliver et al., 2018). The fire culture is unique, and without proper knowledge, a clinician may offend a firefighter, or not completely understand job responsibilities, ultimately decreasing treatment efficacy.

Negative expectations of treatment also prevent firefighters from seeking services (McMahon, 2010). Negative expectations include, perceived lack of usefulness, poor anticipated follow-up by clinicians, and beliefs that family members or co-workers are better resources than professionals. Vogel and colleagues (Vogel, Wester, Wei, & Boysen, 2005) found that an anticipated lack of utility was a barrier to treatment, and those that did not feel as if services would help them, did not get treatment. Gulliver and colleagues (2018) found only 24% of firefighter respondents were confident of adequate follow-up care. Moreover, firefighters in the earlier years of their service prefer seeking support from their spouse, family member, coworker or officer, but more seasoned firefighters prefer seeking help from either a private professional service or EAP (Gulliver et al., 2018).

Structural barriers, including cost and availability of resources are barriers that firefighters report as well. Hom and colleagues (2016) report that cost of treatment was a barrier keeping 35% of their sample from seeking services. Stanley and colleagues (Stanley, Boffa, Hom, Kimbrel, & Joiner, 2017), sampled 525 firefighters and found that volunteer firefighters reported higher numbers of structural barriers compared to career firefighters, and that those barriers accounted for differences in mental health between volunteer and career firefighters.

Logistic barriers, including rotating shifts and a high number of working hours per week, may interfere with a firefighter's ability to access "typical" behavioral health services. An average workday is 8-9 hours for civilians. However, firefighters work in 24-hour shifts. Rotating shift work may result in firefighters being unable to receive services, as their schedules change weekly.

As the number of barriers to treatment seeking increases, a firefighter's likelihood of utilizing behavioral health programs decreases (Bulala, 2013). Gulliver and colleagues (2018) observed that 68% of firefighters would not recommend behavioral health services to their peers. The gap between the rate of behavioral health concerns and the rate of utilization of behavioral health treatments presents a significant issue within this population.

Utility of Peer Support to Address Barriers

Firefighters commonly cope with difficulties by using social support (Fullerton, McCarroll, Ursano, & Wright, 1992), and social support can positively influence recovery from traumatic events (Lyons, 1991; Regehr, Hill, & Glancy, 2000). As such, peer support may be beneficial to firefighters. Peer supporters can relate to firefighters due to shared experiences, perhaps increasing rapport and trust. Peer supporters can provide direct services and support to individuals, advocate on behalf of individuals to ensure the individual's needs are met, and connect individuals to professional services. When delivered in tandem with professional care, peer support programs may also improve satisfaction with professional care (Ashbury, Cameron, Mercer, Fitch, & Nielsen, 1998). Peer supporters can work with both the firefighter and clinician to ensure that the clinician is understanding and addressing the firefighter's needs. As a result, peer supporters can serve as effective connectors or bridges between firefighters and behavioral health treatment, and help reduce lack of clinician familiarity with fire service as a barrier to treatment.

Through the provision of direct support services, peer support may decrease the need for professional health services. Direct services provided by peer supporters include: providing education/information, teaching coping skills, and promoting medication adherence. In studies of peer support within medical and crisis respite settings, peer support has been shown to yield symptom improvement, fewer hospitalizations, and decreased health expenditures (Bouchery et al., 2018; Landers & Zhou, 2011). By reducing the need for professional health services, peer support may play a role in reducing structural and logistic barriers that firefighters report as barriers to treatment.

In the case of clear expert need, peer supporters can play a vital role in facilitating connections to professional services. For example, it is exigent for peer supporters to have a clear understanding of when confidentiality must be broken. Confidentiality is considered the cornerstone of a peer support relationship. In order to enhance trust, a peer supporter should ensure the individual they are working with that they will keep private information confidential. However, in a situation where a firefighter confides that they are a danger to themselves or others, peer supporters must break confidentiality to alert a professional who can address the situation (Shapiro & Galowitz, 2016). Further, fire departments all have different rules and guidelines in which confidentiality must be broken. Firefighters may be hesitant to speak candidly with a professional, without first understanding confidentiality guidelines, thus a peer supporter should have a discussion with the firefighter they are assisting about ethics that informs firefighters of situations in which confidentiality cannot be kept (Davidson, Bellamy, Guy, & Miller, 2012).

Firefighters may not be aware of resources in their community, therefore peer supporters can augment resources available to firefighters. Peer supporters should become familiar with a host of resources available in their community. Greden and colleagues (2010) discuss how connecting veterans to resources that provide assistance with employment, housing, and finance, reduces stress levels. Other examples of resources peer supporters should familiarize themselves with are: crisis hotline numbers, beneficial treatment studies, programs for emergency responders, contact information for specialists and type of insurance taken, employment agencies, food banks, and shelters. Providing firefighters with resources specific to their needs will ensure the resources are able to aid the firefighter; possibly changing firefighters' opinions about negative expectations of treatment.

Peer supporters may also connect firefighters with community groups including Alcoholics Anonymous (AA), Narcotics Anonymous (NA), church groups, parent groups, or veteran groups. Sells, Davidson, Jewell, Falzer, & Rowe, (2006) found that individuals who attended AA or NA meetings regularly self-reported higher treatment motivation for psychiatric, alcohol, and drug use problems. Additionally, participation in community groups may result in decreased self-stigma (Corrigan et al., 2010). Fellowship with a group of individuals who support the firefighter may further strengthen the firefighter's resolve to recovery.

Due to the promise of peer support in helping address behavioral health needs, in 2014 the International Association of Fire Fighters (IAFF) received funding from the Assistance to Firefighters Grant Program (AFG) branch of the Federal Emergency Management Agency (FEMA) to develop an evidence-based, standardized Peer Support Training for fire service. Through an education development, iterative process, a two-day peer-delivered live training was constructed and beta-tested. This program is designed to equip IAFF Trained Peer Supporters to effectively aid their peers, educate the public and colleagues, and bridge the gaps between available resources and those who need them. The training course utilizes interactive methods that improve abilities in multiple areas, including crisis intervention, active listening skills, confidentiality, assessment skills, action planning, engagement, skill building, and awareness of local behavioral health resources. Utilizing the skills taught in the training, IAFF Trained Peer Supporters can build and grow an extensive peer support network. Today, the IAFF has 35 certified Peer Support Trainers delivering training to local Unions throughout the United States and Canada. As of this writing, 3200 individual firefighters have completed the initial training.

Remaining Gaps and Challenges

One of the biggest challenges peer supporters report is finding appropriate clinician partners. According to the General President of the IAFF, there is a shortage of clinicians who understand the mental health disorders and needs of firefighters. In order to effectively engage firefighters in treatment, clinicians should have an understanding of the types of situations firefighters may be exposed to and the behavioral and physical health consequences that subsequently follow. Clinicians also need to be flexible in terms of scheduling due to firefighters' rotating shifts. Perhaps most importantly from an ethics standpoint, clinicians also need to understand the confidentiality policy of each fire department, and be confident in efficient assessment practices for public safety professionals.

Cultural competency is regarded as an important factor in therapeutic relationships and interventions (Asnaani & Hoffman, 2012). As such, it is vital for clinicians working with firefighters to understand fire service culture, including how firefighters interact with their peers and the world around them, how time is typically spent in and out of the fire house, how firefighters respond to emergencies, common behavioral health problems, and prevalent attitudes towards providers. Meyer, Hall-Clark, Hamaoka, & Peterson, (2015) discuss how clinical cultural competence (the integration of cultural knowledge, clinical skills, and awareness of patient attitudes) support treatment outcomes. In the military, many organizations are working to include cultural competence in treatment to obtain desired outcomes among their clients (Meyer et al., 2015). However, culturally competent clinicians are currently lacking within fire service due to lack of research supporting the need in this population.

In addition to unfamiliarity with firefighter culture, another factor constraining the efficacy of provided treatment is the shortage of providers who use evidence-based treatments (EBTs). Use of EBTs enhances therapeutic intervention and effectiveness (American Psychological Association, 2005). EBTs for the mental health challenge most commonly faced by firefighters include Cognitive Processing Therapy (CPT) for PTSD, Motivational Interviewing (MI) and Cognitive Behavioral Therapy (CBT) for alcohol use disorder and other substance-related disorders, and CBT for depression. The Unified Protocol for the

Transdiagnostic Treatment of Emotional Disorders (UP) covers these disorders and is also adaptable to fit other emotional problems commonly faced by firefighters, such as anxiety and irritability.

SOLUTIONS AND RECOMMENDATIONS

Peer support may be used to address the lack of clinician cultural competency for firefighters. By consulting with peer support partners, clinicians can gain better insight into fire service culture and the problems and tribulations firefighters may face. Peer supporters may also work within fire service to reduce negative attitudes towards mental health providers (Dixon, Hackmann, & Lehman, 1997), thus strengthening relationships between firefighters and clinicians. Collaboration between peers and professionals is shown to enhance outcomes for recipients (Klein, Cnaan, & Whitecraft, 1998), which ultimately benefits the firefighter. Collaborations between behavioral health clinicians and peer supporters are mutually beneficial in that clinicians can provide peer supporters with assistance when issues arise that are beyond the scope of peer support, and peer supporters are able to give referrals to clinicians. Strong partnerships between clinicians and peer supporters may lead to better treatment satisfaction and outcomes among firefighters, who tend to underuse behavioral health services.

To address the shortage of clinicians with knowledge of firefighter culture, the authors' team created a Cultural Awareness Training, as part of a federally funded grant awarded by the Assistance to Firefighters Grant Program (AFG) branch of the Federal Emergency Management Agency (FEMA). This training aims to introduce clinicians to fire service culture as well as common presenting problems, diagnoses, and treatments relevant to firefighters. The authors' team presented this training to a series of focus groups: first, a group of clinical psychology graduate students, and then a group of IAFF Trained Peer Supporters. Each focus group completed surveys assessing satisfaction, knowledge acquisition, and feedback for the presenters/authors. The authors' team incorporated feedback from each group and is now in the process of creating a video of this training which will be available for public viewing. Clinicians should ensure proper training in EBTs specific to behavioral health concerns commonly endorsed by firefighters. Depending on where the clinician resides and the resources the clinician has, trainings for EBTs specific to firefighters (CPT, MI, CBT, and UP) can be accessed online or via instructional manual. Some trainings may be offered in person annually. In the name of best practice, clinicians should make sure they have an understanding of both fire service culture as well as EBTs specific to firefighters' needs. Peer supporters may be able to assist firefighters with finding clinicians who use EBTs. Towards this end, peer supporters should have a basic knowledge of available EBTs, and more importantly, awareness of local clinicians who are qualified to provide EBTs.

Case Studies

As noted above, peer supporters can help bridge the gaps between firefighters and clinicians. Often, peer supporters are the first contact for firefighters who are in trouble. It is then the peer supporter's responsibility to discern how to best assist the firefighter. For example, a peer supporter may be able to resolve the issue on his or her own. If this is not possible, a peer supporter may choose to connect the firefighter to resources in the community or to a clinician. If the situation requires a peer supporter to link the firefighter with a clinician, depending on the situation, the clinician's role may differ. The following case studies outline different situations in which peer supporters and clinicians partner to provide services to firefighters. The careful reader can generalize these scenarios to see the extraordinary utility of strong partnerships between professional care providers and peer supporters.

Case Study 1

Peer supporter James is working with a firefighter that recently (6 months ago) suffered the loss of his wife of 3 years in a drunk-driving accident. The firefighter is angry and hostile on the job, and James is seeing his anger grow instead of shrink. James thinks it is time to get the firefighter to see a professional.

James considers whether to send the firefighter to a minister or a professional counselor. James has never heard the firefighter speak about his spiritual beliefs, so he decides that his first step is to engage the firefighter in a discussion about the changes he has noticed and to inquire about the firefighter's wellbeing. As part of the discussion, James asks the firefighter about his grief process, including any faith traditions or spiritual practices. The firefighter jokes that he only attends church "when someone I know is in a tux or in a box." The firefighter mentions that he too has noticed his increased anger, although he had not connected it to his grief and he is surprised and distraught that it has become noticeable at work. James refers the firefighter to a trusted professional counselor. Based on prior interactions, James knows that this counselor is knowledgeable about firefighter culture, has experience treating grief and anger, and will explore relevant cultural factors, including spirituality, in a sensitive way.

Case Study 2

A peer support team is called to help firefighters who responded to a school shooting. Prior to deploying, the team consults with a licensed psychologist to review their support plan. The psychologist provides information about variability of responses to traumas such as community violence and helps the peer support team address any initial questions and concerns. Feeling prepared, the peer support team and the psychologist then develop and agree to a contact plan. The plan outlines when the psychologist will be available to a) provide additional consultation to team members if needed, b) offer direct services for any issues that arise beyond the scope of peer support, and c) to debrief/review after the team returns.

Case Study 3

Maple City, Nostate, USA just experienced the suicide of a respected senior leader within the fire department. The peer support team members, along with many others within the department and the community, are devastated. A few of the peer supporters have been asked to make a statement to the press about the suicide. Fortunately, the peer support team is well-versed in the importance of self-care and self-monitoring the impact of one's personal responses on one's professional capabilities. The peer support team calls in a clinician for a refresher on these topics and to create a plan of action that will not add undue burden to their own grief load. The clinician helps the team voice their concerns about the impact of their grief on their ability to support their community at this time. The clinician encourages the peer supporters to continue self-monitoring their reactions, to adjust their peer support workload appropriately, and to reach out for help if needed. The clinician helps the team review suicide warning signs and safety planning and compiles a list of referral options within and around the community. Additionally, the clinician agrees to speak to the press and works with the peer support team to craft a statement that will respect the deceased, validate the community's sense of loss, and provide information about suicide risk and safety factors.

FUTURE RESEARCH DIRECTIONS

To continue the conversation about how to improve collaborations between peer supporters, clinicians, and others working to support the needs and strengths of emergency responders, future research is needed in the following areas: selection and training of both peers and clinicians, quality and quantity of supervision, for both peers and clinicians, especially in cultural competency and evolving practice guidelines, ongoing educational requirements, and self-care of peer supporters, as well as clinicians that serve them.

Peer support can be a powerful tool in helping firefighters manage their symptoms and get connected with behavioral health services. However, it is important that peer supporters are properly trained in crisis intervention, active listening skills, confidentiality issues and considerations, assessment skills, action planning, peer engagement, skill building, and awareness of local behavioral health resources. Peer supporters must also demonstrate credibility, job competency, and confidence. A lack of skill in these areas could decrease the efficacy of peer support services among firefighters. A simple internet search reveals many organizations offering peer support certification. However, there is limited research on standardized, evidence-based best practices regarding peer support training. Kemp and & Henderson (2012) reported that the main challenge peer supporters endorsed was a lack of understanding of the peer supporter role. Standardized training procedures, like the ones currently being developed and tested by the IAFF, will likely provide clarification on this front, via a common understanding of the peer support role and requisite skills.

Many peer supporters are employed in organizations that understand the utility of supervision and provide peer supporters access to supervisory professionals, such as clinicians or providers (Chinman et al., 2010). Supervisors are tasked with discussing challenges faced by peer supporters, maintaining and reinforcing skills that were learned during training, promoting self-care among peer supporters, advocating for peer support services, and encouraging professional growth. While there is evidence supporting supervision as a useful tool for increasing peer support effectiveness (Crane-Okada, Freeman, Ross, Kiger, & Giuliano, 2010; Giese-Davis et al., 2006; Larimer et al., 2001), there is a dearth of research addressing questions of quality (i.e., what makes for good supervision?) and quantity (i.e., how much supervision is needed?). Future research is needed to establish evidence-based best practices in terms of how, and how much, peer support supervision should be delivered. Further research within fire service is especially needed, as there are no extant evidence-based guidelines for peer support supervision specific to this population.

Prior research demonstrates that both training and supervision are critical for the success of mental health peer support programs (Chapman, Blash, Mayer, & Spetz, 2018). Currently, peer support requirements vary from state to state, and there are no standardized guidelines on how or how often peer supporters should participate in ongoing education requirements. Further research is needed to establish best practice guidelines for ongoing educational requirements to ensure that peer supporters are providing up-to-date services and resources.

Peer supporters are individuals who may also be dealing with their own life stressors. Peer supporters should make sure they are practicing self-care and seeking help if they are experiencing adverse symptoms. Burnout and compassion fatigue are two symptoms of inadequate self-care. At present, the research literature does not adequately outline the importance of self-care among peer supporters in the general population, let alone in fire service specifically. Future research should consider the importance of self-care among firefighter peer supporters.

CONCLUSION

Firefighters are regularly exposed to traumatic events, increasing their risk of developing behavioral and/or physical health concerns. Despite efforts made by fire departments to provide resources to address elevated behavioral health concerns, firefighters report underutilizing these services. Fire service culture promotes brotherhood, and research suggests that social support may reduce adverse symptomology. Thus, peer support services may be beneficial to firefighters, and a good fit for fire service culture. Well-trained and supervised peer supporters may reduce the need for professional services. When situations arise beyond the scope of direct peer support services, peer supporters can connect firefighters to trusted clinicians or other health care professionals that understands the fire service culture. Thus, partnerships between firefighters, peer supporters, and clinicians may be highly valuable in alleviating firefighter concerns and increasing access to needed services. Effective collaboration between peer supporters, clinicians, and others working to support the needs and strengths of firefighters is an aspirational goal and, therefore, an ongoing process. Further research – particularly in the areas of selection and training, supervision, ongoing education, and self-care of peer supporters – will provide insight into how best to harness and promote the power of peer support within fire service.

ACKNOWLEDGMENT

The Warriors Research Institute would like to thank all firefighters past and present who aided in the development and beta testing of the IAFF peer support training. We also would like to thank our clinician partners, peer supporters, and trainers. Thank you to Dr. Claire Cammarata, Dr. Nathan Kimbrel, Capt. Frank Leto, Lt. William Ostiguy, and Lt. Brian Nee for their unwavering support. This chapter was not supported by a specific grant from any funding agency in the public, commercial, or not-for-profit sectors.

REFERENCES

American Psychological Association. (2005, August). *Policy statement on evidence-based practice in psychology.* Meeting of the APA Council of Representatives. Retrieved from http://www.apa.org/practice/guidelines/evidence-based-statement.aspx

Ashbury, F. D., Cameron, C., Mercer, S. L., Fitch, M., & Nielsen, E. (1998). One-on-one peer support and quality of life for breast cancer patients. *Patient Education and Counseling*, *35*(2), 89–100. doi:10.1016/S0738-3991(98)00035-4 PMID:10026552

Asnaani, A., & Hofmann, S. G. (2012). Collaboration in multicultural therapy: Establishing a strong therapeutic alliance across cultural lines. *Journal of Clinical Psychology*, *68*(2), 187–197. doi:10.1002/jclp.21829 PMID:23616299

Bouchery, E. E., Barna, M., Babalola, E., Friend, D., Brown, J. D., Blyler, C., & Ireys, H. T. (2018). The effectiveness of a peer-staffed crisis respite program as an alternative to hospitalization. *Psychiatric Services (Washington, D.C.)*, *69*(10), 1069–1074. doi:10.1176/appi.ps.201700451 PMID:30071793

Bulala, J. (2013). *The Relationship between the utilization of mental health services, coping mechanisms, and reputation in male firefighters* (Doctoral dissertation). Alliant International University, San Francisco, CA.

Byrne, D., & Espnes, G. A. (2008). Occupational stress and cardiovascular disease. *Stress and Health*, *24*(3), 231–238. doi:10.1002mi.1203

Carey, M. G., Al-Zaiti, S. S., Dean, G. E., Sessanna, L., & Finnell, D. S. (2011). Sleep problems, depression, substance use, social bonding, and quality of life in professional firefighters. *Journal of Occupational and Environmental Medicine/American College of Occupational and Environmental Medicine*, *53*(8), 928.

Center for Disease Control and Prevention. (2017). *Firefighter Cancer Rates: The Facts from NIOSH Research*. Retrieved from: https://blogs.cdc.gov/niosh-science blog/2017/05/10/ff-cancer-facts/

Chapman, S. A., Blash, L. K., Mayer, K., & Spetz, J. (2018). Emerging roles for peer providers in mental health and substance use disorders. *American Journal of Preventive Medicine*, *54*(6), S267–S274. doi:10.1016/j.amepre.2018.02.019 PMID:29779551

Chinman, M., Shoai, R., & Cohen, A. (2010). Using organizational change strategies to guide peer support technician implementation in the Veterans Administration. *Psychiatric Rehabilitation Journal*, *33*(4), 269–277. doi:10.2975/33.4.2010.269.277 PMID:20374985

Clossey, L., Solomon, P., Hu, C., Gillen, J., & Zinn, M. (2018). Predicting the job satisfaction of mental health peer support workers (PSWs). *Social Work in Mental Health*, *16*(6), 682–695. doi:10.1080/15332985.2018.1483463

Corneil, W., Beaton, R., Murphy, S., Johnson, C., & Pike, K. (1999). Exposure to traumatic incidents and prevalence of posttraumatic stress symptomatology in urban firefighters in two countries. *Journal of Occupational Health Psychology*, *4*(2), 131–141. doi:10.1037/1076-8998.4.2.131 PMID:10212865

Corrigan, P. W., Morris, S., Larson, J., Rafacz, J., Wassel, A., Michaels, P., ... Rüsch, N. (2010). Self-stigma and coming out about one's mental illness. *Journal of Community Psychology*, *38*(3), 259–275. doi:10.1002/jcop.20363 PMID:23970807

Crane-Okada, R., Freeman, E., Ross, M., Kiger, H., & Giuliano, A. E. (2010). Training senior peer counselors to provide telephone support for newly diagnosed breast cancer survivors. *Journal of Cancer Education*, *25*(2), 174–179. doi:10.100713187-009-0028-7 PMID:20082171

Davidson, L., Bellamy, C., Guy, K., & Miller, R. (2012). Peer support among persons with severe mental illnesses: A review of evidence and experience. *World Psychiatry; Official Journal of the World Psychiatric Association (WPA)*, *11*(2), 123–128. doi:10.1016/j.wpsyc.2012.05.009 PMID:22654945

Dill, J., & Loew, C. (2012). Suicide in the fire and emergency services. *National Volunteer Fire Council*. 1-41. Retrieved from: http://firefighterveteran.com/images/stories/Nationla_Volunteer_Fire_Counsel/Firefight r%2suicide%20report.pdf.

Dixon, L., Hackmann, A., & Lehman, A. (1997). Consumer as staff in assertive community treatment programs. *Administration and Policy in Mental Health*, *25*(2), 199–208. doi:10.1023/A:1022243106341 PMID:9727217

Donahue, M. J. (1977). *Peer counseling for police officers: a program for skill development and personal growth* (Unpublished doctoral dissertation). Boston University, Boston, MA.

Dorgo, S., King, G. A., Bader, J. O., & Limon, J. S. (2013). Outcomes of a peer mentor implemented fitness program in older adults: A quasi-randomized controlled trial. *International Journal of Nursing Studies*, *50*(9), 1156–1165. doi:10.1016/j.ijnurstu.2012.12.006 PMID:23279966

Dorgo, S., King, G. A., & Brickey, G. D. (2009). The application of peer mentoring to improve fitness in older adults. *Journal of Aging and Physical Activity*, *17*(3), 344–361. doi:10.1123/japa.17.3.344 PMID:19799104

Fuhr, D. C., Salisbury, T. T., De Silva, M. J., Atif, N., Van Ginneken, N., Rahman, A., & Patel, V. (2014). Effectiveness of peer-delivered interventions for severe mental illness and depression on clinical and psychosocial outcomes: A systematic review and meta-analysis. *Social Psychiatry and Psychiatric Epidemiology*, *49*(11), 1691–1702. doi:10.100700127-014-0857-5 PMID:24632847

Fullerton, C. S., McCarroll, J. E., Ursano, R. J., & Wright, K. M. (1992). Psychological responses of rescue workers: Fire fighters and trauma. *The American Journal of Orthopsychiatry*, *62*(3), 371–378. doi:10.1037/h0079363 PMID:1497102

Giese-Davis, J., Bliss-Isberg, C., Carson, K., Star, P., Donaghy, J., Cordova, M. J., ... Spiegel, D. (2006). The effect of peer counseling on quality of life following diagnosis of breast cancer: an observational study. *Psycho-Oncology: Journal of the Psychological. Social and Behavioral Dimensions of Cancer*, *15*(11), 1014–1022. PMID:16555366

Greden, J. F., Valenstein, M., Spinner, J., Blow, A., Gorman, L. A., Dalack, G. W., ... Kees, M. (2010). Buddy-to-Buddy, a citizen soldier peer support program to counteract stigma, PTSD, depression, and suicide. *Annals of the New York Academy of Sciences*, *1208*(1), 90–97. doi:10.1111/j.1749-6632.2010.05719.x PMID:20955330

Gulliver, S. B., Pennington, M. L., Torres, V. A., Steffen, L. E., Mardikar, A., Leto, F., ... Kimbrel, N. A. (2018). Behavioral Health Programs in Fire Service: Surveying Access and Preferences. *Psychological Services*; Advance online publication. PMID:29369659

Haddock, C. K., Jahnke, S. A., Poston, W. S. C., Jitnarin, N., Kaipust, C. M., Tuley, B., & Hyder, M. L. (2012). Alcohol use among firefighters in the Central United States. *Occupational Medicine*, *62*(8), 661–664. doi:10.1093/occmed/kqs162 PMID:23064207

Halpern, J., Gurevich, M., Schwartz, B., & Brazeau, P. (2009). Interventions for critical incident stress in emergency medical services: A qualitative study. *Stress and Health*, *25*(2), 139–149. doi:10.1002mi.1230

Hoey, L. M., Ieropoli, S. C., White, V. M., & Jefford, M. (2008). Systematic review of peer support programs for people with cancer. *Patient Education and Counseling*, *70*(3), 315–337. doi:10.1016/j.pec.2007.11.016 PMID:18191527

Hom, M. A., Stanley, I. H., Ringer, F. B., & Joiner, T. E. (2016). Mental health service use among firefighters with suicidal thoughts and behaviors. *Psychiatric Services (Washington, D.C.)*, *67*(6), 688–691. doi:10.1176/appi.ps.201500177 PMID:26927574

International Association for Fire Fighters. (2001). Washington, DC: Developing Fire Service Labor/Employee Assistance Programs.

Javidi, H., & Yadollahie, M. (2012). Post-traumatic stress disorder. *The International Journal of Occupational and Environmental Medicine*, *3*(1), 2–9. PMID:23022845

Kemp, V., & Henderson, A. R. (2012). Challenges faced by mental health peer support workers: Peer support from the peer supporter's point of view. *Psychiatric Rehabilitation Journal*, *35*(4), 337–340. doi:10.2975/35.4.2012.337.340 PMID:22491374

Klein, A., Cnaan, R., & Whitecraft, J. (1998). Significance of peer social support for dually diagnosed clients: Findings from a pilot study. *Research on Social Work Practice*, *8*(5), 529–551. doi:10.1177/104973159800800503

Landers, G. M., & Zhou, M. (2011). An analysis of relationships among peer support, psychiatric hospitalization, and crisis stabilization. *Community Mental Health Journal*, *47*(1), 106–112. doi:10.100710597-009-9218-3 PMID:19551502

Larimer, M. E., Turner, A. P., Anderson, B. K., Fader, J. S., Kilmer, J. R., Palmer, R. S., & Cronce, J. M. (2001). Evaluating a Brief Alcohol Intervention with Fraternities. *Journal of Studies on Alcohol*, *62*(3), 370–380. doi:10.15288/jsa.2001.62.370 PMID:11414347

Løvseth, L. T., & Aasland, O. G. (2010). Confidentiality as a barrier to social support: A crosssectional study of Norwegian emergency and human service workers. *International Journal of Stress Management*, *17*(3), 214–231. doi:10.1037/a0018904

Lyons, J. A. (1991). Strategies for assessing the potential for positive adjustment following trauma. *Journal of Traumatic Stress*, *4*(1), 93–111. doi:10.1002/jts.2490040108

McMahon, C. P. (2010). *A Phenomenological Study of Stress and Coping in the Fire Service* (Doctoral dissertation). Our Lady of the Lake University, San Antonio, TX.

Mead, S., & MacNeil, C. (2006). Peer support: What makes it unique. *International Journal of Psychosocial Rehabilitation*, *10*(2), 29–37.

Melling, B., & Houguet-Pincham, T. (2011). Online peer support for individuals with depression: A summary of current research and future considerations. *Psychiatric Rehabilitation Journal*, *34*(3), 252–254. doi:10.2975/34.3.2011.252.254 PMID:21208865

Meyer, E. G., Hall-Clark, B. N., Hamaoka, D., & Peterson, A. L. (2015). Assessment of military cultural competence: A pilot study. *Academic Psychiatry*, *39*(4), 382–388. doi:10.100740596-015-0328-7 PMID:26054708

Murphy, S. A., Beaton, R. D., Pike, K. C., & Johnson, L. C. (1999). Occupational stressors, stress responses, and alcohol consumption among professional firefighters: A prospective, longitudinal analysis. *International Journal of Stress Management*, *6*(3), 179–196. doi:10.1023/A:1021934725246

National Institute for Mental Health. (2017). *Major Depression.* Retrieved from: https://www.nimh.nih.gov/health/statistics/major-depression.shtml

North, C. S., Tivis, L., McMillen, J. C., Pfefferbaum, B., Cox, J., Spitznagel, E. L., ... Smith, E. M. (2002). Coping, functioning, and adjustment of rescue workers after the Oklahoma City bombing. *Journal of Traumatic Stress: Official Publication of The International Society for Traumatic Stress Studies, 15*(3), 171–175. doi:10.1023/A:1015286909111 PMID:12092908

Pfeiffer, P. N., Heisler, M., Piette, J. D., Rogers, M. A., & Valenstein, M. (2011). Efficacy of peer support interventions for depression: A meta-analysis. *General Hospital Psychiatry, 33*(1), 29–36. doi:10.1016/j.genhosppsych.2010.10.002 PMID:21353125

Regehr, C., Hill, J., & Glancy, G. D. (2000). Individual predictors of traumatic reactions in firefighters. *The Journal of Nervous and Mental Disease, 188*(6), 333–339. doi:10.1097/00005053-200006000-00003 PMID:10890341

Sells, D., Davidson, L., Jewell, C., Falzer, P., & Rowe, M. (2006). The treatment relationship in peer-based and regular case management for clients with severe mental illness. *Psychiatric Services (Washington, D.C.), 57*(8), 1179–1184. doi:10.1176/ps.2006.57.8.1179 PMID:16870970

Shapiro, J., & Galowitz, P. (2016). Peer support for clinicians: A programmatic approach. *Academic Medicine, 91*(9), 1200–1204. doi:10.1097/ACM.0000000000001297 PMID:27355784

Stanley, I. H., Boffa, J. W., Hom, M. A., Kimbrel, N. A., & Joiner, T. E. (2017). Differences in psychiatric symptoms and barriers to mental health care between volunteer and career firefighters. *Psychiatry Research, 247*, 236–242. doi:10.1016/j.psychres.2016.11.037 PMID:27930964

Vogel, D. L., Wester, S. R., Wei, M., & Boysen, G. A. (2005). The Role of Outcome Expectations and Attitudes on Decisions to Seek Professional Help. *Journal of Counseling Psychology, 52*(4), 459–470. doi:10.1037/0022-0167.52.4.459

Watson, A. C., Corrigan, P., Larson, J. E., & Sells, M. (2007). Self-stigma in people with mental illness. *Schizophrenia Bulletin, 33*(6), 1312–1318. doi:10.1093chbulbl076 PMID:17255118

Wu, D., Yin, H., Xu, S., & Zhao, Y. (2011). Risk factors for posttraumatic stress reactions among Chinese students following exposure to a snowstorm disaster. *BMC Public Health, 11*(1), 96. doi:10.1186/1471-2458-11-96 PMID:21314959

ADDITIONAL READING

Gulliver, S. B., Cammarata, C. M., Leto, F., Ostiguy, W. J., Flynn, E. J., Carpenter, G. S. J., ... Kimbrel, N. A. (2015). Project Reach Out: A Training Program to Increase Behavioral Health Utilization Among Professional Firefighters. *International Journal of Stress Management.*

Gulliver, S. B., Pennington, M. L., Torres, V. A., Steffen, L. E., Mardikar, A., Leto, F., ... Kimbrel, N. A. (2018). Behavioral Health Programs in Fire Service: Surveying Access and Preferences. *Psychological Services*; Advance online publication. PMID:29369659

International Association for Fire Fighters. (2001). Washington, DC: Developing Fire Service Labor/ Employee Assistance Programs.

North, C. S., Tivis, L., McMillen, J. C., Pfefferbaum, B., Cox, J., Spitznagel, E. L., ... Smith, E. M. (2002). Coping, functioning, and adjustment of rescue workers after the Oklahoma City bombing. *Journal of Traumatic Stress: Official Publication of The International Society for Traumatic Stress Studies*, *15*(3), 171–175. doi:10.1023/A:1015286909111 PMID:12092908

Shapiro, J., & Galowitz, P. (2016). Peer support for clinicians: A programmatic approach. *Academic Medicine*, *91*(9), 1200–1204. doi:10.1097/ACM.0000000000001297 PMID:27355784

KEY TERMS AND DEFINITIONS

Cultural Awareness Training: A presentation informing clinicians about fire service culture, with the goal of equipping clinicians with working knowledge of duties of the job, common diagnoses, common treatments, and logistics when treating firefighters.

Cultural Competence: Knowledge, awareness, and skills related to working effectively with individuals of various cultures.

Employee Assistance Program (EAP): A workplace program designed to assist work organizations in addressing productivity issues and assist employee clients in identifying and resolving personal concerns, including, health, marital, family, financial, alcohol, drug, legal, emotional, stress, or other personal issues that may affect job performance. An individual's employer typically pays for these services.

Evidence-Based Treatment (EBT): Treatment supported by peer-reviewed scientific evidence.

International Association of Fire Fighters (IAFF): Union consisting of paid full-time firefighters and emergency medical services personnel in the United States and Canada.

Member Assistance Program (MAP): Similar to EAPs, a resource provided to members giving them access to counseling and referral services to assist with problems they may be having which negatively impact job performance. The union or business pays for this service for its members. There is also a difference between governance and reporting structure between EAP and MAPs.

Negative Expectations of Treatment: The belief that treatment will have perceived lack of usefulness, poor anticipated follow-up by clinicians, and beliefs that family members or co-workers are better resources than professionals. Can be a barrier to treatment in fire service.

Peer Support: A program of care in which an individual in recovery supports his or her peers in their recovery and relates to them either by mutual identification or shared responsibility.

Recovery-Oriented Model: The belief that all individuals have the capability to recover and improve their quality of life.

Self-Stigma: Internalized stigma; an individual's belief that their illness makes them weak and/or damaged, leading to diminished self-esteem.

Chapter 12
Evidence-Based Practices to Enhance First Responder Well-Being and Performance

Eamonn Patrick Arble
Department of Psychology, Eastern Michigan University, USA

Bengt B. Arnetz
College of Human Medicine, Michigan State University, USA

ABSTRACT

In this chapter, the authors draw upon a review of the empirical and theoretical literature, as well as their extensive experience developing interventions among law enforcement officers, to provide a commentary on the needs of first responder training. The chapter begins by outlining the need for intervention, highlighting the severe consequences experienced by first responders as a result of their occupational stressors. The chapter then offers a review of the potential structure and timing of first responder training. Finally, specific psychophysiological mechanisms to be targeted during training are reviewed, including summaries of the relevant evidence base supporting their utility.

INTRODUCTION

First responders are called into action during terrifying and unpredictable events, and their lives and the lives of the civilians they serve can be placed at risk should they not execute their duties successfully. Although the needs of first responders as a group are highly divergent, it is clear that training must prepare them to function effectively within a maelstrom of stress and danger, protect their psychobiological health after repeated trauma exposure, and persistently contribute to a culture of organizational effectiveness that citizens can rely upon. These are daunting challenges.

A review of the extant literature suggests that there are numerous potential strategies to foster adaptive coping, including well-established procedures among civilians that may prove useful among first responders as well as military personnel (e.g., Southwick 2015; Fava, 2009; Horn 2016). Furthermore,

DOI: 10.4018/978-1-5225-9803-9.ch012

these interventions have been examined across a breadth of styles and formats, ranging from individual meetings to Internet modules (Castro, 2006; Cohn, Weltman, Ratwani, Chartrand, & McCraty 2010; Gonzalez, 2014; Padesky; 2012). There are mounting data that evidence-based approaches to first responder health can indeed translate to better outcomes across a wide variety of performance and health domains (Andersen & Gustafsberg, 2016; Arble, Lumley, Pole, Blessman, & Arnetz, 2017).

Yet the precise nature of these potential interventions remains elusive, not least in terms of causal mechanisms involved in delivering the desired outcomes. Many of the proposed interventions are derived from principles of clinical psychology, which though potent, were rarely developed with the expected, repeated, and professionally-bound stressors and traumas of first responder work in mind. Furthermore, the targets of intervention among first responders may be quite different than those of other populations. For instance, successful treatment of trauma among civilians emphasizes symptom reduction and a decreased avoidance of aversive stimuli. A man who develops an acute stress reaction subsequent to his house burning down could be seen as having been successfully treated when his daily anxiety decreases, his nightmares abate, and his ability to resume cooking meals on the stove is restored. This is highly distinct from a firefighter being treated for a traumatic experience during a fire, which although involving symptom reduction, must also include an ability to utilize his/her training during the next response call. In addition, while civilian clinical interventions are typically confidential affairs quite distinct from workplace awareness, training among first responders necessarily intersects with professional responsibilities and workplace culture.

BACKGROUND

The Need for Intervention

First responders are faced with a myriad of challenges, ranging from vacillating work hours to demanding bureaucracies, all of which contribute to stress (McCreary & Thompson, 2006). However, perhaps the most unique feature of the work of first responders is the experience of critical incidents (i.e., dangerous and potentially traumatic experiences). Although first responders are a resilient group overall (Galatzer-Levy et al., 2011), they are exposed to threatening and potentially traumatic events at a high frequency (Backman, Arnetz, Levin, & Lublin, 1997; Spielberger, Westberry, Grier, & Greenfield, 1981; Toch et al., 2002). Trauma can be experienced through a direct interaction with critical incidents, but also vicariously, when co-workers, family members, or citizens are threatened or victimized (Kleim & Westphal, 2011).

The heightened exposure to trauma and threat places first responders at increased risk for a wide range of negative outcomes (Violanti et al., 2006), including post-traumatic stress disorder (PTSD). The prevalence of current, duty-related PTSD among first responders far exceeds that of the general population's rate of approximately 4%, with some estimates suggesting a prevalence rate closer to that of Vietnam veterans (approximately 15%; Benedek, Fullerton, & Ursano, 2007; Kessler et al., 2005; Kulka et al., 1990). Moreover, many first responders experience symptoms and behavior problems that fall short of the full diagnostic criteria for PTSD but are nonetheless disturbing or debilitating (Marshall, Spitzer, & Liebowitz, 1999; McMillen, North, & Smith, 2000; Sloan, 1988; Smith, North, McCool, & Shea, 1990). Such post-trauma adjustment problems include acute stress reactions, domestic and other forms of violence, depression, suicidal ideation, and completed suicide (Buchanan, Stephens, & Long, 2001; Rudofossi, 1997; Ursano & McCarroll, 1990; Violanti, 1997; Violanti & Paton, 1999).

The effects of trauma exposure extend beyond psychiatric diagnoses such as PTSD, including first responders' subjective well-being, their social networks, and the departments they serve. The exposure to trauma can result in impaired job performance and attendance problems, decreased job satisfaction, and early retirement (Conrad & Kellar-Guenther, 2006; Norvell et al., 1998; Wright & Saylor, 1991). Worse still, the decrease in performance can lead to injury or death to citizens and other responders, with numerous consequences, including the fiscal repercussions of litigation (Covey, Shucard, Violanti, Lee, & Shucard, 2013). There is also an elevated risk of atherosclerosis and coronary disease in trauma-exposed first responders (Boscarino, 2004; Boscarino & Chang, 1999; Holman et al., 2008). Other common sequelae of trauma exposure are hypervigilance, insomnia, nightmares, difficulty with attention and concentration, somatic symptoms, relationship problems, and substance abuse (McMillen et al., 2000; Rothbaum & Foa, 1993). Finally, spouses and children of exposed individuals may be adversely affected by adjustment disorders following the incident (Boscarino, 2004; Bremner, Afzal, & Vythilingam, 2004; Hoge et al., 2002; Hoge, Terhakopian, Castro, Messer, & Engel, 2007; Schurr, Friedman, & Bernardy, 2002; Vasterling et al., 2002).

The Structure and Timing of First Responder Interventions

The substantial mental, behavioral, and social costs of first responder trauma suggest a strong need for intervention (Amaranto, Steinberg, Castellano, & Mitchell, 2003; Violanti et al., 2006). Yet the unique nature of the work of first responders, the need for organization-level interventions (as opposed to merely individual), and the interplay between professional functioning and well-being, all add to the complexity of identifying best practices.

Currently, interventions among first responders can be organized into three categories: tertiary prevention, secondary prevention, and primary prevention.

Tertiary Prevention

Quite a bit is known about tertiary prevention, or how to treat established psychiatric symptoms and diagnostic issues. For example, prolonged imaginal exposure therapy is an empirically-supported, effective treatment for PTSD (Foa, Keane, & Friedman, 2000). There is great confidence in tertiary prevention, as the evidence base supporting a range of potential treatment interventions continues to grow. Although it is critically important that first responders recognize and have access to these treatment options, tertiary prevention is not an ideal first-line solution. Practically speaking, treatment services are significantly underutilized among some first responder groups, particularly if there is a departmental or professional culture that stigmatizes the expression of emotional difficulties (Amaranto et al., 2003; Barren, 2005). First responders operating within such a culture may view the use of such treatments as a concession of weakness and may further view recommendations that they should engage in such treatments as a kind of condemnation. They may feel as though they are being singled out due to a personal failure or deficiency on their part. An effective but unused treatment is of little value. Furthermore, even successful tertiary methods come with a substantial cost. A police officer who develops and is successfully treated for PTSD has nonetheless suffered greatly. The interventions take time, during which the officer's department is diminished in its functioning due to loss of personnel, and the officer is experiencing severe emotional pain. And even in the case of successful treatment, the officer may not return to premorbid levels of professional functioning.

Secondary Prevention

In contrast to waiting until symptoms arise and addressing them, secondary prevention techniques have been developed to prevent the emergence of stress-related disorders among those who have recently experienced a trauma (Feldner, Monson, & Friedman, 2007). The most widely implemented secondary prevention approach is critical incident stress debriefing (CISD) and its psychological debriefing variants. These techniques typically involve discussion of the traumatic event and associated thoughts and feelings with a supportive facilitator soon after critical incident exposure in an effort to prevent initial symptoms from continuing or worsening. Despite its intuitive appeal and widespread implementation, research suggests that CISD is not only generally ineffective in reducing distress and preventing PTSD, but may cause harm in a few cases (Feldner et al., 2007; Rose, Bisson, & Wessely, 2002; Wessely & Deahl, 2003). Indeed, systematic reviews to date have found no benefits of any one-shot intervention delivered within 30 days after exposure (Rose et al., 2002; Van Emmerick, Kamphuis, Hulsbosch, & Emmelkamp, 2002). Furthermore, the hesitance of first responders to engage in tertiary treatments may apply to secondary prevention as well.

Primary Prevention

Much less is known about how to modify the peri-traumatic risk factors that presage symptom onset - an approach known as primary prevention (Feldner et al., 2007; Violanti & Paton, 1999). Unlike secondary prevention efforts, primary prevention focuses on preparation for traumatic events that have not yet occurred. Primary prevention efforts that aim to bolster resilience among first responders may be viewed as culturally appropriate for this population, because preparation for future events fits the standard training model, does not stigmatize any specific individual, and targets the maintenance of good mental and behavioral health, rather than treatment of mental illness. If successfully implemented, primary prevention techniques equip first responders to successfully navigate critical incidents and their psychological aftermath, both of which may prevent the experience of clinical issues. Ideally, first responders prepared in this way can better endure the demands of their work, while maintaining high levels of emotional and professional functioning.

Among civilians, there is substantial evidence to support the effectiveness of primary prevention. First, there is a substantial body of research on preparation for stressful medical procedures; such programs usually involve informing patients about upcoming experiences, exposing them to the experience either via imagination or video, and teaching them cognitive and behavioral skills (e.g., relaxation, distraction, body positioning) to use during the actual encounter. These approaches have proven useful (Elkins & Roberts, 1983; O'Byrne, Peterson, & Saldana, 1997). Another relevant approach is stress inoculation training (SIT), which has three overlapping phases: conceptualization (includes assessment, rapport, and education), skill acquisition/rehearsal, and finally, application and follow-through. Control-enhancing preparatory interventions such as these have been effective with a variety of stressed and anxious populations (Meichenbaum & Deffenbacher, 1988; Novaco, 1977). Finally, preparatory visualization of adaptive behavior is a technique successfully used in sports psychology to improve performance (Feltz & Landers, 1983; Suinn, 1997).

Comparatively less research has been conducted among first responders and the use of primary prevention techniques, though this trend appears to be changing. Notably, the present authors have developed and assessed a primary prevention training program among police officers, tested in both Sweden and the

United States (Arble et al., 2017; Arnetz, Nevedal, Lumley, Backman, & Lublin, 2009), demonstrating its effectiveness both immediately and longitudinally (Arble et al., 2017; Arnetz et al., 2009; Backman, Arnetz, Levin, & Lublin, 1997). As an illustration of the primary prevention approach, a summary of the program and evidence of its effectiveness will be presented.

Example of Primary Prevention: Mental Imagery Training for Police Trainees

In the present authors' initial studies, 75 Swedish police officers in training were randomly assigned to two gender-matched groups, one receiving a novel mental preparation intervention in addition to the traditional training at the police academy, and the other, police training as usual (Backman et al., 1997). Baseline assessments confirmed that there were no significant differences between the groups on any included measures of emotion or physical functioning.

The training was led by Swedish Special Forces and consisted of 10 weekly 90-minute sessions. There were several aspects of the training, including didactics on the nature of stress and the Jacobsen's (1929) progressive muscle relaxation technique, along with cue-controlled relaxation. The core of the program was the use of guided imagery to facilitate imaginal exposure to potentially stressful on-the-job incidents, and the mental practice of police tactical skills. The group then practiced an abbreviated, 15-minute version of the relaxation techniques. Over the next 60 minutes, two police-relevant stress scenarios were presented. The presentation included exposure to critical incident police work scenarios via narrated, present-tense scenarios and guided imagery, read aloud by the group leader. Direction in adaptive coping skills and police technical/strategic skills was incorporated into the scenario presentation. For example, officers might be instructed to imagine themselves approaching a threatening situation with particular tactical movements, attending to certain stimuli in the environment, and using their weapon appropriately. Each scenario was described in great detail to ensure that participants developed vivid, life-like mental images during the scenario, were emotionally engaged, and physiologically aroused.

This skills training emphasized producing helpful internal states (e.g., using cue-controlled relaxation technique to remain calm and focused), as well as employing proper tactical solutions (e.g., managing one's weapon effectively). The police group leader then debriefed participants' experiences of the imagery exercises and helped to address possible unanticipated effects. To solidify the training's effects, officers were encouraged to practice at home three or four times per week between the sessions. A scripted audiotape was provided to all participants in order to facilitate the imaginal process and to induce cue-controlled relaxation.

The effects of the program were significant and long-lasting. Following completion of the training, as compared to the control group, those in the intervention group reported greater well-being, fewer intestinal issues, and fewer sleep problems. Post-graduation, after one-year of actual police service, 18 of the officers (9 intervention and 9 controls) were randomly selected from the larger pool to participate in an intensive, stressful, critical incident exposure simulation, which consisted of a live reenactment of an armed robbery involving criminal discharge of firearms. Actors portrayed the criminals, and the officers participated fully in the reenactment as if they were responding to a real police work incident. Variables assessed during the simulation included cardiovascular parameters (heart rate recorded continuously and blood pressure assessed pre and post incident), endocrine and other blood-based measures (cortisol, prolactin, LDL-, HDL-, total-cholesterol, and triglycerides, as well as antithrombin were assessed pre and post incident), subjective ratings (mood, self-rated stress appraisal, perceived injury risk, coping, memory of the event), and behavioral measures (self-rated and professionally-judged performance appraisals of the officer during the reenactment).

Self-report data from the officers indicated substantial benefits of the training. Self-rated stress (100-point visual analog scale ratings) during exposure to the reenactment was significantly lower ($p < .01$) in the intervention group than the control group. Whereas controls increased from a pre-scenario mean stress rating of 25.1 (SD = 22.1) to 41.6 (SD = 31.1), the intervention group increased much less from 23.6 (SD = 8.0) to only 26.8 (SD = 14.7). This represents a large effect size (ES = - .80). In addition, participants who, during their first year on the force had experienced any field incident similar to that reenacted in the scenario, reported lower mood disturbance during the reenactment if they had received the imagery training, compared with controls.

The training also resulted in performance-related physiological benefits. Heart rate (HR) was used as the primary indicator of physiological arousal during the scenario, as elevated heart rate predicts the development of post-trauma adjustment problems, especially PTSD. Officers who received training demonstrated a significantly lower HR response compared to non-trained controls ($p <.001$). The improvement due to training (almost 25 BPM) is clinically substantial, with a very large effect size (ES = 1.40). Thus, the lower subjective stress was paralleled by less cardiovascular arousal during a critical maneuver among trained officers. In addition, blood was sampled immediately before and after the reenactment. The groups differed significantly on change in serum cortisol. While the controls' cortisol response decreased over time (pre: M = 515.0, SD = 110.1 nmol/L; post: M = 368.6, SD = 92.7), the intervention group's cortisol level remained consistent (pre: M = 415.1, SD = 129.6; post: M = 400.3, SD = 117.9; group x time interaction, $p = .002$; ES = .89). The inability to sustain cortisol response among controls might indicate deficient physiological coping during a stressful encounter, and low cortisol has been linked with development of PTSD. Thus, the intervention group had a more adaptive cortisol response. Additionally, the training decreased the risk for blood clots during reenactment. Antithrombin plays a central role in countering the body's chemical cascade mechanisms that are involved in creating blood clots during trauma; therefore, increases in antithrombin are desirable during stress. Training counteracted stress-induced blood clot risk due to hemoconcentration (Mohamed et al., 2002) by increasing the levels of antithrombin during the reenactment. No such protective effect was observed for the non-trained controls (significant group x time effect: $p =.045$; ES = 1.03).

Finally, the imaginal exposure training improved police task-specific performance. The intervention also improved actual job-specific behavioral performance among trained officers during reenactment, as rated by objective, blinded special tactics experts. The trained group received higher ratings on professional performance (e.g., control over the suspect, awareness and control over the public), and overall professional performance was rated significantly higher for the imagery trained group (M = 298.8, SD = 36.1) than the control group (M = 253.4, SD = 38.2; $p=.02$; ES = 1.26).

With active support from the Chief of Police of the city of Detroit, the present authors adapted the program to the needs of Detroit, Michigan, a major metropolitan city far removed from the cultural experience of Sweden. The adaptation was done in close collaboration with senior police officers and experienced trainers from the city of Detroit Police Academy. Within this new study, a class of 32 officers in the police academy engaged in the program. In addition to the training detailed above, new aspects were added. Specifically, in addition to visualization and relaxation exercises, coping strategies were discussed by the officers leading the training. These included emotion identification exercises, strategies for help-seeking, and rehearsal of emotional disclosure. Following the training's completion, both the trainers and the participants expressed high satisfaction with the intervention. After their first year of field work, 22 officers were reassessed. Compared to pre-training, these officers showed significant increases in the use of positive reframing coping strategies and significant reductions in anxiety and alcohol use over the year. Most notably, trauma symptoms did not increase during the first year, as would have been expected (Arnetz et al., 2009).

The primary prevention design of the intervention is clear. The training in both countries took place within the context of a traditional police academy setting. Indeed, a key aspect of the intervention is that it is designed to fit within this framework and can be comfortably run by training officers. By incorporating the intervention within standardized training, the participants were not required to be singled out (as might be the case when one is referred for mental health treatment), and the content within the program was likely granted a kind of ecological validity in the mind of the officers. Finally, the participants of these trainings were police cadets who had yet to serve as police officers; thus, the intervention took place well before the experience of the professional stressors. The success of this program across lengthy follow-ups, multiple settings, and with effects on overall officer health and performance in a standardized training scenario, speaks to the potential effectiveness of the primary prevention design.

FUTURE RESEARCH DIRECTIONS

Targets for Intervention

The theoretical and empirical evidence offers a strong case for the use of primary prevention techniques among first responders. Unfortunately, there is no single answer as to the training needs of all first responders. First responder groups experience divergent needs and challenges, resulting in different training requirements (Arble, Daugherty, & Arnetz, 2017). The needs of a fire department in a major metropolitan city may be quite divergent from the needs of a rural police force. Thus, in developing or implementing interventions, key stakeholders should be consulted and actively engaged in the entire process.

Nonetheless, seminal research among first responders and military personnel has identified key structural aspects of developing a training program. As articulated by Driskell and Johnston (1998), knowledge of the intended technique must first be presented in a low-stakes environment, followed by rehearsal of the skills in increasingly realistic and challenging settings. As rehearsal of these dynamic skills continues, the trainees must be given opportunities for feedback and recognition of improvement, thereby increasing their competence, sense of mastery, and confidence. Furthermore, there appear to be several common training foci that are broadly applicable, each of which will be reviewed: Mindfulness; Managing Physiological Reactivity; Emotion Expression and Social Support; and Substance Use.

Mindfulness

The use of mindfulness techniques has increased rapidly in research and clinical practice over the past several years, giving rise to Mindfulness-Based Stress Reduction (MBSR) (Kabat-Zinn, 2003). Mindfulness refers to a state of mind in which the individual is engaging with the full spectrum of momentary experience, both recognizing and accepting one's present reality in a nonjudgmental way (Kabat-Zinn, 1990; Ciarrochi & Godsell, 2005). It is offered as a contrast to a "mindless" state of being, in which an individual is being driven by disengagement, compulsion, or mood states that introduce severe judgment. For example, one might imagine a person at lunch waiting on news that they expect will be quite bad. The person is so anxious that they feel a pain in their stomach and their thoughts are centered upon how their life will change for the worse once this news has been delivered. This individual is so engaged in these anxious thoughts and feelings that they are unaware of the smells and sights around them, and they take their anxious thoughts as proof of the negative outcome they fear: "Something is going to go wrong, I just know it."

For this individual, their anxiety and the hypotheticals surrounding it carry more weight than their immediate surroundings. The awareness and acceptance of one's momentary experience is not present, because in a very real sense, the person is not fully present; they are living in their feared future state. This is likely a relatable experience for many, but it is important to note that mindlessness in this sense need not arise from an anxious state. The person who leaves their home on a cold day without wearing a jacket may do so because they are so focused on a task that they are excited for that the excitement may disrupt the momentary experience of data such as "It's a bit cold outside."

Cultivating a state of mindfulness has proven useful in addressing a wide variety of clinical and subclinical issues, in part, because of its ability to disrupt patterns of internal behavior. Returning to the example of the individual nervously sitting at lunch, cultivating a state of mindfulness could disrupt the cascade of negative thoughts. The individual who would otherwise be focused on the hypothetical future experience, would instead be drawn back to the present, taking in the sights and sounds of their lunch. Relatedly, the mindful state of nonjudgmental acceptance can disrupt psychological defensive and ruminative processes that can prove emotionally taxing. The individual who cannot stop thinking "This is going badly," as well as the individual repeatedly thinking "I must not allow myself to think that way," are both locked in a struggle with their own internal states. Conversely, the mindful stance is one of openness to all psychological content without a prescriptive judgment of its nature. The thought, "This is going badly" is recognized, but one's awareness is expanded beyond the lone perseverative thought to also recognize the numerous other thoughts and experiences. "I must not think that way" is replaced by the recognition that thoughts are transient mental events that are to be recognized but not controlled. Indeed, the attempt to control them may be the very thing that empowers them. Mindfulness based interventions have proven effective in stress reduction, lowering levels of mood disturbance, and overall promoting wellbeing (Brown & Ryan, 2003; Segal, Teasdale, Williams, & Gemar, 2002; Teasdale, Segal, & Williams, 1995).

Mindfulness techniques are of great potential use to first responders. Not only can mindfulness disrupt the experience of mood related disturbances and improve health outcomes, but the emphasis on awareness can prove quite significant. In the present authors' training (detailed above), the state of mindful awareness was offered as a contrast to the experience that police officers colloquially refer to as "tunnel vision." Tunnel vision refers to the experience of physiological arousal in which the officers' perceptual awareness becomes hyper-focused, obscuring peripheral information. One can imagine the experience of a vehicular pursuit, wherein an officer becomes hyper-focused on the pursued vehicle, but neglects to consider the movements of other vehicles on the road. The results of such a lack of mindfulness can be tragic.

Empirical Evidence of Mindfulness Intervention

Research supports the use of mindfulness techniques among first responders. The application of mindfulness-based training among first responders has been shown to be associated with a reduction in PTSD symptoms such as intrusive thoughts, avoidance, and hyperarousal (Chopko & Schwartz, 2013).

Other research among first responders has documented improvements in emotional regulation, decreased fatigue, lower levels of stress, and improved sleep (Christopher, et al., 2015).

Mindfulness has also shown positive results in a military context, a population which bears a great many similarities to first responders. For example, the Master Resilience Training (MRT) program is part of the United State's military's Comprehensive Solider Fitness program (de Vissier et al., 2016). This program, in addition to other features, teaches soldiers mindfulness skills such as self-regulation in the context of stressful scenarios. Trials of the program have been positive thus far, indicating that participants who received the training demonstrate improved resilience as compared to soldiers who did not receive the training (Lester, Harms, Herian, Krasikova, & Beal, 2011). Similarly, the Mind Fit Training (M-FIT) has demonstrated some effectiveness among military personnel. In a study involving a detachment of the United States Marines Corps receiving classroom instruction and mindfulness homework, engagement with the activity correlated with lower self-reported stress and higher mindfulness (Stanley, Schaldach, Kiyonaga, & Jha, 2011).

Managing Physiological Reactivity

There is ample research to suggest that physiological responsiveness during critical incidents can have a large effect on first responder performance, which will in turn affect the ultimate outcome of the event (Arnetz, Arble, Backman, Lynch, & Lublin, 2013; Covey et al., 2013; Violanti, 2010). To understand importance of physiological reactivity in first responders, a brief comment on the biological mechanisms and their performance effects should be considered.

During a critical incident in which an individual is exposed to a potential threat, there is a cascade of physiological responses. The sympathetic nervous system is activated, while the parasympathetic nervous system retreats. In moderate amounts, and depending upon the task being engaged in, this activation of the sympathetic nervous system can prove beneficial: sensory perception can be enhanced, alertness can be increased, and some procedural memory can be more easily accessed (Cahill & Alkire, 2013; Jamieson, Mendes, Blackstock, & Schmader, 2010). In short, this activation is theoretically a source of intensity and energy, that if harnessed, can translate to superior momentary readiness (Kalisch, Müller, & Tüscher, 2015).

However, if this sympathetic nervous system activation becomes excessive, or if the task facing the first responder requires cognitively complex and unrehearsed behaviors, performance during the critical incident can be significantly diminished. The experience of this so-called "fight or flight" response has been well documented (Lovallo, 2016). In response, the adrenal gland begins to release epinephrine, which in turn increases respiration and heart rate, as the individual is primed to either flee or engage in a struggle (Lundberg, 2011). The hypothalamic-pituitary-adrenal (HPA) axis is also activated, generating a hormonal response that will sustain the enhanced readiness as long as the threat is present.

There are numerous deficits that potentially follow from this internal sequence of events. The previously discussed notion of tunnel vision may literally occur, as sympathetic nervous system activation can result in reduced peripheral vision, resulting from alterations in blood flow to the eyes and eye muscle contractions (Klinger & Brunson, 2009; Olson, 1998). This disrupted vision is accompanied by attentional biases, namely, individuals can become focused on the perceived threats to the exclusion of other relevant data. The resulting visual distortions can lead to failure to observe subtle movements and visual cues, decreased reaction time in response to figures in the periphery, and decreased firearm accuracy (Johnson, 2007; Klinger & Brunson, 2009; Olson, 1998). Similarly, although gross motor skills may benefit from increased blood flow and respiration (e.g., one's ability to run fast may be increased), vasoconstriction in the extremities can disrupt more fine motor skills, such as attaching a fire hose to a hydrant (Johnson, 2007).

Cognitive processes are also affected during fight or flight activation. Adrenal hormones (e.g., cortisol) engage vascular processes meant to facilitate more instinctual and reactive responding (i.e., fighting or fleeing). Conversely, these same hormones prompt blood vessel restriction and subsequent diminished oxygen levels in the prefrontal cortex, the region of the brain that is prominently involved in strategic planning, decision making, and logic (Goldstein, Rasmusson, Bunney, & Roth, 1996; Takamatsu et al., 2003), leading to disruptions in these key processes, as well as increased difficulties in some aspects of memory retrieval (Lipton, 2008). These effects are compounded by the reactions of the individual. Due to physical strain, anxiety, or a combination of the two, individuals are likely to begin to breathe rapidly. This may lead to hyperventilation and its associated detriments, and unfortunately, the rapid intake of air is a prompt for continued sympathetic activation (Brown & Gerbarg, 2009; Cacioppo & Tassinary, 1998).

These processes create a clear dilemma for first responders. The evolved neurochemical mechanisms are geared towards rapid and broad responses in the face of threat. However, for first responders, these mechanisms can prove detrimental to the critical features of successful performance; namely, situational awareness, tactical maneuvering, and clear thinking. Fortunately, although the fight or flight response is physiological in nature, malleable psychological and physical processes mediate a number of the relevant sequelae (Kalisch et al., 2015). By managing one's physiological arousal, the noted detriments may be abated, and the responders may be able to perform their duties successfully.

Empirical Evidence of Interventions to Control Physiological Arousal

There is evidence to suggest that with proper training, physiological control can be enhanced. The most straightforward example of modifying these processes is through the practice of muscle relaxation and controlled respiration. As detailed above, the present authors' research among police officers has demonstrated the performance and health benefits that may be derived from cue-controlled relaxation and breathing. Similarly, in a procedure developed by McCraty and colleagues (McCraty, Atkinson, Tomasino, & Bradley, 2009; McCraty & Atkinson, 2012), first responders were trained in skills to reduce physiological reactivity and enhance self-regulation. For example, participants were taught "heart focused breathing" to reduce acute and chronic stress. After a 16-week course, those in the training group reported improvements in a variety of domains, including increased positive emotions, increased vitality, and improved self-regulation in response to stress.

The United States Naval Stress Resilience Training System (STRS) also demonstrates the potential for managing physiological responsiveness via biofeedback training (Rose et al., 2013). In addition to elements of psychoeducation and cognitive therapy, this electronically-delivered program consists of heart rate variability (HRV) exercises (Cohn et al., 2010; Reivich, Seligman, & McBride, 2011). Heart rate variability is the variation in time between heart beats, with high HRV indicating flexible and healthy autonomic nervous system functioning, which is associated with better heath and resilience (Cohn et al., 2010). In this 8-week training program, supplemented at times by phone or electronic consultation, trainees progress through exercises in which they practice until they achieve a predetermined standard of HRV control. Evidence thus far suggests that the training is effective in enhancing the resilience of military personnel (de Vissier, 2016; Smith, 2013).

Recently, Andersen and Gustafsberg (2016) developed a psychobiological intervention named the "international performance resilience and efficiency program" (iPREP). The training is specifically designed to disrupt the features responsible for excessive sympathetic nervous system arousal. The training includes a variety of elements, including psychoeducation about the physiology of stress and training on visualization and focus. Participants are also trained in the use of biofeedback as a mechanism to rehearse controlled breathing, thereby managing sympathetic nervous system response (McCraty & Atkinson, 2012). As noted by the authors, the use of controlled breathing is not a relaxation exercise, but rather, a means of maintaining beneficial levels of arousal during stress, while avoiding the detriments of fight or flight responding. Participants proceed through dynamic training scenarios in which they are taught to recognize their own physiological responses during the scenario. When excessive arousal is noted, the participants rehearse psychological and physiological control techniques (e.g., controlled breathing), and are then asked to apply them during subsequent scenarios. Results from the randomized controlled trial evaluating the iPREP suggest that it can produce enhanced physiological control, increased situational awareness, and improved use of force decision making.

Emotional Expression and Social Support

Successful coping in the face of stress and emotional difficulty can be organized by two primary self-regulatory techniques (Fauerbach et al., 2009): approach strategies and avoidance strategies. Approach strategies are identified through the individual's willingness to experience and engage with their own internal states. These strategies can be described as agentic, because they seek to increase the individual's knowledge, facilitate the direct experience of emotional states, and challenge maladaptive patterns of thought or behavior (Affleck & Tennen, 1996; Davis, Nolen-Hoeksema & Larson, 1998). Conversely, avoidance coping is undertaken as a means of not experiencing threatening internal states by avoiding relevant stimuli, distracting oneself, or denying the existence of such feelings (Anshel, 1996; Roth & Cohen, 1986). Although the majority of the research identifying this distinction has been conducted among civilian populations, research has suggested that this same basic division may be applicable to first responders as well (e.g., Anshel, 2000; Arble & Arnetz, 2016; Dowdall-Thomae, Gilkey, Larson & Arend-Hicks, 2012).

The effectiveness of these contrasting strategies is complex and varies based upon the individual's personality and history, the nature of the stressor, and the specific coping strategies employed (Kashdan & Rottenberg, 2010). Furthermore, although these strategies are distinct, an individual can utilize both strategies at different times, and there is some evidence that flexibility in the application of coping strategies may be quite useful (Park, Chang & You, 2015). These findings seem to suggest that defining ideal coping strategies requires some idiographic considerations (Schuettler & Boals, 2011; Weinberg, Gil, & Gilbar, 2014). Nonetheless, the extant literature demonstrates that avoidance strategies, when used in isolation or when applied too rigidly, can prove harmful (Anshel, 2000; Brown & Campbell, 1994; Joseph, Murphy & Regel, 2012; Littleton, Horsley, John & Nelson, 2007; Suls & Fletcher, 1985).

This coping distinction bears great relevance for first responder groups. Researchers have often speculated that some aspects of first responder culture pull for the use of avoidant coping strategies (Lennings, 1997). Professional and institutional culture may dictate that first responders communicate a sense of strength and self-reliance, which may translate to the minimization of emotional reactions, particularly if such reactions could be seen as "weak" (Hart & Cotton, 2003). For example, a firefighter becoming tearful could be perceived as communicating that he or she is unable to handle the pressures of the work, thereby resulting in a loss of respect or confidence. While becoming tearful in the middle of a critical incident would likely be harmful, a generalized prohibition against tearfulness represents a form of emotional avoidance. Research suggests that first responder subcultures can sometimes give rise to an emotionally repressive style, with the avoidance of emotional content being noted across a wide domain of relationships and contexts (Amaranto et al., 2003).

Unfortunately, the avoidance of emotions as a long-term strategy not only blunts well-being (Arble & Arnetz, 2016), but likely contributes to negative outcomes. Individuals who have difficulty identifying emotions perform worse in the face of stressors and experience greater distress (Salovey, Mayor, Goldman, Turvey, & Palfai, 2002). Furthermore, confusion about one's own internal states predicts negative emotionality (Kerr, Johnson, Gans, & Krumrine, 2004), worse mental health outcomes (Ciarrochi, Chan, Caputi, & Roberts, 2001), and increases in psychosomatic disorders (Taylor, 2000).

This culture of first responders and emotions is inexorably tied to social relationships. The behavior modeled by senior and training personnel can directly begin to structure the coping strategies adopted by junior first responders (Violanti, 1993). Research suggests that a culture of avoidant coping can begin to take hold in less than two years of work experience, with first responders quickly adopting detached and cynical dispositions (Robinson, Sigman, & Wilson, 1997; Violanti, Marshall, & Howe, 1985).

Empirical Evidence of Emotional Response and Social Support Interventions

It thus appears that creating a culture of socially-accepted approach-based coping is ideal. Early research identified that the experience of work stress could be partially mitigated by the experience of social support (e.g., Karasek 1979). Social support is associated with better functioning following a crisis, physical activity, and better mood (Holahan and Moos 1990; LaRocco, House, & French, 1980; Rodin and Salovey 1989). In a meta-analysis conducted by Viswesvaran, Sanchez, and Fisher (1999), a review of 68 studies identified a triune effect of social support on experienced work stress. Increased social support led to lower levels of experienced distress, attenuated the severity of experienced stressors and moderated the relationship between work stress and experienced strain. Prati and Pietrantoni (2010) conducted a meta-analytic review of 37 studies investigating the connection between perceived social support and mental health among first responders specifically, finding that among this population, the mental health benefits of social support were significant.

Several interventions, including those of the present authors, have been based upon this recognition. If a culture of emotional expression and recognition is developed, the benefits of social support can be entwined with the benefits of approach-based coping (Arble & Arnetz, 2016; Arble, Daugherty, & Arnetz, 2018). The same pathological mechanisms that communicate emotional avoidance can instead be used to communicate emotional expression. The aforementioned Master Resilience Training (MRT) program in the United States Army is an example of this, as it explicitly includes modules on relationship building skills (Cornum, 2011). The present researchers' use of the "train the trainers" model is an explicit demonstration of this principle. By having respected senior officers lead junior cadets in exercises involving communication and emotional expression, officers communicate their belief in approach-based coping (Arble et al., 2017).

Substance Use

A particularly harmful avenue of avoidant coping is substance use; substances can be used to blunt emotional experiences, disrupt thoughts, or induce a mood state. Among first responders, alcohol use is noted as the most prominent of substances, as the excessive intake of alcohol to help reduce stress and improve psychological well-being is a common strategy (e.g., Dietrich & Smith, 1986). In a large-scale study of first responder coping, the present authors surveyed a random sample totaling 3,656 Swedish first responders from the following occupations: coast guard, customs control, military, emergency medical services, fire department and police services. In a structural equation modeling framework, a model of first responder coping was developed. Avoidant coping was directly related to a decrease in well-being, and both an increase in exposure to stress and avoidant coping were associated with a greater incidence of substance use. The consumption of alcohol as a means to cope with stress increases the risk to develop alcoholism, obesity, marital conflict, low self-esteem, emotional dysregulation, depression, poor sleep, chronic fatigue and reduced quality of work performance (Peele, 1991; Roskies, 1991).

In a follow-up study (Arble et al., 2018), the present authors examined the role of substance use among police officers specifically, as there is reason to suggest that police officers may uniquely struggle with this issue (Brough, 2004; Hart & Cotton, 2003). Again using a structural equation modelling framework, the survey data of 917 police officers was used to create a path model highlighting the role of substance use among police officers. Within the model, avoidant coping was related to worse wellbeing, in a fashion similar to that of other first responders. However, police officers significantly diverged from other first responders in that substance use appeared more detrimental. A staggering 38% of variability in well-being among police officers was accounted for by substance use alone. Thus, although the role of substance use among all first responders is significant, the following will highlight the role of alcohol among police officers, as it has been the most robustly studied.

The rate of alcohol consumption among police officers has been of interest to researchers for the past several decades, with early studies of alcohol use suggesting that approximately 25% of police reported experiencing problems related to alcohol consumption (Arrigo & Garsky, 1997; Dietrich & Smith, 1986). The use of alcohol among police was so prominent that some scholars came to regard problematic alcohol consumption as an element of police lifestyle itself (Violanti, 1999). Contemporary investigations have offered evidence that problematic alcohol use among police remains an issue in modern law enforcement (Stinson, Liederbach, Brewer, & Todak, 2014), finding that the excessive consumption of alcohol may occur in as many as 40% of police officers. For example, in a study of multiple police departments, nearly 40% of officers reported the experience of binge drinking within the past month (Ballenger et al., 2010).

Police alcohol use has been linked with a variety of negative outcomes, including poor job performance, marital difficulties, emotional dysregulation, and suicide (Loo, 1986; Peele, 1991; Roskies, 1991). Health difficulties are also common among officers; for example, police officers are twice as likely to die from alcoholic liver disease than the general population (McNeil, 1986; McNeil & Wilson, 1993). Unfortunately, the disruption of the health processes of police officers places them and the general public in danger. Some studies suggest that many police officers have consumed alcohol while on duty, the potential outcomes of which could prove deadly (VanRaalte, 1979). Police officers themselves have expressed concern over this data; a study of over 2,000 police officers found that 23% of the officers investigated reported having peers with serious drinking problems (Hurrell et al., 1984). In a particularly powerful demonstration of the dangers of police alcohol consumption, recent research has found that when examining the arrest records of both male and female officers in the United States, DUI and public intoxication were identified as the most frequent causes for arrest (Stinson, Liederbach, & Freiburger, 2012; Stinson, Todak, & Dodge, 2015).

To some extent, these findings cross national boundaries, though there is clear evidence of cultural differences (Richmond, Wodak, Kehoe, & Heather, 1998). For example, a recent study of 4,193 Australian police officers found that 33% of male officers and 24% of female officers reported elevated scores on the AUDIT, a popular measure of alcohol consumption. Other research conducted with Australian officers suggested that approximately 30% of police officers consumed troubling levels of alcohol (Davey, Obst, & Sheehan, 2001), although sex-related differences in consumption were reported, and this appears consistent with other reports (Richmond et al., 1998). Research among police officers in Wales produced similarly alarming results (Richmond et al., 1998). However, a study of 2,372 Norwegian police officers demonstrated a significantly lower rate of problematic alcohol use on a brief version of the AUDIT (Sterud, Hem, Ekeberg, & Lau, 2007).

Empirical Evidence of Substance Use Treatment

Thus, although all first responders should have an awareness of the severe consequences of substance use as an avoidance strategy, police officers should be particularly mindful of this concern. The treatment of substance use is complex and difficult. However, as evidenced by the results of the present researcher's intervention, the primary prevention methodology can prove helpful in reducing substance use (Arble et al., 2017). The means of intervention in this regard are twofold. First, the experience of psychiatric issues such as PTSD and depression is highly predictive of first responder substance use (Chopko, Palmieri, & Adams, 2013). Thus, if interventions are successful in disrupting the development of these symptoms, the use of substances to cope will likely also decrease. Second, the use of substances appears to operate as a coping strategy (Violanti et al., 2011). If the applied training identifies alternative and superior means of emotion regulation and coping (e.g., seeking adaptive social support), the use of substances as a coping mechanism should decline.

CONCLUSION

For all the challenges and responsibilities facing first responders, there is nonetheless cause for optimism. As has been reviewed, a philosophy of primary prevention aimed at addressing specific psychophysiological mechanisms can yield critical health and performance benefits. Furthermore, the successful implementation of intervention protocols across multiple countries, professions, and with different training styles and foci, strongly suggests that first responders as a whole are amenable to novel training methods.

As this research literature progresses, it will benefit from several methodological advances. First, many research designs are hampered by small samples, lack of randomization, and sole reliance of "treatment as usual" comparison groups. Although it is difficult to implement, larger samples, true randomization, and comparison against robust training alternatives can elevate many of the noted interventions from promising, to efficacious. Second, much intervention research among first responders is limited to laboratory settings, including exciting developments in the use of virtual training environments. Although this allows for advanced measurement and experimental control, it is also recognized that performance in a controlled setting is not equivalent to performance in the field. Whenever possible, intervention outcomes should be linked to real-world performance data, such as response time and supervisor evaluations. Finally, more longitudinal designs are required. Tracking performance data longitudinally will offer an important validation of an intervention's effectiveness; it is an understandable concern that an intervention's benefits may attenuate or disappear in the face of first responders' repeated exposure to stressors and critical incidents. Additionally, longitudinal data analysis will allow for a retrospective examination of the factors that ultimately predicted better outcomes, including both performance and health.

REFERENCES

Affleck, G., & Tennen, H. (1996). Construing benefits from adversity: Adaptational significance and dispositional underpinnings. *Journal of Personality*, *64*(4), 899–922. doi:10.1111/j.1467-6494.1996.tb00948.x PMID:8956517

Amaranto, E., Steinberg, J., Castellano, C., & Mitchell, R. (2003). Police stress interventions. *Brief Treatment and Crisis Intervention*, *3*(1), 47–54. doi:10.1093/brief-treatment/mhg001

Andersen, J. P., & Gustafsberg, H. (2016). A training method to improve police use of force decision making: A randomized controlled trial. *SAGE Open*, *6*(2). doi:10.1177/2158244016638708

Anshel, M. H. (2000). A conceptual model and implications for coping with stressful events in police work. *Criminal Justice and Behavior*, *27*(3), 375–400. doi:10.1177/0093854800027003006

Arble, E., & Arnetz, B. B. (2016). A model of first-responder coping: An approach/avoidance bifurcation. *Stress and Health: Journal of the International Society for the Investigation of Stress*. doi:10.1002mi.2692

Arble, E., Daugherty, A. M., & Arnetz, B. B. (2018). Models of first responder coping: Police officers as a unique population. *Stress and Health*, *34*(5), 612–621. doi:10.1002mi.2821 PMID:29882624

Arble, E., Lumley, M. A., Pole, N., Blessman, J., & Arnetz, B. B. (2017). Refinement and preliminary testing of an imagery-based program to improve coping and performance and prevent trauma among urban police officers. *Journal of Police and Criminal Psychology*, *32*(1), 1–10. doi:10.100711896-016-9191-z PMID:28439149

Arnetz, B. B., Arble, E., Backman, L., Lynch, A., & Lublin, A. (2013). Assessment of a prevention program for work-related stress among urban police officers. *International Archives of Occupational and Environmental Health*, *86*(1), 79–88. doi:10.100700420-012-0748-6 PMID:22366986

Arnetz, B. B., Nevedal, D. C., Lumley, M. A., Backman, L., & Lublin, A. (2009). Trauma resilience training for police: Psychophysiological and performance effects. *Journal of Police and Criminal Psychology*, *24*(1), 1–9. doi:10.100711896-008-9030-y

Arrigo, B. A., & Garsky, K. (1997). Police suicide: A glimpse behind the badge. In R. Dunham & J. Alpert (Eds.), *Critical issues in policing: Contemporary readings* (3rd ed.). Long Grove, IL: Waveland Press.

Backman, L., Arnetz, B. B., Levin, D., & Lublin, Å. (1997). Psychophysiological effects of mental imaging training for police trainees. *Stress Medicine*, *13*(1), 43–48. doi:10.1002/(SICI)1099-1700(199701)13:1<43::AID-SMI716>3.0.CO;2-6

Ballenger, J. F., Best, S. R., Metzler, T. J., Wasserman, D. A., Mohr, D. C., Liberman, A., ... Marmar, C. R. (2010). Patterns and predictors of alcohol use in male and female urban police officers. *The American Journal on Addictions, 20*(1), 21–29. doi:10.1111/j.1521-0391.2010.00092.x PMID:21175917

Barren, J. R. (2005). Use of existential-phenomenological counseling for police officers. *Policing: An International Journal of Police Strategies & Management, 28*(2), 255–268. doi:10.1108/13639510510597898

Benedek, D. M., Fullerton, C., & Ursano, R. J. (2007). First responders: Mental health consequences of natural and human-made disasters for public health and public safety workers. *Annual Review of Public Health, 28*(1), 55–68. doi:10.1146/annurev.publhealth.28.021406.144037 PMID:17367284

Boscarino, J. A. (2004). Posttraumatic stress disorder and physical illness: Results from clinical and epidemiologic studies. *Annals of the New York Academy of Sciences*, 10. PMID:15677401

Boscarino, J. A., & Chang, J. (1999). Electrocardiogram abnormalities among men with stress-related psychiatric disorders: Implications for coronary heart disease and clinical research. *Annals of Behavioral Medicine, 21*(3), 227–234. doi:10.1007/BF02884839 PMID:10626030

Bremner, J. D., Vermetten, E., Afzal, N., & Vythilingam, M. (2004). Deficits in verbal declarative memory function in women with childhood sexual abuse-related posttraumatic stress disorder. *The Journal of Nervous and Mental Disease, 192*(10), 643–649. doi:10.1097/01.nmd.0000142027.52893.c8 PMID:15457106

Brough, P. (2004). Comparing the influence of traumatic and organizational stressors on the psychological health of police, fire, and ambulance officers. *International Journal of Stress Management, 11*(3), 227–244. doi:10.1037/1072-5245.11.3.227

Brown, J. M., & Campbell, E. A. (1994). *Stress and policing: Sources and strategies*. New York: John Wiley.

Brown, K. W., & Ryan, R. M. (2003). The benefits of being present: Mindfulness and its role in psychological well-being. *Journal of Personality and Social Psychology, 84*(4), 822–848. doi:10.1037/0022-3514.84.4.822 PMID:12703651

Brown, R. P., & Gerbarg, P. L. (2009). Yoga breathing, meditation, and longevity. *Annals of the New York Academy of Sciences, 1172*(1), 54–62. doi:10.1111/j.1749-6632.2009.04394.x PMID:19735239

Buchanan, G., Stephens, C., & Long, N. (2001). Traumatic events of new recruits and serving police. *Australasian Journal of Disaster and Trauma Studies.*

Cacioppo, J. T., & Tassinary, L. G. (1998). *Principles of neurology* (6th ed.). New York, NY: McGraw-Hill.

Cahill, L., & Alkire, M. T. (2003). Epinephrine enhancement of human memory consolidation: Interaction with arousal at encoding. *Neurobiology of Learning and Memory, 79*(2), 194–198. doi:10.1016/S1074-7427(02)00036-9 PMID:12591227

Castro, C. A., Hoge, C. W., & Cox, A. L. (2006). *Battlemind training: Building soldier resiliency*. Walter Reed Army Inst of Research.

Chopko, B. A., Palmieri, P. A., & Adams, R. E. (2013). Associations between police stress and alcohol use: Implications for practice. *Journal of Loss and Trauma*, *18*(5), 482–497. doi:10.1080/15325024.2012.719340

Chopko, B. A., & Schwartz, R. C. (2013). The relation between mindfulness and posttraumatic stress symptoms among police officers. *Journal of Loss and Trauma*, *18*(1), 1–9. doi:10.1080/15325024.2012.674442

Christopher, M. S., Goerling, R. J., Rogers, B. S., Hunsinger, M., Baron, G., Bergman, A. L., & Zava, D. T. (2016). A pilot study evaluating the effectiveness of a mindfulness-based intervention on cortisol awakening response and health outcomes among law enforcement officers. *Journal of Police and Criminal Psychology*, *31*(1), 15–28. doi:10.100711896-015-9161-x

Ciarrochi, J., Chan, A., Caputi, P., & Roberts, R. (2001). Measuring emotional intelligence. *Emotional intelligence in everyday life: A scientific inquiry*, 25-45.

Ciarrochi, J., & Godsell, C. (2005). Mindfulness-based emotional intelligence: A theory and review of the literature. *Emotional intelligence: An international handbook*, 69-90.

Cohn, J., Weltman, G., Ratwani, R., Chartrand, D., & McCraty, R. (2010). *Stress inoculation through cognitive and biofeedback training*. Office of Naval Research.

Conrad, D., & Kellar-Guenther, Y. (2006). Compassion fatigue, burnout, and compassion satisfaction among Colorado child protection workers. *Child Abuse & Neglect*, *30*(10), 1071–1080. doi:10.1016/j.chiabu.2006.03.009 PMID:17014908

Cornum, R., Matthews, M. D., & Seligman, M. E. (2011). Comprehensive soldier fitness: Building resilience in a challenging institutional context. *The American Psychologist*, *66*(1), 4–9. doi:10.1037/a0021420 PMID:21219042

Covey, T. J., Shucard, J. L., Violanti, J. M., Lee, J., & Shucard, D. W. (2013). The effects of exposure to traumatic stressors on inhibitory control in police officers: A dense electrode array study using a Go/NoGo continuous performance task. *International Journal of Psychophysiology*, *87*(3), 363–375. doi:10.1016/j.ijpsycho.2013.03.009 PMID:23528305

Davey, J. D., Obst, P. L., & Sheehan, M. C. (2001). It goes with the job: Officers' insights into the impact of stress and culture on alcohol consumption within the policing occupation. *Drugs Education Prevention & Policy*, *8*, 141–149. doi:10.1080/096876301300101889

Davis, C. G., Nolen-Hoeksema, S., & Larson, J. (1998). Making sense of loss and benefiting from the experience: Two construals of meaning. *Journal of Personality and Social Psychology*, *75*(2), 561–574. doi:10.1037/0022-3514.75.2.561 PMID:9731325

de Visser, E. J., Dorfman, A., Chartrand, D., Lamon, J., Freedy, E., & Weltman, G. (2016). Building resilience with the Stress Resilience Training System: Design validation and applications. *Work (Reading, Mass.)*, *54*(2), 351–366. doi:10.3233/WOR-162295 PMID:27232057

Dietrich, J. F., & Smith, J. (1986). The nonmedical use of drugs including alcohol among police personnel: A critical literature review. *Journal of Police Science and Administration*.

Dowdall-Thomae, C., Gilkey, J., Larson, W., & Arend-Hicks, R. (2012). Elite firefighter/first responder mindsets and outcome coping efficacy. *International Journal of Emergency Mental Health, 14*(4), 269–281. PMID:23980491

Driskell, J. E., & Johnston, J. H. (1998). Stress exposure training. In J. A. Cannon-Bowers & E. Salas (Eds.), *Making decisions under stress: Implications for individual and team training* (pp. 191–217). Washington, DC: American Psychological Association. doi:10.1037/10278-007

Elkins, P. D., & Roberts, M. C. (1983). Psychological preparation for pediatric hospitalization. *Clinical Psychology Review, 3*(3), 275–295. doi:10.1016/0272-7358(83)90016-8

Fauerbach, J. A., Lawrence, J. W., Fogel, J., Richter, L., Magyar-Russell, G., McKibben, J. B., & Mccann, U. (2009). Approach–avoidance coping conflict in a sample of burn patients at risk for posttraumatic stress disorder. *Depression and Anxiety, 26*(9), 838–850. doi:10.1002/da.20439 PMID:19170120

Fava, G. A., & Tomba, E. (2009). Increasing psychological well-being and resilience by psychotherapeutic methods. *Journal of Personality, 77*(6), 1903–1934. doi:10.1111/j.1467-6494.2009.00604.x PMID:19807860

Feldner, M. T., Monson, C. M., & Friedman, M. J. (2007). A critical analysis of approaches to targeted PTSD prevention: Current status and theoretically derived future directions. *Behavior Modification, 31*(1), 80–116. doi:10.1177/0145445506295057 PMID:17179532

Feltz, D. L., & Landers, D. M. (1983). The effects of mental practice on motor skill learning and performance: A meta-analysis. *Journal of Sport Psychology, 5*(1), 25–57. doi:10.1123/jsp.5.1.25

Foa, E. B., Keane, T. M., & Friedman, M. J. (2000). Guidelines for treatment of PTSD. *Journal of Traumatic Stress: Official Publication of The International Society for Traumatic Stress Studies, 13*(4), 539–588. doi:10.1023/A:1007802031411 PMID:11109232

Galatzer-Levy, I. R., Madan, A., Neylan, T. C., Henn-Haase, C., & Marmar, C. R. (2011). Peritraumatic and trait dissociation differentiate police officers with resilient versus symptomatic trajectories of posttraumatic stress symptoms. *Journal of Traumatic Stress, 24*(5), 557–565. doi:10.1002/jts.20684 PMID:21898602

Goldstein, L. E., Rasmusson, A. M., Bunney, B. S., & Roth, R. H. (1996). Role of the amygdala in the coordination of behavioral, neuroendocrine, and prefrontal cortical monoamine responses to psychological stress in the rat. *The Journal of Neuroscience, 16*(15), 4787–4798. doi:10.1523/JNEUROSCI.16-15-04787.1996 PMID:8764665

Gonzalez, G. C., Singh, R., Schell, T. L., & Weinick, R. M. (2014). An evaluation of the implementation and perceived utility of the airman resilience training program. *Rand Health Quarterly, 4*(2).

Hart, P. M., & Cotton, P. (2003). Conventional wisdom is often misleading: Police stress within an organisational health framework. In M. F. Dollard, A. H. Winefield, & H. R. Winefield (Eds.), *Occupational stress in the service professions* (pp. 103–141). London: Taylor & Francis. doi:10.1201/9780203422809.ch4

Hoge, C. W., Lesikar, S. E., Guevara, R., Lange, J., Brundage, J. F., Engel, C. C. Jr, ... Orman, D. T. (2002). Mental disorders among US military personnel in the 1990s: Association with high levels of health care utilization and early military attrition. *The American Journal of Psychiatry*, *159*(9), 1576–1583. doi:10.1176/appi.ajp.159.9.1576 PMID:12202280

Hoge, C. W., Terhakopian, A., Castro, C. A., Messer, S. C., & Engel, C. C. (2007). Association of posttraumatic stress disorder with somatic symptoms, health care visits, and absenteeism among Iraq war veterans. *The American Journal of Psychiatry*, *164*(1), 150–153. doi:10.1176/ajp.2007.164.1.150 PMID:17202557

Holahan, C. J., & Moos, R. H. (1990). Life stressors, resistance factors, and improved psychological functioning: An extension of the stress resistance paradigm. *Journal of Personality and Social Psychology*, *58*(5), 909–917. doi:10.1037/0022-3514.58.5.909 PMID:2348376

Holman, E. A., Silver, R. C., Poulin, M., Andersen, J., Gil-Rivas, V., & McIntosh, D. N. (2008). Terrorism, acute stress, and cardiovascular health: A 3-year national study following the September 11th attacks. *Archives of General Psychiatry*, *65*(1), 73–80. doi:10.1001/archgenpsychiatry.2007.6 PMID:18180431

Horn, S. R., Charney, D. S., & Feder, A. (2016). Understanding resilience: New approaches for preventing and treating PTSD. *Experimental Neurology*, *284*, 119–132. doi:10.1016/j.expneurol.2016.07.002 PMID:27417856

Hurrell, J. J., Pate, A., Kliesmet, R., Bowers, R. A., Lee, S., & Burg, J. (1984). *Stress among police officers*. Cincinnati, OH: National Institute of Occupational Safety and Health.

Jacobsen, E. (1929). *Progressive relaxation*. Academic Press.

Jamieson, J. P., Mendes, W. B., Blackstock, E., & Schmader, T. (2010). Turning the knots in your stomach into bows: Reappraising arousal improves performance on the GRE. *Journal of Experimental Social Psychology*, *46*(1), 208–212. doi:10.1016/j.jesp.2009.08.015 PMID:20161454

Johnson, B. R. (2007). *Crucial elements of police firearms training*. Looseleaf Law Publications.

Johnson, D. R., Feldman, S., & Lubin, H. (1995). Critical interaction therapy: Couples therapy in combat-related posttraumatic stress disorder. *Family Process*, *34*(4), 401–412. doi:10.1111/j.1545-5300.1995.00401.x PMID:8674521

Joseph, S., Murphy, D., & Regel, S. (2012). An affective–cognitive processing model of post-traumatic growth. *Clinical Psychology & Psychotherapy*, *19*(4), 316–325. doi:10.1002/cpp.1798 PMID:22610981

Kabat-Zinn, J. (1990). *Full catastrophe living: The program of the stress reduction clinic at the University of Massachusetts Medical Center*. Academic Press.

Kabat-Zinn, J. (2003). Mindfulness-based stress reduction (MBSR). *Constructivism in the Human Sciences*, *8*(2), 73.

Kalisch, R., Müller, M. B., & Tüscher, O. (2015). A conceptual framework for the neurobiological study of resilience. *Behavioral and Brain Sciences*, 38. PMID:25158686

Karasek, R. A. Jr. (1979). Job demands, job decision latitude, and mental strain: Implications for job redesign. *Administrative Science Quarterly*, *24*(2), 285–308. doi:10.2307/2392498

Kashdan, T. B., & Rottenberg, J. (2010). Psychological flexibility as a fundamental aspect of health. *Clinical Psychology Review*, *30*(7), 865–878. doi:10.1016/j.cpr.2010.03.001 PMID:21151705

Kerr, S., Johnson, V. K., Gans, S. E., & Krumrine, J. (2004). Predicting adjustment during the transition to college: Alexithymia, perceived stress, and psychological symptoms. *Journal of College Student Development*, *45*(6), 593–611. doi:10.1353/csd.2004.0068

Kessler, R. C., Berglund, P., Demler, O., Jin, R., Merikangas, K. R., & Walters, E. E. (2005). Lifetime prevalence and age-of-onset distributions of DSM-IV disorders in the National Comorbidity Survey Replication. *Archives of General Psychiatry*, *62*(6), 593–602. doi:10.1001/archpsyc.62.6.593 PMID:15939837

Kleim, B., & Westphal, M. (2011). Mental health in first responders: A review and recommendation for prevention and intervention strategies. *Traumatology*, *17*(4), 17–24. doi:10.1177/1534765611429079

Klinger, D. A., & Brunson, R. K. (2009). Police officers' perceptual distortions during lethal force situations: Informing the reasonableness standard. *Criminology & Public Policy*, *8*(1), 117–140. doi:10.1111/j.1745-9133.2009.00537.x

Kulka, R. A., Schlenger, W. E., Fairbank, J. A., Hough, R. L., Jordan, B. K., Marmar, C. R., & Weiss, D. S. (1990). *Trauma and the Vietnam war generation: Report of findings from the National Vietnam Veterans Readjustment Study* (Vol. 18). New York: Brunner/Mazel.

LaRocco, J. M., House, J. S., & French, J. R. P. (1980). Social support, occupational stress, and health. *Journal of Health and Social Behavior*, *21*(3), 202–218. doi:10.2307/2136616 PMID:7410798

Lennings, C. J. (1997). Police and occupationally related violence: A review. *Policing: An International Journal of Police Strategies & Management*, *20*(3), 555–566. doi:10.1108/13639519710180222

Lester, P. B., Harms, P. D., Herian, M. N., Krasikova, D. V., & Beal, S. J. (2011). The comprehensive soldier fitness program evaluation. *Longitudinal analysis of the impact of master resilience training on self-reported resilience and psychological health data (Report# 3).*

Lipton, B. H. (2008). *The biology of belief: Unleashing the power of consciousness, matter, and miracles* (1st ed.). London: Hay House.

Littleton, H., Horsley, S., John, S., & Nelson, D. V. (2007). Trauma coping strategies and psychological distress: A meta-analysis. *Journal of Traumatic Stress: Official Publication of the International Society for Traumatic Stress Studies*, *20*(6), 977–988. doi:10.1002/jts.20276 PMID:18157893

Loo, R. (1986). Suicide among police in a federal force. *Suicide & Life-Threatening Behavior*, *16*(3), 379–388. doi:10.1111/j.1943-278X.1986.tb01019.x PMID:3765001

Lovallo, W. R. (2015). *Stress and health: Biological and psychological interactions*. Sage publications.

Lundberg, U. (2011). Neuroendocrine measurements. In R. J. Contrada & A. Baum (Eds.), *The handbook of stress science* (pp. 531–542). New York, NY: Springer.

Marshall, R. D., Spitzer, R., & Liebowitz, M. R. (1999). Review and critique of the new DSM-IV diagnosis of acute stress disorder. *The American Journal of Psychiatry, 156*(11), 1677–1685. PMID:10553729

McCraty, R., & Atkinson, M. (2012). Resilience training program reduces physiological and psychological stress in police officers. *Global Advances in Health and Medicine: Improving Healthcare Outcomes Worldwide, 1*(5), 44–66. doi:10.7453/gahmj.2012.1.5.013 PMID:27257532

McCraty, R., Atkinson, M., Tomasino, D., & Bradley, R. T. (2009). The Coherent Heart Heart-Brain Interactions, Psychophysiological Coherence, and the Emergence of System-Wide Order. *Integral Review: A Transdisciplinary & Transcultural Journal for New Thought, Research, & Praxis, 5*(2).

McCreary, D. R., & Thompson, M. M. (2006). Development of two reliable and valid measures of stressors in policing: The operational and organizational police stress questionnaires. *International Journal of Stress Management, 13*(4), 494–518. doi:10.1037/1072-5245.13.4.494

McMillen, J. C., North, C. S., & Smith, E. M. (2000). What parts of PTSD are normal: Intrusion, avoidance, or arousal? Data from the Northridge, California, earthquake. *Journal of Traumatic Stress, 13*(1), 57–75. doi:10.1023/A:1007768830246 PMID:10761174

McNeill, M. (1996). *Alcohol and the police workplace-factors associated with excessive intake (Rep. Series No. 119.1)*. Payneham, South Australia: National Police Research Unit.

McNeill, M., & Wilson, C. (1993). *Alcohol and the police workplace (Rep. Series No. 119)*. Adelaide, South Australia: National Police Research Unit.

Meichenbaum, D. H., & Deffenbacher, J. L. (1988). Stress inoculation training. *The Counseling Psychologist, 16*(1), 69–90. doi:10.1177/0011000088161005

Novaco, R. W. (1977). A stress inoculation approach to anger management in the training of law enforcement officers. *American Journal of Community Psychology, 5*(3), 327–346. doi:10.1007/BF00884700 PMID:910754

O'Byrne, K. K., Peterson, L., & Saldana, L. (1997). Survey of pediatric hospitals' preparation programs: evidence of the impact of health psychology research. *Health Psychology: Official Journal of the Division of Health Psychology, American Psychological Association, 16*(2), 147-154.

Olson, D. T. (1998). Deadly force decision making. *FBI Law Enforce Bulletin, 67*, 1–9.

Padesky, C. A., & Mooney, K. A. (2012). Strengths-based cognitive–behavioural therapy: A four-step model to build resilience. *Clinical Psychology & Psychotherapy, 19*(4), 283–290. doi:10.1002/cpp.1795 PMID:22653834

Park, M., Chang, E. R., & You, S. (2015). Protective role of coping flexibility in PTSD and depressive symptoms following trauma. *Personality and Individual Differences, 82*, 102–106. doi:10.1016/j.paid.2015.03.007

Peele, S. (1991). Out of the habit trap. In A. Monat & R. S. Lazarus (Eds.), *Stress and coping: An anthology* (3rd ed.; pp. 475–482). New York: Columbia University. doi:10.7312/mona92982-033

Prati, G., & Pietrantoni, L. (2010). The relation of perceived and received social support to mental health among first responders: A meta-analytic review. *Journal of Community Psychology*, *38*(3), 403–417. doi:10.1002/jcop.20371

Reivich, K. J., Seligman, M. E., & McBride, S. (2011). Master resilience training in the US Army. *The American Psychologist*, *66*(1), 25–34. doi:10.1037/a0021897 PMID:21219045

Richmond, R., Heather, N., Holt, P., & Hu, W. (1993). *Workplace policies and programs for tobacco, alcohol and other drug abuse in Australia: National campaign against drug abuse (National Campaign Against Drug Abuse Monograph No. 24)*. Canberra: Australian Government Publishing Services.

Robinson, H. M., Sigman, M. R., & Wilson, J. P. (1997). Duty-related stressors and PTSD symptoms in suburban police officers. *Psychological Reports*, *81*(3), 835–845. doi:10.2466/pr0.1997.81.3.835 PMID:9400075

Rodin, J., & Salovey, P. (1989). Health psychology. *Annual Review of Psychology*, *40*(1), 533–579. doi:10.1146/annurev.ps.40.020189.002533 PMID:2648984

Rose, R. D., Buckey, J. C. Jr, Zbozinek, T. D., Motivala, S. J., Glenn, D. E., Cartreine, J. A., & Craske, M. G. (2013). A randomized controlled trial of a self-guided, multimedia, stress management and resilience training program. *Behaviour Research and Therapy*, *51*(2), 106–112. doi:10.1016/j.brat.2012.11.003 PMID:23262118

Rose, S. C., Bisson, J., Churchill, R., & Wessely, S. (2002). Psychological debriefing for preventing post traumatic stress disorder (PTSD). *Cochrane Database of Systematic Reviews*, 2. PMID:12076399

Roskies, E. (1991). Stress management: A new approach to treatment. In A. Monat & R. S. Lazarus (Eds.), *Stress and coping: An anthology* (3rd ed.; pp. 411–431). New York: Columbia University Press. doi:10.7312/mona92982-031

Roth, S., & Cohen, L. J. (1986). Approach, avoidance, and coping with stress. *The American Psychologist*, *41*(7), 813–819. doi:10.1037/0003-066X.41.7.813 PMID:3740641

Rothbaum, B. O., & Foa, E. B. (1993). Subtypes of posttraumatic stress disorder and duration of symptoms. *Posttraumatic stress disorder: DSM-IV and beyond*, 23-35.

Rudofossi, D. C. (1998). *The impact of trauma and loss on affective profiles of police officers*. Academic Press.

Salovey, P., Mayor, J. D., Goldman, S. L., Turvey, C., & Palfai, T. P. (2002). Emotional attention, clarity, and repair: exploring emotional intelligence using the trait meta-mood scale. In J. W. Pennebaker (Ed.), *Emotion, disclosure, and health* (pp. 125–154). Washington, DC: American Psychological Association.

Schnurr, P. P., Friedman, M. J., & Bernardy, N. C. (2002). Research on posttraumatic stress disorder: Epidemiology, pathophysiology, and assessment. *Journal of Clinical Psychology*, *58*(8), 877–889. doi:10.1002/jclp.10064 PMID:12115712

Schuettler, D., & Boals, A. (2011). The path to posttraumatic growth versus posttraumatic stress disorder: Contributions of event centrality and coping. *Journal of Loss and Trauma*, *16*(2), 180–194. doi:10.1080/15325024.2010.519273

Segal, Z. V., Teasdale, J. D., Williams, J. M., & Gemar, M. C. (2002). The mindfulness-based cognitive therapy adherence scale: Inter-rater reliability, adherence to protocol and treatment distinctiveness. *Clinical Psychology & Psychotherapy*, *9*(2), 131–138. doi:10.1002/cpp.320

Sloan, P. (1988). Post-traumatic stress in survivors of an airplane crash-landing: A clinical and exploratory research intervention. *Journal of Traumatic Stress*, *1*(2), 211–229. doi:10.1002/jts.2490010208

Smith, B. W., Epstein, E. M., Ortiz, J. A., Christopher, P. J., & Tooley, E. M. (2013). The foundations of resilience: What are the critical resources for bouncing back from stress? In *Resilience in children, adolescents, and adults* (pp. 167–187). New York, NY: Springer. doi:10.1007/978-1-4614-4939-3_13

Smith, E. M., North, C. S., McCool, R. E., & Shea, J. M. (1990). Acute postdisaster psychiatric disorders: Identification of persons at risk. *The American Journal of Psychiatry*, *147*(2), 202–206. doi:10.1176/ajp.147.2.202 PMID:2301660

Southwick, S. M., Pietrzak, R. H., Charney, D. S., & Krystal, J. H. (2015). Resilience: The role of accurate appraisal, thresholds, and socioenvironmental factors. *Behavioral and Brain Sciences*, , 38. PMID:26786005

Spielberger, C. D., Westberry, L. G., Grier, K. S., & Greenfield, G. (1981). *The police stress survey: Sources of stress in law enforcement*. National Institute of Justice.

Stanley, E. A., Schaldach, J. M., Kiyonaga, A., & Jha, A. P. (2011). Mindfulness-based mind fitness training: A case study of a high-stress predeployment military cohort. *Cognitive and Behavioral Practice*, *18*(4), 566–576. doi:10.1016/j.cbpra.2010.08.002

Sterud, T., Hem, E., Ekeberg, Ø., & Lau, B. (2007). Occupational stress and alcohol use: A study of two nationwide samples of operational police and ambulance, personnel in Norway. *Journal of Studies on Alcohol and Drugs*, *68*(6), 896–904. doi:10.15288/jsad.2007.68.896 PMID:17960308

Stinson, P. M., Liederbach, J., Brewer, S. L., & Todak, N. E. (2014). Drink, drive, go to jail? A study of police officers arrested for drunk driving. *Journal of Criminal Justice*, *37*, 356–376.

Stinson, P. M., Liederbach, J., Brewer, S. L., & Todak, N. E. (2014). Drink, drive, go to jail? A study of police officers arrested for drunk driving. *Journal of Criminal Justice*, *37*, 356–376.

Stinson, P. M. Sr, Liederbach, J., & Freiburger, T. L. (2012). Off-duty and under arrest: A study of the crimes perpetuated by off-duty police. *Criminal Justice Policy Review*, *23*(2), 139–163. doi:10.1177/0887403410390510

Stinson, P. M., Todak, N. E., & Dodge, M. (2015). An exploration of crime by policewomen. *Police Practice and Research*, *16*(1), 79–93. doi:10.1080/15614263.2013.846222

Suinn, R. M. (1997). Mental practice in sport psychology: Where have we been, where do we go? *Clinical Psychology: Science and Practice*, *4*(3), 189–207. doi:10.1111/j.1468-2850.1997.tb00109.x

Suls, J., & Fletcher, B. (1985). The relative efficacy of avoidant and nonavoidant coping strategies: A meta-analysis. *Health Psychology*, *4*(3), 249–288. doi:10.1037/0278-6133.4.3.249 PMID:4029107

Takamatsu, H., Noda, A., Kurumaji, A., Murakami, Y., Tatsumi, M., Ichise, R., & Nishimura, S. (2003). A PET study following treatment with a pharmacological stressor, FG7142, in conscious rhesus monkeys. *Brain Research*, *980*(2), 275–280. doi:10.1016/S0006-8993(03)02987-1 PMID:12867268

Taylor, G. T. (2000). Recent developments in alexithymia theory and research. *Canadian Journal of Psychiatry*, *45*(2), 134–142. doi:10.1177/070674370004500203 PMID:10742872

Teasdale, J. D., Segal, Z., & Williams, J. M. G. (1995). How does cognitive therapy prevent depressive relapse and why should attentional control (mindfulness) training help? *Behaviour Research and Therapy*, *33*(1), 25–39. doi:10.1016/0005-7967(94)E0011-7 PMID:7872934

Toch, H. (2002). *Stress in policing*. American Psychological Association. doi:10.1037/10417-000

Ursano, R. J., & McCarroll, J. E. (1990). The nature of a traumatic stressor: Handling dead bodies. *The Journal of Nervous and Mental Disease*, *178*(6), 396–398. doi:10.1097/00005053-199006000-00010 PMID:2348196

Van Emmerick, A. A. P., Kamphuis, J. H., Hulsbosch, A. M., & Emmelkamp, P. M. G. (2002). Single session debriefing following psychotrauma, help or harm: A metaanalysis. *Lancet*, *360*, 766–771. PMID:12241834

VanRaalte, R. C. (1979). Alcohol as a problem among officers. *The Police Chief*, *46*(2), 38–39.

Vasterling, J. J., Duke, L. M., Brailey, K., Constans, J. I., Allain, A. N. Jr, & Sutker, P. B. (2002). Attention, learning, and memory performances and intellectual resources in Vietnam veterans: PTSD and no disorder comparisons. *Neuropsychology*, *16*(1), 5–14. doi:10.1037/0894-4105.16.1.5 PMID:11853357

Violanti, J. M. (1993). What does high stress police training teach recruits? An analysis of coping. *Journal of Criminal Justice*, *21*(4), 411–417. doi:10.1016/0047-2352(93)90022-F

Violanti, J. M. (1997). Residuals of police occupational trauma. *Australasian Journal of Disaster and Trauma Studies*.

Violanti, J. M. (1999). Alcohol abuse in policing: Prevention strategies. *FBI Law Enforcement Bulletin*, *68*, 16–18.

Violanti, J. M. (2010). Dying for work. Stress and health in policing. *Gazette*, *72*(1), 20–21.

Violanti, J. M., Burchfiel, C. M., Miller, D. B., Andrew, M. E., Dorn, J., Wactawski-Wende, J., & Sharp, D. S. (2006). The buffalo cardio-metabolic occupational police stress (BCOPS) pilot study: Methods and participant characteristics. *Annals of Epidemiology*, *16*(2), 148–156. doi:10.1016/j.annepidem.2005.07.054 PMID:16165369

Violanti, J. M., Marshall, J. R., & Howe, B. (1985). Stress, coping, and alcohol use: The police connection. *Journal of Police Science and Administration*.

Violanti, J. M., & Paton, D. (1999). *Police trauma: Psychological aftermath of civilian combat*. Charles C Thomas Publisher.

Violanti, J. M., Slaven, J. E., Charles, L. E., Burchfiel, C. M., Andrew, M. E., & Homish, G. G. (2011). Police and alcohol use: A descriptive analysis and associations with stress outcomes. *American Journal of Criminal Justice*, *36*(4), 344–356. doi:10.100712103-011-9121-7

Viswesvaran, C., Sanchez, J. I., & Fisher, J. (1999). The role of social support in the process of work stress: A meta-analysis. *Journal of Vocational Behavior*, *54*(2), 314–334. doi:10.1006/jvbe.1998.1661

Weinberg, M., Gil, S., & Gilbar, O. (2014). Forgiveness, coping, and terrorism: Do tendency to forgive and coping strategies associate with the level of posttraumatic symptoms of injured victims of terror attacks? *Journal of Clinical Psychology*, *70*(7), 693–703. doi:10.1002/jclp.22056 PMID:24353169

Wessely, S., & Deahl, M. (2003). Psychological debriefing is a waste of time. *The British Journal of Psychiatry*, *183*(1), 12–14. doi:10.1192/bjp.183.1.12 PMID:12835237

KEY TERMS AND DEFINITIONS

Evidence-Based Practices: Interventions, training procedures, and policies that are derived from, and supported by, empirical investigations.

First Responder: An individual whose professional duties involve responding in the face of disasters and emergencies. Common first responder groups include: police officers, firefighters, and paramedics.

Mindfulness: A state of mind in which an individual is fully and nonjudgmentally engaged with their current sensory and internal experiences.

Physiological Reactivity: A broad term capturing the range of physiological responses (e.g., elevated heart rate) an individual demonstrates in a given situation or in response to a stimulus.

Primary Prevention: An intervention that takes place before an adverse event occurs, designed to prevent the emergence of negative consequences as a result of experiencing the event.

Secondary Prevention: An intervention that takes places after an adverse event occurs, but before symptoms have arisen.

Tertiary Prevention: Treatment of an existing pathology or difficulty.

Chapter 13
Trauma Management Therapy for First Responders

Madeline Marks
University of Central Florida, USA

Annelise Cunningham
University of Central Florida, USA

Clint Bowers
University of Central Florida, USA

Deborah Beidel
University of Central Florida, USA

ABSTRACT

Mental health professionals are only recently beginning to understand the risks for stress-related disorders experienced by first responders. For example, it is clear that first responders are at increased risk for Post-Traumatic Stress Disorder. Unfortunately, clinicians currently have a limited repertoire with which to treat these disorders. Treatments for PTSD have been developed for use with military patients, for the most part. It is not clear that these treatments are appropriate, and effective, for first responders. In this chapter, the authors describe a pilot study designed to evaluate whether one specific treatment approach creates similar clinical outcomes for first responders as have been observed for a military sample. The results indicate that clinical outcomes for first responders were nearly identical as those obtained with military personnel. The results are discussed in terms of future directions for research in this area.

INTRODUCTION AND BACKGROUND

First responders risk their lives to protect the community and this profession is considered to be one of the most dangerous and stressful occupations in the United States (Del Ben, Scotti, Chen, & Fortson, 2006; U.S. Department of Labor, 2007). Society has long recognized the physical demands of first responders; however, what is less formally acknowledged are the negative psychological outcomes. The Oklahoma

DOI: 10.4018/978-1-5225-9803-9.ch013

City Bombing and the September 11, 2001 terrorist attack on the World Trade Center (WTC) were the two earliest large-scale critical incidents that illuminated the numerous negative mental health consequences experienced by first responders (Corrigan et al., 2009; North et al., 2002). More recent studies have identified comparable mental health consequences to those of large-scale critical incidents among first responders with exposure to more routinely encountered potentially traumatic events (PTEs) (see Johnson, 2010; Paulus, Vujanovic, Schuhmann, Smith, & Tran, 2017; Stanley, Boffa, Hom, Kimbrel, & Joiner, 2017).

Most notable among these negative mental health consequences is posttraumatic stress disorder (PTSD). The hallmark of a PTSD diagnosis is that symptoms result from exposure to a traumatic event. Traumatic events are those that include exposure to actual or threatened death, serious injury, or sexual violence (American Psychiatric Association, 2013). First responders encounter these traumatic events repeatedly with high frequency as a function of their daily job requirements (Hartley, Violanti, Sarkisian, Andrew, & Burchfiel, 2013; Marmar et al., 2006). Documented prevalence rates for Posttraumatic Stress Disorder (PTSD) among United States police officers range from 6.2% to 15% (Hartley et al., 2013; Pietrzak et al., 2012), and from 6.3% to 22% (Bernard, Driscoll, Kitt, West, & Tak, 2006; DeLorme, 2014) among United States firefighters. Although varied, most studies observe PTSD rates in excess of the general population (6.8%, Kessler et al., 2005) and observe PTSD rates similar to the prevalence rate observed in OEF/OIF veterans (12%, Hoge, Riviere, Wilk, Herrell, & Weathers, 2014). It is estimated that there are at minimum 250,000 first responders in need of treatment for PTSD (Haugen, Evces, & Weiss, 2012); however, there is little scientific literature to guide clinicians in the selection of an effective treatment for PTSD in these patients.

Given the comparable rates of PTSD among first responders and OEF/OIF veterans, the treatment literature on PTSD and veterans may help guide clinicians' clinical practice. Both intensive outpatient programs (IOP) and traditional outpatient programs (OP) have been effective in the treatment of PTSD for veterans (Beidel, Frueh, Neer, Bowers, et al., 2019; Beidel, Frueh, Neer, & Lejuez, 2017). Among veterans that participated in one IOP, the relapse (1%) and dropout (2%) rates for the program were lower than other PTSD treatments and RCTs. In addition to the improved relapse and dropout rates, treatment effects were large ($d = 2.06$). Of the 100 participants that completed treatment, 65.9% no longer met DSM-IV-TR criteria for PTSD, 72% experienced clinically significant symptom improvement, and 94.6% met the VA designated benchmark for symptom improvement. Among veterans that participated in the OP, the relapse (4.5%) and dropout (26%) rates for the exposure portion of the program were compatible with other PTSD treatments and RCTs. Treatment effects were large ($d = 2.06$). Of the 49 participants that completed treatment across groups, 65.9% no longer met DSM-IV-TR criteria for PTSD, 42% experienced clinically significant symptom improvement, and 94.6% met the VA designated benchmark for symptom improvement.

Given these promising outcomes among veterans, the models employed by Beidel, Frueh, Neer, Bowers, et al. (2019) and Beidel, Frueh, Neer, and Lejuez (2017) are worth investigating among a group of treatment seeking first responders. However, it remains unclear if extrapolating treatment practices from the empirical literature with veterans will translate well to other populations, including first responders. It is unclear if similar success can be achieved. There are two specific points that merit consideration. First, unlike active duty personnel who can attend treatment by assignment to a temporary duty status (TDY), no such formal mechanism is in place for first responders. In order to take advantage of an IOP, first responders would need to utilize workman's compensation, personal sick time, vacation time, or Family Medical Leave Act (FMLA). Traditional outpatient therapy is also a challenge when working with first responders. Different from their military counterparts, many first responders work a shift schedule of 24-hours on-duty followed by 48-hours off-duty; therefore, clinicians require flexibility to capitalize on off-duty availability for scheduling purposes.

Second, the extant literature (see Lang & McTeague, 2011) reports concerns about the feasibility of exposure therapy for individuals with a history of multiple exposures to trauma. Several researchers argue that there may be differences in neurophysiological reactivity among individuals with exposure to multiple traumatic events in comparison to single-discrete traumatic events (Diamond, Lipsitz, Fajerman, & Rozenblat, 2010; Eagle & Kaminer, 2013; Kaminer, Eagle, & Crawford-Browne, 2016; Nuttman-Shwartz & Shoval-Zuckerman, 2016). Previous research (Cuthbert et al., 2003; D'Andrea, Pole, DePierro, Freed, & Wallace, 2013; Hagenaars, Stins, & Roelofs, 2012; Lang & McTeague, 2011; McTeague et al., 2010) identified a dulled level of reactivity among individuals with exposure to multiple traumatic events, which may be beneficial for coping with recurrent and chronic stress. This decreased reactivity may work in assistance with coping; however, it may also disrupt the effectiveness of exposure therapy. Specifically, weakened emotional reactivity may decrease the ability to repair the disrupted fear-extinction mechanisms at work in individuals with PTSD.

To our knowledge, this study is the first to evaluate the efficacy and feasibility of Trauma Management Therapy for PTSD among first responders. We examined its efficacy through retrospective record review of first responders treated for occupational-related PTSD from December 2016 to August 2018. PTSD symptoms, as measured by the Clinician Administered PTSD Scale for DSM-5 (CAPS-5) and the PTSD Checklist for DSM-5 (PCL-5) were assessed at pre and post-treatment

METHODS

Participants

Participants (n=29) were firefighter/emergency medical service personnel (FF/EMS; hereafter termed as FF) and law enforcement officers (LEO). All had sought treatment at the University of Central Florida RESTORES Clinic in Orlando, Florida for negative emotional reactions/behaviors related to traumatic events. All patients gave informed consent for treatment. Data were deidentified and amalgamated for this report. Information was obtained from medical records with respect to diagnosis, age, gender, type of responder, scores on the PCL-5 and the CAPS-5 at the beginning and end of treatment. Of the total participants, 48.6% qualified for a single diagnosis of posttraumatic stress disorder (PTSD), whereas 51.4% had comorbid diagnoses in addition to PTSD (e.g., Alcohol Use Disorder (AUD), Major Depressive Disorder (MDD), Generalized Anxiety Disorder (GAD, amongst other DSM-5 mental disorders). Therapists were licensed clinical psychologists or advanced clinical psychology doctoral students who received didactic training in the theory and implementation of all treatment components. See Table 1 for further descriptive information regarding the sample.

Table 1. Demographic Information

		n	%
Relationship Status	Married	12	50.0
	Separated	5	20.8
	Divorced	2	8.3
	Single	5	20.8
Occupation	Firefighter/EMS	21	72.4
	Law Enforcement	8	27.6
Gender	Female	3	10.3
	Male	26	89.7
Age		M	SD
Years of Service		41.0	8.27

Assessment

Clinician-Administered PTSD Scale for DSM-5 (CAPS-5)

The CAPS-5 (CAPS-5; Weathers et al., 2017) is a clinician-administered diagnostic interview used to assess PTSD diagnosis and symptom severity. The CAPS-5 consists of 30 items that assess the 20 DSM-5 diagnostic criteria for PTSD. Each item is scored for symptom severity (scale 0 = "absent" to 4 = "extreme/incapacitating"). A total score is calculated by summing the items that reflect the DSM-5 PTSD criteria. Individual severity scores are calculated by summing the corresponding cluster items. At least one re-experiencing symptom (Criterion B), one avoidance symptom (Criterion C), two negative alterations in cognitions and mood symptoms (Criterion D), and two hyperarousal symptoms (Criterion E) must be rated as "moderate/threshold" (score of 2 on the scale of 0 to 4) or higher to meet DSM-5 PTSD diagnostic criteria. Further, symptoms must have persisted for greater than one month (Criterion F), and clinically significant distress or impairment (Criterion F) is present. The CAPS-5 was administered at pre and post-treatment.

PTSD Checklist (PCL-5)

The PCL-5 (Weathers et al., 2013) is a 20-item self-report measure that corresponds with the 20 symptoms listed in the DSM-5. The PCL-5 is scored by calculating a total severity score (range = 0 - 80) by summing all items. Cluster scores can also be calculated by summing the items within a cluster (Cluster B, items 1-5; Cluster C, items 6-7; Cluster D, items 8-14; Cluster E, items 15-20). Items are rated from 0 "not at all" to 4 "extremely." The PCL-5 was administered at pre and post-treatment.

Trauma Management Therapy is a multi-component behavioral treatment program that combines individual imaginal and in vivo exposure therapy (to address the primary symptoms of PTSD) and a group therapy component that addresses other behaviors that often are present when PTSD exists. The group treatment includes anger management training, behavioral activation for depression, social reintegration, and sleep hygiene training. We deliver the treatment in one of two formats. In our traditional outpatient program, imaginal exposure is delivered first, followed by in vivo exposure, followed by the group treatment. This is a total of 29 treatment sessions delivered over a 16-17-week time period, distributed as follows. Following a psychoeducation session, exposure sessions (typically 14 sessions total) occur two to three times per week. This is followed by group therapy, which occurs once weekly (12 sessions).

In our innovative Intensive Outpatient Program (IOP), we deliver the 29 treatment sessions over a 3-week period. Three sessions per day are delivered (imaginal exposure, in vivo exposure, and group treatment), Monday through Friday for three weeks. Both formats have been demonstrated to be highly effective. Additionally, data from the 17-week program demonstrate the specificity of the individual components – when delivered separately, the group treatment does not result in further significant decreases in CAPS or PCL scores, indicating that change in primary PTSD symptoms occurs as a result of exposure therapy (Beidel, Frueh, Uhde, Wong, & Mentrikoski, 2011; Beidel et al., 2019).

In this pilot study, 31% of the first responders received exposure therapy only, whereas 69% of the first responders participated in the three-week IOP. Because these different components work on different parts of the PTSD syndrome, we can examine the efficacy of exposure therapy for PTSD in first responders, regardless of the specific treatment delivery format.

With respect to the specifics of the exposure therapy delivery, the first session involves a collaborative effort between the clinician and the patient to construct an imaginal exposure scene, based on the specific trauma. Each patient's trauma scene is unique, and includes attention to the sights, sounds, and smells that were present during the traumatic event as well as attention to how the patient was behaving, thinking, and feeling. Below is an example of an imaginal scene:

You are called out for a motor vehicle accident. You are coming to the scene through afternoon traffic via the highway. There are cars everywhere, fi ret rucks, ambulances, traffic stopped, one car is on its side, debris everywhere, people everywhere. You begin to smell the smell of death (use actual smells of coolant/ oil/ transmission/battery acid, if available). You are thinking "Okay, what's my first move, I cannot let these people die." You announce to the scene commander, "medic 161 on scene requesting assignment." He replies, "Pickup truck, passenger seat would be your patient." You start to sweat, and your throat tightens. You are wondering what you will find when you arrive at the pick-up truck. Will you be able to save this person?

You grab the stretcher, which has the heart monitors and jump bag. Your partner grabs the seat collar and backboard. You go to the truck and announce yourself, " Hey, my name is Rick, I'm paramedic, where are you hurting?" He's a kid – he can't be more than 12 years old. You see his eyes move and do not get any other response. You immediately see that he is severely injured. You see cuts around his head, a large laceration across his neck. You pull him out of the truck, lay him on the backboard. He starts bleeding out. Your heart is racing, you are sweating, your throat is tight. You are thinking – damn, what's happening? I am not going to lose this kid. This kid is not going to die.

You yell to your partner "I need the airway bag. I've got to intubate him." You do the intubation, put him on the stretcher and get him into the back of the truck. You get in the back with him. "Code 3" (siren sounds) to the hospital. You do a secondary assessment. You think "He's just a kid. I can't lose him. He hasn't even had a chance to be a teenager." You get on the radio and say, "Approximately 12 year old boy, motor vehicle accident, severe trauma to neck, obvious trachea and esophagus laceration, working a trauma code." You arrive at hospital and get out of the truck. You see people everywhere as you wheel him to trauma room. You say to the physician, "he was sitting in seat, he was conscious, he had eye movement, I moved him, he bled out. I reassessed the lacerations, found trachea severed." The physician looks at you with a puzzled expression. You feel your stomach do a flip. What did you miss? Why is she looking at you like that? You assist others lifting him to the hospital bed. The physician grabs his chin and lifts up. You see the kid is cut ear from ear, almost reaching his spine. The physician says, "There is nothing we can do" and pronounces him dead. You exit the room. You start thinking "what did I miss?" "what did I do wrong?" "I was too late…too late to help this kid." You start to cry, you see the nursing staff crying. The physician starts talking to you. She says, "you did all you can do." You think to yourself, "yeah, but I didn't save him. I'm supposed to save them." You feel helpless, your stomach is in a know as you think about your own kids.

What is important for clinicians to note about this scene is that it is not just a description of events. It included drawing the patient's attention to his emotions, thoughts and physiological responses. Introducing the actual sounds and smells into the scene increases the likelihood of immersion into the scene. Furthermore, as these sights and sounds now may serve as cues (sometimes called triggers) that may elicit responses such as anxiety, flashbacks, or nightmares. Through the process of exposure, these cues will lose their ability to elicit these responses, thereby extinguishing the fear. For more information about the rationale behind exposure therapy and the specifics of implementation, the reader is referred to Beidel, Frueh, Neer, and Lejuez, (2017).

Beginning with session 2, patients engaged in imaginal exposure therapy using the individualized exposure scene. Prior to beginning the session, the therapist asked the patient to estimate their baseline level of arousal using a 9 point (0-8) subjective units of distress scale (SUDS). As the scenario was presented, the patient should experience an increase in anxiety. As the patient continued to imagine the scene, anxiety peaked and subsequently decreased. The exposure continued until within-session habituation (WSH) was achieved. WSH was indicated by a minimum 50% reduction from highest reported SUDS level during that session and the clinician's behavioral observations. Imaginal exposure was conducted for up to 14 sessions and was terminated after evidence of between-session habituation (BSH). BSH was indicated by the absence of SUDS increase following imaginal scene exposure.

RESULTS

Differences Among First Responder Type

Independent sample t-tests were conducted to assess for differences in PTSD symptom severity by first responder type (e.g., FF vs. LEO; see Figures 1 and 2 for pre-treatment scores). No group differences were found on the CAPS-5 ($t = 0.25$, df = 11.97 $p = .81$) or PCL-5 (t = 1.37, df = 21.51, $p = .18$).

Changes in PTSD Symptoms

CAPS-5

To examine changes on the CAPS from pre to post-treatment a paired samples t-test was used and the results revealed a statistically significant decrease in CAPS score ($t = 11.13$, df = 19, $p < 0.001$), resulting in a large effect size ($d = 2.49$), similar to the previous effect sizes identified by Beidel, Frueh, Neer, Bowers, et al. (2017) and Beidel, Frueh, Neer, and Lejuez (2017). See Figure 1.

PCL-5

Changes on the PCL scores from pre to post-treatment were also examined. Results of the paired samples t-test revealed a statistically significant decrease in PCL scores ($t = 14.55$, df = 25, $p < 0.001$), resulting in a large effect size ($d = 2.85$) similar to the previous effect sizes identified by Beidel, Frueh, Neer, Bowers, et al. (2017) and Beidel, Frueh, Neer, and Lejuez (2017). See Figure 2.

DISCUSSION

With minimum estimates as high as 250,000, first responders need PTSD treatment, in the United States. Responding to their need for evidenced-based treatment for PTSD is immediate and necessary (Haugen, Evces, & Weiss, 2012). Despite the points of consideration offered by the authors of the present study that PTSD treatment with first responders may not be feasible, the findings of the current study give no such indication. The present study highlights that the IOP and OP treatment models used with veterans (Beidel, Frueh, Neer, Bowers, et al., 2017; Beidel, Frueh, Neer, & Lejuez, 2017) also are effective treatments for PTSD among first responders. At post-treatment, first responders demonstrated significant decreases from pre- to post-treatment in clinician rated (CAPS-5) and self-reported (PCL-5) symptoms

Figure 1. Pre-treatment and Post-treatment CAPS-5 scores

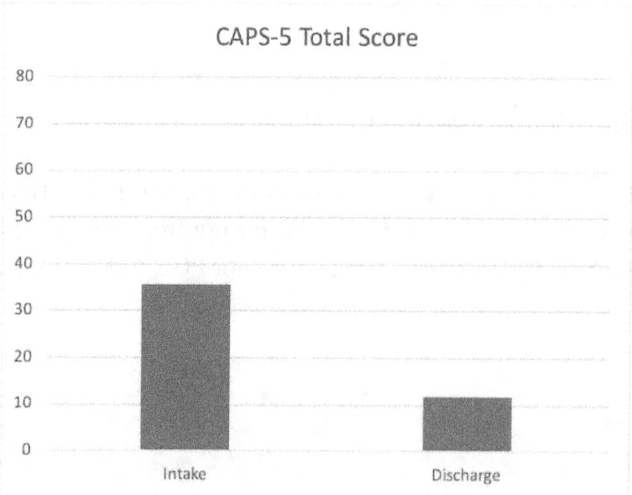

Figure 2. Pre-treatment and Post-treatment PCL-5 scores

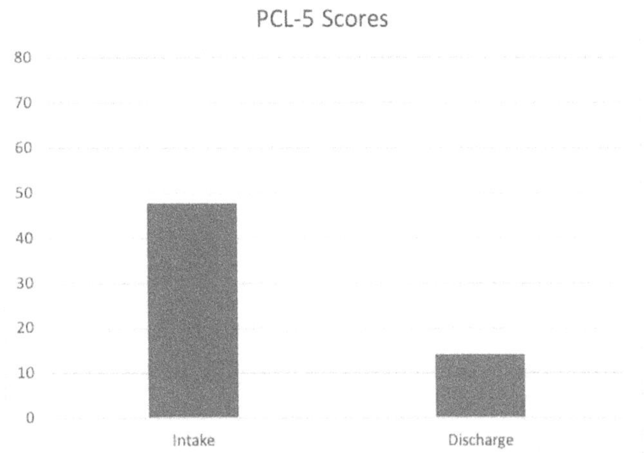

of PTSD. The results demonstrate that exposure therapy is a feasible treatment for PTSD among first responders; therefore, clinicians that work with first responders should consider the use of exposure therapy for treatment of PTSD symptoms.

With regard to scheduling, the first responders in this study maintained attendance at a minimum of two sessions per week, although most participants were able to participate in the IOP three week intensive treatment program. The decrease in reported symptoms highlight the viability of treatment gains within the context scheduling barriers for first responders. A cornerstone of effective treatment is consistent attendance (Reardon, Cukrowicz, Reeves, & Joiner, 2010). The rotating shift schedule of first responders may appear as a deterrent for clinicians to choose exposure therapy. While clinicians working with first responders should be cognizant of their rotating shift schedule it should not deter clinicians from choosing exposure therapy as a treatment modality. The present study was able to work around scheduling barriers to obtain commitment to treatment attendance.

FUTURE RESEARCH DIRECTIONS

The findings raise an interesting point of consideration with regard to the development of PTSD. The hallmark predisposition to the development of PTSD requires exposure to or witness of a life-threatening event (National Center for PTSD, 2018). First responders present as a unique population in that, while employed, they continuously experience or are witnesses to such events. Thus, the risk for maintaining or increasing symptoms of PTSD while continuing to work during a course of treatment could potentially be high. This study demonstrates that exposure therapy serves as an effective treatment modality for first responders, even in the face of continuous exposure to criterion A events. That is, even though first responders remained active in their employment, engaging in exposure therapy simultaneously resulted in a decrease in symptoms reported on the CAPS-5 and PCL-5. The authors originally posed the point of consideration of the impact of exposure to multiple traumas and the potential for weakened emotional reactivity and subsequent decreased ability to repair the disrupted fear-extinction mechanisms involved in PTSD. The results of the present study serve as preliminary evidence against this concern for treatment disruption; however, additional resources should be dedicated to further elucidating the relationship between exposure to multiple traumas, emotional reactivity, and effectiveness of exposure therapy. Future research must focus on the development of treatment recommendations (e.g., session length, number of sessions) specific to first responders. This should include the examination of therapy process variables (i.e., between- and within-session habituation) and differences in response to treatment between first responder occupations.

CONCLUSION

Ultimately, large-scale multi-site randomized controlled trials will be needed to for translating research data into clinical practice. The present findings serve as a foundation to the development of a standard of care for first responders suffering from PTSD. Exposure therapy resulted in the successful and significant reduction of PTSD symptoms in first responders on both the CAPS-5 and PCL-5. Provision of services to this unique and underserved population should include exposure therapy

ACKNOWLEDGMENT

The authors would like to thank the clinicians for their dedication and efforts to providing evidenced based treatment to our hometown heroes.

This research was supported by Department of Justice Antiterrorism and Emergency Assistance Program (2017-RF-GX-0003) through a grant to the Attorney General, state of Florida.

REFERENCES

American Psychiatric Association. (2013). *Diagnostic and Statistical Manual of Mental Disorders* (5th ed.). Washington, DC: Author.

Beidel, D. C., Frueh, B. C., Neer, S. M., Bowers, S. M., Bowers, C. A., Trachik, B., ... Grubaugh, A. (2019). Trauma Management Therapy with virtual-reality augmented exposure therapy for combat-related PTSD: A randomized controlled trial. *Journal of Anxiety Disorders*, *61*, 64–74. doi:10.1016/j.janxdis.2017.08.005 PMID:28865911

Beidel, D. C., Frueh, B. C., Uhde, T. W., Wong, N., & Mentrikoski, J. (2011). Multicomponent behavioral treatment for chronic combat-related posttraumatic stress disorder: A randomized controlled trial. *Journal of Anxiety Disorders*, *25*(2), 224–231. doi:10.1016/j.janxdis.2010.09.006 PMID:20951543

Beidel, D. C., Frueh, C. B., Neer, S. M., & Lejuez, C. W. (2017). The efficacy of Trauma Management Therapy: A controlled pilot investigation of a three-week intensive outpatient program for combat-related PTSD. *Journal of Anxiety Disorders*, *50*(May), 23–32. doi:10.1016/j.janxdis.2017.05.001 PMID:28545005

Bernard, B., Driscoll, R., Kitt, M., West, C., & Tak, S. (2006). Health hazard evaluation of police officers and firefighters after hurricane Katrina - New Orleans, Louisiana, October 17-28 and November 30 - December 5, 2005. *Morbidity and Mortality Weekly Report*, *55*(16), 456–458. PMID:16645571

Corrigan, M., McWilliams, R., Kelly, K. J., Niles, J., Cammarata, C., Jones, K., ... Prezant, D. J. (2009). A computerized, self-administered questionnaire to evaluate posttraumatic stress among firefighters after the World Trade Center collapse. *American Journal of Public Health*, *99*(S3Suppl 3), 702–709. doi:10.2105/AJPH.2008.151605 PMID:19890176

Cuthbert, B. N., Lang, P. J., Strauss, C., Drobes, D., Patrick, C. J., & Bradley, M. M. (2003). The psychophysiology of anxiety disorder: Fear memory imagery. *Psychophysiology*, *40*(3), 407–422. doi:10.1111/1469-8986.00043 PMID:12946114

D'Andrea, W., Pole, N., DePierro, J., Freed, S., & Wallace, D. B. (2013). Heterogeneity of defensive responses after exposure to trauma: Blunted autonomic reactivity in response to startling sounds. *International Journal of Psychophysiology*, *90*(1), 80–89. doi:10.1016/j.ijpsycho.2013.07.008 PMID:23896169

Del Ben, K. S., Scotti, J. R., Chen, Y.-C., & Fortson, B. L. (2006). Prevalence of posttraumatic stress disorder symptoms in firefighters. *Work and Stress*, *20*, 37–48. doi:10.1080/02678370600679512

DeLorme, J. (2014). *The investigation of repeated trauma exposure and psychological adjustment in Firefighters*. California School of Professional Psychology, Alliant International University.

Diamond, G. M., Lipsitz, J. D., Fajerman, Z., & Rozenblat, O. (2010). Ongoing Traumatic Stress Response (OTSR) in Sderot, Israel. *Professional Psychology, Research and Practice*, *41*(1), 19–25. doi:10.1037/a0017098

Eagle, G., & Kaminer, D. (2013). Continuous traumatic stress: Expanding the lexicon of traumatic stress. *Peace and Conflict*, *19*(2), 85–99. doi:10.1037/a0032485

Hagenaars, M. A., Stins, J. F., & Roelofs, K. (2012). Aversive life events enhance human freezing responses. *Journal of Experimental Psychology. General*, *141*(1), 98–105. doi:10.1037/a0024211 PMID:21767043

Hartley, T. A., Violanti, J. M., Sarkisian, K., Andrew, M. E., & Burchfiel, C. M. (2013). PTSD symptoms among police officers: Associations with frequency, recency, and types of traumatic events. *International Journal of Emergency Mental Health*, *15*(4), 241–253. doi:10.1038/nbt.3121.ChIP-nexus PMID:24707587

Haugen, P. T., Evces, M., & Weiss, D. S. (2012). Treating posttraumatic stress disorder in first responders: A systematic review. *Clinical Psychology Review*, *32*(5), 370–380. doi:10.1016/j.cpr.2012.04.001 PMID:22561967

Hoge, C. W., Riviere, L. A., Wilk, J. E., Herrell, R. K., & Weathers, F. W. (2014). The prevalence of post-traumatic stress disorder (PTSD) in US combat soldiers: A head-to-head comparison of DSM-5 versus DSM-IV-TR symptom criteria with the PTSD checklist. *The Lancet. Psychiatry*, *1*(4), 269–277. doi:10.1016/S2215-0366(14)70235-4 PMID:26360860

Johnson, J. (2010). *Understanding Differences in Stress and Coping Between Full-Time and Paid-On-Call Firefighters*. Walden University.

Kaminer, D., Eagle, G., & Crawford-Browne, S. (2016). Continuous traumatic stress as a mental and physical health challenge: Case studies from South Africa. *Journal of Health Psychology*. doi:10.1177/1359105316642831 PMID:27091760

Kessler, R. C., Berglund, P., Delmer, O., Jin, R., Merikangas, K. R., & Walters, E. E. (2005). Lifetime prevalence and age-of-onset distributions of DSM-IV disorders in the National Comorbidity Survey Replication. *Archives of General Psychiatry*, *62*(6), 593–602. doi:10.1001/archpsyc.62.6.593 PMID:15939837

Lang, P. J., & McTeague, L. M. (2011). Discrete and Recurrent Traumatization in PTSD: Fear vs. Anxious Misery. *Journal of Clinical Psychology in Medical Settings*, *18*(2), 207–209. doi:10.100710880-011-9252-5 PMID:21626350

Marmar, C. R., McCaslin, S. E., Metzler, T. J., Best, S., Weiss, D. S., Fagan, J., ... Neylan, T. (2006). Predictors of posttraumatic stress in police and other first responders. *Annals of the New York Academy of Sciences*, *1071*(1), 1–18. doi:10.1196/annals.1364.001 PMID:16891557

McTeague, L. M., Lang, P. J., Laplante, M.-C., Cuthbert, B. N., Shumen, J. R., & Bradley, M. M. (2010). Aversive Imagery in Posttraumatic Stress Disorder: Trauma Recurrence, Comorbidity, and Physiological Reactivity. *Biological Psychiatry*, *67*(4), 346–356. doi:10.1016/j.biopsych.2009.08.023 PMID:19875104

North, C. S., Tivis, L., McMillen, J. C., Pfefferbaum, B., Cox, J., Spitznagel, E. L., ... Smith, E. M. (2002). Coping, functioning, and adjustment of rescue workers after the Oklahoma City bombing. *Journal of Traumatic Stress*, *15*(3), 171–175. doi:10.1023/A:1015286909111 PMID:12092908

Nuttman-Shwartz, O., & Shoval-Zuckerman, Y. (2016). Continuous Traumatic Situations in the Face of Ongoing Political Violence: The Relationship Between CTS and PTSD. *Trauma, Violence & Abuse*, *17*(5), 562–570. doi:10.1177/1524838015585316 PMID:25966968

Paulus, D. J., Vujanovic, A. A., Schuhmann, B. B., Smith, L. J., & Tran, J. (2017). Main and interactive effects of depression and posttraumatic stress in relation to alcohol dependence among urban male firefighters. *Psychiatry Research*, *251*, 69–75. doi:10.1016/j.psychres.2017.02.011 PMID:28189939

Pietrzak, R. H., Schechter, C. B., Bromet, E. J., Katz, C. L., Reissman, D. B., Ozbay, F., ... Southwick, S. M. (2012). The burden of full and subsyndromal posttraumatic stress disorder among police involved in the World Trade Center rescue and recovery effort. *Journal of Psychiatric Research*, *46*(7), 835–842. doi:10.1016/j.jpsychires.2012.03.011 PMID:22464942

Stanley, I. H., Boffa, J. W., Hom, M. A., Kimbrel, N. A., & Joiner, T. E. (2017). Differences in psychiatric symptoms and barriers to mental health care between volunteer and career firefighters. *Psychiatry Research*, *247*, 236–242. doi:10.1016/j.psychres.2016.11.037 PMID:27930964

U.S. Department of Labor. (2007). *2007 census of fatal occupational injuries (revised data)*. Author.

Weathers, F. W., Bovin, M. J., Lee, D. J., Sloan, D. M., Schnurr, P. P., Kaloupek, D. G., ... Marx, B. P. (2017). The Clinician-Administered PTSD Scale for DSM–5 (CAPS-5): Development and Initial Psychometric Evaluation in Military Veterans. *Psychological Assessment*, *30*(3), 383–395. doi:10.1037/pas0000486 PMID:28493729

Weathers, F. W., Litz, B. T., Keane, T. M., Palmieri, P. A., Marx, B. P., & Schnurr, P. P. (2013). *The PTSD Checklist for DSM-5 (PCL-5)*. Academic Press.

ADDITIONAL READING

Beidel, D. C., Frueh, C. B., Neer, S. M., Bowers, C., & Rizzo, A. (2014). *Using Virtual Reality as Part of an Intensive Treatment Program for PTSD* (pp. 1–10). I/ITSEC.

Beidel, D. C., Frueh, C. B., Neer, S. M., Bowers, C., Trachik, B., Uhde, T. W., & Grubaugh, A. (2017). Trauma management therapy with virtual-reality augmented exposure therapy for combat-related PTSD: A randomized controlled trial. *Journal of Anxiety Disorders*, 1–11. doi:10.1016/j.janxdis.2017.08.005 PMID:28865911

Beidel, D. C., Frueh, C. B., Neer, S. M., & Lejuez, C. W. (2017). The efficacy of Trauma Management Therapy: A controlled pilot investigation of a three-week intensive outpatient program for combat-related PTSD. *Journal of Anxiety Disorders*, *50*(May), 23–32. doi:10.1016/j.janxdis.2017.05.001 PMID:28545005

Del Ben, K. S., Scotti, J. R., Chen, Y.-C., & Fortson, B. L. (2006). Prevalence of posttraumatic stress disorder symptoms in firefighters. *Work and Stress*, *20*(March), 37–48. doi:10.1080/02678370600679512

Gramlich, M. A., & Neer, S. M. (2018). Firefighter-Paramedic With Posttraumatic Stress Disorder, Horrific Images, and Depression: A Clinical Case Study. *Clinical Case Studies*, *17*(3), 150–165. doi:10.1177/1534650118770792

Lanza, A., Roysircar, G., & Rodgers, S. (2018). First responder mental healthcare: Evidence-based prevention, postvention, and treatment. *Professional Psychology, Research and Practice*, *49*(3), 193–204. doi:10.1037/pro0000192

Marks, M. R., Bowers, C., Trachik, B., James, N. T., & Beidel, D. (2017). Differences in PTSD Symptomatology Between Combat Veterans and Emergency Dispatchers. *Annals of Emergency Dispatch & Response*, *5*(2), 15–21. Retrieved from https://www.aedrjournal.org/differences-in-ptsd-symptomatology-between-combat-veterans-and-emergency-dispatchers/

Moffitt, J., Bostock, J., & Cave, A. (2014). Promoting well-being and reducing stigma about mental health in the fire service. *Journal of Public Mental Health*, *13*(2), 103–113. doi:10.1108/JPMH-02-2013-0004

Richards, D. A., & Rose, J. S. (1991). Exposure Therapy for Post-traumatic Stress Disorder: Four Case Studies. *The British Journal of Psychiatry*, *158*(6), 836–840. doi:10.1192/bjp.158.6.836 PMID:1678664

Sripada, R. K., Rauch, S. A. M., & Liberzon, I. (2016). Psychological Mechanisms of PTSD and Its Treatment. *Current Psychiatry Reports*, *18*(11), 99. doi:10.100711920-016-0735-9 PMID:27671916

Tolin, D. F., & Foa, E. B. (1999). Treatment of a police officer with PTSD using prolonged exposure. *Behavior Therapy*, *30*(3), 527–538. doi:10.1016/S0005-7894(99)80023-9

KEY TERMS AND DEFINITIONS

Exposure Therapy: Behavioral treatment modality that consists of confronting an individual's core fear to elicit anxiety.

First Responder: Occupation related to individuals trained in emergency response.

Imaginal Exposure Scene: Unique account of the patient's index trauma that includes attention to the sights, sounds, and smells that were present during the traumatic event as well as attention to how the patient was behaving, thinking, and feeling.

Intensive Outpatient Program (IOP): Treatment schedule consisting of increase frequency of attendance in comparison to traditional outpatient services. Schedule includes 29 sessions over a three-week period. Incorporates individual, group, and in vivo sessions.

Posttraumatic Stress Disorder: Clinical diagnosis identified by the DSM-5, consisting of intrusion symptoms, avoidance, negative alterations in mood and cognitions, changes in arousal and reactivity following a traumatic event. Traumatic event can be directly experienced, witnessed, or learned about.

Psychoeducation: Information provided to patients about the causes, symptoms, and treatments of mental health conditions.

Trauma Management Therapy: A multi-component behavioral treatment program to address the primary symptoms of PTSD.

Chapter 14

Narrative Therapy to Address Trauma for Emergency Medical Services and Firefighters

Amanda C. DeDiego
https://orcid.org/0000-0003-2270-5813
University of Wyoming, USA

Isabel C. Farrell
https://orcid.org/0000-0002-7836-9284
Wake Forest University, USA

Andrea M. McGrath
University of Wyoming, USA

ABSTRACT

First responders, including Emergency Medical Services personnel and firefighters, support community members in times of crisis. When responding to emergencies, first responders often experience both direct and vicarious trauma. Over time, the pace and intensity of a career as a first responder leads to poor health habits and high risk for mental health issues including posttraumatic stress disorder. Due to concern about peer perception and mental health stigma, these professionals are less likely to seek mental health supports to manage and process trauma. This chapter explores Narrative Therapy as an ideal option for mental health treatment of first responder trauma, providing a collaborative approach to therapy using the natural coping strategy of storytelling.

INTRODUCTION

First responders, including Emergency Medical Services (EMS) personnel and firefighters, have increased risk of mental health issues due to exposure to trauma over a career (Jones, 2017). More specifically, first responders have increased risk of mental illness symptoms including PTSD, depression, anxiety, sleep

DOI: 10.4018/978-1-5225-9803-9.ch014

issues, substance use, and suicidal ideation as compared to other helping professionals and the general public (Martin, Tran, & Buser, 2017). Risk for such symptoms increase for first responders located in rural areas, working longer shifts, and those without social supports at home (Jones, Nagel, McSweeney, Curran, 2018). Mental health supports, such as Employee Assistance Programs (EAPs) are critical for addressing the high risk for Posttraumatic Stress Disorder (PTSD) and suicide among first responders (Heightman, 2016). This chapter explores storytelling as a natural coping strategy for first responders, and proposes use of Narrative Therapy as means of trauma-informed mental health counseling for this population.

BACKGROUND

Emergency Medical Services (EMS) includes Emergency Medical Technicians (EMTs) and Paramedics. The scope of practice outlined by the National Highway Traffic Safety Administration defines the roles and training of EMS (USDOT, 2007). In this scope of practice, EMTs focus on basic life support (BLS) services which encompass treating and transporting stable patients not in imminent harm of death or disability. Beyond the training of EMTs, Paramedics represent the highest level of certification for EMS. Paramedics oversee the work of EMTs and direct firefighters on scene in the interest of prioritizing patient health outcomes. Paramedics perform invasive medical procedures for advanced life support (ALS) services addressing life-threatening emergencies during patient treatment and transport (USDOT, 2007). Nationally, 70% of EMS personnel are EMTs, and only 24% are Paramedics (USDHS, 2017).

EMS as a field is generally young. The Highway Safety Act of 1966 established the Department of Transportation (DOT; NHTSA, n.d). This marks early organization and development of the EMS system as represented today, with DOT tasked with regulation and implementation of training standards (NHTSA, 2011). Mainstream media representation of EMS dating back to the 1970s, primarily with the television show *Emergency,* began to create both public awareness of 911 services, as well as public misconceptions about emergency support in communities (NHTSA, n.d). EMS often work closely with, or cross train as firefighters. Nationally, 40% of EMS work directly with fire departments (NHTSA, 2011).

Early firefighters in the 1800s in the US were largely volunteers (Kenlon, 1913). Later, through central government regulation, firefighters established a fraternal order or "brotherhood" still recognized today in response to early rivalries between volunteer firefighting communities. In modern firefighting, the United States Fire Administration (USFA) trains, supports, and governs firefighters as a division of the Federal Emergency Management Agency (FEMA), first established in 1973 to address fire prevention (Kruger, 2018). Firefighters focus on fire prevention and response in the community (USDHS, 2017). Training for firefighters includes Firefighter I and Firefighter II certifications (NFPA, 2019). Both levels of certification include foundational training including response to alarms, tools and equipment for fire management, navigating environments safely to address fires, and helping rescue fire victims. The Firefighter II certification includes further skills training with a wider variety of equipment than Firefighter I.

Nationally, 71% of fire departments are staffed by volunteers, and as such, 56% of all firefighters in the US are volunteers (USDHS, 2017). While less common, 17 states also use volunteer EMS (USDOT, 2007). Volunteer first responders often receive no pay for their services or are paid per call (NVFC, 2014). While volunteers still experience camaraderie and the culture of first responders, they may experience this culture differently than career first responders. Further, volunteer first responders experience trauma and stress without as many supports and benefits. For example, it is rare for volunteer first responders to have access to benefits, including EAPs (Heightman, 2016). As such, volunteers may be more likely to experience mental health issues with greater barriers to treatment in coping with exposure to trauma inherent in emergency support services (Stanley, Boffa, Hom, Kimbrel, & Joiner, 2017).

IMPACT OF CAREER ON FIRST RESPONDER WELLNESS

First responders experience high risk for various health issues as a result of their career. Some risk for physical and mental health issues relate to the inherent stress of supporting community crisis. For example, prolonged stress and exposure to fire-related incidents creates high risk for heart disease for firefighters, with nearly half of deaths while on duty caused by cardiovascular events (Kales, Soteriades, Christophi, & Christiani, 2007). EMS routinely experience risk of harm including exposure to communicable diseases, and performing medical procedures in a vehicle traveling at high speed without wearing a seatbelt (Blau, Eggerichs-Purcell, & Bentley, 2012; Weaver et al., 2015). For first responders, the unpredictable nature of a typical shift, when it is unknown when the next "call" will come, does not support much focus on personal wellness. As a result, EMS and fire personnel report poor overall personal health habits both at work and during personal time including speeding, smoking, drinking, and poor eating habits (Pirrallo, Levine, & Dickison, 2005). Further, alcohol and tobacco use represent significant health risks for first responders (Carey, Al-Zaiti, Dean, Sessanna, & Finnell, 2011). For example, firefighters use smoke-less tobacco products at a higher rate than the national average, many of whom only starting use after becoming a firefighter (Jitnarin et al., 2017). Beyond high stress, sleep deprivation, poor health habits, and the unpredictable nature of a typical shift, trauma experienced during community crisis represents perhaps the highest health risk for first responders.

Trauma and Mental Health Stigma

First responders experience trauma both directly through potential for physical or emotional harm, or through repeated exposure to traumatic experiences of patients and their families known as vicarious trauma (Trippany, Kress, & Wilcoxon, 2004). This exposure to trauma is inherent during routine job duties responding to community crisis for both firefighters and EMS. Sleep disturbances due to shift work and unpredictable calls represent high risk for mental health issues, suicidal ideation, and unhealthy alcohol use (NEMSMA, 2016; Vargas de Barros, Martins, Saitz, Bastos, & Ronzani, 2013). Routine and repeated exposure to trauma also increases risk of PTSD for firefighters and EMS personnel (Klimley, Van Hasselt, & Stripling, 2018). In response to training and experience, first responders focus on the needs of patients and victims on the scene, disregarding the impact of the chaotic and emotionally charged environment in the moment to fulfill the responsibility of supporting community members (Palm, Polusny, & Follette, 2004). Further, as part of first responder training, experienced personnel often haze or push new EMS and firefighters to "toughen up" and not react to trauma exposure on the job. Thus following these traumatic events, firefighters and EMS often experience thoughts and mental images (e.g. flashbacks, dreams) related to vicarious trauma but may not have a supportive outlet to process them (Jahnke, Poston, Haddock, & Murphy, 2016). Over time, repeated exposure to trauma without adequate mental health supports leads to increased risk of PTSD and suicide among the first responder population (Martin et al., 2017; Stanley, Hom, & Joiner, 2016).

First responders experience a strong camaraderie, which encourages fire and EMS personnel to depend mainly on peers for support (Regehr, Hill, Goldberg, & Hughes, 2002; Stanley et al., 2016). While common coping for work-related stress and trauma are social supports, due to stigma and first responder culture, there is aversion to using peers as supports in interest of preserving a reputation and image at work (Lanza, Roysircar, & Rodgers, 2018). To address critical incidents experienced in the field, the first responder population can benefit from mental health treatment conducive to the unique population and impact of experiences in the field (Jones, 2017). Prevention focusing on locus of control and developing resilience to promote healthy coping can help mitigate risk factors. Also, interventions that are trauma-informed are critical (Kleim & Westphal, 2011). Mental health stigma and barriers to mental health treatment prevent first responders from seeking supports for mental health issues. First responders experience fear in seeking mental health supports, as counseling carries a perception weakness by coworkers (Vogel, Cohen, Habib, & Massey, 2004). Further barriers include scheduling appointments around shifts and lack of knowledge about supports available (Haugen, McCrillis, Smid, & Nijdam, 2017). First responders often believe mental health practitioners do not understand first responder culture, or the experiences of EMS and firefighters which deters them from seeking professional support (Heightman, 2016).

First responders experience critical events in the field, which represent direct and vicarious trauma (Martin et al., 2017). This experience occurs throughout a career, as typical work duties include attending to community crises. For example, Jahnke (2018) described the typical shift as attending to community members on the worst day of their life. Over time, first responders become desensitized and cynical as means of coping (Jahnke et al., 2016). Tempered emotional reactions become even more difficult when having to navigate expressing compassion and empathy for victims on scene, but avoiding emotional reaction after the emergency is over (Boyle & Healy, 2003). While peer supports represent a protective factor, fear of retribution or tarnishing of reputation deter first responders from processing trauma within the first responder community (Stanley et al, 2016). With no safe outlet, eventually, emotional avoidance becomes a survival tactic leading to burnout and compassion fatigue (Regehr, Goldberg, Glancy, & Knott, 2002). Often first responders turn to use of alcohol as a socially acceptable means of coping with trauma (Gallyer et al., 2018). Substance use, especially alcohol, to cope with trauma leads to high rates of addiction within the first responder community (Fjeldheim et al., 2014; Jahnke, 2012; Poston, 2012). Dark humor represents another commonly accepted means of catharsis to manage emotional reaction to vicarious trauma (Scott, 2007; Tangherlini, 2000). Along with dark humor, first responders often use storytelling as a natural coping strategy to process experiences with peers (Tangherlini, 2000).

SOLUTIONS AND RECOMMENDATIONS

Created by White and Epston, Narrative Therapy's premise is that clients build narratives based from their perceptions of self and others (White, 2007). These narratives, referred to as dominant narratives, are socially constructed, based on language, and are a way that clients' construct their reality (Combs & Freedman, 2012; White, 1995; 2007). Dominant narratives, often confirmed or modified based on interactions with environment, become clients' absolute truth regardless if they are positive or problematic (White, 2007). Problematic dominant narratives are socially, culturally, and politically induced and are the cause for clients' problematic behavior and/or mental health concerns, especially when are incongruent with their lived experiences (Brown & Augusta-Scott, 2007). In Narrative Therapy, clients are the owners, authors, and experts of their own subjective narrative and counselors are the experts in Narrative Therapy (Combs & Freedman, 2012). Narrative Therapy involves four non-linear, free flowing cyclical steps that requires active collaboration between the client and the counselor (White, 1995).

The first step in Narrative Therapy is identifying the problematic dominant narrative that is causing the client distress (White, 1995; 2007). During identification, clients also determine their memberships and association with the dominant narratives in the past, present, and future (Vorster & Phipps, 2009; White, 1995; 2007). Counselors' role in this stage is to provide the space for clients to tell their story. The second step is deconstructing the dominant story. During the deconstruction process, clients break down their dominant story into manageable parts and explore what parts contradict or support each other (Payne, 2006; White, 2007). Counselors support this process by inquiring about their culture and experiences that support the dominant narrative and determining the conception of the problematic narrative (Carr, 1998; Payne, 2006). During the deconstruction process, counselors also help clients to externalize the problem. White (1995) believed that a problematic narrative is powerful because it becomes entrenched in clients' identity; thus, clients become unable to separate themselves between their selfhood and the problem. Clients externalize the problem by objectifying it as something outside of themselves, and often assigning a name to this problem (Carr, 1998; White, 2007). After assigning a name to the problem, clients explore the problems' power and influence over their lives (White, 2007). Externalizing the problem helps empower clients to take control of the problem and visualize the problem as something more manageable (Payne, 2006).

The third step involves reauthoring and re-membering the dominant narrative. In this stage clients revise their problematic dominant stories into stories that are more congruent with their lived experiences (White, 2007). Parts of the problematic dominant narratives either neglected or conflicting, represent "unique outcomes" or "exceptions" (White, 2007, p. 61). White (2007) described that clients are often fascinated by unique outcomes and by placing emphasis on the exceptions or neglected parts, counselors can start the process of reauthoring (Combs & Freedman, 2012). Clients also revise their membership and re-engage in neglected identities and resources that clients want to re-integrate into their narratives (White, 2007).

The fourth step includes performing definitional ceremonies. Definitional ceremonies involves a ritual where clients can share their new and more congruent narrative (White, 2007). Some ceremony options include letter writing (Combs & Freeman, 2012), performance in group therapy (Duba, Kindsvatter, & Priddy, 2010), or the use creative arts such as artwork (Bennett, 2008), music or video recordings (Combs & Freeman, 2012). Definitional ceremonies thicken and strengthen the new narrative and provide meaningful connections to the future (Combs & Freeman, 2012).

Narrative Therapy has gained momentum as a holistic and widely used intervention for diverse populations. In a simple literature search, there are over 5000 articles on Narrative Therapy, and almost 3000 in the last 10 years alone. Narrative Therapy has been proposed to treat trauma (e.g., Bullen, 2015; Cloitre, Garvert, & Weiss, 2017; Lee, 2017), grief (e.g., Hedtke, 2014; Turns & Macey, 2015), anxiety (e.g., Horner & Tully, 2016), and depression (e.g., Lopes, Gonçalves, Fassnacht, Machado, & Sousa, 2014; Rodríguez Vega, Bayón Pérez, PalaoTarrero, & Fernández Liria, 2014). These issues represent key mental health concerns for EMS and firefighters (Martin et al., 2017).

First responders possess a number of natural coping skills, including the use of storytelling as a means of processing and understanding experiences (Tangherlini, 2000). Narrative therapy similarly utilizes storytelling to deconstruct and reconstruct experiences (White, 2007). By starting with the telling of stories, Narrative Therapy draws on the existing coping skills of first responders and can aid in the building of trust and rapport with the first responder population. Given the enduring stigma of help-seeking behavior among the first responder population (Vogel et al., 2004), it is critical to utilize trauma-informed practices that reduce stigma. Narrative Therapy emphasizes the externalization of the problem, highlighting the idea that the person seeking services is not weak or broken, but is a healthy person faced with a problem (White, 2007). The attribution of problems to experience rather than to the person can help to destigmatize the help-seeking experience. The first responder occupation is often an integral part of the first responder's identity and the first responder culture undoubtedly impacts the perception of self and others. Narrative Therapy considers and identifies how the role of culture and context impact the dominant discourse (White, 2007). The emphasis on the constructed narrative and the role of cultural context may help to mitigate the feeling that mental health professionals do not understand first responders. The following example provides illustration of Narrative Therapy with the first responder population to support trauma while addressing stigma.

Example of Narrative Therapy

Marc is a 28-year-old, Caucasian, cisgender male who is currently working as a firemedic in an urban setting. In this role, he has cross trained as a firefighter and a paramedic, providing primarily medical support for patients but fire support as needed during calls. He has worked as a firemedic for approximately 4 years. Marc lives with his girlfriend of two years and identifies this relationship as supportive.

Recently, Marc experienced a traumatic call in which a young child died after drowning in a swimming pool. Marc performed CPR at the scene but was unable to resuscitate the child. Marc's supervisor, per department protocol, required him to see a counselor after the critical incident on his last shift. At first, Marc reports he feels fine, and that events like the child's death is simply "part of the job." After some prodding from the counselor, and reminding about the confidentiality of their discussion, Marc reluctantly shared he has been having trouble sleeping and had a few nightmares about the event in the week since the call. He has noticed feeling more irritable and is dreading returning for his next shift, which is unusual as Marc takes great pride in his identity as a first responder. Marc's girlfriend had also encouraged him to use the counseling supports provided by his county benefits, as she noticed an increase in arguments with Marc since this most recent incident. He reports that he is coming to therapy to appease his girlfriend and supervisor but is reluctant to talk about the recent traumatic event. He acknowledges that he has been more irritable lately but feels that he needs to just "get over it" when asked about vicarious trauma. Marc reports he had seen a counselor in the past under recommendation from his job after another instance of trauma but did not find it helpful. He felt that the counselor did not understand him and wanted to give him a diagnosis, which he worried would impact his job or his coworkers' perceptions of him.

Identifying the Narrative

In initial therapy sessions, the counselor focuses on building rapport and highlighting the therapy process as non-judgmental and collaborative. The counselor shows genuine interest in Marc's experiences in the field, and asks questions about what it is like to be a firemedic. Marc, feeling passionate about his career, answers her questions and then naturally begins to tell her about different calls he has experienced during his career. Drawing on his natural coping strategy of storytelling, the counselor invites Marc to further share his storied experiences as a firemedic. Marc is initially reluctant to talk about negative work experiences but speaks of his positive relationships with coworkers and sense of camaraderie in his work. Marc discusses how his family supported his desire to become a firemedic, and talks about looking up to his father, who worked as a police officer. After building a foundation of trust and collaboration in early sessions, Marc begins to open up about some of the trauma he has witnessed, including the most recent incident with the child's death.

Even as Marc tells stories of being a witness to significant and intense trauma, the counselor notices that he tends to shy away from emotional language when describing his experiences. When the counselor asks about this disconnect, Marc responds by explaining that expressing emotions is not helpful, and that his he is more effective in his job when disconnected emotionally from patients. He expresses a need to "get over" and laugh about his experiences rather than discuss his feelings. From discussion of how Marc has responded to repeated exposure to trauma, Marc and his counselor are able to identify a dominant narrative in his life in which he feels he must shut down his emotional responses and act as though the traumatic events he witnesses do not impact him.

Deconstructing the Dominant Story

Finding that he enjoys telling stories with the counselor, Marc continues to see the counselor. He asks the counselor not to tell his supervisor that he continued to come to sessions after his required "check-in" following the critical incident with the child. In the process of deconstructing the dominant narrative of emotional detachment and being "tough", Marc is able to recognize that the culture of first responders as well as the culture in his family of origin shape this narrative. Marc discusses his father's career as a police officer and his stoicism. Marc finds that his father instilled the idea that men did not express emotions related to traumatic events, especially men who served the community. Men who serve the community must be strong and tough for others who need them. In remembering how his father interacted with other police officers, he remembered their jokes with each other and habit of getting together for a beer after shifts and telling stories. Marc learned from his father that, as a man, the way to deal with trauma was through isolation, dark humor, and alcohol use; these coping strategies further reinforced through his own work as a first responder.

A critical piece of the deconstruction process of Marc's narrative was the externalization of his response to vicarious trauma. Marc believed that his emotional response to vicarious trauma indicated that something was wrong with him or that he was too weak to handle his work. The feelings of helplessness he experienced as a result of being unable to save a child led Marc to view himself as inadequate for his work. Through the process of externalization, the counselor helped Marc to readjust his view of himself and the issue of trauma, emphasizing that the problem was the ongoing trauma experienced as a result of his occupation, rather than a personal weakness in not being able to cope with the trauma. The counselor highlighted normal responses to vicarious trauma and emphasized how Marc's reaction to trauma was common. Over time, Marc was able to distance his concept of self from his response behaviors to trauma and was able to recognize that his experiences were a typical response to a problematic experience, the frequent exposure to trauma. He found validation in knowing that he was not broken or unable to serve his community because of these trauma responses.

Reauthoring and Re-Membering

In the reauthoring process, the counselor encouraged Marc to identify how he would like to see himself respond to ongoing stressors and create a narrative of healthier coping mechanisms and support. In his original dominant narrative, Marc saw himself as inadequate, weak, and helpless when he struggled to deal with ongoing vicarious trauma. Through the restorying and reauthoring process, he was able to identify exceptions to these feelings; remembering times when he performed his work capably, helped others, and gained a sense of purpose and gratification from his work. Marc was able to identify how he ideally wanted to deal with stressors, including involving his girlfriend in his coping rather than pulling away from her. Marc identified wellness activities he would like to use to cope, including fishing with his father. Rather than conceptualizing his inability to tolerate ongoing trauma as a personal weakness, Marc was able to alter his narrative to highlight his strength in caring for others and engaging in emotionally and physically challenging work. As the original problematic narrative was prominent at work and often exacerbated by work culture and peers' coping mechanisms, Marc and the counselor talked about how his new narrative would fit with his peers at the fire station. He processed that although he feared that his peers would not accept his new narrative, in time, he could model for them better coping mechanisms and help them seek support when he saw signs of trauma.

Definitional Ceremony

As Marc and his counselor approached the end of their work together, the counselor asked Marc to engage in a definitional ceremony, celebrating and sharing his new narrative. Marc elected to write a letter to his future self, who would undoubtedly encounter more trauma throughout his work. In this letter, Marc reminded his future self of his inherent strength and ability to cope with the trauma he would encounter. He highlighted the positive aspects of his work and his stories of strength and caring for others. Marc encouraged his future self to utilize healthy coping strategies and seek support from those around him. Marc asked his girlfriend to attend a therapy session with him and shared this letter with her, inviting her to share in his experience and identifying how she could continue to support him. Through the Narrative Therapy process, Marc came to view himself through a preferred narrative in which he encountered problems but did not ascribe the problems nor his reactions to them as an inherent weakness. Marc was able to utilize storytelling, a natural medium, to tell new stories about himself, his world, and his experience. Through the therapy process, Marc felt respected and empowered as the author of his experiences rather than pathologized and stigmatized. In terminating therapy, the counselor reminded Marc she was always available to him if he needed to come back. Marc left feeling the counselor genuinely cared and was interested in his work, comfortable with returning if his trauma again became overwhelming in his career.

FUTURE RESEARCH DIRECTIONS

The previous example provides an outline for how the principles and processes of Narrative Therapy integrate specifically with the work of first responders. Though the first responder population could undoubtedly benefit from mental health care to address the effects of exposure to ongoing trauma, stigma around help-seeking behavior creates a significant barrier to receiving care (Vogel et al., 2004). When first responders have received treatment that has felt ineffective, this can further dissuade them from seeking therapy. As in the example, many first responders may feel that practitioners do not understand their experiences and may feel judged (Heightman, 2016). Further, first responders often feel misunderstood and unappreciated by community members (NHTSA, n.d). The collaborative and non-judgmental experience and the emphasis on the client as the expert and author of experience may help to engage first responders in the therapy process. This collaborative process using a natural coping skill of storytelling may also help overcome the perception that community members do not care about first responders.

After establishing a foundation of trust and collaboration, the four-step process of Narrative Therapy can unfold. The above example illustrates how a first responder client may engage in Narrative Therapy. By beginning with the telling of stories, Narrative Therapy taps into the innate storytelling mechanism that many first responders use to process and understand experiences (Tangherlini, 2000). By creating a comfortable space for the client to tell stories, the counselor allows for the expression of positive and negative stories as a dominant narrative emerges regarding the work, culture, and experiences unique to first responders. Through the process of deconstructing the dominant narrative, first responders are able to externalize the problem, mitigating the stigma of trauma responses and the tendency to attribute typical reactions to personal weakness (Lanza et al., 2018). Externalizing the problem can also involve naming the problem to help separate the problem from the client's personhood. In Marc's example, he could have named the problem "*get over it*". In further deconstructing the narrative, as seen in the example, first responders are able to identify how their experiences and culture may support or contradict the dominant narrative. Additionally, first responder clients could explore exceptions to the dominant narrative as part of the deconstruction process. Although not seen in the example, Marc could have explored when he felt competent at his job, despite patient loss, or when he or his coworkers discussed openly job traumas and their struggles with loss without engaging in avoidant coping mechanisms. Findings exceptions to the dominant narratives helps first responders demystify the strength of dominant narratives and naturally leads to the reauthoring process.

Through the reauthoring process, first responders are able to identify exceptions to the dominant narrative and create new stories of themselves that are more congruent with their lived experiences. Regarding trauma, first responders are better able to conceptualize trauma and trauma reactions as external, no longer tied to internal conceptions of strength or weakness. This helps combat stigma in seeking supports outside of their work community. As seen in the example, first responders are encouraged to identify a new narrative of coping and managing the ongoing trauma encountered in their work. Through definitional ceremonies, the client solidifies these new narratives (White, 2007).

It is important to remember that the deconstruction and reauthoring of experience is a cyclical and non-linear process (White, 1995). Though the above example highlights these steps in a particular order, the therapy process often involves a constant deconstruction and reconstruction of narratives that may intersect and overlap. In examining, deconstructing, and reauthoring experiences through Narrative Therapy, counselors can work to build trusting and collaborative relationships with first responders that may serve to mitigate the stigma of help-seeking and create lasting change in the first responder culture.

CONCLUSION

First responders experience strong stigma against help-seeking behavior, like attending counseling, despite repeated exposure to trauma throughout a career. Without adequate mental health supports, first responders face high risk for compassion fatigue, PTSD, and suicide. Mental health providers have an obligation to find evidence-based and effective ways to reach this population of clients to address trauma experiences. Narrative Therapy as an approach using the natural coping skill of storytelling presents an opportunity to connect with and support the first responder community while addressing underlying mental health stigma.

REFERENCES

Bennett, L. (2008). Narrative methods and children: Theoretical explanations and practice issues. *Journal of Child and Adolescent Psychiatric Nursing*, *21*(1), 13–23. doi:10.1111/j.1744-6171.2008.00125.x PMID:18269408

Blau, G., Eggerichs-Purcell, J., & Bentley, M. A. (2012). Testing the impact of emotional labor on work exhaustion for three distinct emergency medical service (EMS) samples. *Career Development International*, *17*(7), 626–645. doi:10.1108/13620431211283788

Boyle, M. V., & Healy, J. (2003). Balancing mysterium and onus: Doing spiritual work within an emotion-laden organizational context. *Organization*, *10*(2), 351–373. doi:10.1177/1350508403010002010

Brown, C., & Augusta-Scott, T. (Eds.). (2007). *Narrative therapy: Making meaning, making lives*. Thousand Oaks, CA: Sage.

Bullen, E. (2015). Narrative therapy outcomes for women who have experienced domestic violence. *International Journal of Narrative Therapy & Community Work*, (3), 13-27.

Carey, M. G., Al-Zaiti, S. S., Dean, G. E., Sessanna, L., & Finnell, D. S. (2011). Sleep problems, depression, substance use, social bonding, and quality of life in professional firefighters. *Journal of Occupational and Environmental Medicine*, *53*(8), 928–933. doi:10.1097/JOM.0b013e318225898f PMID:21785370

Carr, A. (1998). Michael white's narrative therapy. *Contemporary Family Therapy*, *20*(4), 485–503. doi:10.1023/A:1021680116584

Cloitre, M., Garvert, D. W., & Weiss, B. J. (2017). Depression as a moderator of STAIR narrative therapy for women with post-traumatic stress disorder related to childhood abuse. *European Journal of Psychotraumatology*, *8*(1), 1–7. doi:10.1080/20008198.2017.1377028 PMID:29038682

Combs, G., & Freedman, J. (2012). Narrative, poststructuralist, and social justice: Current practices in narrative therapy. *The Counseling Psychologist*, *40*, 1033–1060. doi:10.1177/0011000012460662

Duba, J. D., Kindsvatter, A., & Priddy, C. J. (2010). Deconstructing the mirror's reflection: Narrative therapy groups for women dissatisfied with their body. *Adultspan: Theory Research & Practice*, *9*(2), 103–116. doi:10.1002/j.2161-0029.2010.tb00075.x

Fjeldheim, C. B., Nöthling, J., Pretorius, K., Basson, M., Ganasen, K., Heneke, R., ... Seedat, S. (2014). Trauma exposure, posttraumatic stress disorder and the effect of explanatory variables in paramedic trainees. *BMC Emergency Medicine*, *14*(11), 1–7. PMID:24755358

Gallyer, A. J., Dougherty, S. P., Gai, A. R., Stanley, I. H., Hom, M. A., Rogers, M. L., ... Joiner, T. E. (2018). Problematic alcohol use and suicidal ideation among firefighters: A multi-study investigation of the explanatory roles of perceived burdensomeness and thwarted belongingness. *Journal of Affective Disorders*, *238*, 281–288. doi:10.1016/j.jad.2018.05.045 PMID:29898427

Haugen, P. T., McCrillis, A. M., Smid, G. E., & Nijdam, M. J. (2017). Mental health stigma and barriers to mental health care for first responders: A systematic review and meta-analysis. *Journal of Psychiatric Research*, *94*, 218–229. doi:10.1016/j.jpsychires.2017.08.001 PMID:28800529

Hedtke, L. (2014). Creating stories of hope: A narrative approach to illness, death and grief. *Australian and New Zealand Journal of Family Therapy*, *35*(1), 4–19. doi:10.1002/anzf.1040

Heightman, A. J. (2016). EMS agencies need to have eap resources to address stress and reduce suicides. *Journal of Emergency Medical Services*, *41*(1). Retrieved from https://www.jems.com/articles/print/volume-41/issue-1/departments-columns/from-the-editor/ems-agencies-need-to-have-eap-resources-to-address-stress-and-reduce-suicides.html PMID:26901952

Horner, E., & Tully, P. D. (2016). Divorcing the voice of fear: A collaborative, narrative approach to anxiety. *International Journal of Narrative Therapy & Community Work*, (2), 37-43.

Jahnke, S. A. (2012). Exploring factors associated with problem drinking among firefighters. *Journal of Substance Abuse Treatment*, *43*(3), e25. doi:10.1016/j.jsat.2012.08.118

Jahnke, S. A. (2018). *Your worst day is our every day: The impact of repeated exposure to trauma on the fire service* [Video Webinar]. Retrieved from https://www.iafc.org/events/event/2018/08/30/default-calendar/your-worst-day-is-our-every-day-the-impact-of-repeated-exposure-to-trauma-on-the-fire-service

Jahnke, S. A., Poston, W. S. C., Haddock, C. K., & Murphy, B. (2016). Firefighting and mental health: Experiences of repeated exposure to trauma. *Work (Reading, Mass.)*, *53*(4), 737–744. doi:10.3233/WOR-162255 PMID:26890595

Jitnarin, N., Poston, W. S. C., Haddock, C. K., Jahnke, S. A., Day, R. S., & Severson, H. H. (2017). Prevalence and correlates of late initiation of smokeless tobacco in us firefighters. *Nicotine & Tobacco Research*, *20*(1), 130–134. PMID:27940900

Jones, S. (2017). Describing the mental health profile of first responders: A systematic review. *Journal of the American Psychiatric Nurses Association*, *23*(3), 200–214. doi:10.1177/1078390317695266 PMID:28445653

Jones, S., Nagel, C., McSweeney, J., & Curran, G. (2018). Prevalence and correlates of psychiatric symptoms among first responders in a southern state. *Archives of Psychiatric Nursing*, *32*(6), 828–835. doi:10.1016/j.apnu.2018.06.007 PMID:30454624

Kales, S. N., Soteriades, E. S., Christophi, C. A., & Christiani, D. C. (2007). Emergency duties and deaths from heart disease among firefighters in the United States. *The New England Journal of Medicine*, *356*(12), 1207–1215. doi:10.1056/NEJMoa060357 PMID:17377158

Kenlon, J. (1913). *Fires and fire-fighters: A history of modern fire-fighting with a review of its development from earliest times*. New York, NY: George H. Doran Company.

Kleim, B., & Westphal, M. (2011). Mental health in first responders: A review and recommendation for prevention and intervention strategies. *Traumatology*, *17*(4), 17–24. doi:10.1177/1534765611429079

Klimley, K. E., Van Hasselt, V. B., & Stripling, A. M. (2018). Posttraumatic stress disorder in police, firefighters, and emergency dispatchers. *Aggression and Violent Behavior*, *43*, 33–44. doi:10.1016/j.avb.2018.08.005

Kruger, L. G. (2018). *United state fire administration: An overview* (CRS Report No. RS20071). Retrieved from https://fas.org/sgp/crs/homesec/RS20071.pdf

Lanza, A., Roysircar, G., & Rodgers, S. (2018). First responder mental healthcare: Evidence-based prevention, postvention, and treatment. *Professional Psychology, Research and Practice*, *49*(3), 193–204. doi:10.1037/pro0000192

Lee, J. (2017). Responding to children in situations of family violence: Narrative therapy group work with children. *International Journal of Narrative Therapy & Community Work*, *1*, 57–70.

Lopes, R. T., Gonçalves, M. M., Fassnacht, D. B., Machado, P. P. P., & Sousa, I. (2014). Long-term effects of psychotherapy on moderate depression: A comparative study of narrative therapy and cognitive-behavioral therapy. *Journal of Affective Disorders*, *167*, 64–73. doi:10.1016/j.jad.2014.05.042 PMID:25082116

Martin, C. E., Tran, J. K., & Buser, S. J. (2017). Correlates of suicidality in firefighter/ems personnel. *Journal of Affective Disorders*, *208*, 177–183. doi:10.1016/j.jad.2016.08.078 PMID:27788381

National EMS Management Association (NEMSMA). (2016). *Mental health and stress in emergency medical services*. Platte City, MO: Author.

National Fire Protection Association (NFPA). (2019). *NFPA 1001: Standard for fire fighter professional qualifications*. Quincy, MA: Author.

National Highway Traffic Safety Administration (NHTSA). (n.d.). *Emergency medical services: Agenda for the future*. Retrieved from https://one.nhtsa.gov/people/injury/ems/agenda/emsman.html#EMS%20 CONTENTS

National Highway Traffic Safety Administration (NHTSA). (2011). *Traffic safety facts: EMS research note* (DOT HS Publication No. 812-041). Retrieved from https://www.ems.gov/pdf/National_EMS_Assessment_Demographics_2011.pdf

National Volunteer Firefighter Council (NVFC). (2014). *What to expect: A guide for family member of volunteer firefighters*. Greenbelt, MD: Author.

Palm, K. M., Polusny, M. A., & Follette, V. M. (2004). Vicarious traumatization: Potential hazards and interventions for disaster and trauma workers. *Prehospital and Disaster Medicine*, *19*(1), 73–78. doi:10.1017/S1049023X00001503 PMID:15453162

Payne, M. (2006). *Narrative therapy: An introduction for counsellors* (2nd ed.). London, UK: Sage.

Pirrallo, R. G., Levine, R., & Dickison, P. D. (2005). Behavioral health risk factors of U.S. emergency medical technicians: The LEADS project. *Prehospital and Disaster Medicine*, *20*(4), 235–242. doi:10.1017/S1049023X00002594 PMID:16128471

Poston, W. (2012). Substance use issues among male career firefighters. *Journal of Substance Abuse Treatment*, *43*(3), e24. doi:10.1016/j.jsat.2012.08.115

Regehr, C., Goldberg, G., Glancy, G., & Knott, T. (2002). Posttraumatic symptoms and disability in paramedics. *Canadian Journal of Psychiatry*, *47*(10), 953–958. doi:10.1177/070674370204701007 PMID:12553131

Regehr, C., Hill, J., Goldberg, G., & Hughes, J. (2003). Postmortem inquiries and trauma responses in paramedics and firefighters. *Journal of Interpersonal Violence*, *18*(6), 607–622. doi:10.1177/0886260503251131

Rodríguez Vega, B., Bayón Pérez, C., PalaoTarrero, A., & Fernández Liria, A. (2014). Mindfulness-based narrative therapy for depression in cancer patients. *Clinical Psychology & Psychotherapy*, *21*(5), 411–419. doi:10.1002/cpp.1847 PMID:23716367

Scott, T. (2007). Expression of humour by emergency personnel involved in sudden deathwork. *Mortality*, *12*(4), 350–364. doi:10.1080/13576270701609766

Stanley, I. H., Boffa, J. W., Hom, M. A., Kimbrel, N. A., & Joiner, T. E. (2017). Differences in psychiatric symptoms and barriers to mental health care between volunteer and career firefighters. *Psychiatry Research*, *247*, 236–242. doi:10.1016/j.psychres.2016.11.037 PMID:27930964

Tangherlini, T. R. (2000). Heroes and lies: Storytelling tactics among paramedics. *Folklore*, *111*(1), 43–66. doi:10.1080/001558700360889

Trippany, R. L., Kress, V. E. W., & Wilcoxon, S. A. (2004). Preventing vicarious trauma: What counselors should know when working with trauma survivors. *Journal of Counseling and Development*, *82*(1), 31–37. doi:10.1002/j.1556-6678.2004.tb00283.x

Turns, B., & Macey, P. (2015). Cinema narrative therapy: Utilizing family films to externalize children's 'problems'. *Journal of Family Therapy*, *37*(4), 590–606. doi:10.1111/1467-6427.12098

U.S. Department of Homeland Security (USDHS). (2017). *Emergency services sector profile*. Washington, DC: Author.

U.S. Department of Transportation (USDOT). (2007). *National EMS scope of practice model* (DOT HS Publication No. 810-657). Retrieved from http://www.ems.gov/education/EMSScope.pdf

Vargas de Barros, V., Martins, L. F., Saitz, R., Bastos, R. R., & Ronzani, T. M. (2013). Mental health conditions, individual and job characteristics and sleep disturbances among firefighters. *Journal of Health Psychology*, *18*(3), 350–358. doi:10.1177/1359105312443402 PMID:22517948

Vogel, J. M., Cohen, A. J., Habib, M. S., & Massey, B. D. (2004). In the wake of terrorism: Collaboration between a psychiatry department and a center for emergency medical services (EMS) to support EMS workers and their families. *Families, Systems & Health*, *22*(1), 35–46. doi:10.1037/1091-7527.22.1.35

Vorster, C., & Phipps, W. D. (2009). Narrative therapy: A return to the intrapsychic perspective? *South African Journal of Psychology. Suid-Afrikaanse Tydskrif vir Sielkunde*, *39*(1), 32–45. doi:10.1177/008124630903900103

Weaver, M. D., Patterson, P. D., Fabio, A., Moore, C. G., Freiberg, M. S., & Songer, T. J. (2015). An observational study of shift length, crew familiarity, and occupational injury and illness in emergency medical services workers. *Occupational and Environmental Medicine*, *72*(11), 798–804. doi:10.1136/oemed-2015-102966 PMID:26371071

White, M. (1995). *Re-authoring lives: Interviews and essays*. Adelaide, South Australia, Australia: Dulwich Centre.

White, M. (2007). *Maps of narrative practice*. New York, NY: Norton.

ADDITIONAL READING

Deppa, K. F., & Saltzberg, J. (2016). *Resilience training for firefighters: An approach to prevent behavioral health problems*. New York, NY: Springer. doi:10.1007/978-3-319-38779-6

Ford, J. D., Grasso, D. J., Elhai, J. D., & Courtois, C. A. (2015). *Posttraumtic stress disorder: Scientific and professional dimensions* (2nd ed.). San Diego, CA: Elsevier.

Haugen, P. T., Evces, M., & Weiss, D. S. (2012). Treating posttraumatic stress disorder in first responders: A systematic review. *Clinical Psychology Review*, *32*(5), 370–380. doi:10.1016/j.cpr.2012.04.001 PMID:22561967

Martin, C. E., Tran, J. K., & Buser, S. J. (2017). Correlates of suicidality in firefighter/ems personnel. *Journal of Affective Disorders*, *208*, 177–183. doi:10.1016/j.jad.2016.08.078 PMID:27788381

Regehr, C., & Bober, T. (2005). *In the line of fire: Trauma in the emergency services*. New York, NY: Oxford University Press. doi:10.1093/acprof:oso/9780195165029.001.0001

Trippany, R. L., Kress, V. E. W., & Wilcoxon, S. A. (2004). Preventing vicarious trauma: What counselors should know when working with trauma survivors. *Journal of Counseling and Development*, *82*(1), 31–37. doi:10.1002/j.1556-6678.2004.tb00283.x

White, M. (2004). Working with people who are suffering the consequences of multiple trauma: A narrative perspective. *The International Journal of Narrative Therapy & Community Work*, *1*, 45–76.

White, M., & Epston, D. (1990). *Narrative means to therapeutic ends*. New York, NY: Norton.

KEY TERMS AND DEFINITIONS

Compassion Fatigue: The gradual loss of the capacity to care for the suffering of others after repeated need to support others over time.

Direct Trauma: An unusually stressful event happening directly to an individual.

Dominant Narrative: The common story, lens, or perception of the principal societal group.

Externalization: A mental health tool of imagining issues or symptoms to be an independent idea instead of an ailment or affliction of the individual.

First Responder: A common term for professionals including emergency medical services personnel and firefighters trained to respond to community emergencies.

Posttraumatic Stress Disorder: A stress-related disorder occurring after a traumatic event characterized by symptoms including sleep disturbance, distressing dreams, avoidance of reminders of the traumatic event, negative mood, and emotional reactivity for at least one month after the traumatic event.

Stigma: The shame perceived or expressed by others when an individual is associated with a certain group, need, or condition.

Vicarious Trauma: The impact of exposure to unusually stressful events experienced by others over time.

Chapter 15
Organizational Prevention and Intervention Services:
Beyond the Early Intervention System

Jennifer Kelly
Independent Researcher, Haddonfield, USA

William D. Walsh
Voorhees Police Department, USA

ABSTRACT

Improving the opportunities for enhanced health and wellness in first responders has gained national attention in recent years. Employers and other stakeholders striving to improve employee utilization of available resources will need to increase transparency in the process and improve understanding between first responders and clinicians. One potential process, early warning systems (EWS) are primarily designed to alert management to an at-risk employee. However, the continuing goal of any effort should be to identify and remedy any employee issue before the employee exhibits the predetermined number of events that trigger an early warning alert. Although many organizations are adopting an EWS by either choice or mandate, they are largely separate and distinct from the agency's health and wellness programming. Administrators are not only unsure of what data to consider, but also what to do when an alert is activated. Ideally, agencies move toward early intervention systems that themselves are conceptualized within the larger framework of wellness programming.

ORGANIZATIONAL MENTAL HEALTH SERVICES

First responder organizations vary across disciplines, occupations, and jurisdictions in their handling of the health and wellness of employees. Prevention and response approaches may vary, even among different subdivisions or teams in the same organization. Standardizing prevention and intervention strategies for all first responders would be difficult, given differences in organizational cultures, geography, and individual experiences; however, basic elements of prevention and intervention programming

DOI: 10.4018/978-1-5225-9803-9.ch015

can remain consistent. For example, as a minimum, each organization's preventive measures should include resilience-building training for employees and their families, beginning before a first responder is deployed in the field, and training on improving mental and physical health in response to adversity and stress (Kelly & Hoban, 2016). Recent initiatives such as the President's Task Force on 21st Century Policing (COPS Office, 2015) and the Law Enforcement Mental Health and Wellness Act of 2017, have placed national attention on the need to make mental health a priority. As such, first responders require (a) continuing education, (b) stress management training including adaptive coping strategies throughout their careers, (c) early intervention systems (EISs) that focus on the whole employee (i.e., not just the behavior triggering an alert), (d) responses to early behavioral alerts that promote well-being, and (e) general intervention options to address mental health emergencies. Employee health and wellness and early warning/intervention systems should be designed with the employee, families, the organization, and the service population in mind.

Training and interventions developed to enhance the health and wellness of public safety employees should be evidence-based or at least integrate research findings. Those involved in the research, development, implementation, and assessment of employee health and wellness programs must be properly trained and vetted to ensure they will benefit employee and organizational health. They must also be able to deal with the sensitive nature and confidentiality requirements of this work. Attention must be paid to ensuring that intervention strategies listed in policies are operational, following the agency's plan, prior to any program rollout.

This chapter provides policy makers, researchers, administration and supervisory staff, and clinicians a framework to create policy that fosters prevention and intervention for mental health difficulties in first responders. It demonstrates the need for transparency and collaboration among stakeholders regarding prevention and intervention, discusses benefits of early alert systems, and presents examples of programming for first responders, not only as they begin their careers, but when they have experienced risk factors for impairment and for those exhibiting mental health difficulties.

EARLY WARNING SYSTEMS

Early Warning Systems (EWS) were originally created to detect and address problematic police officer conduct and enable intervention to correct it (Walker, Alpert, & Kenney, 2001). This concept was born out of the 1981 U.S. Commission of Civil Rights recommendation that police agencies create systems to identify "problem officers" that are frequently the subject of citizen complaints (DeCrescenzo, 2005). The original EWSs were designed primarily to alert management about at-risk employees (DeCrescenzo, 2005; Bertoia, 2008). EWSs are widely used in first responder organizations and are mandated in some locations (e.g., the authors' home state of New Jersey). Despite this, many stakeholders, both on the frontlines and in administrations, are still unsure what data to collect or how to respond appropriately.

Arguably, the original concept of an EWS should be reframed and redesigned more broadly to maintain healthy first responders and organizations, with indirect consequences that benefit their organizations and the communities they serve (Amendola & Davis, 2019). Collaboration with all stakeholders, including labor unions, administration, frontline personnel, and mental health professionals, would help to ensure EWSs are used as intended, to both prevent and address alerts, and not as a disciplinary tool. Union leaderships acknowledging the nonpunitive value of a properly administered EWS would promote frontline personnel buy-in (DeCrescenzo, 2005). Any effort should continuously identify and remedy any employee issue before it triggers an early warning alert.

In 1999, at least 39 percent of county and local law enforcement organizations with service populations greater than 50,000 were using or working toward implementing an EWS (Walker et al., 2001). With increasing mandates to adopt such programs, it is safe to assume the agencies are increasing in number and more varied in size. EWS research has typically only measured the number of complaints against employees. It has been suggested that enhanced employee scrutiny could lead to reduced proactivity, which obviously could skew research (Macintyre, Prenzler, & Chapman, 2008). Formal exploration of the EWS' impact on the health and wellness of employees and the overall agency is needed. An EWS can serve as an additional layer of strategy to maintain a healthy and sound workforce. Little research addresses EWSs in public safety.

Weaknesses in the EWS

In the standard EWS, public safety agencies compile data and then wait until the number of events in a given period triggers an early warning alert for a supervisor to address a potential issue with an employee. Some EWSs are designed to treat the symptom and not the whole person, by offering limited interventions or lacking preventative strategies for employees. Underlying causes of symptoms that trigger EWS alerts are typically not explored or addressed, although doing so would help develop intervention strategies. A more proactive approach would benefit the organization as a whole by preventing, mitigating, or reducing the need to react to an early warning trigger.

Improving the EWS

Fortunately, public safety agency leaders and employees are increasingly acknowledging the need to help first responders cope with trauma and stress. The second author was personally affected by the suicides of two friends who were police officers in 2009 and has seen a quarter of his academy class leave police work since graduating from the police academy in 2004, due to injury, domestic violence, felony arrests, and drunk driving, while one member died of a heroin overdose (after being terminated). According to Chae and Boyle (2013), "at least five prominent themes emerged as content domains that were positively associated with police suicide: organizational stress, critical incident trauma, shift work and atypical work hours, relationship problems, and alcohol use and abuse" (p. 92). Along with bolstering support systems, a holistic approach to officer wellness will address, educate, and mitigate these factors. An EWS can help protect employees, since these stressors often present identifiable symptoms and patterns of conduct.

In addition to helping employees, public safety organizations must seek to prevent civil litigation, civil-rights violations, excessive force, accidents, workplace injury, negligence, suicides, substance use disorders, domestic violence, family crises, divorce, public relations crises, and employee turnover through resignations or terminations. An effective system must include education for employees, supervisors, and their families. So, the warning system concept evolved to offer interventions before more serious issues develop (Walker, 2003). A more holistic Early Intervention System (as opposed to an EWS) with comprehensive health and wellness programming embedded may reduce reliance upon formalized warning systems. According to Walker, Milligan, and Berke (2006), an employee's supervisor is the key to successful early interventions. The way the program is framed, and even its title, can positively impact employee views toward it. Walker et al. (2006) elaborate upon the importance of using the proper terminology, along with the logic behind it:

It is important to get the terminology of EIS right. Supervisors must set the right tone from the beginning. When EISs first appeared about 25 years ago, they were usually called early warning systems. Many agencies still use that term, although it does not convey the right message. The word warning has a punitive, negative tone, implying that it is a precursor to discipline. The PERF (Police Executive Research Forum) study revealed that the best EIS emphasize assisting officers, not punishing them. These systems typically include a range of programs designed to help officers recognize and deal with their performance problems because, time and again, it was discovered that performance problems are rooted in stress and personal and family problems. As a result, the more positive term early intervention system is preferred. (Walker et al., 2006, p. 13)

CASE EXAMPLE: EWS MANDATE IN NEW JERSEY

New Jersey mandates EWSs in every law enforcement agency in the state. Although the directive is titled "Early Warning Systems," the explanation recommends that the EWS "assist officers through early intervention" (New Jersey Office of the Attorney General, 2018a). EWSs hold agencies accountable for their officers' ethical behavior and their wellness and ability to protect and serve their respective communities. The New Jersey Attorney General's Office provided the following explanation on the intention of the EWS in New Jersey:

Early warning systems are designed to monitor officer conduct using objective measures that indicate a potentially escalating risk of harm to the public, the agency, and/or the officer. They are intended to increase public safety and public confidence, while assisting officers through early intervention. . . .

Under Directive 2018-2, the following performance indicators are required to be included in all early warning systems:

1. Internal affairs complaints against the officer, whether initiated by another officer or by a member of the public;

2. Civil actions filed against the officer;

3. Criminal investigations of or criminal complaints against the officer;

4. Any use of force by the officer that is formally determined or adjudicated (for example, by internal affairs or a grand jury) to have been excessive, unjustified, or unreasonable;

5. Domestic violence investigations in which the officer is an alleged subject;

6. An arrest of the officer, including on a driving under the influence charge;

7. Sexual harassment claims against the officer;

8. Vehicular collisions involving the officer that are formally determined to have been the fault of the officer;

9. A positive drug test by the officer;

10. Cases or arrests by the officer that are rejected or dismissed by a court;

11. Cases in which evidence obtained by an officer is suppressed by a court;

12. Insubordination by the officer;

13. Neglect of duty by the officer;

14. Unexcused absences by the officer; and

15. Any other indicators, as determined by the agency's chief executive.

(New Jersey Office of the Attorney General, 2018a)

New Jersey Attorney General Directive 2018-3 (2018b) offers more examples than most policies of potential remedial actions in response to an EWS alert. The list provided includes:

1. Training or re-training;

2. Counseling;

3. Intensive supervision;

4. Fitness-for-duty examination;

5. Employee Assistance Program referral; and

6. Any other appropriate remedial or corrective action.

(New Jersey Office of the Attorney General, 2018a, pp. 3–4)

In New Jersey, if an early warning alert is triggered based on the data maintained in the EWS, the officer's agency must notify the county prosecutor's office and provide all the data for review, including the intervention used in response to the alert. This mandate is designed for oversight, to ensure appropriate data collection and interventions in the agencies. In an investigation, the data could lead to adverse consequences for the organization or the employee, including remedial training, a change in employment status, and even an administrative or criminal investigation; agencies may face sanctions, audits, or increased oversight.

EIS BEST PRACTICES

Amedola and Davis (2019) offer an aspirational definition of EIS, which would provide employees with "resources and tools in order to prevent disciplinary action, and to promote officer safety, satisfaction and wellness." They also suggest going beyond the traditional data collection and evaluation followed by intervention, to include monitoring employees and supervisors. As they note, the EIS is designed to be "pre-disciplinary," which shows the primary objective must shift toward officer wellness, not reprimands.

According to Amedola and Davis (2019), this focus on pre-disciplinary interventions means a system should consider indicators beyond those that directly lead to discipline, such as excessive force complaints. An EIS that considers an employees' need for additional knowledge or training, life changes, personal problems, and mental health difficulties, might include indicators such as tardiness, risk-taking behavior, damage to vehicles, complaints by peers, and excessive overtime (indicating potential family or financial difficulties), etc. Best practices warrant thresholds relevant to each employee's position with potential variations depending on the unit, shift, etc. Absolute and comparative approaches to defining thresholds may more accurately reflect an individual employee's difficulties than a simple threshold of occurrences. This may include officers who are subthreshold across several categories of alert or ones who are approaching an alert threshold (Jackson et al., 2016). Reviewing the context of each alert to potentially rule out concern based on prior knowledge about the officer or unit could reduce false positive results. An EIS policy needs clear performance standards and thresholds in order to determine what training is necessary. Responses to alerts should be recorded, including detailed descriptions of the interventions taken and their outcomes. Maintaining historical data is likely to prove useful, not only for quality assurance of the system, but to monitor the success of the intervention as well as the performance of supervisors (Amendola & Davis, 2019).

Perceptions, Misconceptions, and the Need for Transparency

Some government organizations have taken the increased call for transparency in government to heart by publishing online their rules and regulations, reports on use-of-force data, and even body-worn-camera footage. However, government leaders tend to miss the importance of transparency within the organization, particularly in mental health.

Too much mystery and paranoia still surround mental health professionals and their role with first responders in our culture. The only interaction some first responders may have with a mental health professional is during their pre-employment psychological screening. They then spend roughly 25 years of their career trying to avoid being "on the couch" again. The reason? The only thing they know about coworkers going to see "the shrink" is that it never ends well for the employee, which is often a misconception. The first responder community sees fitness-for-duty examinations as career-ending events (Schlosser & Kudrick, Jr., 2019). The perception is that even if the person is cleared to return to duty, they are not promotable, nor will they be considered for any special assignments. Sadly, the same perception holds true for first responders who realize on their own, without an organizational intervention that they should talk with a mental health professional. The employees who do seek help will often do so by paying cash out of pocket and will proceed to their appointments with a cloak-and-dagger approach. Employees do not want the stigma of perceived weakness for speaking with a mental health professional or a diagnosis to follow them around for the rest of their careers.

Public safety personnel experience uncertainty, anxiety, or even fear of mental health professionals and the potential for a diagnosis due to health care coding requirements mandated for mental health clinicians. In consultation with mental health and human resource professionals, leaders of public safety organizations must work together to demystify the preconceived notions prevalent in the first responder community. This attention to internal transparency could send a positive message to agency members regarding the importance of employee health and wellness.

Bridging the Gap Between Employees and Wellness Services

More open dialogue and opportunities to embed the clinician in public safety activities can bridge the gap between first responders, administrations, and mental health clinicians. Some examples include mental health clinicians speaking at in-service training sessions, multidisciplinary police mental health working groups, and mental health professionals participating in ride-along programs with frontline and supervisory personnel. Integrating the mental health professional in this manner will provide an understanding of the culture of the organization the clinician is servicing, common sources of distress and anxiety among employees and their families, and perhaps ways the organization can reduce distress for their employees, all while taking care not to breach confidentiality. Once a person perceives a betrayal of trust, regaining that trust is typically difficult. Opportunities such as the examples listed above would enable first responders to get to know mental health professionals and perhaps break preconceived notions regarding those who choose to serve others through the practice of counseling and psychotherapy.

Standardized Training

In the absence of a closer relationship between first responder agencies and certified mental health clinicians, other (often well-meaning) people or organizations will fill that void. Problems arise when they do not have the appropriate education and experience or become complacent about evaluating new evidence or continuing their education.

Wellness is becoming a popular topic in both the public and the private sectors, with an increase in attention to wellness initiatives, grant availability, and expanding budgets may receive additional funding for health and wellness programs. Demand requires a supply of organizations and instructors offering their services in return for payment. Public safety administrators must use caution when vetting psychoeducational training curricula and instructors. It is wonderful that health and wellness, especially mental health, are finally getting the attention they demand.

However, public safety organizations must make sure not to cause harm in their well-intentioned attempts to address the issues facing our first responder populations. Establishing a standard for certification to provide instruction to first responder communities is something public safety leaders and mental health professionals can work on together, to ensure that what is taught helps first responders, rather than hurting them. This collaborative approach to reviewing and approving programs will further bridge the gap between the agency and trainer/clinician. A peer-reviewed and evidence-based training curriculum for each discipline could be standardized with input from police, corrections, fire, emergency medical services, and emergency-communications communities. At a minimum, the agency should consult with a licensed mental health professional to vet the qualifications of any instructors and the validity of their training programs.

Transparency in Early Interventions

Organizational responses to mental health emergencies should not be a surprise to employees or supervisors. If an employee comes to a supervisor and indicates thinking about suicide, a substance use disorder, or domestic issues, the supervisor should not have to dig out the policy manual. These revelations could even surface during a meeting between the supervisor and employee in response to an EIS alert. Everyone should know before the employee's personal or professional crisis arises how the organization responds and helps.

Internal transparency and collaborative relationships are both components of this topic. For example, the authors' experience in law enforcement is that employees often fear that the organization will take custody of the officer's firearm if the employee relays experiencing a mental health emergency. The likelihood of that scenario should be made clear to all. Effective resilience-building strategies made available to employees and accepted in the employee's life prior to the crisis should work to end the over-identification with title and foster more identification as a human being, so that the loss of symbols of authority does not increase psychological trauma to the already suffering employee. Public safety employees need to know that symbols of their authority are not symbols of their personal identity or humanity.

Common Interventions for Early Alerts

The typical response to an early intervention alert is one of two options: remedial training or counseling (DeCrescenzo, 2005; Walker et al., 2001; Bertoia, 2008). The supervisor or training staff of the agency often orchestrates remedial training and presents it in-house. This response may fail in the absence of formal lesson plans and learning objectives, because of the time constraints of the supervisor, employee, or both, or because an underlying catalyst to the behavior is left unexplored. The training may also take place by sending the employee to an external training course, with the potential drawback being the lack of feedback to the sending organization regarding the employee's reception and retention of the information provided. The focus could be on how to avoid unwanted attention at work, rather than on how to return things to their normal balance in the employee's life.

Counseling sounds like a huge step forward for the public safety community. Traditionally, public safety organizations have resisted mental health counseling or even involvement of mental health professionals with employees following pre-employment psychological screenings. Counseling in first responder jargon is not what it seems to readers coming from the psychological disciplines. The term *counseling* in the public safety realm deals with correcting a specific behavior through discussion and a plan to improve, diminish, or eradicate the flagged employee behavior. In a counseling session that a supervisor organizes, the employee is presented with the problematic behavior and research the supervisor has conducted into that employee's history. The supervisor seeks the employee's acknowledgment of the behavior and the adverse impact it has had or could have on the service population, the organization and its mission, and the employee. Together they try to formulate a performance improvement plan, establish benchmarks to measure improvements, and adopt a timeline for the changes (Walker et al., 2001; Walker et al., 2006). The present authors propose a clearer focus on the underlying difficulty, within both the alert mechanism and intervention, so that employees' mental health is best served.

An agency contemplating developing an EIS should consider consulting its employees and mental health professionals to see if they feel it would be beneficial to share these alerts with a departmentally sanctioned mental health professional. An oversight mechanism like this would help ensure the agency is responding with appropriate intervention strategies based upon the needs of both the organization and the individual employee. In essence, it is consulting with the agency's mental health professional to obtain feedback on potential avenues to best address underlying mental health issues.

The other standard intervention option in an EIS is the referral to an employee assistance program (EAP), whether in-house or contracted to an external provider. A noteworthy concern in this process relates to the level of training and experience the EAP staff have in assisting public safety personnel with their unique stressors and the impact of their careers on family members and support systems. A variation of the existing EIS referral to EAP would be a yet different type of psychological visit from pre-employment screening, annual wellness visit, or fitness-for-duty examination: An automatic EIS alert visit with a mental health professional who specializes in public safety treatment. Akin to the EAP referral, the latter may be much more effective if it precedes the two common traditional responses of remedial training and supervisory counseling in that it will potentially lead to the treatment of the underlying cause(s) of any behavior that triggers early alerts.

When behaviors leading to an early alert or other complaints are too severe or disruptive for the effective and safe provision of services to the community, the fitness-for-duty examination may be the most appropriate intervention. Although a fitness-for-duty examination is listed as a potential intervention strategy in the New Jersey Attorney General's Directive 2018-3 (2018b), it may not always be an appropriate response by a mental health professional. The following list includes potential clinically relevant intervention options once an employee has been identified by the EIS:

- Voluntary referral EAP
- Automatic referral to the department psychologist
- Peer support referral
- Occupational health referral
- Referral to rehabilitation facility
- Sleep specialist referral
- Anger management referral
- Fitness-for-duty examination

Family as an Early Intervention System

Taking the term *Early Intervention System* most literally, a first responder's family and personal support system is where changes and difficulties are first noticed, and training and participation in any meaningful program must not neglect that fact. In most instances, close family members or friends are more likely than a coworker or a supervisor to observe changes in mood, behavior, energy levels, optimism, faith, and happiness.

The first vital step to empowering the employee's family to act as an additional layer of protection involves a trained mental health professional conducting a seminar to educate first responder family members and support systems. There they could learn to recognize warning signs their loved ones may display, realize those signs could correlate with distress from work, and identify ways they can assist their loved one and/or find the resources available to them, should they need more assistance.

Both authors have conducted family education courses for police agencies and academies and have received overwhelmingly positive feedback and expressions of gratitude from those who have attended. Feedback often includes reports of a better understanding of their police officer family member's calling and the unique stressors that come with a career in service, including being under the constant microscope of the media and the general public. Employees must also take personal responsibility for realizing when they need help, seeking it themselves when they are able to do so, and accepting the help. Believing this before it becomes needed is the key. A major factor in ensuring that employees will trust the agency and the process is their knowledge of the steps involved in assisting them prior to their crisis surfacing.

Achieving Greater Buy-In

Public safety leaders must always be mindful of all stakeholders. If an organization has an employee-oversight system to detect potentially problematic behaviors or patterns of behaviors, that organization could be sending a message that it is only interested in sifting out the negative, unless the oversight system is complemented with an awards and recognition program, a health and wellness program, and the ability to offer valid interventions for employees when they are going through a crisis or triggering a confirmed early warning alert. If the organization offers proactive and preventative interventions in addition to a transparent EIS it may prove to be a more accepted management tool.

Transparency and *health and wellness* have recently become popular buzzwords in the public safety leadership community, although rarely, if ever, are these two terms used in the same conversation. Could separating them result in missing a vital link for sustainable health and wellness efforts? In the experience of the authors, the fear and mystery surrounding the mental health profession is real for most first responders. The authors are personally aware of first responders who have experienced substance use disorders or mental health, personal, or family crises and have paid out-of-pocket to see a mental health clinician due to an intense fear of a real or perceived stigma that comes with a diagnosis required to utilize one's health-insurance plan.

Achieving buy-in through education is the key to success in the implementation of effective and meaningful organizational strategies. An early intervention system could be a component of a more comprehensive plan to help the first responder community.

Critical Incident Interventions

While the EIS is meant to look at data sets over a period of time and alert supervisors to potential issues, a critical incident is a triggering event in its own category. A common intervention public safety agencies use is critical-incident stress debriefings that administrators and/or peers typically conduct. In some of the more traumatic cases, a one-on-one appointment would be made for the affected personnel with a licensed mental health clinician who specializes in treating public safety personnel. The lack of standardization and training on which resources to utilize and who decides what defines a true critical incident for a particular employee or group of employees would be an area worthy of further research and collaboration between public safety leaders, researchers, and the mental health community. Organizations must have an open dialogue when considering criteria that would gauge which incidents are traumatic enough to require a one-on-one consultation with a licensed mental health professional, with the possibility that this would best be done on a case-by-case basis. Subjectivity in these decisions and the selection process and decision-maker training or lack thereof are extremely problematic.

Wellness Options for Employees

A multidisciplinary approach to serving the needs of employees and their support systems requires working across paradigms. Integration could include all or some of the following: peer support, critical-incident stress-management teams, EAP staff, chaplains, and mental health clinicians. Each of these groups of professionals can work within the discipline or in concert with others to assist the first responder community in preparation for shiftwork, the disturbing situations and scenes they will encounter, moral injuries, potential shifts in their faith and idealism, dehumanization, gallows humor, and personal family disruptions. Those agencies would achieve this most effectively through resilience training, psychoeducation, early intervention systems, intervention options, and the inclusion of families and support systems in these initiatives. Agency leaders must be aware that individual employees may have different preferences regarding who makes them feel most comfortable in these dialogues. For some employees, a peer support team member may be preferable, others may choose to confide in a chaplain, and some may wish to speak only with a licensed mental health professional. The employee's preference may also vary according to his or her needs or stage in life. Ideally, policies and programs would be designed to allow the employee to control selections for personal counsel and support while ensuring that employees are educated on the services and unique perspectives each discipline may provide. Employees must also be made aware of the confidentiality protections or lack thereof in working with each of these disciplines.

Employees may not always have the level of self-awareness or the ability to overcome obstacles, real or perceived, to seek help during a time of personal and/or professional crisis. Agencies may rely on supervisor or peer observations of changes in an employee's attitude, demeanor, behavior, or personal situation. EISs are one solution being utilized by public safety agencies to aid the organization in identifying employees who may need assistance through interventions.

Pre-Existing EWS Flags

Those in public safety circles commonly know that exposure to trauma, moral distress, moral injury (Papazoglou & Chopko, 2017), substance use disorder (Sack, 2017), post-traumatic stress disorder or injury, cardiac issues, digestive issues, hypertension, and sleep disorders are all prevalent dangers in first responder communities (Violanti, 2014) and should serve as a pre-existing flag for first responders. Action should focus on reducing the dangers associated with what is already known to be hurting or killing our first responders, in addition to causes such as felonious assaults, accidents, disease, and fires. Preventative strategies should be designed with input from mental health professionals, frontline personnel, labor union representatives, supervisors and administrators, and members of first responder families.

The responsibility for the health and wellness of our first responders should not rest solely upon the shoulders of the leaders of public safety organizations. Ideally, labor unions incorporate health and wellness when negotiating for their represented employees. There is a tendency for collective bargaining units to place emphasis on gaining increased salary for employees toward the end of their careers in public safety, in order to increase the take-home amount of their pension, to the exclusion of more present-focused concerns. Health and wellness bargaining items, such as fitness center memberships and/or incentives, more affordable health care plans, education incentives or tuition reimbursement, psychotherapy, maternity/paternity leave, and bereavement leave are often not typical concerns. Public safety leaders and union leaders are in a unique position to guide these conversations so that employees value thriving in the present equally to monthly pension payout calculations that are 30 years or more in the future. This shift in mindset could improve the quality of life for first responders and their families and support systems in the present.

Comfort With the Clinician

In order to ensure a comfortable relationship in which the public safety employee is open to sharing thoughts and feelings with a mental health professional, agencies may want to consider instituting a wellness check-up program with a licensed mental health clinician who specializes in treating the first responder community. Post-critical-incident visits may be the first time employees meet a mental health professional. Perhaps it is the second time, the first being a pre-employment screening, also an uncomfortable situation for a job candidate. The first author has partnered with several police departments in Burlington County, New Jersey, to facilitate annual wellness visits for agency employees. The officers meet to discuss anything they wish or simply to receive psychoeducation. Benefits to this approach include an opportunity for the employee to discuss with a professional in a secure environment the operational and organizational stressors, family difficulties, coping skills, critical-incident and cumulative stress, and any other topics that benefit their overall wellness. Other advantages include the opportunity for individual education on resilience, coping skills, and self-care. One of the most beneficial aspects of this program is the familiarity between the officer and the clinician. The building of trust and rapport can be achieved early, which could greatly assist if the officer automatically attends a counseling session in response to a critical incident or an EIS alert.

Agency leaders, along with their respective organizations, would benefit greatly from familiarizing themselves with some of the resources currently being used, such as resource phone numbers, training programs, and critical-incident stress debriefings, and the research available on such programs. Critical-incident stress debriefings have contradictory or little evidence gleaned from studies. The studies that evaluated critical-incident stress debriefings did not specifically address a sample that was exclusively public safety personnel to prove efficacy in that population (Mitchell & Dorian, 2017). The selection of a critical-incident stress management (CISM) team to service the organization should be vetted with a mental health professional. There are numerous resource phone numbers available in the first responder community for employees to make a cold call for help. These services can be evaluated by offering anonymous surveys to first responders to determine how effective or detrimental the sources whose services they attempted to use were to their health and wellness.

FUTURE DIRECTIONS

Policies dictating responses to the needs of first responders' mental health would best be written with the counsel of mental health professionals to ensure the correct message is being sent to public safety personnel. A commonly discussed nuance in the language is the use of the word *mandatory* versus *automatic* intervention. The two terms may seem synonymous to a policy writer, but something as simple as word choice could make or break buy-in of a well-intentioned organizational intervention strategy. This example is just one of many that could be listed to illustrate the importance of multidisciplinary collaboration in policy and procedure development.

Organizational interventions for public safety agencies must be carefully planned with the assistance and counsel of mental health professionals, buy-in from the rank and file and administration, and support of the community served. The interventions should cover all phases and facets of the public safety employee's career and ensure support for their personal lives as well. An organization's opportunity to show the priority placed on health and wellness begins in the hiring process. Training programs in academies for both new employees and their family regarding critical-incident and cumulative stress, organizational stress, sleep disorders, resilience-building techniques, nutrition, physical fitness, financial wellness, spiritual wellness, and resources available to help the employee and the family in times of crisis are critical. These training sessions and face-to-face visits should not be a "checkbox" completed one time in a career of 30 years or more; rather, they should continue as an ongoing open dialogue between the employees and mental health professionals throughout an employee's entire career.

EIS conceptualization can be broadened to capture a greater variety of potentially problematic behaviors. In New Jersey, while the list of circumstances requiring documentation is extensive, it is focused on behavior suggestive of illegal or at the very least overly aggressive behavior. However, other circumstances could aid in monitoring the well-being of public safety personnel, such as a noticeable increase in overtime and secondary employment shifts, avoidance of going home after work or arriving for work extremely early, isolation from coworkers, complaints of pain, increased sick time usage, complaints of changes in sleeping habits or lack of sleep, unexplained weight gain or loss, changes in eating habits, or changes in marital or family residence status. These suggested factors that a supervisor could monitor may not necessarily be part of a formal EIS; nonetheless, they could provide an early alert to trigger a supervisor's probing questions. They are likely not dissimilar from the facts that down the road would trigger an alert or employee assistance program referral. The best case scenario would result in helping an employee before a formal EIS alert mandates an intervention; the worst case scenario would be that nothing is wrong, and the employee perceives their supervisor's care for his or her welfare (given the conversation is framed appropriately)—obviously, a win-win situation. As such, the EIS needs to remain flexible and continually reviewed to ensure any policy changes are reflected.

In addition to training supervisors on the goal of the EIS and the manner in which to assess employees close to alert status or already flagged, organizational staff in other fields may also play a role. The agency's human resource professionals can further enlighten personnel about their available insurance and relevant health care plans, including any employee assistance programs available to them and their support systems. The human resources representative could also have conversations with employees regarding logistical issues, such as sick time, administrative leave, the Family and Medical Leave Act, temporary disability, and worker's compensation, to name a few.

REFERENCES

Amendola, K. L., & Davis, R. C. (2019). *Best practices in early intervention system implementation and use in law enforcement agencies*. Washington, DC: National Police Foundation.

Bertoia, T. (2008). Developing an early intervention system for police misconduct in a law enforcement agency. *New South Wales Police Integrity Commission Research and Issues Papers*, *1*, 1–31.

Brucia, E., Cordova, M., & Ruzek, J. (2016). Critical Incident Interventions: Crisis Response and Debriefings. In C. Mitchell & E. Dorian (Eds.), *Police psychology and its growing impact on modern law enforcement* (pp. 119–139). Hershey, PA: IGI Global.

Chae, M. H., & Boyle, D. J. (2013). Police suicide: Prevalence, risk, and protective factors. *Policing: An International Journal of Police Strategies & Management*, *36*(1), 91–118. doi:10.1108/13639511311302498

DeCrescenzo, D. (2005). Early detection of the problem officer. *FBI Law Enforcement Bulletin*, *74*(7), 14–17.

Jackson, B. A., Towe, V. L., Wagner, L., Hunt, P., Greathouse, S., & Hollywood, J. S. (2016). Managing officer behavioral risk using early intervention systems: Addressing system design challenges for Law Enforcement and corrections environments. *Policing: Journal of Policy Practice*, *11*(1), 103–117.

Kelly, J., & Hoban, J. E. (2016). Health and wellness programming: The added contribution of an ethical mindset. In C. L. Mitchell & E. H. Dorian (Eds.), *Police psychology and its growing impact on modern law enforcement*. Hershey, PA: IGI Global.

Macintyre, S., Prenzler, T., & Chapman, J. (2008). Early intervention to reduce complaints: An Australian Victoria police initiative. *International Journal of Police Science & Management*, *10*(2), 238–250. doi:10.1350/ijps.2008.10.2.77

New Jersey Office of the Attorney General. (2018a, March 20). *Attorney General Grewal announces two new law enforcement policies designed to ensure law enforcement safety and promote public trust* [Press release]. Retrieved from https://nj.gov/oag/newsreleases18/pr20180320c.html

New Jersey Office of the Attorney General. (2018b). Attorney general law enforcement directive 2018-3. Trenton, NJ: Author.

Papazoglou, K., & Chopko, B. (2017). The role of moral suffering (moral distress and moral injury) in police compassion fatigue and PTSD: An unexplored topic. *Frontiers in Psychology*, *8*, 1999. doi:10.3389/fpsyg.2017.01999 PMID:29187830

Sack, D. (2017, January 31). *Trauma and first responders: When the helpers need help*. Retrieved from https://www.psychologytoday.com/us/blog/where-science-meets-the-steps/201701/trauma-and-first-responders-when-the-helpers-need-help

Schlosser, L. Z., & Kudrick, A. A. Jr. (2019, May). You have to see the psych: Reducing the stigma of mental health treatment among police personnel. *The Police Chief*, *86*(5), 50–56.

U.S. Commission on Civil Rights. (1981). *Who is guarding the guardians?* Washington, DC: U.S. Commission on Civil Rights.

Violanti, J. M. (2014). *Dying for the job: police work exposure and health*. Springfield, IL: Charles C Thomas Publishers.

Walker, S. (2003). *Early intervention systems for law enforcement agencies (United States Department of Justice, Office of Community Oriented Policing Services)*. Washington, DC: Police Executive Research Forum.

Walker, S., Alpert, G. P., & Kenney, D. J. (2001, July). Early warning systems: Responding to the problem police officer. *National Institute of Justice Research in Brief, 1–8*. Retrieved from https://www.ncjrs.gov/pdffiles1/nij/grants/188565.pdf

Walker, S., Milligan, S. O., & Berke, A. (2006). *Strategies for intervening with officers through early intervention systems: A guide for front-line supervisors (United States Department of Justice, Office of Community Oriented Policing Services)*. Washington, DC: Police Executive Research Forum.

Chapter 16
"More Than Peer Support: Organizational and Relational Intervention Model": First Responder Assistance Program (F.R.A.P.)

Mario Jose Gonzalez
Independent Researcher, USA

Marie Guma
Independent Researcher, USA

Bernardo Jose Gonzalez
https://orcid.org/0000-0002-4102-2893
Boundless Leadership Consulting, USA

ABSTRACT

The chapter describes a replicable and innovative approach designed to assist first responder communities through the mental health challenges they face in their personal and professional lives. The First Responder Assistance Program (FRAP) strives to create a healthy environment, through a unified structure, three tiered organizational and relational intervention approach, inclusive of peer support, peer chaplaincy support, and clinician involvement. The FRAP Model establishes a direct correlation between organizational wellness, and the individual health of its members. It emphasizes a "top to bottom" organizational intervention, with the understanding that no matter how much help is provided to the individual, the environment must be addressed in order to obtain sustainable results. It stresses a "holistic" approach to healing with a focus on post traumatic growth and the systematic building of individual and organizational resilience.

DOI: 10.4018/978-1-5225-9803-9.ch016

THE QUESTION

I was sitting in the Fire Chief's Office making a presentation about the needed expansion of our Peer Chaplaincy Program, when he asked a question for which I had no comprehensive answer, at least none that was satisfying to my own mind. "Why are we having more problems with first responder mental health now than we have ever had in the past?" The Chief continued with his line of questioning, not necessarily seeking an answer from me, but more in a rhetorical fashion, externally processing something that obviously he had been wondering for quite some time. He said, "The calls haven't changed. We used to run difficult trauma calls back in the day." As the conversation continued, some obvious possibilities, all with some merit, were posed as reasonable answers:

- Awareness has been heightened, so perhaps what was once hidden, now has come to light
- Maybe the stigma has lessened because we are talking more openly about mental health
- The advent of social media may not allow for a space to disconnect
- Perhaps it is the increase in the sheer volume and intensity of calls
- Or maybe the pace of present-day living is affecting our ability to cope

Now it is here that I must interject that neither the Fire Chief nor I (Chaplain Mario Gonzalez)_are sociologists or researchers, but with over 60 years of combined experience as first responders, I think there is some merit and validity to our suppositions.

As we moved on to the task at hand, deciding we were not going to find a definitive answer in the time allotted for our meeting, the question continued to roam in my mind. Are traumatic calls truly adversely affecting and wounding first responders more today than they did in the past? Were former generations of first responders just tougher and more resilient than us, or were they just better at hiding their emotional pain and woundedness? The more I thought, meditated, and prayed about this, the more convinced I became that the answer to both questions is "yes". Perhaps first responders of yester-year, were both tougher and better at hiding their emotional pain than their contemporary brothers and sisters.

Now before I'm taken out to the woodshed by my fellow first responders for having made such a statement, let me just say that I believe we are plenty tough. A lot of what came out of my short impromptu brain storming session with the Fire Chief raised more questions than provided answers. I happen to believe that this is actually good. It is always in the space where hard questions are asked with integrity, that good answers are birthed. Yes, some good work is being done in the area of breaking down the ingrained culture of invincibility and stigma associated with seeking assistance in our first responder community. But are we being shortsighted in what we mean by changing the culture?

Yes, in most Departments, peer support is now considered as an important component in the battle for first responder mental health. But do we have measurable outcomes that our inventions are effective? Although PTSD and other anxiety driven mental health challenges are now topics of conversation in most first responder communities, are we looking at these topics from the most appropriate and helpful perspectives? Are Department administrations "being forced" to take reactionary measures due to new laws and incidents within their organizations? Are they willing to take the necessary steps to not only implement but institutionalize well thought-out support programs? Is their willingness to intervene, truly motivated by a desire to improve the lives of their most precious asset…their people?

In this chapter we will attempt to address some of these questions and provide the best answers from our optic, based on the many years of experience helping the public as well as then pivoting to help our own. In doing this, we believe that a replicable model of organizational and individual relational assistance will begin to appear as the best "wholistic" approach to helping our own.

THE CULTURE

Whenever the topic of changing the first responder community culture arises, the conversation inevitably defaults to the ingrained mindset of invincibility that comes with the uniform, and the stigma attached to seeking assistance. The firefighter, the police officer, and the alarm office call taker are at the receiving end of the most recognizable number in our country…"911". When that number is dialed, the expectation is that the cavalry is coming and help is on the way. But not only help--whatever the emergency at hand--that help had better be prepared to show up ready to have all the answers and provide appropriate assistance in a timely and professional manner. It is expected that the help is strong, courageous, and ready-to-respond at any hour of the day; immutable in the face danger; infallible in split second decisions, and lest we forget, courteous and level headed when faced with individuals who might be unruly because they are quite possibly going through the worst day of their life. Repeat that countlessly over a 25-30 year career, and is it any wonder that most first responders carry an imaginary "S" tattooed on their chest underneath the uniform? Expect Superman or Wonder Woman--that is who had better be showing up. For most of us, it doesn't take long to realize that these expectations are unattainable. However illusory avatars don't die easily, because the ingrained stigma attached to seeking help as mere mortals persists.

There is no denying that addressing this mindset needs to be a component of changing first responder culture, but to stop there would not only be short-sighted but ineffective. First Responder culture is a subculture of two other parent cultures; the organizational culture fostered in each individual Department, and the culture at large from which it draws its members. Together, these shape First Responder culture.

In addressing organizational culture, we must first asses from a management and training perspective, whether the organization is fostering a culture of authority and power or a culture of service. Foundationally at its core, first responder work is about service. The purpose of our profession is service. Service is what we are paid to do, and an attitude of service is what is expected of us. This being the case, it would stand to reason that internally we should be fostering and modeling a culture of service and self-care, for, and by each other. This congruence of expected external behavior and internal culture could be described as "Organizational Wellness". We consider this to be an integral and necessary function in the pursuit of the well-being of the individuals that make up the whole. We are indeed "our brother's keeper", and this attitude should permeate the entire culture of the organization from its highest levels and across all ranks.

This can only be accomplished by an absolute commitment from the administrative and training hierarchy, to implement and adhere to policies that foster this culture of care and service. It is also imperative to hold all positions of authority within the organization accountable to this higher calling of leadership. Sadly, in most organizations, this is not the case. In the day to day "battle" of running a para-military organization, too often pride, ego, and undisciplined behavior in need of adjustment, get in the way of the best intended efforts of creating and maintaining an internal organizational culture of service and care.

In an authority and power-driven culture, management tends to look at its members as unruly children who only respond to the hard line of punishment. Conversely, the rank and file look at management as uncaring parents. This antagonistic mentality leads to a mutual lack of trust and a feeling of administrative betrayal from the rank and file. This will always stand in the way and damage any attempt to create a healthy culture of internal service. The very real and valid administrative challenge of holding its members accountable to appropriate discipline when needed, should never offer up as collateral damage its attempt to create an internal culture of care and service.

On the other hand, a culture of administrative service and care looks at discipline as a constructive tool for improvement. It understands that the well-being of the one leads to the betterment of the whole. It stands by the principle of assistance before discipline and it holds all of its members accountable on an individual basis without using a shotgun approach to disciplinary policy. Organizationally, this is by far not only the harder road, but also the road less traveled. Nevertheless, if we are to truly address the needed change of culture within our industry, we must first endeavor to honestly asses, and then be willing to take the hard steps to improve this aspect of our organizational culture.

Turning our focus to the influence the culture at large is having on first responder culture, it doesn't take long to identify the advent of social media and the rapid growth of portable technology as a major contributor to decreasing interpersonal and relational connection. Fire Station dining rooms and day rooms are not the bevy of relational interaction that they used to be. In fire stations, breaking bread as a family used to be commonplace. Although you can still find pockets of this important tradition in many of our houses, we are slowly experiencing its demise, much in the same way we have witnessed it in the American home. Even when we manage to get together for meals, the unwelcomed presence of technology alarmingly interferes with and disconnects us from being present with each other.

Increasingly, the conversations--when they do happen--are not about our personal lives, so much as they are about the popular entertainment choices of the day. We are becoming so comfortable with the imaginary worlds presented to us by our own inventions, that connecting to the reality of being present is becoming increasingly difficult. From a completely non-clinical and anecdotal evidential perspective, this to me cannot be conducive to the well-being of our mental health, especially when it is challenged by the harsh realities of our profession. I am not saying that technology and entertainment are the root of all our mental health challenges, but we ignore this topic to our own detriment.

Another area where cultural thinking seems to have shifted, and is also affecting the first responder sub-culture, is the notion that life should be easy, and that problems when they come should be resolved at the drop of a hat. Hardship somehow has become an interruption, rather than a normal possibility. The ease and rapid access to all things comfortable inclusive of service, information, and climate control, to name just a few, have made us an extremely impatient society when it comes to dealing with hardship or discomfort.

In our chosen profession, the first responder is regularly confronted with the disruption of these expectations in the life of those he or she is sworn to protect. The constant exposure to these events can begin to intrude into an idyllic expectation of life, especially when it touches too close to home. For example, the death of a child, ran by a paramedic who is a new parent himself; a deadly assault on an elderly couple handled by a police officer dealing with the death of his or her parents; or a nursing home call handled by a rescue crew in which one of its members just placed their mom in an assisted living facility.

This collision of worlds accentuates and opens our eyes to the reality that we have little to no control over the outcome of most things happening around us. This "reality check" to someone who has been living under the illusion that their life journey should always go as they expect or have planned can be terrifying. Again, I am not saying that first responders live in some sort of unrealistic panacea, but the fact is that the culture we live in tends to expect and almost demands quick solutions to problems and ease of life. Accept it or not, our personnel are made up of a microcosm of the society surrounding us. We must do a better job educating our internal culture as to the normalcy of pain and hardship, and the opportunity for growth when confronted with both of these challenges in our everyday life. If we fail to understand what changing first responder culture should look like and miss the mark in truly making a difference in this important task, we will constantly be in a reactionary mode when it comes to the mental health of our people.

With respect to changing the culture, in an organization, education and awareness can become the fertile ground where culture change is plausible. But for this to happen, it must occur in the context of Departmental support and participation across all ranks. Any educational intervention must be accompanied by an administrative/leadership modeling of the behavior being promoted. The educational focus should also address the wider topic of how the culture at large is affecting the internal first responder community as just described.

THE SPIRITUALITY OF HEALING

It has been said that we are all recovering from something. The wisdom of this statement is at once both humbling and sobering. No one goes through this life without experiencing pain, disappointment, or heartache in some way. Our journey to healing and wholeness invariably has its starting place from a realization that we have been broken. Like participants in a high-speed game of bumper cars, we are constantly in need of forgiveness either given or received. Acceptance of brokenness, gratitude for where we are in the journey, and our need of forgiveness are prerequisites for healing.

This involves two important linchpins needed on the road to healing; humility and vulnerability. If humility and vulnerability start us on the road, the unflinching search for truth, in our need for love, is where the hard work is done. We are all relational beings. We are in a relationship with ourselves, our present situation, our past events, the world around us, each other, and if we are open to it, the existence of the spiritual and the source of all things created...God. We share the same world, but with each of us experiencing different and unique realities. Our experiences color and filter the way we see the world, but the one constant, whether we are able or willing to see it, is truth.

The addict trapped by his or her addiction, experiences the reality of transient relief through their substance or behavior of choice, but the truth is that they are on the road to deepening their pain. In the mind of a person feeling the paralyzing anxiety which connects a past event to a possible future, nothing could be more real, but is it truth? Recorded in the eighteen chapter of the Book of James, a 1st Century Roman Precept in Judea asked a very important question, but his pride and impatience did not let him wait for the answer...What is truth? It is in the answer to this question, and our alignment with this most elusive concept, where the proverbial rubber meets the very real road in our journey to wholeness.

Indeed, whether you ascribe to his claims of divinity, are a follower of his way, or think he was just a historical anomaly, that most famous of all Galilean carpenters truly put His finger on the pulse of the question of healing and wholeness when he made the following statement. "And you shall know the truth and the truth shall set you free." In meditating on the intersection between spirituality and healing, I decided to pose the question to a trusted friend with a long career of helping people on their road to healing as a successful therapist. I am grateful to my friend, Flora del Cueto LMHC, for her thoughtful and insightful answer to this question. How then do healing and spirituality relate to each other?

"My experience as a clinician has revealed that those who have a relationship with God, a spiritual leaning, are more likely to surrender in the process of recovery and healing particularly from significant traumatic events. That is, those people with a spiritual leaning, or close relationship with God, are less likely to have emotional resistance as they explore the thoughts and memories associated with trauma and or abuse. In contrast, persons who have animosity towards God and or no spiritual leanings, tend to have a greater resistance to emotional healing and the exploration of those events that are emotionally painful" - Marie Guma MS. PsyD (ABD)

THE NEED

In order to try to answer the chief's rhetorical question that spontaneously created quite a conversation between him and Mario, I (Marie Guma MS. PsyD (ABD)) must dive a bit into the history of behavioral health or synonymously coined, mental health. According to the World Health Organization, mental health is:

... a state of well-being in which the individual realizes his or her own abilities, can cope with the normal stresses of life, can work productively and fruitfully, and is able to make a contribution to his or her community.1

Mental health is no longer solely defined as the absence of mental illness. Neither of these concepts are new to modern society. As early as 1500 BC the Egyptians depicted emotional turmoil in their drawings. They believed that mental illness was due to spirit possessions. The Greeks attributed mental illnesses as rage inflicted by the gods. During the Dark Ages, the cause of mental illness was ties to being possessed by the devil. During these times, a person who did not get better was thought to have weakness in their faith.

Witchcraft was thought to be the cause of mental abnormalities during the 15th and 16th centuries. The chosen treatments during this era were purging, bloodletting and removal of organs that the doctors believed could get infected. Mentally ill citizens were placed in mental hospitals that were primitive and the care was brutal. The patients were mixed with criminals and given the same treatments, where punishment was meant to sway their behaviors. They did not have adequate food, beds or toilets. The patients were placed in isolation or chained. They were not cared for by doctors or nurses but by warders.

During the 18th century, Philippe Pinel reformed the care for the mentally ill. Asylums were directed by doctors and nurses. Kindness replaced the penalizations administered in caring for this community. By the 19th century sedatives came into the picture as did Freud with concepts of mental processes and development. In the 1920's shock therapy and insulin comas were being administered in asylums. In the mid 1940's Moniz began the practice of lobotomies in treating mental illness. By the time Moniz passed in 1972, lobotomies were still in practice.

As is evidenced, the concept of mental health is not new but understanding it as another physiological system in our body and how to treat it, is. In fact, in 1949 the lobotomy won the medical Nobel Prize for treating mental health. This is significant because it explains the current attached stigma on anything related to mental health and mental health treatment in society. If we add to this stigma Mario's perspective on the first responder's personality, culture, and the stress levels inherent to the career, one can clearly understand why these ingredients have been a recipe for disaster. The disaster we are seeing today, where every 18 hours a firefighter is completing suicide in the United States. First responders are signing up and accepting the fact that these careers are dangerous and have high probabilities of death; but first responders' suicide rates are doubling and even tripling line of duty deaths. This is a disaster and an injustice for these men and women.

RESILIENCE AND POST TRAUMATIC GROWTH

Recently, I asked a group of firefighters who have been retired a minimum of 18 years, to define *resilience* in the fire service. They were all in agreement that resilience was synonymous with being tough, not allowing things to affect you, being able to suck it up and do your job and do it well. I poised the rhetorical question, "So if you feel that you need to suck it up and not allow things to affect you, are you also admitting that the possibility of things affecting you are part of the job?" They all smiled as if I had caught them with their hand in the cookie jar and finally one said, "We saw things no one should ever have to see. Letting it affect us, or letting others know it affected us made us weak."

I explained to the group that what they were calling "weak" was being human. They understood that being human was equivalent to having feelings, both negative and positive feelings. They understood that asking firemen, police officers, EMT, correctional officers, dispatchers or soldiers to not let things affect them was also asking them to not be human, to go against their nature. I went a bit further, I wanted them to fully grasp the understanding that being human is not just a pretty concept to excuse a crying grown man but an actual physiological process in their body over which they have absolutely no control.

I began by explaining our command center: the brain, how it controls both physical movements and emotional responses. I described how the brain gets information from the external world and how it reacts with neurochemicals. I described feelings in terms of some of these neurochemicals for them to understand that feelings are not an abstract concept but an actual neurobiological reaction in our bodies. They finally understood that creating a culture in an entire industry where you are deemed "successful" if you go against your nature, over which you have no control, was asking for more than anyone could truly handle.

One of these great men said, Marie, we did not tolerate the ones perceived as weak and teased them because sometimes it was all we could do to keep from being weak ourselves. Keeping the attention on others kept it off me. We did do somethings right though. We weren't lazy. We shared as a family at the kitchen table. Now a day's guys at the station are on their phones and barely know their brothers' names. They all have separate rooms and only see each other during a call. Pardon my French but I knew who had farted just by the smell.

After this group understood what is meant by being human as a physical concept, I went on to correct their definition of resilience. I validated some of their definitions in order to avoid having them leave the conversation. I confirmed that it was definitely about mental toughness, but not by denying what they felt but instead by accepting it and being able to recover or bounce back from it. Resilience is the ability to recuperate functioning after setbacks, barriers, trauma, or difficulties. They were able to understand that if a first responder is spending his or her energy on hiding their human nature, fighting their normal reactions, or not accepting that it is ok not to be ok, than they are wasting time in which they could be getting the assistance they need to be able to bounce back in the arena they love so much.

It's like a pulled muscle or broken leg injury of a football player during a game. What if for years football players traditionally had "sucked it up" and continued playing injured? What if they did not get the rest, physical therapy and assistance they needed to be able to make a full recovery? They would be playing in pain, their careers would be shortened dramatically, their injuries would progressively get worse, their self-confidence and abilities would suffer, and they would begin to cope with numbing agents to be able to get through a day.

Today first responders are numbing their expected reactions to what they see and do every day with alcohol, drugs, sex, gambling just to name a few. When we are fighting something we have no control over and is a normal process within our bodies, we are setting ourselves up for failure. Accepting these processes in and of itself is a sign of resilience as well as the first step in being resilient or recovering from misfortune.

Post traumatic growth (PTG) is the next step above resiliency. PTG is the ability to bounce back from a traumatic event but land in a higher, happier, and more appreciative state then previously in. It is becoming more self-actualized. According to Abraham Maslow, self-actualization represents growth of an individual toward fulfillment of the highest needs. The needs that give meaning to life. Thankfully, after a traumatic event, it has been found that most people are resilient and bounce back to their prior state. It is a small subset that never recovers or grows to a higher level of resiliency or PTG.

What if I were to say to you that first responders have the highest ability to be the most self-actualized humans on earth? It is said that an average person experiences 5 traumatic events in their entire life. First responders, depending what areas you serve, at the very minimum experience at least 5 traumatic events a week, thus giving these industries the experiences needed to find more meaning and more happiness in one's life.

When two holocaust survivors were interviewed together, one stated, *"It is indecent to ever be happy again after going through what I went through and watching the suffering of those in concentration camps." The other replied, "I feel it is indecent to never be happy again. To appreciate that we are still alive and have the ability to keep living."* Post traumatic growth has been found to increase maturity, meaning in life and happiness in individuals that achieve it. So why is the opinion of these two survivors so different? An underlying characteristic in PTG is the ability to recalibrate the experience and your perception of it. For example, being able to change a first responder's opinion of their job from being a thankless, tiresome, traumatic filled, bureaucratic, soul crushing experience to the luckiest job in the world where you have the ability to experience things that are the paths to more fulfilling and happier lives, it recalibrates their perception of the inherent trauma surrounding their careers.

Factors that have been found to affect the possibility of experiencing post traumatic growth include the person's personality pre-trauma. Costa and McCrae's five factor model of personality (FFM;1992) consists of extraversion, neuroticism, openness, agreeableness and conscientiousness dimensions. In 2015, a study found that neuroticism is correlated to a pathogenic outcome after a traumatic event, whereas extraversion was highly associated to positive post-traumatic outcomes.

Those who exhibit openness use cognitive strategies that correlate to PTG. Individuals who were agreeable were more likely to perceive positive changes after a traumatic event and conscientious individuals were characterized with more self-control, more meticulous and pursued goals with tenacity thus facilitating PTG. Another factor that influences PTG is the levels of psychological resilience of the individual as well as the amount of psychological damage caused by the event.

People who have attained PTG have reported that being in relationships where they felt nurtured and validated were essential to their growth. Being able to connect with people who can give them professional assistance during this time and feel genuinely accepted by them were two other factors that highly contributed to PTG. It is important to mention here that post traumatic growth is not only an outcome but also a process. One can experience distress as well as growth simultaneously. A professional placing emphasis on PTG too soon may cause the individual to feel like their trauma is being minimized. Professionals dealing with individuals who have experienced trauma need to understand that PTG is not always an outcome and need the mention of growth to initially come from the person struggling.

Post traumatic growth comes at a big price. Following a traumatic event, one must experience high levels of distress, vulnerability, and an increased awareness of one's mortality. The price is counterbalanced with the rewards. A firefighter from San Diego Fire Rescue experienced multiple stabbings from a homeless man while he was trying to assist the homeless man's friend on a call. This firefighter states that what shocked him the most was the speed in which the attacker took his knife out and stabbed him multiple times. This firefighter now knows how fast he can be attacked and feels much better prepared where and how he places himself in relation to others on a call. Another reward of gaining PTG is an increase in self-confidence. Individuals who bounce back or attain growth after a traumatic event gain insight into their strength, become proud of themselves and what they have been able to overcome, and become confident in being able to prosper against any obstacle.

Those who attain post traumatic growth also experience more fulfillment in their relationships, clarity in their purpose and meaning, and are grateful for what they have. It has been reported that growth creates a new resistance or resilience, individuals are more prepared for future traumas, they bounce back quicker, feel they have stronger minds, can assess current situations better by using their past. Many who attained post traumatic growth have reported they worry less because they know things can be a lot worse.

Going back to the conversation between Mario and his chief and the big question as to why mental health issues seem to be more prominent in today's first responder industry, I am reminded of my conversation with the retired firefighters. I agree with the driver engineer who boasted, they did some things better back then. He admitted they did not understand mental health nor give it any creditability. He admitted that the culture accepted and even required the men to remain silent and suffer alone, but he says confidently, *"We knew each other. We talked. We connected. The kitchen table was our family, therapist, judge and jury."*

The word "connected" brought me back to my doctoral education, where we are taught that social connection can strengthen one's immune system, helps you recover from disease faster and may even lengthen one's life. Connectedness reduces depression and anxiety, increases self-esteem, increases empathy, trust, and cooperation with others which in turn causes others to cooperate and trust, generating a positive feedback loop of social, emotional and physical well-being.

The lack of connection has shown to be a greater detriment to our health than obesity, smoking, and high blood pressure. The lack of connection leaves us more vulnerable to anxiety, depression, antisocial behaviors and suicidal behaviors which create a further negative loop of isolation. Reports of connectedness in the United States are dropping in alarming rates. In 1985, Americans were asked how many people in their lives they felt they could turn to or feel comfortable sharing a personal problem. At that time, Americans claimed an average of three people they could confide in. The same study was repeated in 2004 and this time Americans reported having an average of zero people they could confide in.

One could be bewildered by these numbers and question how this could be in our current society where our ability to reach someone is the easiest it has ever been. It does not matter where you are, you can reach someone by pressing one button. We are in an era where you don't just talk to someone by pressing one button, but you can see them as well—a technology easily accessible to most in the world.

The issue with these devices is they have created delusion of connection. When we send text messages that include an emoji to replace an entire paragraph, not only are we allowing for misinterpretation, but we are going back to an era of communicating through pictures. We are also excluding the ability to express ourselves, read body language, listen to tone. What we see of our outside world are the fake superficial lives on our devices of those around us. The worlds they have created through pictures that are cropped and filtered to make us look the way we wished we looked. Notifications on our phones have conditioned our brains to abnormal amounts of increased dopamine, thus creating the need for constant hits which you try to attain by constantly checking your phone while you are in the outside world where you would've been connecting to someone, but instead looking at your phone for a dopamine fix.

Recently, Microsoft admitted that our attention span in the digital world has dropped to less than 8 seconds. That is less than a goldfish. We no longer analyze and interpret information giving depth and meaning to our lives, instead we have opted for practicality in our devices that also cause shallow thinking.

In the fire industry, the inclusion of personal smart devices is not the only cause of the decreased sense of connectedness within the fire houses. Fire stations' layouts have changed. Private rooms with TVs have replaced the large room with cots. Kitchen tables are used just for meals, they are no longer the safe base after a tough call or a good cry in your brother or sister's arms. The private rooms give firefighters the ability to suffer alone while social media helps them escape their reality or numb their pain. The layouts, lack of kitchen table talks and the use of smart phones all attribute to the lack of connection in the fire industry.

They are also responsible for the increase of post-traumatic stress disorder (PTSD) in this service. PTSD is simply defined by the treatable malfunction of certain biological, specifically neurobiological, mechanisms. To simplify this even more, without minimizing the disorder's ability to absolutely render someone to the point of being debilitated, it is a glitch in your brain. In order to be functioning first responders, the stress reaction of fight, flight or freeze must be automatically triggered while doing your job. This reaction is what allows first responders to be cool, calm and collected to do their jobs in crisis situations.

Physically what this reaction looks like is: the primal part of the first responder's brain is revved up to 100%, specifically the hypothalamic, pituitary and adrenal systems (HPA). This signals the first responder's body to be in survival mode, focused and ready to go, thus heart rate increases, breathing increases and glucose increases through the release of norepinephrine, adrenaline and cortisol. As the HPA is ignited, the prefrontal cortex area of your brain shuts down for efficiency and survival. The prefrontal cortex of your brain is the last to develop (between the ages of 23-25 years old) and is responsible for all our executive functions like planning, judgement and impulse control. Since this area of the brain shuts off, first responders train extensively in order to make all their procedures instinctual.

The glitch that occurs in PTSD is when that trauma, event or call is not processed into the thinking part of our brains and it remains stuck in the primal brain, which is why someone with PTSD reacts to triggers as if the event is occurring at that very moment because the brain has not processed it or brought it to the part of the brain where it can rationalize it. It is why virtual reality therapy, EMDR and exposure therapy have been so successful in treating PTSD, because these treatments eliminate the firewall or glitch not allowing the event to be processed in your cortex. Going on a traumatic call, not sitting at the kitchen table to allow the call to be processed, isolating oneself in a private room, escaping into social media, and lack of connectedness have contributed to PTSD.

Although the battle against the stigma of mental health is in full force and the culture is changing through education and awareness, the lack of connection needs to be addressed further within the first responder industries. Peer support has played a monumental role in connection but usually it is with first responders that are already suffering. Listening to the retired first responders, getting back to some of the roots of connection in the firehouse, incorporating the systems they were using to keep each other healthy may be a great start.

ORGANIZATIONAL AND RELATIONAL INTERVENTION MODEL

First Responder Assistance Program (FRAP)

I (Dr. Bernardo Gonzalez) believe the failure to address systemic conditions within a First Responder's organizational culture can have substantial negative effects within the First Responder community (First Responder personnel and family). Equally important is the fact that the negative impact created also directly influences and shapes a First Responder's on the job behavior and level of service. More specifically, how First Responders connect and relate to the people and communities they serve.

The heartbreaking reality is that First Responders are not only impacted by on the job stressors, but also the scars, experiences, and in cases deep unresolved trauma carried from their past. With this in mind, most First Responder Departments address these issues in a reactive manner, sending employees to Employee Assistance Programs (EAP) for help, only when the situation or behavior is flagged by someone (usually a supervisor), or when the employee acts out in a manner that puts in question their mental wellness.

In most situations, whether medical or when dealing with mental wellness, the earlier we address a situation the greater the chance for healing. Using a simple analogy, one does not wait to treat an injury from a fall until there is an acute infection in the body. If one does, this delay in treatment severely impacts the healing process and also increases the level of pain and suffering for the person. In the same manner, a reactionary position when treating the mind can produce the same level of increased pain and suffering for the individual who is left untreated.

Equally important, the organization's response to these situations can set in motion a negative cause and effect scenario, as it relates to employee and management relationships. The employee perceives that they are not being valued by the organization and commences to isolate themselves and mistrusts the administration. From my professional experience, this reactionary response and delay in providing assistance can obstruct constructive growth and healing for the organization and individual.

Organizational Intervention

As we examine the existing organizational culture, we can see the incredible impact stress (both on the job and personal) has on the First Responder Community. Anyone having any experience in the field (First Responders) can also attest to the fact that First Responders are already coming with, and are significantly affected by, trauma and stressors caused by Adverse Childhood Experiences (ACE). Unfortunately, as noted, most First Responder Departments fail to proactively engage with this reality and for the most part are solely connecting with on the job stressors relating to Post Traumatic Stress Disorders (PTSD). Interestingly enough some of the work and research accomplished in the military (Ken Falke and others) point to a significant connection existing with Adverse Childhood Experiences and PTSD.

This is an important point to understand due to the reactionary response and focus of most First Responder Departments. Although not a clinician myself, I can attest from my academic, personal, and professional experiences, that First Responders create mental frameworks or elaborations that screen out rational cognition. These elaborations if not properly processed internally, can create negative projections of the future. When these negative projections are left unchecked, the First Responder utilizes these self-created elaborations, that are now separated from facts and the original situation, to shape their values, plans, and actions. If organizations fail to address the negative elaborations being created, the behavior generated from these unhealthy mental constructs can commence to erode and poison the health of an organization.

Moreover, the organizational culture in directly dependent and is built on the thoughts, mental framework, and behavior of its employees. Further, if left unrestrained these unhealthy thoughts and elaborations in time are passed on as unhealthy values and behavior, becoming fused and part of the informal and at times formal organizational culture. This is why, in my professional opinion, it is important for First Responder Departments to be proactive regarding the mental health and wellbeing of their personnel.

As an example, a First Responder Department may very well have a formal culture that has respect and fairness as two of their organizational values, while unfortunately at the same time the informal culture is living and breathing values of unhealthy competition, unfairness, and ruthlessness. It is imperative for First Responder Departments to assess the health and overall wellness of their formal and informal cultures, as well as their people. How are our employees shaping their internal values, plans, and actions? What thinking process is influencing their decision-making practices? The root of an action is directly connected to one's thinking process.

That being said, all professional behavior (healthy or unhealthy) is also connected to this process. For First Responder Departments to proactively engage and positively influence this thinking process would not only help to modify and enhance employee behavior but also heal the organizational culture, and in the process help to preserve its future. In my professional opinion organizations make a grave mistake if their main attention to wellness is centered around PTSD, solely focused as it relates to on the job stressors.

The following example demonstrates my assertion. A Fire Rescue personnel commences his/her career with a past history of family abuse and alcoholism. Unknown to himself/herself and the organization, the scars from his/her childhood experiences commence to affect personal and on the job relationships, as well as negatively impact his/her behavior on the field. Additionally, the barrier and self-defense mechanism created is so ingrained that he/she fails to see the erosion occurring inside. For years his supervisors have counseled him/her as to his discourteous comments and lack of empathy while servicing the community.

However, being a good test taker, he/she makes rank and progresses through the ranks encouraging unhealthy behavior. His/her behavior, now as a supervisor and leader, commence to advance and advocate a dysfunctional and unhealthy informal organizational culture. One can see how ignoring these types of situations can produce negative outcomes for the health of an organization. Equally important, the negative impact for the organization is dependent on how many individuals are affected by significant past experiences that are left untreated. If that number is high, and these types of situations are left untreated, then the impact on the organization, especially the informal culture, will be serious. From my optic, organizations pay a heavy price ignoring this reality.

FRAP Model

The First Responder Assistance Program/Model (FRAP) encompasses the following three Foundational Pillars:

1. Organizational and Individual Inner Healing
2. Positive and Constructive Organizational and Individual Growth
3. Fostering of Organizational and Individual Relationships and Resiliency

With this in mind, FRAP's mission is to help transform First Responder Communities (Organizations and Individuals) from a culture of isolation, distrust, fear, and unhealthy behavior, to a culture of organizational and individual healing, positive and constructive growth, and fostering of healthy relationships and resiliency.

Methodology

- In order to change a resistant culture, one must transform and modify the system from within (Organizational Intervention)
- The FRAP will first help identify unhealthy institutional and behavioral patterns hampering positive growth within First Responder Communities (Assessment of Formal and Informal Cultures)
- The FRAP will work hand in hand with First Responder Communities to implement and institutionalize a systemic progression of care that focuses on Pre-Situational, Situational, and Post-Situational responses, structured within a unified framework and system:
  - Peer Response and Follow-Through
  - Faith-Based Chaplaincy Support
  - Integration of Mental Health and Substance Abuse (Clinicians)

FRAP Modules

The FRAP Modules were created to ensure that First Responder Departments implementing the model understand the necessity to utilize the modules in support of enhancing the formal and informal organizational culture. The FRAP believes that an organizational intervention is not only the best manner in which to change the organizational culture, but also to provide the assistance and support needed to First Responders on the field. The FRAP Modules is comprised of the following:

1. Educational Module

The Educational Model facilitates awareness, understanding, and learning to the following stakeholders:

1. Executive Level Personnel
2. Operational Personnel
3. Support Personnel
4. Families and other Support Groups

The Awareness and Understanding Component of the Educational Module is composed of drills and interactive learning, utilized to retain knowledge and develop pertinent skills and good habits, as it relates to Peer Response, Chaplaincy, and Mental Health Clinicians participating in the FRAP.

The Informational Component of the Educational Module focuses on the importance of communication. The FRAP will work with First Responder Departments to create newsletters, videos, and online communication aimed to facilitate learning and reinforce skills related to Peer Response, Chaplaincy, and Mental Health Clinicians working within FRAP. The most critical element of the Educational Module is to enhance the existing organizational culture (both formal and informal).

2. Training Module

The Training Module facilitates organizational efforts to develop or enhance skills, improve performance, and inculcate individual self-fulfillment for the following stakeholders:

1. Executive Level Personnel
2. Operational Personnel
3. Support Personnel

The Formal Training Module utilizes best practices in the field to provide quality training at the Basic Level (all Departmental personnel), Intermediate Level (Peer Response Personnel), and Advance Level (Chaplaincy Personnel and Mental Health Clinicians). Chaplains and Mental Health Clinicians participating in the FRAP are required to also attend the Basic and Intermediate Levels of training to have a thorough understanding of the mindset and training received by Departmental personnel and peers.

3. Process Module

The Process Module examines the formal and informal organizational culture to determine systemic areas needing enhancement. The Process Module focuses on the following organizational and systemic areas:

- Assessment of Organizational Culture
    - Formal and Informal Culture
- Enhancement of Organizational Culture
    - Formal Culture
        - Enhancement of Policies, Procedures, Guidelines, Strategic Plans, Selection Process, Evaluation Process, Discipline Structure, and Promotional Process
    - Informal Culture
        - Fostering a healthy thinking process and modification of employee behavior
- Implementation and Institutionalization of FRAP
    - Critical Incident Peer Response and Follow-Through
    - Faith-Based Chaplaincy Support
    - Integration of Mental Health and Substance Abuse (Clinicians)

4. Mental Health Module

The Mental Health Module provides oversight and a sense of security and confidence to ensure that internal and external Clinicians are adhering to clinical best practices. Equally important the FRAP utilizes clinical oversight to seamlessly integrate the work being done by peers and chaplains. With this in mind, Clinical Oversight focuses on the following two areas:

- Clinician integration to Peers and Chaplains
- Check and balance related to therapeutic practices
- Clinician awareness training of First Responder culture

FRAP Step by Step Process and Methodology

FRAP personnel will work hand in hand with First Responder Departments to fully implement and institutionalize the FRAP Model within their internal organizational framework. FRAP personnel will also assist the Departments to fully implement **the four** FRAP modules (Educational, Training, Process, and Mental Health Oversight). The following depicts the implementation methodology utilized by the FRAP:

1. Assessment of organizational formal and informal culture
2. Work with stakeholder community (First Responder Department) to individualize the FRAP Model and reach a final consensus of the areas to be implemented and institutionalized
3. If desired by First Responder Department, selection of Pilot Project (Organizational Department, Section, or Entity)
4. Commence to work with selected department/organization to set up their own internal model integrated with best practices, as it relates to the progression of care (Chaplaincy Program, Critical Incident Peer Response System, Chaplaincy support, and Mental Health and Substance Abuse Clinician integration
5. Ensure selected department, section, or entity is incorporating Post Traumatic Growth (PTG) components within Pre-Crisis, Crisis Response, and Post-Crisis First Responder progression of care
6. Fully implement the FRAP Model in Pilot Project (organizational department, section, or entity)
7. Evaluate model as well as the Pre-Crisis, Crisis Response, and Post-Crisis Follow-up system of care (Pilot Project)
8. Fine tune any areas needing enhancement
9. Implement the model Department-wide
10. Fully institutionalize the model
11. Replicate model and implementation within other First Responder Departments and communities

FRAP Organizational Pillars

Foundational Pillar:

- Organizational and Individual Inner Healing
- Positive and Constructive Organizational and Individual Growth
- Fostering of Organizational and Individual Relationships and Resiliency

Structural Pillar:

- Peer Response System, Faith-Based Chaplaincy Support, and Mental Health and Substance Abuse Progression of Care fused within FRAP's Foundational Pillars (Organizational and Individual Inner Healing, Positive and Constructive Organizational and Individual Growth, and Fostering of Organizational and Individual Relationships and Resiliency)

Supporting Pillar of FRAP:

- Pre-Situational
  - Building Resiliency through Education, Communication, and Awareness aimed at enhancing organizational formal and informal cultures
- Situational Response
  - A response that is Timely, Appropriate and accomplished by Trained personnel
- Post Situational Response
  - Continuum of Care and Follow-Through at the Organizational and Individual Levels inclusive of possible clinician participation when needed or requested

Reinforcing Pillar:

- FRAP's Peer Response, Faith-Based Chaplaincy, and Mental Health and Substance Abuse Clinicians provide a continuum of care encompassing:
  - Education
  - Training
  - Experiential Involvement
  - Support Groups
  - Processes (Policies, Procedures, Guidelines, Strategic Plans)

SUMMARY

As has been shown, the organizational culture, both formal and informal, can produce both positive and negative effects on First Responders. In part, a First Responder's inner healing and growth is directly impacted by their organizational reality. If a First Responder's organizational reality demonstrates a culture of isolation, distrust, fear, and unbalanced behavior, it would be logical and expected for the First Responder's inner healing and growth to be severely impacted.

If one compounds this reality with a First Responder's past experiences and childhood significant events, as well as on the job meaningful stressors, it should not surprise anyone to see the data reflect a high percentage of suicides, substance abuse, domestic violence, and divorce from the First Responder Community. It is also prudent to deduce that if a First Responder's behavior reflects this type of pain and suffering (based on the data) in their personal life, one should not be surprised to find their quality

Figure 1. Organizational and relational intervention model First Responder Assistance Program (FRAP)

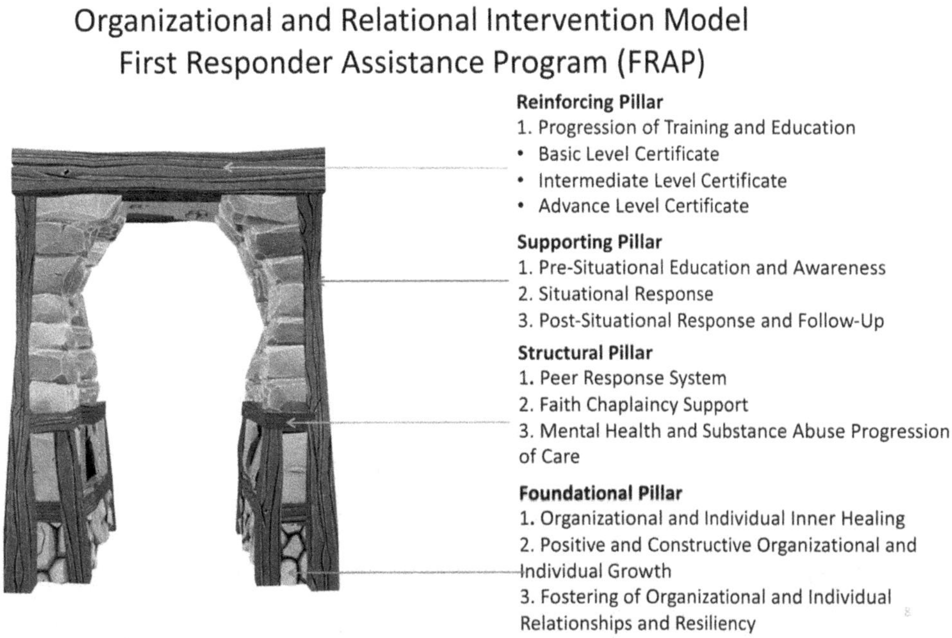

of service as it relates to their profession also diminishing in return. The FRAP focuses on the organization, with its overall mission to:

1. Foster Organizational and Individual Inner Healing
2. Foster Positive and Constructive Organizational and Individual Growth
3. Foster Organizational and Individual Relationships and Resiliency

The FRAP Model if properly implemented and institutionalized can greatly enhance an organization's formal and informal culture. Additionally, by integrating a unified structure and progression of care encompassing Peer Response, Chaplaincy, and mental health clinicians within the formal organizational culture of First Responder Departments, the FRAP can go a long way in bridging the gap that exists among management and First Responders. The implementation and institutionalization of FRAP clearly display an organizational culture that values its First Responders. FRAP's overall mission is to enhance the organizational culture of First Responders as well as to validate the values associated with the First Responder profession.

REFERENCES

Argyris, C. (1970). *Intervention Theory and Method: A Behavioral Science View*. Reading, MA: Addison-Wesley Publishing Company.

Carter, S. L. (1996). *Integrity*. Harper Collins Publishers.

Deming, W. E. (1982). *Out of the Crisis*. Massachusetts Institute of Technology.

Drucker, P. (1985). *Innovation and Entrepreneurship*. New York: Harper Row Publishing.

Harvard Business Review. (1997). *The Work of Leadership*. Author.

Hersey, P., & Blanchard, K. (2000). *Management of Organizational Behavior*. Prentice Hall Inc.

Jensen, R. A. (2000). *Mass Fatality and Casualty Incidents*. CRC Press LLC.

Kouzes, J., & Posner, B. (1997). *The Leadership Challenge*. San Francisco, CA: Jossey Bass.

Management Review. (1998). *Invigorating Change Initiatives*. Author.

McGregor, D. (1960). *The Human Side of Enterprise*. New York: McGraw-Hill Book Company.

Nations Business. (1998). *The Way of the Warrior: Leadership Lessons from History's Top Twelve Military Masters*. Author.

Peters, T., & Austin, N. (1985). *A Passion for Excellence – The Leadership Difference*. Random House, Inc.

Senge, P. (1994). *The Fifth Discipline – The Art & Practice of The Learning Organization*. Doubleday Dell Publishing.

Territo, L., & Vetter, H. J. (1981). *Stress and Police Personnel*. Allyn and Bacon, Inc.

Training & Development. (1998). *Leadership Lessons from the Magic Kingdom*. Author.

Training & Development. (1998). *The Teaching Organization*. Author.

Transformational leadership or effective managerial practices? (1998). *Group & Organization Management, 23*(3), 220-237.

Chapter 17
Changing Hearts and Minds: Getting Administrative Support for Delivery of Care

Kimberly Neisler
University of Central Florida, USA

Nancy Rosado
University of Central Florida, USA

Deborah C. Beidel
University of Central Florida, USA

ABSTRACT

By the nature of their occupation, first responders witness numerous traumatic events. Most of the time, their training and desire to help others allows them to respond professionally and appropriately. However, there are certain events that, for whatever reason, affect first responders in a more dramatic way, leading to emotional and behavioral changes that affect their interpersonal relationships and occupational functioning. Even if they recognize the need, first responders often are hesitant to reveal their distress and/or seek professional help to superiors, believing that they will be perceived as unfit for duty. In this chapter, the need for administrators to understand and accept the severe impact of traumatic events is discussed. Consistent with the individualized nature of traumatic responses, a tiered strategy of intervention is proposed. Finally, drawing from an occupational health perspective, a model that conceptualizes and responds to exposure to traumatic events as an occupational hazard is discussed.

INTRODUCTION

As you read this chapter, thousands of first responders are handling calls, hoping to positively impact the lives of perfect strangers who have called for help. Some of those calls will be life changing for the responder due to the intense nature of the event.

DOI: 10.4018/978-1-5225-9803-9.ch017

The occupation of a first responder is first and foremost to protect the community. This is a multifaceted occupation, with physical requirements and cognitive demands, and often needing to work in challenging environmental conditions. Throughout this book, there has been significant attention to the challenges that first responders face as they go about their jobs:

- A job that most people cannot do.
- A job that requires individuals to tolerate what is intolerable to others.
- A job that provides a front row seat for some of life's ugliest moments (i.e., overexposure to violence, death, extreme physical injury and life or death decision making).

Although, for the most part, first responders cope with their jobs well, there should never be any underestimation of the emotional toll that this constant exposure to traumatic events can take on someone. The effects of this cumulative stress can create a breaking point. Then, there are those events from which no one should just be able to walk away: The mass shootings that result in dozens of lives lost, the child who drowns in the family swimming pool, the horrific car accident where one of the victims is a first responder's family member or friend. As one first responder shared, "I'm retiring. I've seen one too many homicides, one too many suicides, one too many car wrecks."

BACKGROUND

First responders are exposed to traumatic events and stressors on a regular basis (Substance Abuse and Mental Health Services Administration, 2018). Not every event produces traumatic stress, and it is often not possible to predict which event will be "the one." Among 215 first responders requesting treatment at a University of Central Florida Posttraumatic Stress Disorder treatment clinic (UCF RESTORES), the traumatic events that precipitated the request for treatment are presented in Table 1.

Despite the type of event, the cumulative nature of exposure to trauma can result in high rates of depression, substance abuse, acute stress disorder, posttraumatic stress disorder (PTSD), and suicidal ideation/suicide. As to the latter, each year, more firefighters and law enforcement officers commit suicide than are killed in the line of duty (Heyman, Dill, & Douglas, 2018).

First responder suicides are serious events, and, in some cases, one suicide can give permission to others to do the same. A study of police officers in New York City (O'Neill, 2001) revealed that the mixture of a failed relationship, alcohol consumption, and accessibility of firearms was a deadly combination. When suicides occur, urging from upper level administrations to "ask for help" is common; yet, many first responders worry that admitting that they are experiencing emotional distress leaves them open to judgment by peers (can they be trusted to have their partner's back?), judgment by administration that could lead to negative career repercussions (should they be taken off the road because they may be a liability?) and self-doubt (can I trust myself to react).

Table 1. Types of traumatic event that precipitated a request for treatment

Traumatic Event	Percentage
Pediatric call	22%
Mass shooting	16%
Multiple events	13%
Death of family member or friend	11%
Motor vehicle accident with death	10%
Gory/graphic/dramatic death	8%
Near death experience	7%
Shooting	6%
Suicide calls	4%
Trauma not related to work	4%
Trauma during military service	3%
Sexual assault	1%

What is necessary is not an isolated response in a time of crisis, but a continuous recognition of the stressful nature of these occupations. In other words:

- First responders are equipped with a myriad of tools, techniques, and training to handle the physical aspects of the jobs.
- However, the protective gear does not protect them from the emotional distress as a result of dealing with traumatic events.
- Past culture encouraged a "suck it up, buttercup" environment. "You knew what you were getting into."
- It is time to bring the emotional impact of these jobs out of the shadows.
- Administrators must create an environment that allows that, while first responders protect, serve, and care for others as part of the profession, the same approach exists for those who are part of this profession.

PROMOTING A BEHAVIORAL HEALTH ASSISTANCE PROGRAM

Despite the acknowledgment that first responders are constantly exposed to traumatic events the general public seldom witnesses, attitudinal barriers often prevent someone from seeking help. One attitudinal barrier is the misconceptualization regarding the goal of a comprehensive behavioral health program, which is to return the first responder to full duty. However, in order for such a program to be effective, all of the elements should be in place in advance, not after someone steps forward and asks for help. First, it is important that the agency be able to provide a professional contact to make a competent assessment of the first responder's needs. When perceived favorably by personnel, this individual may be part of an Employee Assistance Program (EAP) or a private, culturally competent practitioner. An alternative contact to the agency's EAP is strongly recommended, in cases where feedback from first responders suggests that they are reluctant to trust, and therefore contact, the EAP. This person should also be able to provide any needed referrals. Second, although expertise in treating trauma is key, not every employee exhibiting impairment will be in need of treatment for PTSD. First responders are people and, in addition to trauma, face the same life challenges as every other member of the community. Thus, this individual and any referral sources should be able to provide counseling for common family and parenting issues as well as marital and relationships problems. Third, the agency must be prepared to deal quickly and effectively with stressors and issues that pose immediate difficulties for the first responder. This last point relates to crisis intervention and may require the need for individuals specifically trained in critical incident stress management (CISM) or psychological first aid.

The most effective Behavioral Health Assistance Programs have levels of intervention that are deployed consistently with the first responders' need. These different groups may operate independently or, in the case of a mass violence event, may be deployed simultaneously, and first responders in need are triaged based upon their response to the trauma.

Paraprofessional Services

One level of intervention is specialty trained peers. At most agencies, these peers are known as CISM teams. CISM is a procedure which is developed specifically to assist first responders who deal with a critical incident event. The goals of the CISM team are defusing and/or debriefing. Defusing is a short intervention that occurs typically within 24 hours of an event. Its goal is to allow people who are involved in the incident to learn about stress reactions and discuss their emotions. Debriefing is a more structured version of the same process and is typically conducted by a team of peers and professionals, again typically within 24-72 hours after the event. Defusing and debriefing are conducted separately, one session each with the goal of stabilization.

Other peer support teams represent a more extensive approach to stress management that can be called out during a critical incident or to deal with ongoing stressors first responders face. The idea behind peer support is that individuals in the military or first responder profession are very reluctant to seek treatment from a behavioral health professional or to reveal a mental health challenge, out of concern that doing so could be the end to a career. They are more likely to speak to peers who have similar experiences, background, and history. However, even here, there are concerns about confidentiality when the trained peer is part of the agency's peer support team. Unless there is an agreement with the agency, that conversations with a peer support team member are considered confidential, individuals in distress may be reluctant to be completely honest because the agency may require the team member to reveal shared information based on concerns about liability.

One peer support training program, which is known as REACT (Recognize, Evaluate, Advocate, Coordinate, and Track) (Marks et al., 2017), trains peers how to identify signs of stress and distress in their peers. Additionally, REACT teaches how to deliver emotional support, how to ask the difficult questions ("Are you thinking about hurting yourself?"), and how to effectively respond to the answers they receive ("Yeah, they are all better off without me"). Finally, peers who are trained in REACT learn when and how to reach out, and how to function as a resource for first responders and their families using the following training modules:

- Provide a mental schema for diagnosable disorders and familiarize attendees with available treatment options.
- Identify stress injuries.
- Initiate and maintain conversations and motivate peers to follow through with help-seeking behaviors.
- Facilitate acute stress management, including anger management and cognitive restructuring principles.

Throughout the workshop, it is repeatedly stressed that this training is not designed to train peers to diagnose or treat mental health disorders, but to recognize signs and assist peers in finding the appropriate remedies. Finally, in addition to providing support during and after traumatic events that result from work-related events, peer support teams can provide the first level of support for first responders experiencing personal and work-related stress.

Peer support and CISM teams are popular programs, but often face administrative concerns about agency liability, if the peer is acting as a therapist and concerns about "hiding" an impaired employee from superiors. These concerns are not always easy to overcome, although careful explanation and the high success rate of peer support teams to get impaired first responders into treatment will often assuage administrative fears.

Chaplaincy Programs

A second level of intervention are chaplaincy/spiritual programs. Originally used for department ceremonies or hospital visits, these individuals can be used for crisis response, if they are trained appropriately, and as members of peer support teams. Most individuals in the chaplaincy program are also employed as first responders, again allowing them to bridge the "culture gap" that sometimes plagues therapists or behavioral health specialists who do not understand the challenges and stressors of the profession. Disclosures to a chaplain (by the nature of their profession) are considered confidential, providing assurance that information will not be shared with administration.

Behavioral Health Professionals

The third level of intervention involves the use of behavioral health professionals (i.e., trained and licensed psychologists, social workers, mental health counselors, or psychiatrists who can provide intensive treatment). An important consideration is that the referral should be to a clinician who is experienced in the treatment of first responders–both in terms of understanding the culture and in treating the traumatic experiences that will be discussed. This is not always the therapist whose office is physically closest to their residence or place of work. Many first responders tell stories of finally asking for help and then being "fired" by the therapist, who revealed that the events the first responder described were "too traumatizing" for the therapist. This lack of cultural competency and the ability to hear and work with the traumas that first responders describe presents a major barrier to finding appropriate care. Administrators need to understand that not all therapists have the necessary therapeutic skills and to assist their agency in securing appropriate therapeutic resources.

In order to address this need for cultural competence, the Florida Firefighters Safety and Health Collaborative (www.floridafirefightersafety.org) has developed a two-day immersion course for mental health clinicians. This course is designed to teach firefighter culture and allow clinicians to more effectively treat firefighters. The two-day course includes the following topics and activities:

- Four hours of didactics on topics such as firefighter lingo, rescuer personality, firefighter family, retirees, and behavioral health challenges brought on by traumatic stress.
- Four hours of simulated firefighting in bunker gear, including live fire and smoke drill simulation.
- Four hours of fire station visits to understand the fire station layout and a typical day, and see the response to a call.
- Four hours of discussions of traumatic events firefighters have faced and facilitation of discussion.

In addition to the two-day course, clinicians must complete 10 hours of ride time at a fire rescue department. If it is successfully completed, the clinicians are included in a database (which is administered by the Florid Firefighters Safety and Health Collaborative) of culturally competent therapists. According to the collaborative, these courses have been very popular across the state of Florida and, hopefully, will lead to therapists who are better able to understand and assist firefighters seeking behavioral health treatment. Should this program prove successful, as determined by an increase in the number of culturally competent therapists delivering evidence-based treatments with positive therapeutic outcomes, these classes could serve as a model for cultural training for other first responders.

A COMPREHENSIVE STANDARD OF CARE FOR FIRST RESPONDERS

The types of intervention represent only the first steps to get administrative support for addressing the traumatic effects of stress in first responders. They all represent actions that should be taken after the traumatic injury has occurred. As the recognition of the potential long-term psychological impact upon the career of first responders becomes more apparent, several states have passed legislation to include a primary diagnosis of PTSD as a recognized condition that must be addressed by Workman's Compensation. Standard of care is defined as the "degree of care (watchfulness, attention, caution, and prudence) that a reasonable person should exercise under the circumstances. Individuals who do not meet the standard of care could be liable for negligence" ("Standard of care," 2019). To date, no recognized standard of care exists for the treatment of PTSD in first responders. The subsection below presents the critical components of a comprehensive standard of care.

Necessary Attitudes for Implementing a Standard of Care

This chapter is subtitled *Getting Administrative Support for Delivery of Care* because, without support at the administrative level, first responders will continue to hide in the shadows (or be hidden by their colleagues), believing that requesting treatment for PTSD and other trauma disorders will be the end of their career. Thus, hearing from the administration that "it's OK to ask for help" is an important attitude that must be communicated from the top level of the administration, but there is a need for more than simple worlds. One approach toward prevention of suicide among police officers could be easily adapted to deal more broadly with first responder mental health. The approach, based on an occupational-health assessment protocol (Fein, 1998, cited in Amsel, Placidi, Hendin, O'Neill, & Mann, 2001), begins by acknowledging that traumatic stress is an occupational hazard for first responders. The next subsection analyzes the specific steps to implement this occupational health model and the required resources to do so. However, prior to that discussion, other basic attitudinal changes are necessary.

Administrators are charged with responsibility for running operations and being aware of what is happening within their command. This responsibility often clashes with the need for confidentiality. In fact, maintaining confidentiality is key to first responders deciding to seek treatment. Although for administrative and manpower purposes supervisors may need to know that someone needs time off from work to attend appointments, the specifics of the problem do not need to be shared. The exception is when the first responder is in danger of harming him/herself or another person. Then, supervisors, and in fact anyone aware of such a threat, must act. A voluntary commitment is always preferable, but, at times, involuntary evaluation and treatment may be necessary. Again, preparation and forethought are critical. First responders take others to the emergency room all the time, meaning that they are known at mental health receiving facilities. Having a standing arrangement with a mental health service facility in another jurisdiction or county (where the first responder is not known) can prevent embarrassment or anger, when it is the first responder who is escorted by police officers into an emergency room because of the need for involuntary hospitalization.

Often, supervisors (i.e., chief, sheriff, or lieutenant) are unwilling to give up the control or uncomfortable with not knowing the details of the first responder's mental health treatment. It is important to train a supervisor as well as the team, and give them the necessary tools, directions, and discretion to carry out their assignment. Certainly, supervisors must hold the team accountable, but only the team supervisors should be aware of the nature and reason for intervention. The goal is to get first responders (any department's most valuable assets) the help that they need to perform at optimal level and provide the needed community service. These conversations need to involve human resources, employee assistance program personnel, worker's compensation carriers, legal offices, and government officials.

Undoubtedly, providing this level of care and maintaining a "hands-off" attitude is easier in smaller municipalities than it is in larger districts or major cities, where there is more media scrutiny when something "goes wrong." Similarly, situations become more complicated when employees are represented by a union. Despite the intricacies that are involved in any particular department, the overall goal remains the same (i.e., creating an atmosphere where a first responder can step forward and ask for help as the result of traumatic experiences), whether a singular horrific incidence or the cumulative effect of years of responding to community events occurs.

A Comprehensive Model for Building a First Responder Standard of Care

Returning to the idea of traumatic stress as an occupational hazard for first responders, below, the authors detail a protocol for the implementation of occupational-health assessment, modified for mental health (Amsel et al., 2001; Kahn 1993, cited in Amsel et al., 2001):

1. Identify a health problem with an elevated incidence in the occupation.
2. Identify the risk factors for the problem.
3. Identify which of the established risk factors has elevated exposure in the population.
4. Modify work processes to reduce exposure to the hazard, where possible.
5. Introduce protective factors.

6. Monitor and treat sequelae of exposure.

Identify a Health Problem

At least 20 years of evidence show that more first responders die as a result of suicide than in the line of duty. Although the primary reason for suicide in police officers appears to be failed relationships, the reasons for the failed relationships may be varied, but certainly includes PTSD in the first responder. With mass violence events such as 9/11/2001 and mass shootings in communities across the nation, there is now general acknowledgement that "stuff it away" is no longer appropriate and that traumatic stress responses represent an occupational health problem.

Identify Risk Factors for the Problem

As defined by the *Diagnostic and Statistical Manual of Mental Disorders (5th edition)* (American Psychiatric Association, 2013), the onset PTSD and other trauma-related disorders is the existence of a traumatic event. Thus, traumatic events represent the primary risk factor. Other factors include family and personal history, prior exposure to traumatic events, economic factors, and other personal risk factors, such as sex.

Identify Which of the Established Risk Factors Has Elevated Exposure in the Population

Exposure to a traumatic event, such as witnessing the violent death or severe bodily injury of another person, is an unlikely event for most individuals, perhaps occurring once or twice in a lifetime. For others, such as those in the military and first responders, it is a common and, for some first responders, almost daily event. Thus, the primary risk factor for traumatic stress is one to which first responders are exposed to repeatedly. This heightens their risk for negative emotional responses, which can include, but are not necessarily limited to, PTSD.

Modify Work Processes to Reduce Exposure to the Hazard Where Possible

It is unlikely that the nature of the work of the first responder allows the modification of work processes to reduce exposure to traumatic events. First responders who seek treatment do not want to return to a "desk job." They want to return to full duty. Although a standard of care should carefully examine procedures and best practices that might lower the risk of exposure, more effort should be spent introducing protective factors and monitoring and treating the sequelae of exposure.

Introduce Protective Factors

The first responder community can take a myriad of actions to serve as protective factors. First, the topics of trauma, traumatic stress, the aftermath of trauma, resiliency, and the various behavioral and emotional disorders that can result from trauma should be an integral part of every recruit's training. The introduction of these topics prior to beginning the actual job will not inoculate someone against the effects of trauma, but, when the new recruit does have a "bad call" and is feeling typical posttraumatic stress, the recruit may at least recall that such effects are common after such an event and do not indicate weakness. Education about these issues should also be part of any family orientation that occurs at this time. Additionally, continuing education of all officers regarding, for example, mental health topics, the biology of trauma, stress and stress management, sleep hygiene, anger management, interpersonal relationships, and financial stressors would be a potential potent protective factor. To date, no agreed-upon standardized or even "sample" curriculum are available, even though such standards would be welcomed by the field.

Although education is an important first step, a successful standard of care cannot end there. CISM and peer support teams are another type of protective factor that contribute to a complete standard of care. Earlier in this chapter, the authors noted the composition and purpose of CISM teams (i.e., defusings and debriefings). Defusings are conducted as brief conversations by the team to assess, triage and mitigate symptoms and occur within hours after a critical incident. Debriefings use a 7-phase model, are more in depth and occur up to 10 days out from incident and even later if the incident involved large numbers of responders (Sept. 11th is a good example). Good practice among CISM teams will include a licensed mental health professional, in order to assure confidentiality of the discussions. It is critical that, while attendance in these defusings and debriefings may be mandatory, speaking in the sessions must always be voluntary. Forcing people to speak during these meetings has been demonstrated to create psychological harm.

Peer support teams fulfill many functions as CISM teams, but often also function in situations outside of a critical incident. Not all administrations embrace peer support programs, but, when there is administrative support, peer support becomes a critical part of first responder culture. Peer support is useful when first responders have limited opportunities to access formal mental health treatment or when first responders have concerns about the stigma or negative changes in job duties or pay should they engage in mental health treatment. Data suggest that first responders who receive early regular peer support report (a) significant gains in cognitive functioning, (b) improved social and over all functioning, and (c) decrease in psychiatric symptoms (e.g., Repper &Carter, 2011).

Finally, prevention may include an overall focus on general wellness and well-being. Having easy access to gym facilities, educational classes/workshops on health topics, wellness tips delivered via email or text, and health fairs are examples of methods to promote wellness, decrease stress, and reduce vulnerability to traumatic stress. If administrators lead by example and encourage the use of these opportunities, that culture of "taking care of our own" will permeate through the agency.

Monitor and Treat Sequelae of Exposure

Not everyone responds to trauma in the same fashion. It is a mistake to assume that, after even the most horrific mass casualty event, *everyone* will develop PTSD or that *no one* will develop PTSD. Part of developing a standard of care is acknowledging that not everyone reacts to an event in the same fashion, and that immediately rushing in to provide treatment can create more damage than good. In some individuals, temporary symptoms may be present immediately after an event, but decrease over a period of weeks. In instances where many members of a department may be impacted by the same traumatic event, establishing a voluntary monitoring program over 30 to 60 days will help determine those whose symptoms are remitting vs. those whose symptoms are stable or worsening.

However, there comes a time when even the best education and prevention strategies are not enough to prevent the onset of behavioral health disorders such as depression, anxiety, PTSD, or substance abuse. Various appropriate treatment options exist. The key is finding therapists who are culturally competent and use evidence-based interventions.

FUTURE DIRECTIONS

As the number of states who consider PTSD as a workman's compensation issue continues to grow, to date, there is minimal vetting of potential providers by Employee Assistance Programs, who typically accept a therapist's self-declaration as "experienced in treating trauma." Unfortunately, many therapists who claim that distinction have had no experience with either first responder culture or the type of traumas that they experience. As the authors noted above, first responders often describe being "fired" as patients by therapists who indicate that the traumas the first responders revealed were too upsetting for the therapist to handle. Given the reluctance of most first responders to seek treatment, having a bad experience with an ill-prepared and improperly trained therapist will discourage many of them from seeking further treatment. Thus, imperative for any standard of care are clinicians who have been trained and certified as culturally competent (i.e., they understand first responder culture) and well-versed in evidence-based treatments for trauma disorders. Cultivating such therapists will require collaboration between the first responders community and university-based training clinics.

CONCLUSION

This chapter addressed the issues and challenges in implementing behavioral health programs for first responders, especially getting substantive support from departmental administrations. Support is more than just a statement that "It is ok to not be ok." It requires the establishment and support of programs that are put in place with initial training and continue throughout the life of the first responder, including first responders who have retired. The authors hope that this chapter will motivate others to work with the administrative arms of their organizations to develop a comprehensive standard of care to address the psychological occupational hazards that are an integral part of the career of a first responder.

ACKNOWLEDGMENT

This research was supported in part by the Department of Justice Antiterrorism and Emergency Assistance Program [2017-RF-GX-0003].

REFERENCES

American Psychiatric Association. (2013). *Diagnostic and statistical manual of mental disorders* (5th ed.). Washington, DC: American Psychiatric Association Press.

Amsel, L., Placidi, G., Hendin, H., O'Neill, M., & Mann, J. J. (2001). An evidence-based educational intervention to improve evaluation and preventive services for officers at risk for suicidal behaviors. In D. C. Sheehan (Ed.), *Suicide and law enforcement* (pp. 17–30). Quantico, VA: Department of Justice.

Heyman, M., Dill, J., & Douglas, R. (2018). *Ruderman white paper on mental health and suicide of first responders*. Boston, MA: Ruderman Family Foundation.

Marks, M. R., Bowers, C., DePesa, N. S., Trachik, B., Deavers, F. E., & James, N. T. (2017). REACT: A paraprofessional training program for first responders – A pilot study. *Bulletin of the Menninger Clinic, 81*(2), 150–165. doi:10.1521/bumc.2017.81.2.150 PMID:28609149

O'Neill, M. (2001). Police suicides in the New York City Police Department: Causal factors and remedial measures. In D. C. Sheehan & J. I. Warren (Eds.), *Suicide and Law Enforcement* (pp. 139–149). Quantico, VA: U.S. Department of Justice.

Repper, J., & Carter, T. (2011). A review of the literature on peer support in mental health services. *Journal of Mental Health (Abingdon, England), 20*(4), 392–411. doi:10.3109/09638237.2011.583947 PMID:21770786

Standard of Care. (2019). In *Nolo*. Retrieved from https://www.nolo.com/dictionary/standard-of-care-term.html

Substance Abuse and Mental Health Services Administration. (2018). *First responders: Behavioral health concerns, emergency response, and trauma*. Washington, DC: SAMHSA.

KEY TERMS AND DEFINITIONS

Behavioral Health: A field of study that examines how emotions and behavior affect psychological and physical well-being.

Cultural Competence: In healthcare, it is the ability to deliver care to someone with an understanding of their unique perspective, values, and needs.

First Responder: An individual uniquely trained and responsible for going to a place where there is a need for emergency assistance.

Occupational Health Assessment: An examination conducted by a professional to determine environmental adjustments that might be made to promote a healthy working environment.

Peer Support: The use of specially trained individuals to provide emotional and behavioral support to their colleagues.

Standard of Care: A process, procedure, or course of treatment that clinicians follow and that is accepted as an appropriate approach by their professional community.

Trauma: An experience that creates deep emotional distress for an individual.

Compilation of References

Adams, K., Shakespeare-Finch, J., & Armstrong, D. (2015). An interpretative phenomenological analysis of stress and well-being in emergency medical dispatchers. *Journal of Loss and Trauma*, *20*(5), 430–448. doi:10.1080/15325024.2014.949141

Adler, A., Bliese, P. D., McGurk, D., Hoge, C. W., & Castro, C. A. (2009). Battlemind debriefing and battlemind training as early interventions with soldiers returning from Iraq: Randomization by platoon. *Journal of Consulting and Clinical Psychology*, *77*(5), 928–940. doi:10.1037/a0016877 PMID:19803572

Adler, A., Litz, B., Castro, C. A., Suvak, M., Thomas, J. L., Burrell, L., ... Bliese, P. D. (2008). A group randomized trial of critical incident stress debriefing provided to U.S. peacekeepers. *Journal of Traumatic Stress*, *21*(3), 253–263. doi:10.1002/jts.20342 PMID:18553407

Affleck, G., & Tennen, H. (1996). Construing benefits from adversity: Adaptational significance and dispositional underpinnings. *Journal of Personality*, *64*(4), 899–922. doi:10.1111/j.1467-6494.1996.tb00948.x PMID:8956517

Agaibi, C. E., & Wilson, J. P. (2005). Trauma, PTSD, and resilience: A review of the literature. *Trauma, Violence & Abuse*, *6*(3), 195–216. doi:10.1177/1524838005277438 PMID:16237155

Agnew, J., McDiarmid, M. A., Lees, P. S. J., & Duffy, R. (1991). Reproductive hazards of firefighting. I. Non-chemical hazards. *American Journal of Industrial Medicine*, *19*(4), 433–445. doi:10.1002/ajim.4700190403 PMID:2035545

Air Line Pilots Association (ALPA). (1997). *Critical Incident Response Program Guide*. Herndon, VA: ALPA.

Alkus, S., & Padesky, C. (1983). Special problems of police officers: Stress-related issues and interventions. *The Counseling Psychologist*, *11*(2), 55–64. doi:10.1177/0011000083112010

Allen, C. E., Mercer, M. C., & Lilly, M. M. (2016). Duty-related posttraumatic stress symptoms in 911 telecommunicators: The roles of childhood trauma exposure and emotion-focused coping. *Journal of Aggression, Maltreatment & Trauma*, *25*(7), 686–701. doi:10.1080/10926771.2016.1175534

Alvord, M. K., & Grados, J. J. (2005). Enhancing resilience in children: A proactive approach. *Professional Psychology, Research and Practice*, *36*(3), 238–245. doi:10.1037/0735-7028.36.3.238

Amani, R., & Gill, T. (2013). Shift working, nutrition and obesity: Implications for workforce health- a systematic review. *Asia Pacific Journal of Clinical Nutrition*, *22*(4), 505–515. PMID:24231009

Amaranto, E., Steinberg, J., Castellano, C., & Mitchell, R. (2003). Police stress interventions. *Brief Treatment and Crisis Intervention*, *3*(1), 47–54. doi:10.1093/brief-treatment/mhg001

Amendola, K. L., & Davis, R. C. (2019). *Best practices in early intervention system implementation and use in law enforcement agencies*. Washington, DC: National Police Foundation.

American Counseling Association. (2005). *ACA Code of Ethics*. Alexandria, VA: Author.

American Psychiatric Association. (1954). *First Aid for Psychological Reactions in Disasters*. Washington, DC: American Psychiatric Association.

American Psychiatric Association. (2013). *Diagnostic and statistical manual of mental disorders* (5th ed.). Arlington, VA: Author.

American Psychiatric Association. (2013). *Diagnostic and Statistical Manual of Mental Disorders* (5th ed.). Washington, DC: Author.

American Psychological Association. (2002). Ethical principles of psychologists and code of conduct. *The American Psychologist*, *57*(12), 1060–1073. doi:10.1037/0003-066X.57.12.1060 PMID:12613157

American Psychological Association. (2005, August). *Policy statement on evidence-based practice in psychology.* Meeting of the APA Council of Representatives. Retrieved from http://www.apa.org/practice/guidelines/evidence-based-statement.aspx

American Psychological Association. (2017) *Multicultural Guidelines: An ecological approach to context, identity, and intersectionality*. Retrieved from http://www.apa.org/about/policy/multicultural-guidelines.aspx

Amir, M., Weil, G., Kaplan, Z., Tocker, T., & Witzum, E. (1998). Debriefing with group psychotherapy in a homogenous group of non-injured victims of a terrorist attack: A prospective study. *Acta Psychiatrica Scandinavica*, *98*(3), 237–242. doi:10.1111/j.1600-0447.1998.tb10074.x PMID:9761413

Amsel, L., Placidi, G., Hendin, H., O'Neill, M., & Mann, J. J. (2001). An evidence-based educational intervention to improve evaluation and preventive services for officers at risk for suicidal behaviors. In D. C. Sheehan (Ed.), *Suicide and law enforcement* (pp. 17–30). Quantico, VA: Department of Justice.

Andersen, J. P., & Gustafsberg, H. (2016). A training method to improve police use of force decision making: A randomized controlled trial. *SAGE Open*, *6*(2). doi:10.1177/2158244016638708

Anshel, M. H. (2000). A conceptual model and implications for coping with stressful events in police work. *Criminal Justice and Behavior*, *27*(3), 375–400. doi:10.1177/0093854800027003006

Antecol, H., & Cobb-Clark, D. (2006). The sexual harassment of female active-duty personnel: Effects on job satisfaction and intentions to remain in the military. *Journal of Economic Behavior & Organization*, *61*(1), 55–80. doi:10.1016/j.jebo.2004.11.006

Appel, J. W., Beebe, G. W., & Hilgardner, D. W. (1946). Comparative incidence of neuropsychiatric casualties in World War I and World War II. *The American Journal of Psychiatry*, *102*(2), 196–199. doi:10.1176/ajp.103.2.196 PMID:21001991

Arble, E., & Arnetz, B. B. (2016). A model of first-responder coping: An approach/avoidance bifurcation. *Stress and Health: Journal of the International Society for the Investigation of Stress.* doi:10.1002mi.2692

Arble, E., Daugherty, A. M., & Arnetz, B. B. (2018). Models of first responder coping: Police officers as a unique population. *Stress and Health*, *34*(5), 612–621. doi:10.1002mi.2821 PMID:29882624

Arble, E., Lumley, M. A., Pole, N., Blessman, J., & Arnetz, B. B. (2017). Refinement and preliminary testing of an imagery-based program to improve coping and performance and prevent trauma among urban police officers. *Journal of Police and Criminal Psychology*, *32*(1), 1–10. doi:10.100711896-016-9191-z PMID:28439149

Arbona, C., & Schwartz, J. P. (2016). Posttraumatic stress disorder symptom clusters, depression, alcohol abuse, and general stress among Hispanic male firefighters. *Hispanic Journal of Behavioral Sciences*, *38*(4), 507–522. doi:10.1177/0739986316661328

Argyris, C. (1970). *Intervention Theory and Method: A Behavioral Science View*. Reading, MA: Addison-Wesley Publishing Company.

Arnett, J. (2008). The neglected 95%: Why American psychology needs to become less American. *The American Psychologist*, *63*(70), 602–614. doi:10.1037/0003-066X.63.7.602 PMID:18855491

Arnetz, B. B., Arble, E., Backman, L., Lynch, A., & Lublin, A. (2013). Assessment of a prevention program for work-related stress among urban police officers. *International Archives of Occupational and Environmental Health*, *86*(1), 79–88. doi:10.100700420-012-0748-6 PMID:22366986

Arnetz, B. B., Nevedal, D. C., Lumley, M. A., Backman, L., & Lublin, A. (2009). Trauma resilience training for police: Psychophysiological and performance effects. *Journal of Police and Criminal Psychology*, *24*(1), 1–9. doi:10.100711896-008-9030-y

Arrigo, B. A., & Garsky, K. (1997). Police suicide: A glimpse behind the badge. In R. Dunham & J. Alpert (Eds.), *Critical issues in policing: Contemporary readings* (3rd ed.). Long Grove, IL: Waveland Press.

Artiss, K. (1963). Human behavior under stress: From combat to social psychiatry. *Military Medicine*, *128*(10), 1011–1015. doi:10.1093/milmed/128.10.1011 PMID:14055063

Ashbury, F. D., Cameron, C., Mercer, S. L., Fitch, M., & Nielsen, E. (1998). One-on-one peer support and quality of life for breast cancer patients. *Patient Education and Counseling*, *35*(2), 89–100. doi:10.1016/S0738-3991(98)00035-4 PMID:10026552

Asmundson, G. J., & Stapleton, J. A. (2008). Associations between dimensions of anxiety sensitivity and PTSD symptom clusters in active-duty police officers. *Cognitive Behaviour Therapy*, *37*(2), 66–75. doi:10.1080/16506070801969005 PMID:18470738

Asnaani, A., & Hofmann, S. G. (2012). Collaboration in multicultural therapy: Establishing a strong therapeutic alliance across cultural lines. *Journal of Clinical Psychology*, *68*(2), 187–197. doi:10.1002/jclp.21829 PMID:23616299

Backman, L., Arnetz, B. B., Levin, D., & Lublin, Å. (1997). Psychophysiological effects of mental imaging training for police trainees. *Stress Medicine*, *13*(1), 43–48. doi:10.1002/(SICI)1099-1700(199701)13:1<43::AID-SMI716>3.0.CO;2-6

Back, S. E., Foa, E. B., Killeen, T. K., Mills, K. L., Teesson, M., Dansky Cotton, B., & Brady, K. T. (2015). *Treatments that work. Concurrent treatment of PTSD and substance use disorders using prolonged exposure (COPE): Therapist guide*. New York, NY: Oxford University Press.

Badge of Life. (2018). *Psychological survival for police officers*. Retrieved from https://www.badgeoflife.org

Bailey, W., & Hightower, S. (1996). *Critical Incident Response Program*. Dallas, TX: Southwest Airlines Pilots' Association, Transport Workers Union.

Baird, S., & Jenkins, S. (2003). Vicarious traumatization, secondary traumatic stress, and burnout in sexual assault and domestic violence agency staff. *Violence and Victims*, *18*(1), 71–86. doi:10.1891/vivi.2003.18.1.71 PMID:12733620

Bakker, A. B., Demerouti, E., & Euwema, M. C. (2005). Job resources buffer the impact of job demands on burnout. *Journal of Occupational Health Psychology*, *10*(2), 170–180. doi:10.1037/1076-8998.10.2.170 PMID:15826226

Ballenger, J. F., Best, S. R., Metzler, T. J., Wasserman, D. A., Mohr, D. C., Liberman, A., ... Marmar, C. R. (2011). Patterns and predictors of alcohol use in male and female urban police officers. *The American Journal on Addictions*, *20*(1), 21–29. doi:10.1111/j.1521-0391.2010.00092.x PMID:21175917

Bandura, A. (1977). Self-efficacy: Toward a unifying theory of behavioral change. *Psychological Review*, *84*(2), 191–215. doi:10.1037/0033-295X.84.2.191 PMID:847061

Bandura, A. (1997). *Self-efficacy: The exercise of Control*. New York, NY: W.H. Freeman and Company.

Bandura, A. (1997). *Self-efficacy: The exercise of control*. New York: Freeman.

Bandura, A. (2005). The evolution of social cognitive theory. In K. G. Smith & M. A. Hitt (Eds.), *Great minds in management: The process of theory development* (pp. 9–35). New York, NY: Oxford University Press.

Bandura, A. (2007). An agentic perspective on positive psychology. In S. J. Lopez (Ed.), *Positive psychology: Expecting the best in people* (pp. 167–196). Westport, CT: Greenwood Publishing Company.

Barnard, L. K., & Curry, J. F. (2011). Self-compassion as a mechanism of change in mindfulness and acceptance-based treatments. In R. A. Baer (Ed.), *Assessing mindfulness and acceptance processes in clients: Illuminating the theory and practice of change* (pp. 135–153). Oakland, CA: New Harbinger Publications.

Barren, J. R. (2005). Use of existential-phenomenological counseling for police officers. *Policing: An International Journal of Police Strategies & Management*, *28*(2), 255–268. doi:10.1108/13639510510597898

Bartel, A. P. (1981). Race differences in job satisfaction: A reappraisal. *The Journal of Human Resources*, *16*(2), 294–303. doi:10.2307/145514

Başoğlu, M., & Mineka, S. (1992). The role of uncontrollable and unpredictable stress in post-traumatic stress responses in torture survivors. In M. Başoğlu (Ed.), *Torture and Its Consequences: Current Treatment Approaches* (pp. 182–225). New York, NY: Cambridge University Press.

Beaton, R. D., & Murphy, S. A. (1993). Sources of occupational stress among firefighters/EMTs and firefighters/paramedics and correlations with job-related outcomes. *Prehospital and Disaster Medicine*, *8*(2), 140–150. doi:10.1017/S1049023X00040218 PMID:10155458

Beaton, R. D., & Murphy, S. A. (1995). Working with people in crisis: Research implications. In C. R. Figly (Ed.), *Compassion fatigue: Coping with secondary traumatic stress disorder in those who treat the traumatized* (pp. 51–81). Philadelphia, PA: Brunner/Mazel.

Beck Institute for Cognitive Behavior Therapy. (2015). Retrieved from https://beckinstitute.org/

Behr, R. (2000). *Under the headset: Surviving dispatcher stress*. Wildomar, CA: Staggs.

Beidel, D. C., Frueh, B. C., Neer, S. M., Bowers, S. M., Bowers, C. A., Trachik, B., ... Grubaugh, A. (2019). Trauma Management Therapy with virtual-reality augmented exposure therapy for combat-related PTSD: A randomized controlled trial. *Journal of Anxiety Disorders*, *61*, 64–74. doi:10.1016/j.janxdis.2017.08.005 PMID:28865911

Beidel, D. C., Frueh, B. C., Uhde, T. W., Wong, N., & Mentrikoski, J. (2011). Multicomponent behavioral treatment for chronic combat-related posttraumatic stress disorder: A randomized controlled trial. *Journal of Anxiety Disorders*, *25*(2), 224–231. doi:10.1016/j.janxdis.2010.09.006 PMID:20951543

Beidel, D. C., Frueh, C. B., Neer, S. M., & Lejuez, C. W. (2017). The efficacy of Trauma Management Therapy: A controlled pilot investigation of a three-week intensive outpatient program for combat-related PTSD. *Journal of Anxiety Disorders*, *50*(May), 23–32. doi:10.1016/j.janxdis.2017.05.001 PMID:28545005

Belsher, B. E., Ruzek, J. I., Bongar, B., & Cordova, M. J. (2012). Social constraints, posttraumatic cognitions, and posttraumatic stress disorder in treatment-seeking trauma survivors: Evidence for a social-cognitive processing model. *Psychological Trauma: Theory, Research, Practice, and Policy*, *4*(4), 386–391. doi:10.1037/a0024362

Bendix, J. (2019). The real reason docs burn out. *Medical Economics*, *96*(2), 14–25.

Benedek, D. M., Fullerton, C., & Ursano, R. (2007). First responders: Mental health consequences of natural and human-made disasters for public health and public safety workers. *Annual Review of Public Health*. doi:10.1146/annurev.publichealth.28.021406.144037 PMID:17367284

Benight, C. C., & Harper, M. L. (2002). Coping self-efficacy perceptions as a mediator between acute stress response and long-term distress following natural disasters. *Journal of Traumatic Stress: Official Publication of The International Society for Traumatic Stress Studies*, *15*(3), 177–186. doi:10.1023/A:1015295025950 PMID:12092909

Benner, A. (1982, August). *Concerns cops have about shrinks*. Paper presented at the annual meeting of the American Psychological Association, San Francisco, CA.

Bennett, L. (2008). Narrative methods and children: Theoretical explanations and practice issues. *Journal of Child and Adolescent Psychiatric Nursing*, *21*(1), 13–23. doi:10.1111/j.1744-6171.2008.00125.x PMID:18269408

Berg, A. M., Hem, E., Lau, B., Haseth, K., & Ekeberg, O. (2005). Stress in the Norwegian police service. *Occupational Medicine*, *55*(2), 113–120. doi:10.1093/occmed/kqi023 PMID:15757985

Berger, W., Coutinho, E. S., Figueira, I., Marques-Portella, C., Luz, M. P., Neylan, T. C., ... Mendlowicz, M. V. (2012). Rescuers at risk, a systematic literature review and meta-regression analysis of the worldwide current prevalence and correlates of PTSD in rescue workers. *Social Psychiatry and Psychiatric Epidemiology*, *47*(6), 1001–1011. doi:10.100700127-011-0408-2 PMID:21681455

Berger, W., Figueira, I., Maurat, A. M., Bucassio, E. P., Vieira, I., Jardim, S. R., ... Mendlowicz, M. V. (2007). Partial and full PTSD in Brazilian ambulance workers: Prevalence and impact on health and on quality of life. *Journal of Traumatic Stress*, *20*(4), 637–642. doi:10.1002/jts.20242 PMID:17721969

Bergin, A. J., & Pakenham, K. I. (2016). The stress-buffering role of mindfulness in the relationship between perceived stress and psychological adjustment. *Mindfulness*, *7*(4), 928–939. doi:10.100712671-016-0532-x

Bergman, A. L., Christopher, M. S., & Bowen, S. (2016). Changes in facets of mindfulness predict stress and anger outcomes for police officers. *Mindfulness*, *7*(4), 851–858. doi:10.100712671-016-0522-z

Bergman, H. E., Przeworski, A., & Feeny, N. C. (2016). Rates of subthreshold PTSD among U.S. military veterans and service members: A literature review. *Military Psychology*, *29*(2), 117–127. doi:10.1037/mil0000154 PMID:28630531

Bernard, B., Driscoll, R., Kitt, M., West, C., & Tak, S. (2006). Health hazard evaluation of police officers and firefighters after hurricane Katrina - New Orleans, Louisiana, October 17-28 and November 30 - December 5, 2005. *Morbidity and Mortality Weekly Report*, *55*(16), 456–458. PMID:16645571

Berne, E. (1985). *Games people play: The basic handbook of transactional analysis*. New York: Ballantine Books.

Bernert, R. A., Kim, J. S., Iwata, N. G., & Perlis, M. L. (2015). Sleep disturbances as an evidence-based suicide risk factor. *Current Psychiatry Reports*, *17*(3), 15. doi:10.100711920-015-0554-4 PMID:25698339

Berninger, A., Webber, M. P., Cohen, H. W., Gustave, J., Lee, R., Niles, J. K., ... Prezant, D. J. (2010). Trends of elevated PTSD risk in firefighters exposed to the World Trade Center disaster: 2001-2005. *Public Health Reports*, *125*(4), 556–566. PMID:20597456

Berninger, A., Webber, M. P., Niles, J. K., Gustave, J., Lee, R., Cohen, H. W., ... Prezant, D. J. (2010). Longitudinal study of probable post-traumatic stress disorder in firefighters exposed to the World Trade Center disaster. *American Journal of Industrial Medicine*, *53*(12), 1177–1185. PMID:20862700

Bertoia, T. (2008). Developing an early intervention system for police misconduct in a law enforcement agency. *New South Wales Police Integrity Commission Research and Issues Papers*, *1*, 1–31.

Bisson, J. I., Jenkins, P. L., Alexander, J., & Bannister, C. (1997). Randomised controlled trial of psychological debriefing for victims of acute burn trauma. *The British Journal of Psychiatry*, *171*(1), 78–81. doi:10.1192/bjp.171.1.78 PMID:9328501

Bisson, J. I., McFarlane, A. C., Rose, S., Ruzek, J. I., & Watson, P. J. (2009). Psychological debriefing for adults. In E. B. Foa, T. M. Keane, M. J. Friedman, & J. A. Cohen (Eds.), *Effective treatments for ptsd (pp. 83 - 104)*. New York, NY: The Guilford Press.

Blau, G., Eggerichs-Purcell, J., & Bentley, M. A. (2012). Testing the impact of emotional labor on work exhaustion for three distinct emergency medical service (EMS) samples. *Career Development International*, *17*(7), 626–645. doi:10.1108/13620431211283788

Blevins, C. A., Weathers, F. W., Davis, M. T., Witte, T. K., & Domino, J. L. (2015). The posttraumatic stress disorder checklist for DSM-5 (PCL-5): Development and initial psychometric evaluation. *Journal of Traumatic Stress*, *28*(6), 489–498. doi:10.1002/jts.22059 PMID:26606250

Block, J., & Kremen, A. M. (1996). IQ and ego-resiliency: Conceptual and empirical connections and separateness. *Journal of Personality and Social Psychology*, *70*(2), 349–361. doi:10.1037/0022-3514.70.2.349 PMID:8636887

Boffa, J. W., Stanley, I. H., Hom, M. A., Norr, A. M., Joiner, T. E., & Schmidt, N. B. (2017). PTSD symptoms and suicidal thoughts and behaviors among firefighters. *Journal of Psychiatric Research*, *84*, 277–283. doi:10.1016/j.jpsychires.2016.10.014 PMID:27810667

Bogstrand, S. T., Skogstad, L., & Ekeberg, O. (2016). The association between alcohol, medicinal drug use and post-traumatic stress symptoms among Norwegian rescue workers after the 22 July twin terror attacks. *International Emergency Nursing*, *28*, 29–33. doi:10.1016/j.ienj.2016.03.003 PMID:27068750

Bohl, N. (1995). Measuring the effectiveness of CISD. *Fire Engineering,* 125-126.

Bohl, N. (1991). The effectiveness of brief psychological interventions in police officers after critical incidents. In J. T. Reese, J. Horn, & C. Dunning (Eds.), *Critical Incidents in Policing, Revised* (pp. 31–38). Washington, DC: Department of Justice.

Bohl, N. (1995). Measuring the effectiveness of CISD: A study. *Fire Engineering.*, *148*(8), 125–126.

Bohl-Penrod, N. K., & Clark, D. W. (2017). Peer support in public safety organizations. In C. L. Mitchell & E. H. Dorian (Eds.), *Police psychology and its growing impact on modern law enforcement* (pp. 237–251). Hershey, PA: IGI Global.

Boland, L. L., Kinzy, T. G., Myers, R. N., Fernstrom, K. M., Kamrud, J. W., Mink, P. J., & Stevens, A. C. (2018). Burn-out and exposure to critical incidents in a cohort of emergency medical services workers from Minnesota. *The Western Journal of Emergency Medicine*, *19*(6), 987–995. doi:10.5811/westjem.8.39034 PMID:30429931

Bonanno, G. A. (2004). Loss, Trauma, and Human Resilience: Have We Underestimated the Human Capacity to Thrive After Extremely Aversive Events? *The American Psychologist*, *59*(1), 20–28. doi:10.1037/0003-066X.59.1.20 PMID:14736317

Boscarino, J. A. (2004). Posttraumatic stress disorder and physical illness: Results from clinical and epidemiologic studies. *Annals of the New York Academy of Sciences*, 10. PMID:15677401

Boscarino, J. A., Adams, R. E., & Figley, C. R. (2005). A Prospective Cohort Study of the Effectiveness of Employer-Sponsored Crisis Interventions after a Major Disaster. *International Journal of Emergency Mental Health*, *7*(1), 31–44. PMID:15869077

Boscarino, J. A., Adams, R. E., & Figley, C. R. (2011). Mental health service use after the world trade center disaster: Utilization trends and comparative effectiveness. *The Journal of Nervous and Mental Disease*, *199*(2), 91–99. doi:10.1097/NMD.0b013e3182043b39 PMID:21278537

Boscarino, J. A., & Chang, J. (1999). Electrocardiogram abnormalities among men with stress-related psychiatric disorders: Implications for coronary heart disease and clinical research. *Annals of Behavioral Medicine*, *21*(3), 227–234. doi:10.1007/BF02884839 PMID:10626030

Bouchery, E. E., Barna, M., Babalola, E., Friend, D., Brown, J. D., Blyler, C., & Ireys, H. T. (2018). The effectiveness of a peer-staffed crisis respite program as an alternative to hospitalization. *Psychiatric Services (Washington, D.C.)*, *69*(10), 1069–1074. doi:10.1176/appi.ps.201700451 PMID:30071793

Boudreau, M. (2015). Africentric Resilience Training: A Prevention Program for African American Soldiers. *Dissertations & Theses*. 229. Retrieved from https://aura.antioch.edu/etds/229

Bowbrow, B., Panczyk, M., Stolz, U., Sotelo, M., Vadeboncoeur, T., Sutter, J., ... Spaite, D. (2014). Statewide implementation of a standardized prearrival telephone CPR program is associated with increased bystander CPR and survival from out-of-hospital cardiac arrest. *Circulation*, *130*(22), A1.

Bowman, S., & Roysircar, G. (2011). Training and practice in trauma, catastrophes, and disaster counseling. *The Counseling Psychologist*, *39*(8), 1160–1181. doi:10.1177/0011000010397934

Boyle, M. V., & Healy, J. (2003). Balancing mysterium and onus: Doing spiritual work within an emotion-laden organizational context. *Organization*, *10*(2), 351–373. doi:10.1177/1350508403010002010

Bradley, R., Greene, J., Russ, E., Dutra, L., & Westen, D. (2005). A multidimensional meta-analysis of psychotherapy for PTSD. *The American Journal of Psychiatry*, *162*(2), 214–227. doi:10.1176/appi.ajp.162.2.214 PMID:15677582

Brauer, B. R. (2016). The fire and emergency services culture: Can it be changed? *Fire Engineering*. Retrieved from https://www.fireengineering.com/articles/print/volume-169/issue-8/features/the-fire-and-emergency-services-culture-can-it-be-changed.html

Bremner, J. D., Vermetten, E., Afzal, N., & Vythilingam, M. (2004). Deficits in verbal declarative memory function in women with childhood sexual abuse-related posttraumatic stress disorder. *The Journal of Nervous and Mental Disease*, *192*(10), 643–649. doi:10.1097/01.nmd.0000142027.52893.c8 PMID:15457106

Bresge, A. (2016). *Halifax police chief making mental health, PTSD a priority*. Retrieved from https://www.ctvnews.ca/canada/halifax-police-chief-making-mental-health-ptsd-a-priority-1.2849866

Brewin, C. R., Andrew, B., & Valentine, J. D. (2000). Meta-analysis of risk factors for posttraumatic stress disorder in trauma-exposed adults. *Journal of Consulting and Clinical Psychology*, *68*(5), 748–766. doi:10.1037/0022-006X.68.5.748 PMID:11068961

Brisbon, N. M., & Lachman, M. E. (2017). Dispositional mindfulness and memory problems: The role of perceived stress and sleep quality. *Mindfulness*, *8*(2), 379–386. doi:10.100712671-016-0607-8 PMID:28344682

Broadbent, M., Gardett, I., Knight, C., Scott, G., Clawson, J. J., & Olola, C. (2018b). Persons description reported to emergency police dispatch. *Annals of Emergency Dispatch & Response*, *6*(3), 21–27.

Broadbent, M., Knight, C., Warner, D., Williams, N., Scott, G., Clawson, J. J., ... Olola, C. (2018a). Weapons reported on-scene by callers to emergency police dispatch. *Annals of Emergency Dispatch & Response*, *6*(1), 19–25.

Brodeur, M. D. (2009). *Assessment of resilience and its protective factors in disaster volunteers* (Doctoral dissertation). Retrieved from ProQuest Dissertations and Theses database. (UMI No. 3385340)

Bromet, E. J., Hobbs, M. J., Clouston, S. A., Gonzalez, A., Kotov, R., & Luft, B. J. (2016). DSM-IV post-traumatic stress disorder among World Trade Center responders 11-13 years after the disaster of 11 September 2001 (9/11). *Psychological Medicine*, *46*(4), 771–783. doi:10.1017/S0033291715002184 PMID:26603700

Brondolo, E., Wellington, R., Brady, N., Libby, D., & Brondolo, T. J. (2008). Mechanism and strategies for preventing post-traumatic stress disorder in forensic workers responding to mass fatality incidents. *Journal of Forensic and Legal Medicine*, *15*(2), 78–88. doi:10.1016/j.jflm.2007.04.007 PMID:18206823

Brough, P. (2004). Comparing the influence of traumatic and organizational stressors on the psychological health of police, fire, and ambulance officers. *International Journal of Stress Management*, *11*(3), 227–244. doi:10.1037/1072-5245.11.3.227

Brown, C., & Augusta-Scott, T. (Eds.). (2007). *Narrative therapy: Making meaning, making lives*. Thousand Oaks, CA: Sage.

Brown, J. M., & Campbell, E. A. (1994). *Stress and policing: Sources and strategies*. New York: John Wiley.

Brown, J., & Campbell, E. A. (1990). Sources of occupational stress in the police. *Work and Stress*, *4*(4), 305–318. doi:10.1080/02678379008256993

Brown, K. W., & Ryan, R. M. (2003). The benefits of being present: Mindfulness and its role in psychological well-being. *Journal of Personality and Social Psychology*, *84*(4), 822–848. doi:10.1037/0022-3514.84.4.822 PMID:12703651

Brown, L. A., Wiley, J. F., Wolitzky-Taylor, K., Roy-Byrne, P., Sherbourne, C., Stein, M. B., ... Craske, M. G. (2014). Changes in self-efficacy and outcome expectancy as predictors of anxiety outcomes from the calm study. *Depression and Anxiety*, *31*(8), 678–689. doi:10.1002/da.22256 PMID:24619599

Brown, R. P., & Gerbarg, P. L. (2009). Yoga breathing, meditation, and longevity. *Annals of the New York Academy of Sciences*, *1172*(1), 54–62. doi:10.1111/j.1749-6632.2009.04394.x PMID:19735239

Brucia, E. (2018). *The effects of residential treatment at the West Coast Post-trauma Retreat on police officers with PTSD* (Unpublished doctoral dissertation). Palo Alto University, Palo Alto, CA.

Brucia, E., Cordova, M. J., & Ruzek, J. I. (2017). Critical incident interventions: Crisis response and debriefings. In C. Mitchell & E. H. Dorian (Eds.), *Police psychology and its growing impact on modern law enforcement* (pp. 119–142). Hershey, PA: IGI Global. doi:10.4018/978-1-5225-0813-7.ch006

Brucia, E., Cordova, M., & Ruzek, J. (2016). Critical Incident Interventions: Crisis Response and Debriefings. In C. Mitchell & E. Dorian (Eds.), *Police psychology and its growing impact on modern law enforcement* (pp. 119–139). Hershey, PA: IGI Global.

Brunet, A., Weiss, D. S., Metzler, T. J., Best, S. R., Neylan, T. C., Rogers, C., ... Marmar, C. R. (2001). The Peritraumatic Distress Inventory: A proposed measure of PTSD criterion A2. *The American Journal of Psychiatry*, *158*(9), 1480–1485. doi:10.1176/appi.ajp.158.9.1480 PMID:11532735

Bryant, R. A. (2007). Early intervention for post-traumatic stress disorder. *Early Intervention in Psychiatry*, *1*(1), 19–26. doi:10.1111/j.1751-7893.2007.00006.x PMID:21352105

Bryant, R. A., & Guthrie, R. M. (2005). Maladaptive appraisals as a risk factor for posttraumatic stress: A study of trainee firefighters. *Psychological Science, 16*(10), 749–752. doi:10.1111/j.1467-9280.2005.01608.x PMID:16181434

Bryant, R. A., Harvey, A. G., Dang, S. T., Sackville, T., & Basten, C. (1998). Treatment of acute stress disorder: A comparison of cognitive-behavioral therapy and supportive counseling. *Journal of Consulting and Clinical Psychology, 66*(5), 862–866. doi:10.1037/0022-006X.66.5.862 PMID:9803707

Brymer, M., Jacobs, A., Layne, C., Pynoos, R., Ruzek, J., Steinberg, A., & Watson, P. (2006). *Psychological First Aid: Field Operations Guide* (2nd ed.). National Child Traumatic Stress Network and National Center for PTSD.

Buchanan, G., Stephens, C., & Long, N. (2001). Traumatic events of new recruits and serving police. *Australasian Journal of Disaster and Trauma Studies.*

Bulala, J. (2013). *The Relationship between the utilization of mental health services, coping mechanisms, and reputation in male firefighters* (Doctoral dissertation). Alliant International University, San Francisco, CA.

Bullen, E. (2015). Narrative therapy outcomes for women who have experienced domestic violence. *International Journal of Narrative Therapy & Community Work*, (3), 13-27.

Bureau of Labor Statistics, U. S. Department of Labor. (2017). *Occupational outlook handbook.* Retrieved from http://bls.gov

Burgess, D. (2015). *Firefighter breastmilk pilot study summary.* Report to the Arizona Fire Department.

Burke, T. W. (1995). Dispatcher stress. *FBI Law Enforcement Bulletin, 64*(10), 1. Retrieved from https://paloaltou.idm.oclc.org/login?url=https://search.ebscohost.com/login.aspx?direct=true&db=a9h&AN=9510252868

Burke, T. W. (1995). Dispatcher stress. *FBI Law Enforcement Bulletin, 64*(10), 1–6.

Burke, T. W. (2005). Dispatch. In L. E. Sullivan & M. Simonetti (Eds.), *Encyclopedia of law enforcement* (Vol. 1, pp. 137–139). California: Sage.

Byrne, D., & Espnes, G. A. (2008). Occupational stress and cardiovascular disease. *Stress and Health, 24*(3), 231–238. doi:10.1002mi.1203

C.O.P.S. (2018). *Concerns of police survivors.* Retrieved from https://www.concernsofpolicesurvivors.org

Cacioppo, J. T., Berntson, G. G., Malarkey, W. B., Kiecolt-Glaser, J. K., Sheridan, J. F., Poehlmann, K. M., ... Glaser, R. (1998). Autonomic, neuroendocrine, and immune responses to psychological stress: The reactivity hypothesisa. *Annals of the New York Academy of Sciences, 840*(1), 664–673. doi:10.1111/j.1749-6632.1998.tb09605.x PMID:9629293

Cacioppo, J. T., Burleson, M. H., Poehlmann, K. M., Malarkey, W. B., Kiecolt-Glaser, J. K., Berntson, G. G., ... Glaser, R. (2000). Autonomic and neuroendocrine responses to mild psychological stressors: Effects of chronic stress on older women. *Annals of Behavioral Medicine, 22*(2), 140–148. doi:10.1007/BF02895778 PMID:10962707

Cacioppo, J. T., & Tassinary, L. G. (1998). *Principles of neurology* (6th ed.). New York, NY: McGraw-Hill.

Cahill, L., & Alkire, M. T. (2003). Epinephrine enhancement of human memory consolidation: Interaction with arousal at encoding. *Neurobiology of Learning and Memory, 79*(2), 194–198. doi:10.1016/S1074-7427(02)00036-9 PMID:12591227

Campbell, I., & Kodz, J. (2011). What makes great police leadership? What research can tell us about the effectiveness of different leadership styles, competencies and behaviours. A Rapid Evidence Review. *National Policing Improvement Agency, 11*, 1–27.

Campbell, R. (2017). *Patterns of female firefighter injuries on the fireground*. Quincy, MA: National Fire Protection Association.

Campfield, K., & Hills, A. (2001). Effect of timing of critical Incident Stress Debriefing (CISD) on posttraumatic symptoms. *Journal of Traumatic Stress*, *14*(2), 327–340. doi:10.1023/A:1011117018705 PMID:11469160

Caplan, G. (1961). *An approach to Community Mental Health*. New York: Grune and Stratton.

Caplan, G. (1964). *Principles of Preventive Psychiatry*. New York: Basic Books.

Caplan, G. (1969). Opportunities for school psychologists in the primary prevention of mental health disorders in children. In A. Bindman & A. Spiegel (Eds.), *Perspectives in Community Mental Health* (pp. 420–436). Chicago: Aldine.

Carey, M. G., Al-Zaiti, S. S., Dean, G. E., Sessanna, L., & Finnell, D. S. (2011). Sleep problems, depression, substance use, social bonding, and quality of life in professional firefighters. *Journal of Occupational and Environmental Medicine/ American College of Occupational and Environmental Medicine, 53*(8), 928.

Carey, M. G., Al-Zaiti, S. S., Dean, G. E., Sessanna, L., & Finnell, D. S. (2011). Sleep problems, depression, substance use, social bonding, and quality of life in professional firefighters. *Journal of Occupational and Environmental Medicine*, *53*(8), 928–933. doi:10.1097/JOM.0b013e318225898f PMID:21785370

Carleton, R. N., Afifi, T. O., Taillieu, T., Turner, S., El-Gabalawy, R., Sareen, J., & Asmundson, G. J. G. (2018a). Anxiety-related psychopathology and chronic pain comorbidity among public safety personnel. *Journal of Anxiety Disorders*, *55*, 48–55. PMID:29566981

Carleton, R. N., Afifi, T. O., Turner, S., Taillieu, T., Duranceau, S., LeBouthillier, D. M., ... Asmundson, G. J. G. (2018). Mental disorder symptoms among public safety personnel in Canada. *Canadian Journal of Psychiatry*, *63*(1), 54–64. doi:10.1177/0706743717723825 PMID:28845686

Carleton, R. N., Afifi, T. O., Turner, S., Taillieu, T., LeBouthillier, D. M., Duranceau, S., ... Hozempa, K. (2018). Suicidal ideation, plans, and attempts among public safety personnel in Canada. *Canadian Psychology*, *59*(3), 220–231. doi:10.1037/cap0000136

Carlier, I. V. E., Lamberts, R. D., Van Uchelen, A. J., & Gersons, B. P. (1998). Disaster-related posttraumatic stress in police officers: A field study of the impact of debriefing. *Stress Medicine*, *14*(3), 143–148. doi:10.1002/(SICI)1099-1700(199807)14:3<143::AID-SMI770>3.0.CO;2-S

Carlier, I. V. E., Voerman, A. E., & Gersons, B. P. R. (2000). The influence of occupational debriefing on post-traumatic stress symptomatology in traumatized police officers. *The British Journal of Medical Psychology*, *73*(1), 87–98. doi:10.1348/000711200160327 PMID:10759053

Carlier, I. V., Lamberts, R. D., & Gersons, B. P. (1997). Risk factors for posttraumatic stress symptomology in police officers: A prospective analysis. *The Journal of Nervous and Mental Disease*, *195*(8), 498–506. doi:10.1097/00005053-199708000-00004 PMID:9284863

Carlson Neil, R. (2013). *Physiology of behavior*. Boston: Pearson.

Carr, A. (1998). Michael white's narrative therapy. *Contemporary Family Therapy*, *20*(4), 485–503. doi:10.1023/A:1021680116584

Carroll, L., Gilroy, P. J., & Murra, J. (1999). The moral imperative: Self-care for women psychotherapists. *Women & Therapy*, *22*(2), 133–143. doi:10.1300/J015v22n02_10

Carter, S. L. (1996). *Integrity*. Harper Collins Publishers.

Cassan, D. (2010). Police and socialisation in France and in England: How do they stand towards the community policing model? *Journal of Police Studies*, *3*(16), 243–260.

Castro, C. A., & Adler, A. B. (2011). Re-conceptualizing combat-related posttraumatic stress disorder as an occupational hazard. In A. B. Adler, P. B. Bliese, & C. A. Castro (Eds.), *Deployment Psychology: Evidence-Based Strategies to Promote Mental Health in the Military* (pp. 217–242). Washington, DC: American Psychological Association. doi:10.1037/12300-009

Castro, C. A., Hoge, C. W., & Cox, A. L. (2006). *Battlemind training: Building soldier resiliency*. Walter Reed Army Inst of Research.

Center for Disease Control and Prevention. (2017). *Firefighter Cancer Rates: The Facts from NIOSH Research*. Retrieved from: https://blogs.cdc.gov/niosh-science blog/2017/05/10/ff-cancer-facts/

Centers for Disease Control and Prevention (CDC). (2015). *Adult obesity facts*. Retrieved from http://www.cdc.gov/obesity/data/adult.html

Centers for Disease Control and Prevention (CDC). (2018). *Physical Activity: Why it matters*. Retrieved from https://www.cdc.gov/physicalactivity/about-physical-activity/why-it-matters.html

Centre for Occupational and Environmental Health. (2000). *Occupational Physicians Reporting Activity. Quarterly Report*. Manchester, UK: University of Manchester.

Chae, M. H., & Boyle, D. J. (2013). Police suicide: Prevalence, risk, and protective factors. *Policing: An International Journal of Police Strategies & Management*, *36*(1), 91–118. doi:10.1108/13639511311302498

Chang, E. C., Downey, C. A., Hirsch, J. K., & Lin, N. J. (Eds.). (2016). *Cultural, racial, and ethnic psychology book series. Positive psychology in racial and ethnic groups: Theory, research, and practice*. Washington, DC: American Psychological Association; doi:10.1037/14799-000

Chang, J. H., Kim, D., Jang, E., Park, J. E., Bae, H., Han, C. W., & Kim, S. H. (2016). Reliability and validity of the Korean version of the Symptom Checklist Post Traumatic Stress Disorder Scale. *Journal of Korean Medical Science*, *31*(5), 777–782. doi:10.3346/jkms.2016.31.5.777 PMID:27134501

Chapman, S. A., Blash, L. K., Mayer, K., & Spetz, J. (2018). Emerging roles for peer providers in mental health and substance use disorders. *American Journal of Preventive Medicine*, *54*(6), S267–S274. doi:10.1016/j.amepre.2018.02.019 PMID:29779551

Charbotel, B., Croidieu, S., Vohito, M., Guerin, A. C., Renaud, L., Jaussaud, J., ... Bergeret, A. (2009). Working conditions in call-centers, the impact on employee health: A transversal study. Part II. *International Archives of Occupational and Environmental Health*, *82*(6), 747–756. doi:10.100700420-008-0351-z PMID:18704480

Chaves, C., Lopez-Gomez, I., Hervas, G., & Vazquez, C. (2019). The Integrative Positive Psychological Intervention for Depression (IPPI-D). *Journal of Contemporary Psychotherapy*, 1–9. doi:10.100710879-018-9412-0

Chemtob, C., Tomas, S., Law, W., & Cremniter, D. (1997). Post disaster psychosocial intervention. *The American Journal of Psychiatry*, *134*, 415–417. PMID:9054792

Chenault, S., Martin, J., & Matusiak, R. E. (2016). The Ripple Effect: Empathy Statements of Participants of an Impact of Crime on Victims Class. *Corrections: Policy, Practice and Research*, *1*(3), 196–214. doi:10.1080/23774657.2016.1210994

Chen, Y. S., Chen, M. C., Chou, F. H. C., Sun, F. C., Chen, P. C., Tsai, K. Y., & Chao, S. S. (2007). The relationship between quality of life and posttraumatic stress disorder or major depression for firefighters in Kaohsiung, Taiwan. *Quality of Life Research: An International Journal of Quality of Life Aspects of Treatment, Care and Rehabilitation, 16*(8), 1289–1297. doi:10.100711136-007-9248-7 PMID:17668289

Cherpitel, C. J. (2000). A brief screening instrument for problem drinking in the emergency room: The RAPS4. Rapid Alcohol Problems Screen. *Journal of Studies on Alcohol, 61*(3), 447–449. doi:10.15288/jsa.2000.61.447 PMID:10807217

Chesnais, J. (1996). Fertility, family, and social policy in contemporary Western Europe. *Population and Development Review, 22*(4), 729. doi:10.2307/2137807

Chinman, M., Shoai, R., & Cohen, A. (2010). Using organizational change strategies to guide peer support technician implementation in the Veterans Administration. *Psychiatric Rehabilitation Journal, 33*(4), 269–277. doi:10.2975/33.4.2010.269.277 PMID:20374985

Chiu, S., Niles, J. K., Webber, M. P., Zeig-Owens, R., Gustave, J., Lee, R., ... Prezant, D. J. (2011). Evaluating risk factors and possible mediation effects in posttraumatic depression and posttraumatic stress disorder comorbidity. *Public Health Reports, 126*(2), 201–209. PMID:21387950

Chopko, B. A., Facemire, V. C., Palmieri, P. A., & Schwartz, R. C. (2016). Spirituality and health outcomes among police officers: Empirical evidence supporting a paradigm shift. *Criminal Justice Studies, 29*(4), 363–377. doi:10.1080/1478601X.2016.1216412

Chopko, B. A., Palmieri, P. A., & Adams, R. E. (2013). Associations between police stress and alcohol use: Implications for practice. *Journal of Loss and Trauma, 18*(5), 482–497.

Chopko, B. A., Palmieri, P. A., & Adams, R. E. (2015). Correlates of career traumatization and symptomology among active duty police officers. *Criminal Justice Studies, 25*(1), 83–95. doi:10.1080/1478601X.2012.657905

Chopko, B. A., Palmieri, P. A., & Adams, R. E. (2015). Critical incident history questionnaire replication: Frequency and severity of trauma exposure among officers from small and midsize police agencies. *Journal of Traumatic Stress, 28*(2), 157–161. doi:10.1002/jts.21996 PMID:25808672

Chopko, B. A., Palmieri, P. A., & Facemire, V. C. (2014). Prevalence and predictors of suicidal ideation among U.S. law enforcement officers. *Journal of Police and Criminal Psychology, 29*(1), 1–9.

Chopko, B. A., & Schwartz, R. C. (2013). The relation between mindfulness and posttraumatic stress symptoms among police officers. *Journal of Loss and Trauma, 18*(1), 1–9. doi:10.1080/15325024.2012.674442

Chow, H. M., Mar, R. A., Xu, Y., Liu, S., Wagage, S., & Braun, A. R. (2014). Embodied comprehension of stories: Interactions between language regions and modality-specific neural systems. *Journal of Cognitive Neuroscience, 26*(2), 279–295. doi:10.1162/jocn_a_00487 PMID:24047383

Christopher, M. S., Goerling, R. J., Rogers, B. S., Hunsinger, M., Baron, G., Bergman, A. L., & Zava, D. T. (2015). A pilot study evaluating the effectiveness of a mindfulness-based intervention on cortisol awakening response and health outcomes among law enforcement officers. *Journal of Police and Criminal Psychology, 31*(1), 15–28. doi:10.100711896-015-9161-x

Ciarrochi, J., & Godsell, C. (2005). Mindfulness-based emotional intelligence: A theory and review of the literature. *Emotional intelligence: An international handbook*, 69-90.

Ciarrochi, J., Chan, A., Caputi, P., & Roberts, R. (2001). Measuring emotional intelligence. *Emotional intelligence in everyday life: A scientific inquiry*, 25-45.

Cicognani, E., Pietrantoni, L., Palestini, L., & Prati, G. (2009). Emergency workers' quality of life: The protective role of sense of community, efficacy beliefs and coping strategies. *Social Indicators Research*, *94*(3), 449–463. doi:10.100711205-009-9441-x

Cieslak, R., Luszczynska, A., Shoji, K., Douglas, A., Melville, E., & Benight, C. C. (2014). A meta-analysis of the relationship between job burnout and secondary traumatic stress among workers with indirect exposure to trauma. *Psychological Services*, *11*(1), 75–86. doi:10.1037/a0033798 PMID:23937082

Ci, S., Lan, Y., Zhang, Q., Zhou, D., & De, J. (2015). Analysis of posttraumatic stress disorder in rescuers and firefighters. *Zhonghua Lao Dong Wei Sheng Zhi Ye Bing Za Zhi*, *33*(6), 448–450. PMID:26653381

Clark, A. E. (1997). Job satisfaction and gender: Why are women so happy at work? *Labour Economics*, *4*(4), 314–372. doi:10.1016/S0927-5371(97)00010-9

Clawson, J. J., Dernocoeur, K. B., & Murray, C. (2015). *Principles of Emergency Medical Dispatch.* Salt Lake City, UT: Priority Press.

Clawson, J. J., Gardett, I., Scott, G., Fivaz, C., Barron, T., Broadbent, M., & Olola, C. (2018, February). Hospital-confirmed acute myocardial infarction: Prehospital identification using the Medical Priority Dispatch System. *Prehospital and Disaster Medicine*, *33*(1), 29–35. doi:10.1017/S1049023X1700704X PMID:29223194

Clawson, J. J., Scott, G., Gardett, I., Youngquist, S., Taillac, P., Fivaz, C., & Olola, C. (2016). Predictive ability of an emergency medical dispatch stroke diagnostic tool in identifying hospital-confirmed strokes. *Journal of Stroke and Cerebrovascular Diseases*, *25*(8), 2031–2042. doi:10.1016/j.jstrokecerebrovasdis.2016.04.021 PMID:27256173

Clawson, J., Scott, G., Gardett, I., Patterson, B., Barron, T., & Olola, C. (2014). Ability of a diabetic problems protocol to predict patient severity indicators determined by on-scene EMS crews. *Resuscitation*, *85*(s1), S111.

Cloitre, M., Garvert, D. W., & Weiss, B. J. (2017). Depression as a moderator of STAIR narrative therapy for women with post-traumatic stress disorder related to childhood abuse. *European Journal of Psychotraumatology*, *8*(1), 1–7. doi:10.1080/20008198.2017.1377028 PMID:29038682

Clossey, L., Solomon, P., Hu, C., Gillen, J., & Zinn, M. (2018). Predicting the job satisfaction of mental health peer support workers (PSWs). *Social Work in Mental Health*, *16*(6), 682–695. doi:10.1080/15332985.2018.1483463

Cohen, K., & Collens, P. (2013). The impact of trauma work on trauma workers: A metasynthesis on vicarious trauma and vicarious posttraumatic growth. *Psychological Trauma: Theory, Research, Practice, and Policy*, *5*(6), 570–580. doi:10.1037/a0030388

Cohen, S., Tyrrell, D. A., & Smith, A. P. (1991). Psychological stress and susceptibility to the common cold. *The New England Journal of Medicine*, *325*(9), 606–612. doi:10.1056/NEJM199108293250903 PMID:1713648

Cohn, J., Weltman, G., Ratwani, R., Chartrand, D., & McCraty, R. (2010). *Stress inoculation through cognitive and biofeedback training*. Office of Naval Research.

Combs, G., & Freedman, J. (2012). Narrative, poststructuralist, and social justice: Current practices in narrative therapy. *The Counseling Psychologist*, *40*, 1033–1060. doi:10.1177/0011000012460662

Conrad, D., & Kellar-Guenther, Y. (2006). Compassion fatigue, burnout, and compassion satisfaction among Colorado child protection workers. *Child Abuse & Neglect*, *30*(10), 1071–1080. doi:10.1016/j.chiabu.2006.03.009 PMID:17014908

Corneil, W., Beaton, R., Murphy, S., Johnson, C., & Pike, K. (1999). Exposure to traumatic incidents and prevalence of posttraumatic stress symptomatology in urban firefighters in two countries. *Journal of Occupational Health Psychology*, *4*(2), 131–141. doi:10.1037/1076-8998.4.2.131 PMID:10212865

Cornum, R., Matthews, M. D., & Seligman, M. E. (2011). Comprehensive soldier fitness: Building resilience in a challenging institutional context. *The American Psychologist*, *66*(1), 4–9. doi:10.1037/a0021420 PMID:21219042

Corrigan, M., McWilliams, R., Kelly, K. J., Niles, J., Cammarata, C., Jones, K., ... Prezant, D. J. (2009). A computerized, self-administered questionnaire to evaluate posttraumatic stress among firefighters after the World Trade Center collapse. *American Journal of Public Health*, *99*(S3Suppl 3), 702–709. doi:10.2105/AJPH.2008.151605 PMID:19890176

Corrigan, P. W., Morris, S., Larson, J., Rafacz, J., Wassel, A., Michaels, P., ... Rüsch, N. (2010). Self-stigma and coming out about one's mental illness. *Journal of Community Psychology*, *38*(3), 259–275. doi:10.1002/jcop.20363 PMID:23970807

Corrigan, P. W., Watson, A. C., & Barr, L. (2006). The self-stigma of mental illness: Implications for self-esteem and self-efficacy. *Journal of Social and Clinical Psychology*, *25*(8), 875–884. doi:10.1521/jscp.2006.25.8.875

Covey, T. J., Shucard, J. L., Violanti, J. M., Lee, J., & Shucard, D. W. (2013). The effects of exposure to traumatic stressors on inhibitory control in police officers: A dense electrode array study using a Go/NoGo continuous performance task. *International Journal of Psychophysiology*, *87*(3), 363–375. doi:10.1016/j.ijpsycho.2013.03.009 PMID:23528305

Coxon, A., Cropley, M., Schofield, P., Start, K., Horsfield, C., & Quinn, T. (2016). "You're never just making one decision": Exploring the lived experiences of ambulance Emergency Operations Centre personnel. *Emergency Medicine Journal*, *33*(9), 645–651. PMID:27002162

Crane-Okada, R., Freeman, E., Ross, M., Kiger, H., & Giuliano, A. E. (2010). Training senior peer counselors to provide telephone support for newly diagnosed breast cancer survivors. *Journal of Cancer Education*, *25*(2), 174–179. doi:10.100713187-009-0028-7 PMID:20082171

Critchley, H. D. (2002). Electrodermal responses: What happens in the brain. *The Neuroscientist*, *8*(2), 132–142. doi:10.1177/107385840200800209 PMID:11954558

Crocq, L. (1999). *Les Traumatismes psychiques de guerre*. Paris, France: Odile Jacob.

Crocq, L., Dalligand, L., Villerbu, L., Tarquinio, C., Duchet, C., Coq, J. M., ... Vitry, M. (2007). *Traumatismes psychiques: Prise en charge psychologique des victims*. Paris, France: Elsevier-Masson.

Crosby, F. (2007). *The Real Meaning of Brotherhood. Fire Engineering*. Retrieved from http://www.fireengineering.com/index/articles

Cuthbert, B. N., Lang, P. J., Strauss, C., Drobes, D., Patrick, C. J., & Bradley, M. M. (2003). The psychophysiology of anxiety disorder: Fear memory imagery. *Psychophysiology*, *40*(3), 407–422. doi:10.1111/1469-8986.00043 PMID:12946114

D'Andrea, W., Pole, N., DePierro, J., Freed, S., & Wallace, D. B. (2013). Heterogeneity of defensive responses after exposure to trauma: Blunted autonomic reactivity in response to startling sounds. *International Journal of Psychophysiology*, *90*(1), 80–89. doi:10.1016/j.ijpsycho.2013.07.008 PMID:23896169

Daas-Brailsford, P. (2010). Secondary trauma among disaster responders. In P. Daas-Brailsford (Ed.), *Crisis and disaster counseling* (pp. 213–228). Thousand Oaks, CA: SAGE. doi:10.4135/9781452275093.n14

Dattilio, F. M. (2010). *Cognitive-behavioral therapy with couples and families: A comprehensive guide for clinicians*. New York: Guilford Press.

Davey, J. D., Obst, P. L., & Sheehan, M. C. (2001). It goes with the job: Officers' insights into the impact of stress and culture on alcohol consumption within the policing occupation. *Drugs Education Prevention & Policy*, *8*, 141–149. doi:10.1080/096876301300101889

Davidson, L., Bellamy, C., Guy, K., & Miller, R. (2012). Peer support among persons with severe mental illnesses: A review of evidence and experience. *World Psychiatry; Official Journal of the World Psychiatric Association (WPA)*, *11*(2), 123–128. doi:10.1016/j.wpsyc.2012.05.009 PMID:22654945

Davis, C. G., Nolen-Hoeksema, S., & Larson, J. (1998). Making sense of loss and benefiting from the experience: Two construals of meaning. *Journal of Personality and Social Psychology*, *75*(2), 561–574. doi:10.1037/0022-3514.75.2.561 PMID:9731325

de Jong, J. T. V. M. (1995). Prevention of the consequences of man–made or natural disaster at the (inter)national, the community, the family and the individual level. In S. E. Hobfoll & M. W. de Vries (Eds.), *Extreme stress and communities: Impact and intervention* (pp. 207–229). Boston: Kluwer. doi:10.1007/978-94-015-8486-9_9

de Jong, J. T. V. M. (Ed.). (2002). *Trauma, war and violence: Public mental health in sociocultural context*. New York, NY: Plethnum-Kluwer. doi:10.1007/b109606

De Terte, I., Stephens, C., & Huddleston, L. (2014). The development of a three part model of psychological resilience. *Stress and Health*, *30*(5), 416–424. doi:10.1002mi.2625 PMID:25476966

de Visser, E. J., Dorfman, A., Chartrand, D., Lamon, J., Freedy, E., & Weltman, G. (2016). Building resilience with the Stress Resilience Training System: Design validation and applications. *Work (Reading, Mass.)*, *54*(2), 351–366. doi:10.3233/WOR-162295 PMID:27232057

Deahl, M., Srinivasan, M., Jones, N., Thomas, J., Neblett, C., & Jolly, A. (2000). Preventing psychological trauma in soldiers. The role of operational stress training and psychological debriefing. *The British Journal of Medical Psychology*, *73*(1), 77–85. doi:10.1348/000711200160318 PMID:10759052

DeAngelis, T. (2019). The legacy of trauma. *Monitor on Psychology*, *50*, 36–43.

DeCrescenzo, D. (2005). Early detection of the problem officer. *FBI Law Enforcement Bulletin*, *74*(7), 14–17.

Del Ben, K. S., Scotti, J. R., Chen, Y. C., & Fortson, B. L. (2006). Prevalence of posttraumatic stress disorder symptoms in firefighters. *Work and Stress*, *20*(1), 37–48.

DeLorme, J. (2014). *The investigation of repeated trauma exposure and psychological adjustment in Firefighters*. California School of Professional Psychology, Alliant International University.

Deming, W. E. (1982). *Out of the Crisis*. Massachusetts Institute of Technology.

Devilly, G. J., Gist, R., & Cotton, P. (2006). Ready! Fire! Aim! The status of psychological debriefing and therapeutic interventions: In the workplace and after disasters. *Review of General Psychology*, *10*(4), 318–345. doi:10.1037/1089-2680.10.4.318

Diamond, G. M., Lipsitz, J. D., Fajerman, Z., & Rozenblat, O. (2010). Ongoing Traumatic Stress Response (OTSR) in Sderot, Israel. *Professional Psychology, Research and Practice*, *41*(1), 19–25. doi:10.1037/a0017098

Dickerson, S. S., & Kemeny, M. E. (2004). Acute stressors and cortisol responses: A theoretical integration and synthesis of laboratory research. *Psychological Bulletin*, *130*(3), 355–391. doi:10.1037/0033-2909.130.3.355 PMID:15122924

Dicks, R. L. H. (2014). *Prevalence of PTSD Symptoms in Canadian 911 Operators* (Unpublished master's thesis). University of the Fraser Valley, Canada.

Dietrich, J. F., & Smith, J. (1986). The nonmedical use of drugs including alcohol among police personnel: A critical literature review. *Journal of Police Science and Administration*.

DiGangi, J. A., Gomez, D., Mendoza, L., Jason, L. A., Keys, C. B., & Koenen, K. C. (2013). Pretrauma risk factors for posttraumatic stress disorder: A systematic review of the literature. *Clinical Psychology Review*, *33*(6), 728–744. doi:10.1016/j.cpr.2013.05.002 PMID:23792469

Dill, J., & Loew, C. (2012). Suicide in the fire and emergency services. *National Volunteer Fire Council*. 1-41. Retrieved from: http://firefighterveteran.com/images/stories/Nationla_Volunteer_Fire_Counsel/Firefight r%2suicide%20report.pdf.

Dillard, M. B., Warm, J. S., Funke, G. J., Nelson, T., Finomore, V. S., McClernon, C. K., ... Funke, M. E. (2019). Vigilance tasks: Unpleasant, mentally demanding, and stressful even when time flies. *Human Factors*, *61*(2), 225–242. doi:10.1177/0018720818796015 PMID:30216088

Dimeff, L. A., & Koerner, K. (2017). *Dialectical Behavior Therapy in clinical practice: Applications across disorders and settings*. New York: Guilford Press.

Dixon, H. C., & Overall, N. C. (2016). Dispositional mindfulness attenuates the link between daily stress and depressed mood. *Journal of Social and Clinical Psychology*, *35*(3), 255–268. doi:10.1521/jscp.2016.35.3.255

Dixon, L., Hackmann, A., & Lehman, A. (1997). Consumer as staff in assertive community treatment programs. *Administration and Policy in Mental Health*, *25*(2), 199–208. doi:10.1023/A:1022243106341 PMID:9727217

Donahue, M. J. (1977). *Peer counseling for police officers: a program for skill development and personal growth* (Unpublished doctoral dissertation). Boston University, Boston, MA.

Donnelly, E. (2012). Work-related stress and posttraumatic stress in emergency medical services. *Prehospital Emergency Care*, *16*(1), 76–85. doi:10.3109/10903127.2011.621044 PMID:22128908

Dorgo, S., King, G. A., Bader, J. O., & Limon, J. S. (2013). Outcomes of a peer mentor implemented fitness program in older adults: A quasi-randomized controlled trial. *International Journal of Nursing Studies*, *50*(9), 1156–1165. doi:10.1016/j.ijnurstu.2012.12.006 PMID:23279966

Dorgo, S., King, G. A., & Brickey, G. D. (2009). The application of peer mentoring to improve fitness in older adults. *Journal of Aging and Physical Activity*, *17*(3), 344–361. doi:10.1123/japa.17.3.344 PMID:19799104

Dowdall-Thomae, C., Gilkey, J., Larson, W., & Arend-Hicks, R. (2012). Elite firefighter/first responder mindsets and outcome coping efficacy. *International Journal of Emergency Mental Health*, *14*(4), 269–281. PMID:23980491

Driscoll, R. J., Tubbs, R. L., & Habes, D. J. (2007). *NIOSH health hazard evaluation report*. Retrieved from: https://www. cdc.gov/niosh/hhe/reports/pdfs/1997-0137-3026.pdf

Driskell, J. E., & Johnston, J. H. (1998). Stress exposure training. In J. A. Cannon-Bowers & E. Salas (Eds.), *Making decisions under stress: Implications for individual and team training* (pp. 191–217). Washington, DC: American Psychological Association. doi:10.1037/10278-007

Drucker, P. (1985). *Innovation and Entrepreneurship*. New York: Harper Row Publishing.

Duba, J. D., Kindsvatter, A., & Priddy, C. J. (2010). Deconstructing the mirror's reflection: Narrative therapy groups for women dissatisfied with their body. *Adultspan: Theory Research & Practice*, *9*(2), 103–116. doi:10.1002/j.2161-0029.2010.tb00075.x

Dunnigan, R. (2012). *Emergency responders' trauma symptoms following the west coast post- trauma retreat recovery program* (Unpublished doctoral dissertation). Alliant International University, San Francisco, CA.

Durand, G., Tsismenakis, A. J., Jahnke, S. A., Baur, D. M., Christophi, C. A., & Kales, S. A. (2011). Firefighters physical activity: Relation to fitness and cardiovascular disease risk. *Medicine and Science in Sports and Exercise*, *43*(9), 1752–1759. doi:10.1249/MSS.0b013e318215cf25 PMID:21364484

Dyregrov, A. (1998). Psychological debriefing: An effective method? *TRAUMATOLOGYe, 4*(2), Article 1.

Eagle, G., & Kaminer, D. (2013). Continuous traumatic stress: Expanding the lexicon of traumatic stress. *Peace and Conflict*, *19*(2), 85–99. doi:10.1037/a0032485

Ehlers, A., & Clark, D. M. (2000). A cognitive model of posttraumatic stress disorder. *Behaviour Research and Therapy*, *38*(4), 319–345. doi:10.1016/S0005-7967(99)00123-0 PMID:10761279

Ehrenreich, J. H., & Elliott, T. L. (2004). Managing stress in humanitarian aid workers. *Peace and Conflict*, *10*(1), 53–66. doi:10.120715327949pac1001_4

Eid, J., Johnsen, B. H., & Weisaeth, L. (2001). The effects of group psychological debriefing on acute stress reactions following a traffic accident: A quasi-experimental approach. *International Journal of Emergency Mental Health*, *3*, 145–154. PMID:11642192

Elkins, P. D., & Roberts, M. C. (1983). Psychological preparation for pediatric hospitalization. *Clinical Psychology Review*, *3*(3), 275–295. doi:10.1016/0272-7358(83)90016-8

Engelhard, I. M., van den Hout, M. A., Weerts, J., Hox, J. J., & van Doornen, L. J. (2009). A prospective study of the relation between posttraumatic stress and physical health symptoms. *International Journal of Clinical and Health Psychology*, *9*(3).

Evanoff, B., & Rosenstock, L. (1986). Reproductive hazards in the workplace: A case study of women firefighters. *American Journal of Industrial Medicine*, *9*(6), 503–515. doi:10.1002/ajim.4700090602 PMID:3740071

Evans, R., Pistrang, N., & Billings, J. (2013). Police officers' experiences of supportive and unsupportive social interactions following traumatic incidents. *European Journal of Psychotraumatology*, *4*(1), 1–9. doi:10.3402/ejpt.v4i0.19696 PMID:23516046

Evarts, B., & Molis, J. L. (2018). *United States Firefighter Injuries 2017*. Quincy, MA: National Fire Protection Association.

Everly, G. (1989). *A clinical guide to the treatment of the human stress response*. New York, NY: Plenum Press. doi:10.1007/978-1-4613-0741-9

Everly, G. (2019). *Critical Incident Stress Management (CISM) and Psychological Crisis Intervention: a Practical Review of Research.* Severna Park, MD: Resiliency Science Institutes International.

Everly, G. S. Jr, Flannery, R. B. Jr, & Eyler, V. A. (2002). Critical incident stress management (CISM): A statistical review of the literature. *The Psychiatric Quarterly*, *73*(3), 171–182. doi:10.1023/A:1016068003615 PMID:12143079

Everly, G. S. Jr, Flannery, R. B. Jr, Eyler, V., & Mitchell, J. T. (2001). Sufficiency analysis of an integrated multicomponent approach to crisis intervention: Critical Incident Stress Management. *Advances in Mind-Body Medicine*, *17*, 174–183. PMID:11572844

Everly, G. S. Jr, Flannery, R. B. Jr, & Mitchell, J. T. (2000). Critical Incident Stress Management (CISM): A review of the literature. *Aggression and Violent Behavior*, *5*(1), 23–40. doi:10.1016/S1359-1789(98)00026-3

Everly, G. S. Jr, & Mitchell, J. T. (2008). *Integrative Crisis Intervention and Disaster Mental Health.* Ellicott City, MD: Chevron Publishing Corporation.

Everly, G. S., Lating, J. M., & Mitchell, J. T. (2000b). Innovations in group crisis intervention: Critical incident stress debriefing (CISD) and critical incident stress management (CISM). In A. Roberts (Ed.), *Crisis intervention handbook: Assessment, treatment, and research* (pp. 77–97). New York: Oxford University Press.

Everly, G. S., & Mitchell, J. T. (1999). *Critical Incident Stress Management (CISM): A New Era and Standard of Care in Crisis Intervention* (2nd ed.). Chevron Pub.

Fahy, R. F., LeBlanc, P. R., & Molis, J. L. (2018). *Firefighter Fatalities in the United States - 2017*. Quincy, MA: National Fire Protection Association.

Fauerbach, J. A., Lawrence, J. W., Fogel, J., Richter, L., Magyar-Russell, G., McKibben, J. B., & Mccann, U. (2009). Approach–avoidance coping conflict in a sample of burn patients at risk for posttraumatic stress disorder. *Depression and Anxiety*, *26*(9), 838–850. doi:10.1002/da.20439 PMID:19170120

Fava, G. A., & Tomba, E. (2009). Increasing psychological well-being and resilience by psychotherapeutic methods. *Journal of Personality*, *77*(6), 1903–1934. doi:10.1111/j.1467-6494.2009.00604.x PMID:19807860

Fay, J., Kamena, M. D., Benner, A., & Buscho, A. (2006). A residential milieu treatment approach for first-responder trauma. *Traumatology*, *12*(3), 255–262. doi:10.1177/1534765606294991

Fear, N. T., Iversen, A., Meltzer, H., Workman, L., Hull, L., Greenberg, N., & Jones, M. (2007). Patterns of drinking in the UK Armed Forces. *Addiction (Abingdon, England)*, *102*(11), 1749–1759. doi:10.1111/j.1360-0443.2007.01978.x PMID:17935583

Feldmann, T. B., & Johnson, P. W. (1992). The selfobject function of weapons: A self psychology examination. *The Journal of the American Academy of Psychoanalysis*, *20*(4), 561–576. doi:10.1521/jaap.1.1992.20.4.561 PMID:1291544

Feldner, M. T., Monson, C. M., & Friedman, M. J. (2007). A critical analysis of approaches to targeted PTSD prevention: Current status and theoretically derived future directions. *Behavior Modification*, *31*(1), 80–116. doi:10.1177/0145445506295057 PMID:17179532

Feltz, D. L., & Landers, D. M. (1983). The effects of mental practice on motor skill learning and performance: A meta-analysis. *Journal of Sport Psychology*, *5*(1), 25–57. doi:10.1123/jsp.5.1.25

Figley, C. R. (2013). Measuring compassion satisfaction as well as fatigue: Developmental history of the compassion satisfaction and fatigue test. In *Treating Compassion Fatigue* (pp. 115–128). New York, NY: Routledge.

Firefighter Behavioral Health Alliance FF & EMS Suicide Deaths by Year and Type. (n.d.). Retrieved from http://www.ffbha.org/ff-ems-suicide-deaths-by-year-type/

Fjeldheim, C. B., Nothling, J., Pretorius, K., Basson, M., Ganasen, K., Heneke, R., ... Seedat, S. (2014). Trauma exposure, posttraumatic stress disorder and the effect of explanatory variables in paramedic trainees. *BMC Emergency Medicine*, *14*(11), 1–7. PMID:24755358

Flannery, R. B. (2005). *Assaulted Staff Action Program (ASAP): Fifteen years of Empirical Findings*. Paper presented at the 8th World Congress on Stress Trauma and Coping: Crisis Intervention: Best Practices in Prevention, Preparedness and Response, Baltimore, MD.

Flannery, R. B. (2015). Treating psychological trauma in first responders: A multi-modal paradigm. *The Psychiatric Quarterly*, *86*(2), 261–267. doi:10.100711126-014-9329-z PMID:25403791

Foa, E. B., Hembree, E. A., Cahill, S. P., Rauch, S. A. M., Riggs, D. S., Feeny, N. C., & Yadin, E. (2005). Randomized trial of prolonged exposure for posttraumatic stress disorder with and without cognitive restructuring: Outcome at academic and community clinics. *Journal of Consulting and Clinical Psychology*, *73*(5), 953–964. doi:10.1037/0022-006X.73.5.953 PMID:16287395

Foa, E. B., Hembree, E. A., & Rothbaum, B. O. (2007). *Prolonged exposure therapy for PTSD: Emotional processing of traumatic experiences*. Cambridge, UK: Oxford University Press.

Foa, E. B., Hembree, E. A., & Rothbaum, B. O. (2007). *Prolonged exposure therapy for ptsd: Emotional processing of traumatic experiences*. New York, NY: Oxford University Press.

Foa, E. B., Keane, T. M., & Friedman, M. J. (2000). Guidelines for treatment of PTSD. *Journal of Traumatic Stress: Official Publication of The International Society for Traumatic Stress Studies*, *13*(4), 539–588. doi:10.1023/A:1007802031411 PMID:11109232

Foa, E. B., & Kozak, M. J. (1986). Emotional processing of fear: Exposure to corrective information. *Psychological Bulletin*, *99*(1), 20–35. doi:10.1037/0033-2909.99.1.20 PMID:2871574

Foa, E. B., & Rothbaum, B. O. (1998). *Treating the trauma of rape: Cognitive–behavioral therapy for PTSD*. New York: Guilford.

Foa, E. B., Zinbarg, R., & Rothbaum, B. O. (1992). Uncontrollability and unpredictability in post-traumatic stress disorder: An animal model. *Psychological Bulletin*, *112*(2), 218–238. doi:10.1037/0033-2909.112.2.218 PMID:1454893

Forbes, D., Lewis, V., Varker, T., Phelps, A., Andrea, P., O'Donnell, M., ... Creamer, M. (2011). Psychological first aid following trauma: Implementation and evaluation framework for high-risk organizations. *Psychiatry*, *74*(3), 224–239. doi:10.1521/psyc.2011.74.3.224 PMID:21916629

Forslund, K., Kihlgren, A., & Kihlgren, M. (2004). Operators' experiences of emergency calls. *Journal of Telemedicine and Telecare*, *10*, 290–297. PMID:15494088

Forstenzer, A. (1980, July). Stress, the psychological scarring of air crash rescue personnel. *Firehouse*, 50-52.

Fox, J. H., Burkle, F. M. Jr, Bass, J., Pia, F. A., Epstein, J. L., & Markenson, D. (2012). The effectiveness of psychological first aid as a disaster intervention tool: Research analysis of peer-reviewed literature from 1990 - 2010. *Disaster Medicine and Public Health Preparedness*, *6*(3), 247–252. doi:10.1001/dmp.2012.39 PMID:23077267

Fox, J., Desai, M. M., Britten, K., Lucas, G., Luneau, R., & Rosenthal, M. S. (2012). Mental-health conditions, barriers to care, and productivity loss among officers in an urban police department. *Connecticut Medicine*, *76*(9), 525–531. PMID:23155671

Fox, K. A., Hornick, C. W., & Hardin, E. (2006). *International Association of Firefighters Diversity Initiative: Achieving and Retaining a Diverse Fire Service Workforce*. Washington, DC: IAFF.

Frederick, C. J. (Ed.). (1981). *Aircraft Accidents: Emergency Mental Health Problems*. Washington, DC: National Institute of Mental Health, U.S. Department of Health and Human Services.

Freeman, K. (1979). CMHC responses to the Chicago and San Diego airplane disasters. *Technical Assistance Center Report*, *2*(1), 10–12.

Freudenberger, H. J. (1980). *Burnout: The high cost of high achievement*. Garden City, NY: Anchor Press.

Friborg, O., Hjemdal, O., Rosenvinge, J. H., Martinussen, M., Aslaksen, P. M., & Flaten, M. A. (2006). Resilience as a moderator of pain and stress. *Journal of Psychosomatic Research*, *61*(2), 213–219. doi:10.1016/j.jpsychores.2005.12.007 PMID:16880024

Fuehrlein, B. S., Mota, N., Arias, A. J., Trevisan, L. A., Kachadourian, L. K., Krystal, J. H., ... Pietrzak, R. H. (2016). The burden of alcohol use disorders in US military veterans: Results from the National Health and Resilience in Veterans Study. *Addiction (Abingdon, England)*, *111*(10), 1786–1794. doi:10.1111/add.13423 PMID:27061707

Fuhr, D. C., Salisbury, T. T., De Silva, M. J., Atif, N., Van Ginneken, N., Rahman, A., & Patel, V. (2014). Effectiveness of peer-delivered interventions for severe mental illness and depression on clinical and psychosocial outcomes: A systematic review and meta-analysis. *Social Psychiatry and Psychiatric Epidemiology*, *49*(11), 1691–1702. doi:10.100700127-014-0857-5 PMID:24632847

Fullerton, C. S., McCarroll, J. E., Ursano, R. J., & Wright, K. M. (1992). Psychological responses of rescue workers: Fire fighters and trauma. *The American Journal of Orthopsychiatry*, *62*(3), 371–378. doi:10.1037/h0079363 PMID:1497102

Fullerton, C. S., Ursano, R. J., & Wang, L. (2004). Acute Stress Disorder, Posttraumatic Stress Disorder, and Depression in Disaster or Rescue Workers. *The American Journal of Psychiatry*, *161*(8), 1370–1376. doi:10.1176/appi.ajp.161.8.1370 PMID:15285961

Fullerton, C. S., Ursano, R. J., & Wang, L. (2004). Acute stress disorder, posttraumatic stress disorder, and depression in disaster or rescue workers. *The American Journal of Psychiatry*, *161*(8), 1370–1376. PMID:15285961

Gagliano, A. (2014). *Why women leave*. Retrieved from http://fireengineering.com

Gagliano, A., & Gagliano, M. (2018). *Challenges of the firefighter marriage*. Tulsa, OK: Fire Engineering Books & Videos.

Galatzer-Levy, I. R., Madan, A., Neylan, T. C., Henn-Haase, C., & Marmar, C. R. (2011). Peritraumatic and trait dissociation differentiate police officers with resilient versus symptomatic trajectories of posttraumatic stress symptoms. *Journal of Traumatic Stress*, *24*(5), 557–565. doi:10.1002/jts.20684 PMID:21898602

Gallyer, A. J., Dougherty, S. P., Gai, A. R., Stanley, I. H., Hom, M. A., Rogers, M. L., ... Joiner, T. E. (2018). Problematic alcohol use and suicidal ideation among firefighters: A multi-study investigation of the explanatory roles of perceived burdensomeness and thwarted belongingness. *Journal of Affective Disorders*, *238*, 281–288. doi:10.1016/j.jad.2018.05.045 PMID:29898427

Gardett, I., Olola, C., Scott, G., Broadbent, M., & Clawson, J. J. (2017). Comparison of emergency medical dispatcher stroke identification and paramedic on-scene stroke assessment. *Annals of Emergency Dispatch & Response*, *5*(1), 6–10.

Gariepy, G., Honkaniemi, H., & Quesnel-Vallee, A. (2016). Social support and protection from depression: Systematic review of current findings in Western countries. *The British Journal of Psychiatry*, *209*(4), 284–293. doi:10.1192/bjp.bp.115.169094 PMID:27445355

Garmezy, L. B., & Cummins, V. L. (2000). *Preventing police stress through co-training of officers and spouses*. Poster session presented at the meeting of the American Psychological Association, Washington, DC.

Gene-Cos, N. (2006). Post-traumatic stress disorder: The management of PTSD in adults and children in primary and secondary care. *The Psychiatrist*, *30*(9), 357–357.

Gerber, G. L., & Ward, K. C. (2011). Police personality: Theoretical issues and research. In J. Kitaeff (Ed.), *Handbook of police psychology* (pp. 421–436). New York: Routledge.

Germer, C. K., & Neff, K. D. (2013). Self-compassion in clinical practice. *Journal of Clinical Psychology*, *69*(8), 856–867. doi:10.1002/jclp.22021 PMID:23775511

Giese-Davis, J., Bliss-Isberg, C., Carson, K., Star, P., Donaghy, J., Cordova, M. J., ... Spiegel, D. (2006). The effect of peer counseling on quality of life following diagnosis of breast cancer: an observational study. *Psycho-Oncology: Journal of the Psychological. Social and Behavioral Dimensions of Cancer*, *15*(11), 1014–1022. PMID:16555366

Gillespie, E. (2017, May 14). *First responders' selfless service leaves them vulnerable to PTSD's toll: Programs aim to help those who face trauma daily.* Retrieved from https://www.columbian.com/news/2017/may/14/first-responders-selfless-service-leaves-them-vulnerable-to-ptsds-toll/

Gilmartin, K. (2002). *Emotional survival for law enforcement: A guide for officers and their families*. Tucson, AZ: E-S Press.

Gist, R., Taylor, V. H., & Raak, S. (2011). *Suicide surveillance, prevention, and intervention measures for the US Fire Service: Findings and recommendations for the suicide and depression summit.* Baltimore, MD: National Fallen Firefighters Foundation.

Gjefle, A., & Vikari, V. (2012). Training to the rescue: First responders power up skills while cutting costs. *Public Management*, *41*(3), 35–38.

Glicken, M. D. (2006). *Learning from resilient people: Lessons we can apply to counseling and psychotherapy*. Thousand Oaks, CA: Sage Publications.

Goenjian, A. K., Karayan, I., Pynoos, R. S., Minassian, D., Najarian, L. M., Steinberg, A. M., & Fairbanks, L. A. (1997). Outcome of psychotherapy among early adolescents after trauma. *The American Journal of Psychiatry*, *154*(4), 536–542. doi:10.1176/ajp.154.4.536 PMID:9090342

Goenjian, A. K., Walling, D., Steinberg, A. M., Karavan, I., Najarian, L. M., & Pynoos, R. (2005). A prospective study of posttraumatic stress and depressive reactions among treated and untreated adolescents 5 years after a catastrophic disaster. *The American Journal of Psychiatry*, *162*(12), 2302–2308. doi:10.1176/appi.ajp.162.12.2302 PMID:16330594

Golden, L. L., Jones, R. T., & Donlon, K. (2014). Delayed treatment seeking following the April 16th shootings at Virginia Tech: Impact on a first responder. *Clinical Case Studies*, *13*(5), 391–404. doi:10.1177/1534650113512174

Golding, S. E., Horsfield, C., Davies, A., Egan, B., Jones, M., Raleigh, M., ... Cropley, M. (2017). Exploring the psychological health of emergency dispatch centre operatives: A systematic review and narrative synthesis. *PeerJ*, *5*, e3735. doi:10.7717/peerj.3735 PMID:29062596

Goldstein, D. B. (2005). A comparison of utilization of peer support services and perceived stigma within the Vermont State Police. *Forensic Examiner*, *14*(3), 44–48.

Goldstein, L. E., Rasmusson, A. M., Bunney, B. S., & Roth, R. H. (1996). Role of the amygdala in the coordination of behavioral, neuroendocrine, and prefrontal cortical monoamine responses to psychological stress in the rat. *The Journal of Neuroscience*, *16*(15), 4787–4798. doi:10.1523/JNEUROSCI.16-15-04787.1996 PMID:8764665

Gonzalez, G. C., Singh, R., Schell, T. L., & Weinick, R. M. (2014). An evaluation of the implementation and perceived utility of the airman resilience training program. *Rand Health Quarterly, 4*(2).

Graf, F. A. (1986). The relationship between social support and occupational stress among police officers. *Journal of Police Science and Administration*, *14*(3), 178–186.

Grant, B. F., Goldstein, R. B., Saha, T. D., Chou, S. P., Jung, J., Zhang, H., ... Hasin, D. S. (2015). Epidemiology of DSM-5 Alcohol Use Disorder: Results from the National Epidemiologic Survey on Alcohol and Related Conditions III. *Journal of the American Medical Association Psychiatry*, *72*(8), 757–766. PMID:26039070

Grant, L. (2014). Hearts and Minds: Aspects of Empathy and Wellbeing in Social Work Students. *Social Work Education, 33*(3), 338–352. doi:10.1080/02615479.2013.805191

Grauwiler, P., Barocas, B., & Mills, L. G. (2008). Police peer support programs: Current knowledge and practice. *International Journal of Emergency Mental Health, 10*(1), 27–38. PMID:18546757

Greden, J. F., Valenstein, M., Spinner, J., Blow, A., Gorman, L. A., Dalack, G. W., ... Kees, M. (2010). Buddy-to-Buddy, a citizen soldier peer support program to counteract stigma, PTSD, depression, and suicide. *Annals of the New York Academy of Sciences, 1208*(1), 90–97. doi:10.1111/j.1749-6632.2010.05719.x PMID:20955330

Griffith, J. C., Roberts, D. L., & Wakeham, R. T. (2016). Bullying at the Fire Station? Perceptions Based on Gender, Race and Sexual Orientation. *American International Journal of Social Sciences, 5*, 34–44.

Griffiths, K. L., Mackey, M. G., & Adamson, B. J. (2007). The impact of a computerized work environment on professional occupational groups and behavioural and physiological risk factors for musculoskeletal symptoms: A literature review. *Journal of Occupational Rehabilitation, 17*(4), 743–765. doi:10.100710926-007-9108-x PMID:17987369

Grillon, C., Pine, D. S., Lissek, S., Rabin, S., Bonne, O., & Vythilingam, M. (2009). Increased anxiety during anticipation of unpredictable aversive stimuli in posttraumatic stress disorder but not in generalized anxiety disorder. *Biological Psychiatry, 66*(1), 47–53. doi:10.1016/j.biopsych.2008.12.028 PMID:19217076

Gulliver, S. B., Pennington, M. L., Torres, V. A., Steffen, L. E., Mardikar, A., Leto, F., ... Kimbrel, N. A. (2018). Behavioral Health Programs in Fire Service: Surveying Access and Preferences. *Psychological Services*; Advance online publication. PMID:29369659

Gulliver, S. B., Zimering, R., Knight, J., Morissette, S., Kamholz, B., Meyer, E., ... Kimbrel, N. (2018). Tobacco and alcohol use among firefighters during their first 3 years of service. *Psychology of Addictive Behaviors, 32*(3), 255–263. doi:10.1037/adb0000366 PMID:29771556

Gunn, C., Mackus, M., Griffin, C., Munafo, M. R., & Adams, S. (2018). A systematic review of the next-day effects of heavy alcohol consumption on cognitive performance. *Addiction (Abingdon, England), 113*(12), 2181–2193. doi:10.1111/add.14404 PMID:30144191

Gurevich, M., Halpern, J., Brazeau, P., Defina, P. S., & Schwartz, B. (2009). Frontline stress behind the scenes: Emergency medical dispatchers. *Ryerson University, Do Psychology.*

Haase, J., Britt, T., Coward, D., Leidy, N., & Penn, P. E. (1992). Simultaneous concept analysis of spiritual perspective, hope, acceptance, and self-transcendence. *Image--the Journal of Nursing Scholarship, 24*(2), 141–147. doi:10.1111/j.1547-5069.1992.tb00239.x PMID:1601456

Haddock, C. K., Poston, W. S., Jahnke, S. A., & Jitnarin. (2017). Alcohol use and problem drinking among women firefighters. *Women's Health Issues, 27*, 632-638. Retrieved from http://whijournal.com

Haddock, C. K., Day, R. S., Poston, W. S., Jahnke, S. A., & Jitnarin, N. (2015). Alcohol use and caloric intake from alcohol in a national cohort of U.S. career firefighters. *Journal of Studies on Alcohol and Drugs, 76*(3), 360–366. PMID:25978821

Haddock, C. K., Jahnke, S. A., Poston, W. S., Jitnarin, K., Kaipust, C. M., Tuley, B., & Hyder, M. L. (2012). Alcohol use among firefighters in the Central United States. *Occupational Medicine, 62*(8), 661–664. doi:10.1093/occmed/kqs162 PMID:23064207

Haddock, C. K., Poston, W. S. C., Jahnke, S. A., & Jitnarin, N. (2017). Alcohol use and problem drinking among women firefighters. *Women's Health Issues, 27*(6), 632–638. PMID:28822615

Haddock, C. K., Poston, W. S., Jahnke, S. A., & Jitnarin, N. (2017). Alcohol Use and Problem Drinking among Women Firefighters. *Women's Health Issues*, *27*(6), 632–638. doi:10.1016/j.whi.2017.07.003 PMID:28822615

Hagenaars, M. A., Stins, J. F., & Roelofs, K. (2012). Aversive life events enhance human freezing responses. *Journal of Experimental Psychology. General*, *141*(1), 98–105. doi:10.1037/a0024211 PMID:21767043

Hall, M. H., Brindle, R. C., & Buysse, D. J. (2018). Sleep and cardiovascular disease: Emerging opportunities for psychologists. *The American Psychologist*, *73*(8), 994–1006. doi:10.1037/amp0000362 PMID:30394778

Halpern, J., Gurevich, M., Schwartz, B., & Brazeau, P. (2009). Interventions for critical incident stress in emergency medical services: A qualitative study. *Stress and Health*, *25*(2), 139–149. doi:10.1002mi.1230

Hammelman, J. (2013). *Physiological and psychological responses to 911 emergency tapes* (Doctoral dissertation). Retrieved from ProQuest dissertations and theses database. (Order No. 10138220)

Hammond, D. C. (2000). Clinical Corner. *Journal of Neurotherapy*, *4*(3), 93–97. doi:10.1300/J184v04n03_07

Hansen, J. (2017). Night shift work and risk of breast cancer. *Current Environmental Health Reports, 4,* 325-339. Retrieved from http://ncbi.nlm.nih.gov doi/ doi:10.100740572-017-0155-y

Harrison, R. L., & Westwood, M. J. (2009). Preventing vicarious traumatization of mental health therapists: Identifying protective practices. *Psychotherapy (Chicago, Ill.)*, *46*(2), 203–219. doi:10.1037/a0016081 PMID:22122619

Hartley, T. A., Violanti, J. M., Fekedulegn, D., Andrew, M. E., & Burchfiel, C. M. (2007). Associations between major life events, traumatic incidents, and depression among Buffalo police officers. *International Journal of Emergency Mental Health, 9*, 25–35. Retrieved from http:// www.ncbi.nlm.nih.gov/pubmed/11227748

Hartley, T. A., Sarkisian, K., Violanti, J. M., Andrew, M. E., & Burchfiel, C. M. (2013). PTSD symptoms among police officers: Associations with frequency, recency, and types of traumatic events. *International Journal of Emergency Mental Health*, *15*(4), 241. PMID:24707587

Hart, P. M., & Cotton, P. (2003). Conventional wisdom is often misleading: Police stress within an organisational health framework. In M. F. Dollard, A. H. Winefield, & H. R. Winefield (Eds.), *Occupational stress in the service professions* (pp. 103–141). London: Taylor & Francis. doi:10.1201/9780203422809.ch4

Harvard Business Review. (1997). *The Work of Leadership*. Author.

Harvey, S. B., Milligan-Saville, J. S., Paterson, H. M., Harkness, E. L., Marsh, A. M., Dobson, M., ... Bryant, R. A. (2016). The mental health of fire-fighters: An examination of the impact of repeated trauma exposure. *The Australian and New Zealand Journal of Psychiatry*, *50*(7), 649–658. doi:10.1177/0004867415615217 PMID:26607303

Hassling, P. (2000). Disaster management and the Gothenburg fire of 1998: When first responders are blamed. *International Journal of Emergency Mental Health*, *2*(2), 267–273. PMID:11217158

Haugen, P. T., Evces, M., & Weiss, D. (2012). Treating posttraumatic stress disorder in first responders: A systematic review. *Clinical Psychology Review*, *32*(5), 370–380. doi:10.1016/j.cpr.2012.04.001 PMID:22561967

Haugen, P. T., McCrillis, A. M., Smid, G. E., & Nijdam, M. J. (2017). Mental health stigma and barriers to mental health care for first responders: A systematic review and meta- analysis. *Journal of Psychiatric Research*, *94*, 218–229. doi:10.1016/j.jpsychires.2017.08.001 PMID:28800529

Hayes, S. C. (2016). *Acceptance & Action Questionnaire (AAQ) and variations*. Jenison, MI: Association for Contextual Behavioral Science. Retrieved from https://contextualscience.org/acceptance_action_questionnaire_aaq_and_variations

Hayes, S. C., Strosahl, K. D., & Wilson, K. G. (1999). *Acceptance and commitment therapy: An experiential approach to behavior change*. New York, NY: Guilford Press.

Haynes, H. J., & Stein, G. P. (2017). *US Fire Department Profile 2015*. Quincy, MA: National Fire Protection Association.

Hedtke, L. (2014). Creating stories of hope: A narrative approach to illness, death and grief. *Australian and New Zealand Journal of Family Therapy*, *35*(1), 4–19. doi:10.1002/anzf.1040

Heightman, A. J. (2016). EMS agencies need to have eap resources to address stress and reduce suicides. *Journal of Emergency Medical Services*, *41*(1). Retrieved from https://www.jems.com/articles/print/volume-41/issue-1/departments-columns/from-the-editor/ems-agencies-need-to-have-eap-resources-to-address-stress-and-reduce-suicides.html PMID:26901952

Hem, E., Berg, A. M., & Ekberg, O. (2001). Suicide in police – a critical review. *Suicide & Life-Threatening Behavior*, *31*(2), 224–233. doi:10.1521uli.31.2.224.21513 PMID:11459255

Henderson, S. N., Van Hasselt, V. B., LeDuc, T. J., & Couwels, J. (2016). Firefighter suicide: Understanding cultural challenges for mental health professionals. *Professional Psychology, Research and Practice*, *47*(3), 224–230. doi:10.1037/pro0000072

Hersey, P., & Blanchard, K. (2000). *Management of Organizational Behavior*. Prentice Hall Inc.

Hetrick, S. E., Purcell, R., Garner, B., & Parslow, R. (2010). Combined pharmacotherapy and psychological therapies for post traumatic stress disorder (PTSD). *Cochrane Database of Systematic Reviews*. doi:10.1002/14651858.CD007316.pub2 PMID:20614457

Heyman, M., Dill, J., & Douglas, R. (2018). *Ruderman white paper on mental health and suicide of first responders*. Boston, MA: Ruderman Family Foundation.

Heyman, M., Dill, J., & Douglas, R. (2018). *The Ruderman White Paper on Mental Health and Suicide of First Responders*. Boston, MA: Ruderman Foundation.

Heyman, M., Dill, J., & Douglas, R. (2018). *The Ruderman White Paper on Mental Health and Suicide of First Responders*. Ruderman Family Foundation.

Hobfoll, S. E., Briggs-Phillips, M., & Stines, L. R. (2003). Fact or artifact: The relationship of hope to a caravan of resources. In R. Jacoby & G. Keinan (Eds.), *Between stress and hope: From a disease-centered to a health-centered perspective* (pp. 81–104). Westport, CT: Praeger.

Hobfoll, S. E., Spielberger, C. D., Breznitz, S., Figley, C., Folkman, S., Lepper-Green, B., ... van der Kolk, B. (1991). War-related stress: Addressing the stress of war and other traumatic events. *The American Psychologist*, *46*(8), 848–855. doi:10.1037/0003-066X.46.8.848 PMID:1928937

Hobfoll, S., Watson, P., Bell, C., Bryant, R., Brymer, M. J., Friedman, M. J., ... Ursano, R. J. (2007). Five essential elements of immediate and mid-term mass trauma intervention: Empirical evidence. *Psychiatry*, *70*(4), 283–315. doi:10.1521/psyc.2007.70.4.283 PMID:18181708

Hoey, L. M., Ieropoli, S. C., White, V. M., & Jefford, M. (2008). Systematic review of peer support programs for people with cancer. *Patient Education and Counseling*, *70*(3), 315–337. doi:10.1016/j.pec.2007.11.016 PMID:18191527

Hoge, C. W., Grossman, S. H., Auchterlonie, J. L., Riviere, L. A., Milliken, C. S., & Wilk, J. E. (2014). PTSD treatment for soldiers after combat deployment: Low utilization of mental health care and reasons for dropout. *Psychiatric Services (Washington, D.C.)*, *65*(8), 997–1004. doi:10.1176/appi.ps.201300307 PMID:24788253

Hoge, C. W., Lesikar, S. E., Guevara, R., Lange, J., Brundage, J. F., Engel, C. C. Jr, ... Orman, D. T. (2002). Mental disorders among US military personnel in the 1990s: Association with high levels of health care utilization and early military attrition. *The American Journal of Psychiatry*, *159*(9), 1576–1583. doi:10.1176/appi.ajp.159.9.1576 PMID:12202280

Hoge, C. W., Riviere, L. A., Wilk, J. E., Herrell, R. K., & Weathers, F. W. (2014). The prevalence of post-traumatic stress disorder (PTSD) in US combat soldiers: A head-to-head comparison of DSM-5 versus DSM-IV-TR symptom criteria with the PTSD checklist. *The Lancet. Psychiatry*, *1*(4), 269–277. doi:10.1016/S2215-0366(14)70235-4 PMID:26360860

Hoge, C. W., Terhakopian, A., Castro, C. A., Messer, S. C., & Engel, C. C. (2007). Association of posttraumatic stress disorder with somatic symptoms, health care visits, and absenteeism among Iraq War veterans. *The American Journal of Psychiatry*, *164*(1), 150–153. doi:10.1176/ajp.2007.164.1.150 PMID:17202557

Holahan, C. J., & Moos, R. H. (1990). Life stressors, resistance factors, and improved psychological functioning: An extension of the stress resistance paradigm. *Journal of Personality and Social Psychology*, *58*(5), 909–917. doi:10.1037/0022-3514.58.5.909 PMID:2348376

Hollerbach, B. S., Heinrich, K. M., Poston, W. S., Haddock, C. K., Kehler, A. K., & Jahnke, S. A. (2017). Current Female Firefighters' Perceptions, Attitudes, and Experiences with Injury. *International Fire Service Journal of Leadership & Management*, (11).

Holman, E. A., Silver, R. C., Poulin, M., Andersen, J., Gil-Rivas, V., & McIntosh, D. N. (2008). Terrorism, acute stress, and cardiovascular health: A 3-year national study following the September 11th attacks. *Archives of General Psychiatry*, *65*(1), 73–80. doi:10.1001/archgenpsychiatry.2007.6 PMID:18180431

Hom, M. A., Stanley, I. H., Ringer, F. B., & Joiner, T. E. (2016). Mental health service use among firefighters with suicidal thoughts and behaviors. *Psychiatric Services (Washington, D.C.)*, *67*(6), 688–691. doi:10.1176/appi.ps.201500177 PMID:26927574

Hom, M. A., Stanley, I. H., Spencer-Thomas, S., & Joiner, T. E. (2017). Women firefighters and workplace harassment: Associated suicidality and mental health sequelae. *The Journal of Nervous and Mental Disease*, *205*(12), 910–917. doi:10.1097/NMD.0000000000000759 PMID:29088006

Horner, E., & Tully, P. D. (2016). Divorcing the voice of fear: A collaborative, narrative approach to anxiety. *International Journal of Narrative Therapy & Community Work*, (2), 37-43.

Horn, S. R., Charney, D. S., & Feder, A. (2016). Understanding resilience: New approaches for preventing and treating PTSD. *Experimental Neurology*, *284*, 119–132. doi:10.1016/j.expneurol.2016.07.002 PMID:27417856

Horowitz, M., Wilner, N., & Alvarez, W. (1979). The Impact of Event Scale: A measure of subjective stress. *Psychosomatic Medicine*, *41*(3), 209–218. PMID:472086

Horvath, C. (2013). Same old story: The biggest issues facing women firefighters today. *FireRescue1*. Retrieved from https://www.firerescue1.com/cod-company-officer-development/articles/1453190-Same-old-story-The-biggest-issues-facing-women-firefighters-today/

Howlett, S. L., & Collins, A. (2014). Vicarious traumatization: Risk and resilience among crisis support volunteers in a community organization. *South African Journal of Psychology. Suid-Afrikaanse Tydskrif vir Sielkunde*, *44*(2), 180–190. doi:10.1177/0081246314524387

Hulett, D. M., Bendick, M., Thomas, S. Y., & Moccio, F. (2008). *A national report card on women in firefighting*. Madison, WI: International Association of Women in Fire and Emergency Services. Retrieved from https://www.i-women.org/wp-content/uploads/2014/07/35827WSP.pdf

Hurrell, J. J., Pate, A., Kliesmet, R., Bowers, R. A., Lee, S., & Burg, J. (1984). *Stress among police officers*. Cincinnati, OH: National Institute of Occupational Safety and Health.

Hyland, P., Boduszek, D., Dhingra, K., Shevlin, M., Maguire, R., & Morley, K. (2015). A test of the inventory of attitudes towards seeking mental health services. *British Journal of Guidance & Counselling*, *43*(4), 397–412. doi:10.1080/03069885.2014.963510

IAFC President's Letter: Time to Lead on Diversity and Inclusion. (2016). Retrieved from https://www.iafc.org/on-scene/on-scene-article/president-s-letter-time-to-lead-on-diversity-and-inclusion

Imel, Z. E., Laska, K., Jakupcak, M., & Simpson, T. L. (2013). Meta-analysis of dropout in treatments for posttraumatic stress disorder. *Journal of Consulting and Clinical Psychology*, *81*(3), 394–404. doi:10.1037/a0031474 PMID:23339535

Inglish, P. (2010). *Top 10 Most Dangerous Jobs 2007-2010 Hub Pages Elite Jobs*. Retrieved from Hubpages.com/hub/Most_Dangerous_

Inslicht, S. S., McCaslin, S. E., Metzler, T. J., Henn-Haase, C., Hart, S. L., Maguen, S., ... Marmar, C. R. (2010). Family psychiatric history, peritraumatic reactivity, and posttraumatic stress symptoms: A prospective study of police. *Journal of Psychiatric Research*, *44*(1), 22–31. PMID:19683259

International Association for Fire Fighters. (2001). Washington, DC: Developing Fire Service Labor/Employee Assistance Programs.

International Association of Chiefs of Police (IACP). (2016). *Peer support guidelines*. Retrieved from https://www.theiacp.org/sites/default/files/all/p-r/Psych-PeerSupportGuidelines.pdf

International Association of Firefighters. (2008). *The Fire Service Joint Labor Management Wellness-Fitness Initiative* (3rd ed.). Washington, DC: International Association of Firefighters.

Jackson, B. A., Towe, V. L., Wagner, L., Hunt, P., Greathouse, S., & Hollywood, J. S. (2016). Managing officer behavioral risk using early intervention systems: Addressing system design challenges for Law Enforcement and corrections environments. *Policing: Journal of Policy Practice*, *11*(1), 103–117.

Jacobsen, E. (1929). *Progressive relaxation*. Academic Press.

Jahnke, S. A. (2015). Firefighter divorce: 3 important facts. *FireRescue1*. Retrieved from http://firerescue1.com

Jahnke, S. A. (2018). *Your worst day is our every day: The impact of repeated exposure to trauma on the fire service* [Video Webinar]. Retrieved from https://www.iafc.org/events/event/2018/08/30/default-calendar/your-worst-day-is-our-every-day-the-impact-of-repeated-exposure-to-trauma-on-the-fire-service

Jahnke, S. A. (2012). Exploring factors associated with problem drinking among firefighters. *Journal of Substance Abuse Treatment*, *43*(3), e25. doi:10.1016/j.jsat.2012.08.118

Jahnke, S. A., Haddock, C. K., Jitnarin, N., Kaipust, C., Hollerbach, B. S., & Poston, W. S. C. (Manuscript submitted for publication). The prevalence and health impacts of frequent work discrimination and harassment among women firefighters in the US fire service. *BioMed Research International*. PMID:31016195

Jahnke, S. A., Poston, W. S. C., Haddock, C. K., & Jitnarin, N. (2013). Obesity and incident injury among career firefighters in the central United States. *Obesity (Silver Spring, Md.)*, *21*(8), 1505–1508. PMID:23512940

Jahnke, S. A., Poston, W. S. C., Haddock, C. K., & Murphy, B. (2016). Firefighting and mental health: Experiences of repeated exposure to trauma. *Work (Reading, Mass.)*, *53*(4), 737–744. doi:10.3233/WOR-162255 PMID:26890595

Jahnke, S. A., Poston, W. S., Jitnarin, N., & Haddock, C. K. (2018). Maternal and Child Health Among Female Firefighters in the US. *Maternal and Child Health Journal*, *22*(6), 922–931. PMID:29423588

Jahnke, S.A., Poston, W.C., & Haddock, C.K. (2014). Perceptions of Alcohol use among US Firefighters. *Journal of Substance Abuse and Alcoholism*, *2*(2).

Jahnke, S., Poston, W., Haddock, C., Jitnarin, N., Hyder, M., & Horvath, C. (2012). The health of women in the US fire service. *BMC Women's Health*, *12*(1), 39. doi:10.1186/1472-6874-12-39 PMID:23114186

Jamieson, J. P., Mendes, W. B., Blackstock, E., & Schmader, T. (2010). Turning the knots in your stomach into bows: Reappraising arousal improves performance on the GRE. *Journal of Experimental Social Psychology*, *46*(1), 208–212. doi:10.1016/j.jesp.2009.08.015 PMID:20161454

Janoff–Bulman, R. (1992). *Shattered assumptions: Toward a new psychology of trauma*. New York: Free Press.

Javidi, H., & Yadollahie, M. (2012). Post-traumatic stress disorder. *The International Journal of Occupational and Environmental Medicine*, *3*(1), 2–9. PMID:23022845

Jenkins, S. R. (1996). Social support and debriefing efficacy among emergency medical workers after a mass shooting incident. *Journal of Social Behavior and Personality*, *11*, 447–492.

Jensen, R. A. (2000). *Mass Fatality and Casualty Incidents*. CRC Press LLC.

Jitnarin, N., Poston, W. S. C., Haddock, C. K., Jahnke, S. A., Day, R. S., & Severson, H. H. (2017). Prevalence and correlates of late initiation of smokeless tobacco in us firefighters. *Nicotine & Tobacco Research*, *20*(1), 130–134. PMID:27940900

Jitnarin, N., Poston, W. S., Haddock, C. K., Jahnke, S. A., & Day, R. S. (2015). Tobacco use pattern among a national firefighter cohort. *Nicotine & Tobacco Research*, *17*(1), 66–73. doi:10.1093/ntr/ntu131 PMID:25145378

Johnson, B. R. (2007). *Crucial elements of police firearms training*. Looseleaf Law Publications.

Johnson, D. R., Feldman, S., & Lubin, H. (1995). Critical interaction therapy: Couples therapy in combat-related post-traumatic stress disorder. *Family Process*, *34*(4), 401–412. doi:10.1111/j.1545-5300.1995.00401.x PMID:8674521

Johnson, J. (2010). *Understanding Differences in Stress and Coping Between Full-Time and Paid-On-Call Firefighters*. Walden University.

Johnson, M. D. (2012). Healthy marriage initiatives: On the need for empiricism in policy implementation. *The American Psychologist*, *67*(4), 296–308. doi:10.1037/a0027743 PMID:22468785

Jones, S. (2017). Describing the mental health profile of first responders: A systematic review. *Journal of the American Psychiatric Nurses Association*, *23*(3), 200–214. doi:10.1177/1078390317695266 PMID:28445653

Jones, S. P., Carter, B., Ford, G. A., Gibson, J. M. E., Leathley, M. J., McAdam, J. J., ... Watkins, C. L. (2012). The identification of acute stroke: An analysis of emergency calls. *International Journal of Stroke*, *8*(6), 408–412. doi:10.1111/j.1747-4949.2011.00749.x PMID:22335960

Jones, S., Nagel, C., McSweeney, J., & Curran, G. (2018). Prevalence and correlates of psychiatric symptoms among first responders in a southern state. *Archives of Psychiatric Nursing*, *32*(6), 828–835. doi:10.1016/j.apnu.2018.06.007 PMID:30454624

Joseph, S., Murphy, D., & Regel, S. (2012). An affective–cognitive processing model of post-traumatic growth. *Clinical Psychology & Psychotherapy*, *19*(4), 316–325. doi:10.1002/cpp.1798 PMID:22610981

Kabat-Zinn, J. (1990). *Full catastrophe living: The program of the stress reduction clinic at the University of Massachusetts Medical Center*. Academic Press.

Kabat-Zinn, J. (2003). Mindfulness-based stress reduction (MBSR). *Constructivism in the Human Sciences*, *8*(2), 73.

Kabat-Zinn, J., Lipworth, L., & Burney, R. (1985). The clinical use of mindfulness meditation for the self-regulation of chronic pain. *Journal of Behavioral Medicine*, *8*(2), 163–190. doi:10.1007/BF00845519 PMID:3897551

Kales, S. N., Polyhronopoulos, G. N., Aldrich, J. M., Leitao, E. O., & Christiani, D. C. (1999). Correlates of body mass index in hazardous materials firefighters. *Journal of Occupational and Environmental Medicine*, *41*(7), 589–595. PMID:10412100

Kales, S. N., Soteriades, E. S., Christophi, C. A., & Christiani, D. C. (2007). Emergency duties and deaths from heart disease among firefighters in the United States. *The New England Journal of Medicine*, *356*(12), 1207–1215. doi:10.1056/NEJMoa060357 PMID:17377158

Kalisch, R., Müller, M. B., & Tüscher, O. (2015). A conceptual framework for the neurobiological study of resilience. *Behavioral and Brain Sciences*, 38. PMID:25158686

Kamena, M. D., Gentz, D., Hays, V., Bohl-Penrod, N., & Greene, L. W. (2011). Peer support teams fill an emotional void in law enforcement agencies. *The Police Chief*, *78*(8), 80–84.

Kaminer, D., Eagle, G., & Crawford-Browne, S. (2016). Continuous traumatic stress as a mental and physical health challenge: Case studies from South Africa. *Journal of Health Psychology*. doi:10.1177/1359105316642831 PMID:27091760

Karasek, R. A. Jr. (1979). Job demands, job decision latitude, and mental strain: Implications for job redesign. *Administrative Science Quarterly*, *24*(2), 285–308. doi:10.2307/2392498

Kardiner, A., & Spiegel, H. (1947). *War, Stress, and Neurotic Illness*. New York: Hoeber.

Kashdan, T. B., & Rottenberg, J. (2010). Psychological flexibility as a fundamental aspect of health. *Clinical Psychology Review*, *30*(7), 865–878. doi:10.1016/j.cpr.2010.03.001 PMID:21151705

Kazantzis, N., & Dattilio, F. M. (2010). Definitions of homework, types of homework, and ratings of the importance of homework among psychologists with cognitive behavior therapy and psychoanalytic theoretical orientations. *Journal of Clinical Psychology*, *66*(7), 758–773. doi:10.1002/jclp.20699 PMID:20527055

Kearns, M. C., Ressler, K. J., Zatzick, D., & Rothbaum, B. O. (2012). Early intervention for PTSD: A review. *Depression and Anxiety*, *29*(10), 833–842. doi:10.1002/da.21997 PMID:22941845

Kehler, A., Jahnke, S.A., Haddock, C.K., Poston, W.S., Jitnarin, N., & Heinrich, K.M. (2018). Reproductive Health Concerns Among Female Firefighters. *International Fire Service Journal of Leadership and Management,* 12.

Kelly, J., & Hoban, J. E. (2016). Health and wellness programming: The added contribution of an ethical mindset. In C. L. Mitchell & E. H. Dorian (Eds.), *Police psychology and its growing impact on modern law enforcement*. Hershey, PA: IGI Global.

Kemp, V., & Henderson, A. R. (2012). Challenges faced by mental health peer support workers: Peer support from the peer supporter's point of view. *Psychiatric Rehabilitation Journal*, *35*(4), 337–340. doi:10.2975/35.4.2012.337.340 PMID:22491374

Kenlon, J. (1913). *Fires and fire-fighters: A history of modern fire-fighting with a review of its development from earliest times*. New York, NY: George H. Doran Company.

Kerr, S., Johnson, V. K., Gans, S. E., & Krumrine, J. (2004). Predicting adjustment during the transition to college: Alexithymia, perceived stress, and psychological symptoms. *Journal of College Student Development*, *45*(6), 593–611. doi:10.1353/csd.2004.0068

Kessler, R. C., Berglund, P., Demler, O., Jin, R., Merikangas, K. R., & Walters, E. E. (2005). Lifetime prevalence and age-of-onset distributions of DSM-IV disorders in the National Comorbidity Survey Replication. *Archives of General Psychiatry*, *62*(6), 593–602. doi:10.1001/archpsyc.62.6.593 PMID:15939837

Kessler, R. C., Chiu, W. T., Demler, O., & Walters, E. E. (2005). Prevalence, severity, and comorbidity of twelve-month DSM-IV disorders in the National Comorbidity Survey Replication (NCS-R). *Archives of General Psychiatry*, *62*(6), 617–627. doi:10.1001/archpsyc.62.6.617 PMID:15939839

Kessler, R. C., & Frank, R. G. (1997). The impact of psychiatric disorders on work loss days. *Psychological Medicine*, *27*(4), 861–873. doi:10.1017/S0033291797004807 PMID:9234464

Kessler, R. C., Mickelson, K. D., & Williams, D. R. (1999). The prevalence, distribution, and mental health correlates of perceived discrimination in the United States. *Journal of Health and Social Behavior*, *40*(3), 208–230. PMID:10513145

Kessler, R. C., Sonnega, A., Bromet, E., Hughes, M., & Nelson, C. B. (1995). Posttraumatic stress disorder in the national comorbidity survey. *Archives of General Psychiatry*, *52*(12), 1048–1060. doi:10.1001/archpsyc.1995.03950240066012 PMID:7492257

Khantzian, E. J. (1999). *Treating addiction as a human process*. Northvale, NJ: Jason Aronson.

Khatiban, M., Hosseini, S., Bikmoradi, A., Roshanaei, G., & Karampourian, A. (2015). Occupational burnout and its determinants among personnel of emergency medical services in Iran. *Acta Medica Iranica*, *53*(11), 711–716. PMID:26786993

Khoury, B., Sharma, M., Rush, S. E., & Fournier, C. (2015). Mindfulness-based stress reduction for healthy individuals: A meta-analysis. *Journal of Psychosomatic Research*, *78*(6), 519–528. doi:10.1016/j.jpsychores.2015.03.009 PMID:25818837

Kilpatrick, D. G., Resnick, H. S., Milanak, M. E., Miller, M. W., Keyes, K. M., & Friedman, M. J. (2013). National estimates of exposure to traumatic events and PTSD prevalence using DSM-IV and DSM-5 criteria. *Journal of Traumatic Stress*, *26*(5), 537–547. doi:10.1002/jts.21848 PMID:24151000

Kimbrel, N. A., Steffen, L. E., Meyer, E. C., Kruse, M. I., Knight, J. A., Zimering, R. T., & Gulliver, S. B. (2011). A revised measure of occupational stress for firefighters: Psychometric properties and relationship to posttraumatic stress disorder, depression and substance abuse. *Psychological Services*, *8*(4), 294–306. doi:10.1037/a0025845

Kim, J. E., Dager, S. R., Jeong, H. S., Ma, J., Park, S., Kim, J., ... Lyoo, I. K. (2018). Firefighters, posttraumatic stress disorder, and barriers to treatment: Results from a nationwide total population survey. *PLoS One*, *13*(1), e0190630. doi:10.1371/journal.pone.0190630 PMID:29304155

Kim, J. I., Park, H., & Kim, J. H. (2017). The mediation effect of PTSD, perceived job stress and resilience on the relationship between trauma exposure and the development of depression and alcohol use problems in Korean firefighters: A cross-sectional study. *Journal of Affective Disorders*, *229*, 450–455. doi:10.1016/j.jad.2017.12.055 PMID:29331707

Kim, J. I., Park, H., & Kim, J. H. (2018). Alcohol use disorders and insomnia mediate the association between PTSD symptoms and suicidal ideation in Korean firefighters. *Depression and Anxiety*, *35*(11), 1095–1103. doi:10.1002/da.22803 PMID:30028563

Kira, I., Lewandowski, L., Templin, R., Ramaswamy, V., Ozkan, B., & Mohanesh, J. (2008). Measuring cumulative trauma dose, types and profiles using a development-based taxonomy of trauma. *Traumatology*, *14*(2), 62–87. doi:10.1177/1534765608319324

Kirlin, L., Nichols, J., Rusk, K., Parker, R., & Rauh, M. (2017). The effect of age on fitness among female firefighters. *Occupational Medicine, 67*(7), 528–533. doi:10.1093/occmed/kqx123 PMID:29016908

Kirmeyer, S. L., & Dougherty, T. W. (1988). Work load, tension, and coping: Moderating effects of supervisor support. *Personnel Psychology, 41*(1), 125–139. doi:10.1111/j.1744-6570.1988.tb00635.x

Kirschman, E. (2004). *I love a fire fighter: What the family needs to know*. New York: Guilford Press.

Kirschman, E. (2007). *I love a cop: What police families need to know* (Rev. ed.). New York, NY: The Guilford Press.

Kirschman, E., Kamena, M., & Fay, J. (2014). *Counseling cops: What clinicians need to know*. New York: Guilford Press.

Kleim, B., & Westphal, M. (2011). Mental health in first responders: A review and recommendation for prevention and intervention strategies. *Traumatology, 17*(4), 17–24. doi:10.1177/1534765611429079

Klein, A., Cnaan, R., & Whitecraft, J. (1998). Significance of peer social support for dually diagnosed clients: Findings from a pilot study. *Research on Social Work Practice, 8*(5), 529–551. doi:10.1177/104973159800800503

Klimley, K. E., Van Hasselt, V. B., & Stripling, A. M. (2018). Posttraumatic stress disorder in police, firefighters, and emergency dispatchers. *Aggression and Violent Behavior, 43*, 33–44. doi:10.1016/j.avb.2018.08.005

Klinger, D. A., & Brunson, R. K. (2009). Police officers' perceptual distortions during lethal force situations: Informing the reasonableness standard. *Criminology & Public Policy, 8*(1), 117–140. doi:10.1111/j.1745-9133.2009.00537.x

Knaevelsrud, C., & Maercker, A. (2007). Internet-based treatment for PTSD reduces distress and facilitates the development of a strong therapeutic alliance: A randomized controlled clinical trial. *BMC Psychiatry, 7*(1), 13. doi:10.1186/1471-244X-7-13 PMID:17442125

Knapp, P. H., Levy, E. M., Giorgi, R. G., Black, P. H., Fox, B. H., & Heeren, T. C. (1992). Short-term immunological effects of induced emotion. *Psychosomatic Medicine, 54*(2), 133–148. doi:10.1097/00006842-199203000-00002 PMID:1565752

Kobassa, S. C. (1979). Stressful life events, personality, and health: An inquiry into hardiness. *Journal of Personality and Social Psychology, 37*, 1–11. PMID:458548

Kobassa, S. C., Maddi, S. R., & Kahn, S. (1982). Hardiness and Health: A prospective study. *Journal of Personality and Social Psychology, 42*(1), 168–177. doi:10.1037/0022-3514.42.1.168 PMID:7057354

Komarovskaya, I., Maguen, S., McCaslin, S. E., Metzler, T. J., Madan, A., Brown, A. D., ... Marmar, C. R. (2011). The impact of killing and injuring others on mental health symptoms among police officers. *Journal of Psychiatric Research, 45*(10), 1332–1336. doi:10.1016/j.jpsychires.2011.05.004 PMID:21658717

Kosor, R. (2019, February 9). *The command post: If it feels good, don't say it*. [Audio Podcast].

Kouzes, J., & Posner, B. (1997). *The Leadership Challenge*. San Francisco, CA: Jossey Bass.

Krieger, N. (1999). Embodying inequality: A review of concepts, measures, and methods for studying health consequences of discrimination. *International Journal of Health Services: Planning Administration and Evaluation, 29*(2), 295–352. PMID:10379455

Kruger, L. G. (2018). *United state fire administration: An overview* (CRS Report No. RS20071). Retrieved from https://fas.org/sgp/crs/homesec/RS20071.pdf

Kulka, R. A., Schlenger, W. E., Fairbank, J. A., Hough, R. L., Jordan, B. K., Marmar, C. R., & Weiss, D. S. (1990). *Trauma and the Vietnam war generation: Report of findings from the National Vietnam Veterans Readjustment Study* (Vol. 18). New York: Brunner/Mazel.

Kuyken, W., Padesky, C. A., & Dudley, R. (2009). *Collaborative case conceptualization: Working effectively with patients in cognitive– behavioral therapy*. New York, NY: Guilford Press.

Lamia, M. C., & Krieger, M. J. (2009). *The White Knight Syndrome: Rescuing yourself from your need to rescue others.* Oakland, CA: New Harbinger Publications.

Landers, G. M., & Zhou, M. (2011). An analysis of relationships among peer support, psychiatric hospitalization, and crisis stabilization. *Community Mental Health Journal*, *47*(1), 106–112. doi:10.100710597-009-9218-3 PMID:19551502

Lang, P. J., & McTeague, L. M. (2011). Discrete and Recurrent Traumatization in PTSD: Fear vs. Anxious Misery. *Journal of Clinical Psychology in Medical Settings*, *18*(2), 207–209. doi:10.100710880-011-9252-5 PMID:21626350

Lanza, A., Roysircar, G., & Rodgers, S. (2018). First responder mental healthcare. Evidence-based prevention, postvention, and treatment services. *Professional Psychology, Research and Practice*, *49*(3), 193–204. doi:10.1037/pro0000192

Larimer, M. E., Turner, A. P., Anderson, B. K., Fader, J. S., Kilmer, J. R., Palmer, R. S., & Cronce, J. M. (2001). Evaluating a Brief Alcohol Intervention with Fraternities. *Journal of Studies on Alcohol*, *62*(3), 370–380. doi:10.15288/jsa.2001.62.370 PMID:11414347

LaRocco, J. M., House, J. S., & French, J. R. P. (1980). Social support, occupational stress, and health. *Journal of Health and Social Behavior*, *21*(3), 202–218. doi:10.2307/2136616 PMID:7410798

Larson, S. L., Eyerman, J., Foster, M. S., & Gfroerer, J. C. (2007). *Worker substance use and workplace policies and programs (DHHS Publication No. SMA 07 – 4273, Analytic Series A-29)*. Rockville, MD: Substance Abuse and Mental Health Services Administration, Office of Applied Studies.

Lazarus, R. S. (1966). *Psychological Stress And The Coping Process*. New York: McGraw-Hill.

Lazarus, R. S. (1969). *Patterns of Adjustment and Human Effectiveness*. New York: McGraw-Hill.

Leary, M. R., Tate, E. B., Adams, C. E., Allen, A. B., & Hancock, J. (2007). Self-compassion and reactions to unpleasant self-relevant events: The implication of treating oneself kindly. *Journal of Personality and Social Psychology*, *92*(5), 887–890. doi:10.1037/0022-3514.92.5.887 PMID:17484611

Lee, D. J., Liverant, G. I., Lowmaster, S. E., Gradus, J. L., & Sloan, D. M. (2014). PTSD and reasons for living: Associations with depressive symptoms and alcohol use. *Psychiatry Research*, *219*(3), 550–555. doi:10.1016/j.psychres.2014.06.016 PMID:24984579

Lee, J. (2017). Responding to children in situations of family violence: Narrative therapy group work with children. *International Journal of Narrative Therapy & Community Work*, *1*, 57–70.

Lennings, C. J. (1997). Police and occupationally related violence: A review. *Policing: An International Journal of Police Strategies & Management*, *20*(3), 555–566. doi:10.1108/13639519710180222

Leonhardt, J. (2006). Critical Incident Stress Management (CISM) in Air Traffic Control (ATC). In J. Leonhardt & J. Vogt (Eds.), *Critical Incident Stress Management CISM in Aviation* (pp. 81–91). Aldershot, UK: Ashgate Publishing Company.

Lepore, S. J. (2001). A social–cognitive processing model of emotional adjustment to cancer. In A. Baum & B. L. Andersen (Eds.), *Psychosocial interventions for cancer* (pp. 99–116). Washington, DC: American Psychological Association. doi:10.1037/10402-006

Lepore, S., & Revenson, T. (2007). Social constraints on disclosure and adjustment to cancer. *Social and Personality Psychology Compass*, *1*(1), 313–333. doi:10.1111/j.1751-9004.2007.00013.x

Lester, P. B., Harms, P. D., Herian, M. N., Krasikova, D. V., & Beal, S. J. (2011). The comprehensive soldier fitness program evaluation. *Longitudinal analysis of the impact of master resilience training on self-reported resilience and psychological health data (Report# 3).*

Liao, H., Arvey, R., Butler, R., & Nutting, S. (2001). Correlates of work injury frequency and duration among firefighters. *Journal of Occupational Health Psychology*, *6*(3), 229–242. PMID:11482634

LiBassi, M.D. (1987). Employee Trauma Recovery Program. In Personnel Resources, Local Procedures Manual. Dallas, TX: American Airlines.

Liedenbaum, C. (2011). *Policing between task and implement: A comparative study of the basic police in the Netherlands and North Rhine-Wesphalia*. Nijmegen: WLP.

Lifton, R. J. (1970). *History and Human Survival: Essays on the Young and the Old, Survivors and the Dead, Peace and War, and on Contemporary Psychohistory*. New York: Random House.

Lifton, R. J. (1973). *Home from the War: Vietnam Veterans—Neither Victims nor Executioners*. New York: Simon & Schuster.

Lifton, R. J. (1993). *The Protean Self: Human Resilience in an Age of Fragmentation*. New York: Basic Books.

Lightsey, O. R. Jr. (2006). Resilience, meaning, and well-being. *The Counseling Psychologist*, *34*(1), 96–107. doi:10.1177/0011000005282369

Lilly, M.M., Calhoun, R., Painter, I., & Meischke, H. (under review). Destress 9-1-1: A randomized control trial of an online mindfulness-based intervention in reducing stress among emergency medical dispatchers.

Lilly, M. M., & Allen, C. E. (2015). Psychological inflexibility and psychopathology in 9-1-1 telecommunicators. *Journal of Traumatic Stress*, *28*(3), 262–266. doi:10.1002/jts.22004 PMID:25964163

Lilly, M. M., London, M. J., & Mercer, M. C. (2016). Predictors of obesity and physical health complaints among 911 telecommunicators. *Safety and Health at Work*, *7*(1), 55–62. doi:10.1016/j.shaw.2015.09.003 PMID:27014492

Lilly, M. M., & Pierce, H. (2013). PTSD and depressive symptoms in 911 telecommunicators: The role of peritraumatic distress and world assumptions in predicting risk. *Psychological Trauma: Theory, Research, Practice, and Policy*, *5*(2), 135–141. doi:10.1037/a0026850

Lima Ede, P., Assuncao, A. A., & Barreto, S. M. (2015). Prevalence of depression among firefighters. *Cadernos de Saude Publica*, *31*(4), 733–743. PMID:25945983

Lindemann, E. (1944). Symptomatology and management of acute grief. *The American Journal of Psychiatry*, *101*(2), 141–148. doi:10.1176/ajp.101.2.141 PMID:8192191

Lindy, J. (1985). The trauma membrane and other clinical concepts derived from psychotherapeutic work with survivors of natural disasters. *Psychiatric Annals*, *15*(3), 153–160. doi:10.3928/0048-5713-19850301-06

Lipsky, M. (2010). *Street-level bureaucracy: dilemmas of the individual in public services*. New York, NY: Russell Sage Foundation.

Lipton, B. H. (2008). *The biology of belief: Unleashing the power of consciousness, matter, and miracles* (1st ed.). London: Hay House.

Littleton, H., Horsley, S., John, S., & Nelson, D. V. (2007). Trauma coping strategies and psychological distress: A meta-analysis. *Journal of Traumatic Stress: Official Publication of the International Society for Traumatic Stress Studies*, *20*(6), 977–988. doi:10.1002/jts.20276 PMID:18157893

Litz, B. T. (2008). Early intervention for trauma: Where are we and where do we need to go? A commentary. *Journal of Traumatic Stress*, *21*(6), 503–506. doi:10.1002/jts.20373 PMID:19107726

Litz, B. T., Gray, M. J., Bryant, R. A., & Adler, A. B. (2002). Early intervention for trauma: Current status and future directions. *Clinical Psychology: Science and Practice*, *9*(2), 112–134. doi:10.1093/clipsy.9.2.112

London, M. J., Mercer, M. C., & Lilly, M. M. (2017). Considering the impact of early trauma on coping and pathology to predict posttraumatic growth among 9-1-1 telecommunicators. *Journal of Interpersonal Violence*, *00*(0), 1–23. doi:10.1177/0886260517716942 PMID:29294814

Loo, R. (1986). Suicide among police in a federal force. *Suicide & Life-Threatening Behavior*, *16*(3), 379–388. doi:10.1111/j.1943-278X.1986.tb01019.x PMID:3765001

Lopes, R. T., Gonçalves, M. M., Fassnacht, D. B., Machado, P. P. P., & Sousa, I. (2014). Long-term effects of psychotherapy on moderate depression: A comparative study of narrative therapy and cognitive-behavioral therapy. *Journal of Affective Disorders*, *167*, 64–73. doi:10.1016/j.jad.2014.05.042 PMID:25082116

Lovallo, W. R. (2015). *Stress and health: Biological and psychological interactions*. Sage publications.

Løvseth, L. T., & Aasland, O. G. (2010). Confidentiality as a barrier to social support: A crosssectional study of Norwegian emergency and human service workers. *International Journal of Stress Management*, *17*(3), 214–231. doi:10.1037/a0018904

Lundberg, U. (2011). Neuroendocrine measurements. In R. J. Contrada & A. Baum (Eds.), *The handbook of stress science* (pp. 531–542). New York, NY: Springer.

Luszcynska, A., Benight, C. C., & Cieslak, R. (2009). Self-efficacy and health-related outcomes of collective trauma: A systematic review. *European Psychologist*, *14*(1), 51–62. doi:10.1027/1016-9040.14.1.51

Luthans, F. (2002). The need for and meaning of positive organizational behavior. *Journal of Organizational Behavior*, *23*(6), 695–706. doi:10.1002/job.165

Luthans, F., Avey, J. B., Avolio, B. J., Norman, S. M., & Combs, G. M. (2006). Psychological capital development: Toward a micro-intervention. *Journal of Organizational Behavior*, *27*(3), 387–393. doi:10.1002/job.373

Luthans, F., Avey, J. B., Avolio, B. J., & Peterson, S. J. (2010). The development and resulting performance impact of positive psychological capital. *Human Resource Development Quarterly*, *21*(1), 41–67. doi:10.1002/hrdq.20034

Luthans, F., Youssef, C. M., & Avolio, B. J. (2006). *Psychological Capital: Developing the Human Competitive Edge*. New York: Oxford University Press. doi:10.1093/acprof:oso/9780195187526.001.0001

Lyons, J. A. (1991). Strategies for assessing the potential for positive adjustment following trauma. *Journal of Traumatic Stress*, *4*(1), 93–111. doi:10.1002/jts.2490040108

Ma, C. C., Burchfiel, C. M., Andrew, M. E., Fekedulegn, T. A., Hartley, J. K., Gu, J. K., ... Charles, L. E. (2013). Shift work and work stress among police officers. *Annals of Epidemiology*, *23*(9), 596. doi:10.1016/j.annepidem.2013.06.080

MacBeth, A., & Gumley, A. (2012). Exploring compassion: A meta-analysis of the association between self-compassion & psychopathology. *Clinical Psychology Review*, *32*(6), 545–552. doi:10.1016/j.cpr.2012.06.003 PMID:22796446

Macedonia, M. (2018). *Self-Care and self-compassion of first responders: Predictors of resilience* (Doctoral Dissertation). Antioch University New England. https://aura.antioch.edu/etds/431/

Macintyre, S., Prenzler, T., & Chapman, J. (2008). Early intervention to reduce complaints: An Australian Victoria police initiative. *International Journal of Police Science & Management*, *10*(2), 238–250. doi:10.1350/ijps.2008.10.2.77

Maguen, S., Metzler, T. J., McCaslin, S. E., Inslicht, S. S., Henn-Haase, C., Neylan, T. C., & Marmar, C. R. (2009). Routine work environment stress and PTSD symptoms in police officers. *The Journal of Nervous and Mental Disease*, *197*(10), 754–760. doi:10.1097/NMD.0b013e3181b975f8 PMID:19829204

Mahoney, M. (2010). Shift Work, Jet Lag, and Female Reproduction. *International Journal of Endocrinology*. PMID:20224815

Maier, S. F., & Watkins, L. R. (1998). Cytokines for psychologists: Implications of bidirectional immune-to-brain communication for understanding behavior, mood, and cognition. *Psychological Review*, *105*(1), 83–107. doi:10.1037/0033-295X.105.1.83 PMID:9450372

Makawatsakul, N., & Kleiner, B. H. (2003). The effect of downsizing on morale and attrition. *Management Research News*, *26*(2/3/4), 52–62. doi:10.1108/01409170310783998

Malcolm, A. S., Seaton, J., Perera, A., Sheehan, D. C., & Van Hasselt, V. B. (2005). Critical incident stress debriefing and law enforcement: An evaluative review. *Brief Treatment and Crisis Intervention*, *5*(3), 261–278. doi:10.1093/brief-treatment/mhi019

Management Review. (1998). *Invigorating Change Initiatives*. Author.

Mansfield, A. J., Schaper, K. M., Yanagida, A. M., & Rose, C. S. (2014). One day at a time: The experiences of partners of veterans with posttraumatic stress disorder. *Professional Psychology, Research and Practice*, *45*, 488–495.

Marchand, A., Nadeau, C., Beaulieu-Prévost, D., Boyer, R., & Martin, M. (2015). Predictors of posttraumatic stress disorder among police officers: A prospective study. *Psychological Trauma: Theory, Research, Practice, and Policy*, *7*(3), 212–221. doi:10.1037/a0038780 PMID:25793514

Marier, C. J., & Moule, R. K. (2018). Feeling blue: Officer perceptions of public antipathy predict police occupational norms (Abstract). *American Journal of Criminal Justice*, advance online publication. Retrieved from http://link.springer.com

Marin, A. (2012). *In the line of duty: Investigation into how the Ontario Provincial Police and the Ministry of Community Safety and Correctional Services have addressed operational stress injuries affecting police officers*. Ontario Ombudsman.

Marin, R. A., Christensen, A., & Atkins, D. C. (2014). Infidelity and behavioral couple therapy: Relationship outcomes over 5 years following therapy. *Couple & Family Psychology*, *3*, 1–12.

Marks, M. R., Bowers, C., DePesa, N. S., Trachik, B., Deavers, F. E., & James, N. T. (2017). REACT: A paraprofessional training program for first responders – A pilot study. *Bulletin of the Menninger Clinic*, *81*(2), 150–166. doi:10.1521/bumc.2017.81.2.150 PMID:28609149

Markus, G., Hartmann, T., Brand, S., Holsboer-Trachsler, E., & Puhse, U. (2010). The relationship between shift work, perceived stress, sleep and health in Swiss police officers. *Journal of Criminal Justice*, *38*(6), 1167–1175. doi:10.1016/j.jcrimjus.2010.09.005

Marmar, C. R., McCaslin, S. E., Metzler, T. J., Best, S., Weiss, D. S., Fagan, J., & Neylan, T. (2006). Predictors of posttraumatic stress in police and other first responders. *Annals of the New York Academy of Sciences*, *1071*(1), 1–18. doi:10.1196/annals.1364.001 PMID:16891557

Marshall, R. D., Spitzer, R., & Liebowitz, M. R. (1999). Review and critique of the new DSM-IV diagnosis of acute stress disorder. *The American Journal of Psychiatry*, *156*(11), 1677–1685. PMID:10553729

Martin, C. E., Tran, J. K., & Buser, S. J. (2017). Correlates of suicidality in firefighter/ems personnel. *Journal of Affective Disorders*, *208*, 177–183. doi:10.1016/j.jad.2016.08.078 PMID:27788381

Martin, V., & Paulus, B. (2017). Alcohol use and suicidality in firefighters: Associations with depressive symptoms and posttraumatic stress. *Comprehensive Psychiatry*, *74*, 44–52. doi:10.1016/j.comppsych.2017.01.002 PMID:28092775

Maslach, C., Schaufeli, W., & Leiter, M. (2001). Job burnout. *Annual Review of Psychology*, *52*(1), 397–422. doi:10.1146/annurev.psych.52.1.397 PMID:11148311

Masten, A. S., Best, K. M., & Garmezy, N. (1990). Resilience and development: Contributions from the study of children who overcome adversity. *Development and Psychopathology*, *2*(4), 425–444. doi:10.1017/S0954579400005812

Masten, A. S., & Garmezy, N. (1985). Risk, Vulnerability, and Protective Factors in Developmental Psychopathology. In B. Lahey & A. E. Kazdin (Eds.), *Advances in Clinical Child Psychology* (pp. 1–52). New York: Plenum. doi:10.1007/978-1-4613-9820-2_1

Masten, A. S., & Narayan, A. J. (2012). Child development in the context of disaster, war, and terrorism: Pathways of risk and resilience. *Annual Review of Psychology*, *63*(1), 227–257. doi:10.1146/annurev-psych-120710-100356 PMID:21943168

Mastracci, S. H., Guy, M. E., & Newman, M. A. (2012). *Emotional labor and crisis response: working on the razor's edge*. Armonk, NY: M. E. Sharpe.

Mastrofski, S. D., Rosenbaum, D. P., & Fridell, L. (2011). *Police supervision: A 360-degree view of eight police departments*. National Police Research Platform.

McCanlies, E. C., Mnatsakanova, A., Andrew, M. E., Burchfiel, C. M., & Violanti, J. M. (2014). Positive psychological factors are associated with lower PTSD symptoms among police officers: Post Hurricane Katrina. *Stress and Health*, *30*(5), 405–415. doi:10.1002mi.2615 PMID:25476965

McCann, L., & Pearlman, L. A. (1990). *Psychological trauma and the adult survivor* (Vol. 21). New York, NY: Brunner/Mazel.

McCauley, J. L., Killeen, T., Gros, D. F., Brady, K. T., & Back, S. E. (2012). Posttraumatic stress disorder and co-occurring substance use sisorders: Advances in assessment and treatment. *Clinical Psychologist*, *19*(3), 1–27.

McCoy, S. P., & Aamodt, M. G. (2010). A comparison of law enforcement divorce rates with those of other occupations. *Journal of Police and Criminal Psychology*, *25*, 1–16.

McCrady, B. S., & Epstein, E. E. (2015). Couple therapy and alcohol problems. In A. S. Gurman, J. L. Lebow, & D. K. Snyder (Eds.), *Clinical Handbook of Couple Therapy* (5th ed.; pp. 555–584). New York: Guilford.

McCraty, R., & Atkinson, M. (2012). Resilience training program reduces physiological and psychological stress in police officers. *Global Advances in Health and Medicine: Improving Healthcare Outcomes Worldwide*, *1*(5), 44–66. doi:10.7453/gahmj.2012.1.5.013 PMID:27257532

McCraty, R., Atkinson, M., Tomasino, D., & Bradley, R. T. (2009). The Coherent Heart Heart-Brain Interactions, Psychophysiological Coherence, and the Emergence of System-Wide Order. *Integral Review: A Transdisciplinary & Transcultural Journal for New Thought, Research, & Praxis*, *5*(2).

McCreary, D. R., & Thompson, M. M. (2006). Development of two reliable and valid measures of stressors in policing: The operational and organizational police stress questionnaires. *International Journal of Stress Management*, *13*(4), 494–518. doi:10.1037/1072-5245.13.4.494

McDiarmid, M., Lees, P., Agnew, J., Midzenski, M., & Duffy, R. (1991). Reproductive hazards of firefighting II. Chemical hazards. *American Journal of Industrial Medicine*, *19*(4), 447–472. doi:10.1002/ajim.4700190404 PMID:2035546

McGregor, D. (1960). *The Human Side of Enterprise*. New York: McGraw-Hill Book Company.

McHugh, J. (2019). *Yoga mats in the squad room.* Retrieved from https://psmag.com/magazine/yoga-mats-in-the-squad-room

McIntosh, W. L. (2016). Suicide rates by occupational group – 17 states, 2012. *Morbidity and mortality weekly report*, 65. PMID:27359167

McMahon, C. P. (2010). *A Phenomenological Study of Stress and Coping in the Fire Service* (Doctoral dissertation). Our Lady of the Lake University, San Antonio, TX.

McMillen, J. C., North, C. S., & Smith, E. M. (2000). What parts of PTSD are normal: Intrusion, avoidance, or arousal? Data from the Northridge, California, earthquake. *Journal of Traumatic Stress*, *13*(1), 57–75. doi:10.1023/A:1007768830246 PMID:10761174

McNeil, J. (2008). Diversity in the fire service: A problem or a solution? *Fire Engineering*, *161*(10), 129.

McNeill, M. (1996). *Alcohol and the police workplace-factors associated with excessive intake (Rep. Series No. 119.1).* Payneham, South Australia: National Police Research Unit.

McNeill, M., & Wilson, C. (1993). *Alcohol and the police workplace (Rep. Series No. 119).* Adelaide, South Australia: National Police Research Unit.

McQuerry Tuttle, B., Giano, Z., & Merten, M. J. (2018). Stress spillover and negative relationship functioning for law enforcement marriages. *The Family Journal (Alexandria, Va.)*, *26*(2), 246–252. doi:10.1177/1066480718775739

McTeague, L. M., Lang, P. J., Laplante, M.-C., Cuthbert, B. N., Shumen, J. R., & Bradley, M. M. (2010). Aversive Imagery in Posttraumatic Stress Disorder: Trauma Recurrence, Comorbidity, and Physiological Reactivity. *Biological Psychiatry*, *67*(4), 346–356. doi:10.1016/j.biopsych.2009.08.023 PMID:19875104

Mead, S., & MacNeil, C. (2006). Peer support: What makes it unique. *International Journal of Psychosocial Rehabilitation*, *10*(2), 29–37.

Meichenbaum, D. H., & Deffenbacher, J. L. (1988). Stress inoculation training. *The Counseling Psychologist*, *16*(1), 69–90. doi:10.1177/0011000088161005

Meischke, H., Lilly, M., Beaton, R., Calhoun, R., Tu, A., Stangenes, S., ... Baseman, J. (2018). Protocol: A multi-level intervention program to reduce stress in 9-1-1 telecommunicators. *BMC Public Health*, *18*(1), 570. doi:10.118612889-018-5471-0 PMID:29716576

Meischke, H., Painter, I., Lilly, M., Beaton, R., Revere, D., Calhoun, B., ... Baseman, J. (2015). An exploration of sources, symptoms and buffers of occupational stress in 9-1-1 emergency call centers. *Annals of Emergency Dispatch & Response*, *3*(2), 28–35.

Meischke, H., Painter, I., Lilly, M., Beaton, R., Revere, D., Calhoun, B., ... Baseman, J. (2015). An exploration of sources, symptoms, and buffers of occupational stress in 9-1-1 emergency call centers. *Annals of Emergency Dispatch & Response*, *3*(2), 28–35.

Melling, B., & Houguet-Pincham, T. (2011). Online peer support for individuals with depression: A summary of current research and future considerations. *Psychiatric Rehabilitation Journal*, *34*(3), 252–254. doi:10.2975/34.3.2011.252.254 PMID:21208865

Ménard, K. S., & Arter, M. L. (2013). Police officer alcohol use and trauma symptoms: Associations with critical incidents, coping, and social stressors. *International Journal of Stress Management*, *20*(1), 37–56. doi:10.1037/a0031434

Ménard, K. S., & Arter, M. L. (2014). Stress, coping, alcohol use, and posttraumatic stress disorder among an international sample of police officers: Does gender matter? *Police Quarterly*, *17*(4), 307–327. doi:10.1177/1098611114548097

Meyer, E. C., Zimering, R. T., Daly, E., Knight, J., Kanholz, B. W., & Gulliver, S. B. (2012). Predictors of posttraumatic stress disorder and other psychological symptoms in trauma-exposed firefighters. *Psychological Services*, *9*, 1–15. PMID:22449083

Meyer, E. G., Hall-Clark, B. N., Hamaoka, D., & Peterson, A. L. (2015). Assessment of military cultural competence: A pilot study. *Academic Psychiatry*, *39*(4), 382–388. doi:10.100740596-015-0328-7 PMID:26054708

Milligan-Saville, J., Choi, I., Deady, M., Scott, P., Tan, L., Calvo, R. A., ... Harvey, S. B. (2018). The impact of trauma exposure on the development of PTSD and psychological distress in a volunteer fire service. *Psychiatry Research*, *270*, 1110–1115. doi:10.1016/j.psychres.2018.06.058 PMID:30190167

Milliken, C. S., Auchterlonie, J. L., & Hoge, C. W. (2007). Longitudinal assessment of mental health problems among active and reserve component soldiers returning from the Iraq war. *Journal of the American Medical Association*, *298*(18), 2141–2148. doi:10.1001/jama.298.18.2141 PMID:18000197

Mills, K. L., Teesson, M., Ross, J., & Peters, L. (2006). Trauma, PTSD, and substance use disorders: Findings from the Australian National Survey of Mental Health and Well-Being. *The American Journal of Psychiatry*, *163*(4), 652–658. PMID:16585440

Mills, M. R., Rindfuss, R., McDonald, P., & Te Velde, E. (2011). Why do people postpone parenthood? Reasons and social policy incentives. *Human Reproduction Update*, *17*(6), 848–860. doi:10.1093/humupd/dmr026 PMID:21652599

Mineka, S., Cook, M., & Miller, S. (1984). Fear conditioned with escapable and inescapable shock: Effects of a feedback stimulus. *Journal of Experimental Psychology. Animal Behavior Processes*, *10*(3), 307–323. doi:10.1037/0097-7403.10.3.307

Mineka, S., & Oehlberg, K. (2008). The relevance of recent developments in classical conditioning to understanding the etiology and maintenance of anxiety disorders. *Acta Psychologica*, *127*(3), 567–580. doi:10.1016/j.actpsy.2007.11.007 PMID:18226795

Mitani, S., Masatoshi, F., Keiji, N., & Shirakawa, T. (2006, July). Impact of post-traumatic stress disorder and job-related stress on burnout: A study of fire service workers. *The Journal of Emergency Medicine*, *31*(1), 7–11. doi:10.1016/j.jemermed.2005.08.008 PMID:16798146

Mitchell, J. T. (1982). The psychological impact of the Air Florida 90 Disaster on fire-rescue, paramedic and police officer personnel. In Mass Casualties: a lessons learned approach, accidents, civil disorders, natural disaster, terrorism. Washington, DC: Department of Transportation. (DOT HS 806302)

Mitchell, J.T. (1982, Fall). Recovery from rescue. *Response, the Magazine of Emergency Management*, 7-10.

Mitchell, J. T. (1983). When disaster strikes … The critical incident stress Debriefing process. *Journal of Emergency Medical Services*, *13*(11), 49–52. PMID:10258348

Mitchell, J. T. (1983). When disaster strikes: The critical incident stress debriefing process. *Journal of Emergency Medical Services*, *8*(1), 36–39. PMID:10258348

Mitchell, J. T. (2004). Characteristics of Successful Early Intervention Programs. *International Journal of Emergency Mental Health*, *6*(4), 175–184. PMID:15635898

Mitchell, J. T. (2006). A brief history of Crisis Intervention in Aviation. In J. Vogt & J. Leonhardt (Eds.), *Critical Incident Stress Management in Aviation*. Hampshire, UK: Ashgate Publishing Limited.

Mitchell, J. T. (2007). *Group Crisis Support: Why it works, When and How to Provide It*. Ellicott City, MD: Chevron Publishing.

Mitchell, J. T. (2017). *Critical Incident Stress Management: Group Crisis Intervention* (5th ed.). Ellicott City, MD: International Critical Incident Stress Foundation.

Mitchell, J. T., & Everly, G. S. (2001). *Critical Incident Stress Management: Basic Group Crisis Interventions*. Ellicott City, MD: International Critical Incident Stress Foundation.

Mitchell, J. T., & Everly, G. S. Jr. (2001). *Critical Incident Stress Debriefing: An operations manual for CISD, Defusing and other group crisis intervention services* (3rd ed.). Ellicott City, MD: Chevron.

Mitchell, S. G., & Mitchell, J. T. (2006). Caplan, Community and Critical Incident Stress Management. *International Journal of Emergency Mental Health*, *8*(1), 1–10. PMID:16573247

Mould-Millman, N.-K., Meese, H., Alattas, I., Ido, M., Yi, I., Oyewumi, T., ... Yancey, A. (2018).. . *Prehospital Emergency Care*, *22*(6), 734–742. PMID:29596006

Mumford, E. A., Taylor, B. G., & Kubu, B. (2015). Law enforcement officer safety and wellness. *Police Quarterly*, *18*(2), 111–133.

Munce, S. E., Stansfeld, S. A., Blackmore, E. R., & Stewart, D. E. (2007). The role of depression and chronic pain conditions in absenteeism: Results from a national epidemiologic survey. *Journal of Occupational and Environmental Medicine*, *49*(11), 1206–1211. doi:10.1097/JOM.0b013e318157f0ba PMID:17993924

Murphy, J. G., Yurasek, A. M., Dennhardt, A. A., Skidmore, J. R., McDevitt-Murphy, M. E., MacKillop, J., & Martens, M. P. (2013). Symptoms of depression and PTSD are associated with elevated alcohol demand. *Drug and Alcohol Dependence*, *127*(1-3), 129–136. PMID:22809894

Murphy, S. A., Beaton, R. D., Pike, K. C., & Johnson, L. C. (1999). Occupational stressors, stress responses, and alcohol consumption among professional firefighters: A prospective, longitudinal analysis. *International Journal of Stress Management*, *6*(3), 179–196. doi:10.1023/A:1021934725246

NATCA/FAA. (2003). *You are Not Alone: Critical Incident Stress Management Program*. Washington, DC: NATCA / FAA.

National Center for Women and Policing. (2018). *Police family violence fact sheet*. Retrieved from http://www.womenandpolicing.com/violencefs.asp

National EMS Management Association (NEMSMA). (2016). *Mental health and stress in emergency medical services*. Platte City, MO: Author.

National Fire Protection Association (NFPA). (2019). *NFPA 1001: Standard for fire fighter professional qualifications*. Quincy, MA: Author.

National Fire Protection Association. (2013). NFPA 1582: Standard on Comprehensive Occupational Medical Program for All Fire Departments. Quincy, MA: NFPA, 98.

National Fire Protection Association. (2018). NFPA 1500: Standard on Fire Department Occupational Safety and Health Program. Quincy, MA: NFPA, 37.

National Highway Traffic Safety Administration (NHTSA). (2011). *Traffic safety facts: EMS research note* (DOT HS Publication No. 812-041). Retrieved from https://www.ems.gov/pdf/National_EMS_Assessment_Demographics_2011.pdf

National Highway Traffic Safety Administration (NHTSA). (n.d.). *Emergency medical services: Agenda for the future*. Retrieved from https://one.nhtsa.gov/people/injury/ems/agenda/emsman.html#EMS%20CONTENTS

National Institute for Mental Health. (2017). *Major Depression*. Retrieved from: https://www.nimh.nih.gov/health/statistics/major-depression.shtml

National Institute of Mental Health (NIMH). (2002). *Mental health and mass violence: Evidence-based early psychological intervention for victims/survivors of mass violence. A workshop to reach consensus on best practices. (NIH Publication No. 02- 5138).* Washington, DC: U.S. Government Printing Office.

National Institutes of Health. (n.d.). *Drinking Levels Defined.* Retrieved from https://www.niaaa.nih.gov/alcohol-health/overview-alcohol-consumption/moderate-binge-drinking

National Institutes of Mental Health. (n.d.). *Mental Health Information.* Retrieved from https://www.nimh.nih.gov/health/statistics/major-depression.shtml

National Volunteer Firefighter Council (NVFC). (2014). *What to expect: A guide for family member of volunteer fire-fighters.* Greenbelt, MD: Author.

Nations Business. (1998). *The Way of the Warrior: Leadership Lessons from History's Top Twelve Military Masters.* Author.

Neff, K. D., & Pommier, E. (2012). The relationship between self-compassion and other-focused concern among college undergraduates, community adults, and practicing mediators. *Self and Identity, 12*(2), 160–176. doi:10.1080/15298868.2011.649546

Neff, L. A., & Karney, B. R. (2009). Stress and reactivity to daily relationship experiences: How stress hinders adaptive processes in marriage. *Journal of Personality and Social Psychology, 97*(3), 435–450. doi:10.1037/a0015663 PMID:19686000

Neil, T., Oney, J., DiFonso, L., Thacker, B., & Reichart, W. (1974). *Emotional First Aid.* Louisville: Kemper-Behavioral Science Associates.

New Jersey Office of the Attorney General. (2018a, March 20). *Attorney General Grewal announces two new law enforcement policies designed to ensure law enforcement safety and promote public trust* [Press release]. Retrieved from https://nj.gov/oag/newsreleases18/pr20180320c.html

New Jersey Office of the Attorney General. (2018b). Attorney general law enforcement directive 2018-3. Trenton, NJ: Author.

Newman, A., Ucbasaran, D., Zhu, F., & Hirst, G. (2014). Psychological capital: A review and synthesis. *Journal of Organizational Behavior, 35*(S1), S120–S138. doi:10.1002/job.1916

Neyer, G., & Andersson, G. (2008). *Consequences of Family Policies on Childbearing Behavior: Effects or Artifacts?* (Vol. 34). Oxford, UK: Blackwell Publishing.

Niles, S. G., Yoon, H. J., Balın, E., & Amundson, N. E. (2010). Using A Hope-Centered Model Of Career Development in Challenging Times. *Turkish Psychological Counseling and Guidance Journal, 4.* Retrieved from http://dergipark.gov.tr/download/article-file/200146

Niles, S. G., In, H., & Amundson, N. (2014). Using an Action Oriented Hope-Centered Model of Career Development. *Journal of Asia Pacific Counseling, 4*(1), 1–13. doi:10.18401/2014.4.1.1

Nock, M. K., Borges, G., Bromet, E. J., Alonso, J., Angermeyer, M., Beautrais, A., ... Williams, D. (2008). Cross-national prevalence and risk factors for suicidal ideation, plans and attempts. *Journal of Psychiatry, 192*(2), 98–105. doi:10.1192/bjp.bp.107.040113 PMID:18245022

Nock, M. K., Stein, M. B., Heeringa, S. G., Ursano, R. J., Colpe, L. J., Fullerton, C. S., ... Kessler, R. C. (2014). Prevalence and correlates of suicidal behavior among soldiers. *JAMA Psychiatry, 71*(5), 514–522. doi:10.1001/jamapsychiatry.2014.30 PMID:24590178

Norcross, J. C., & Barnett, J. E. (2007). Self-care as ethical imperative. *National Register of Health Service Psychologists*. Retrieved from https://www.nationalregister.org/pub/the-national-register-report-pub/the-register-report-spring-2008/self-care-as-ethical-imperative/

North, C. S., Tivis, L., McMillen, J. C., Pfefferbaum, B., Cox, J., Spitznagel, E. L., ... Smith, E. M. (2002). Coping, functioning, and adjustment of rescue workers after the Oklahoma City bombing. *Journal of Traumatic Stress*, *15*(3), 171–175. doi:10.1023/A:1015286909111 PMID:12092908

North, C. S., Tivis, L., McMillen, J. C., Pfefferbaum, B., Spitznagel, E. L., Cox, J., ... Smith, E. M. (2002). Psychiatric disorders in rescue workers after the Oklahoma City bombing. *The American Journal of Psychiatry*, *159*(5), 857–859. doi:10.1176/appi.ajp.159.5.857 PMID:11986143

North, C., Tivis, C., McMillen, J., Pfefferbaum, B., Cox, J., Spitznagel, E., ... Smith, E. (2002). Coping, functioning, and adjustment of Rescue workers after the Oklahoma City bombing. *Journal of Traumatic Stress*, *15*, 171–175. PMID:12092908

Novaco, R. W. (1977). A stress inoculation approach to anger management in the training of law enforcement officers. *American Journal of Community Psychology*, *5*(3), 327–346. doi:10.1007/BF00884700 PMID:910754

Nurmi, L. (1999). The sinking of the Estonia: The effects of Critical Incident Stress Debriefing on Rescuers. *International Journal of Emergency Mental Health*, *1*, 23–32. PMID:11227750

Nurminen, T. (1998). Shift work and reproductive health. *Scandinavian Journal of Work, Environment & Health*, *24*, 28–34. PMID:9916814

Nuttman-Shwartz, O., & Shoval-Zuckerman, Y. (2016). Continuous Traumatic Situations in the Face of Ongoing Political Violence: The Relationship Between CTS and PTSD. *Trauma, Violence & Abuse*, *17*(5), 562–570. doi:10.1177/1524838015585316 PMID:25966968

O'Brien, C. P. (2008). The CAGE questionnaire for detection of alcoholism: A remarkably useful but simple tool. *Journal of the American Medical Association*, *300*(17), 2054–2056. doi:10.1001/jama.2008.570 PMID:18984895

O'Hara, A. (2012, August). Badge of life: Police mental health. *Badge of Life Newsletter,* 1–3.

O'Neill, M. (2001). Police suicides in the New York City Police Department: Causal factors and remedial measures. In D. C. Sheehan & J. I. Warren (Eds.), *Suicide and Law Enforcement* (pp. 139–149). Quantico, VA: U.S. Department of Justice.

O'Byrne, K. K., Peterson, L., & Saldana, L. (1997). Survey of pediatric hospitals' preparation programs: evidence of the impact of health psychology research. *Health Psychology: Official Journal of the Division of Health Psychology, American Psychological Association, 16*(2), 147-154.

Ogle, C. M., Rubin, D. C., & Siegler, I. C. (2015). The relation between insecure attachment and posttraumatic stress: Early life versus adulthood traumas. *Psychological Trauma: Theory, Research, Practice, and Policy*, *7*(4), 324–332. doi:10.1037/tra0000015 PMID:26147517

Okechukwu, C. A., Souza, K., Davis, K. D., & de Castro, A. B. (2014). Discrimination, harassment, abuse, and bullying in the workplace: Contribution of workplace injustice to occupational health disparities. *American Journal of Industrial Medicine*, *57*(5), 573–586. doi:10.1002/ajim.22221 PMID:23813664

Olson, D. T. (1998). Deadly force decision making. *FBI Law Enforce Bulletin*, *67*, 1–9.

Osofsky, H. J., Osofsky, J. D., Arey, J., Kronenberg, M. E., Hansel, T., & Many, M. (2011). Hurricane Katrina's first responders: The struggle to protect and serve in the aftermath of the disaster. *Disaster Medicine and Public Health Preparedness*, *5*(S2Suppl 2), S214–S219. doi:10.1001/dmp.2011.53 PMID:21865490

Oxley, J. C. (2011). The Moral Dimensions of Empathy: Limits and Applications in Ethical Theory. New York, NY: Palgrave Macmillan.

Ozer, E. J., Best, S. R., Lipsey, T. L., & Weiss, D. S. (2003). Predictors of posttraumatic stress disorder and symptoms in adults: A meta-analysis. *Psychological Bulletin, 129*(1), 52–73. doi:10.1037/0033-2909.129.1.52 PMID:12555794

Ozer, E. J., Best, S. R., Lipsey, T. L., & Weiss, D. S. (2008). Predictors of posttraumatic stress disorder and symptoms in adults: A meta-analysis. *Psychological Trauma: Theory, Research, Practice, and Policy, S*(1), 3–36. doi:10.1037/1942-9681.S.1.3

Padesky, C. A. (2006). *The next phase: Building positive qualities with cognitive therapy.* Invited address presented at the International Congress of Cognitive Psychotherapy, Göteborg, Sweden.

Padesky, C. A., & Mooney, K. A. (2012). Strengths-Based Cognitive-Behavioural Therapy: A Four-Step Model to Build Resilience. *Clinical Psychology & Psychotherapy, 19*(4), 283–290. doi:10.1002/cpp.1795 PMID:22653834

Palmer, C. G. (2014). Stress and coping in wildland firefighting dispatchers. *Journal of Emergency Management (Weston, Mass.), 12*(4), 303–314. PMID:25069024

Palm, K. M., Polusny, M. A., & Follette, V. M. (2004). Vicarious traumatization: Potential hazards and interventions for disaster and trauma workers. *Prehospital and Disaster Medicine, 19*(1), 73–78. doi:10.1017/S1049023X00001503 PMID:15453162

Papazoglou, K., & Chopko, B. (2017). The role of moral suffering (moral distress and moral injury) in police compassion fatigue and PTSD: An unexplored topic. *Frontiers in Psychology, 8*, 1999. doi:10.3389/fpsyg.2017.01999 PMID:29187830

Papazoglou, K., & Tuttle, B. M. (2018). Fighting police trauma: Practical approaches to addressing psychological needs of officers. *SAGE Open, 8*(3). doi:10.1177/2158244018794794

Pappas, S. (2019). APA issues first-ever guidelines for practice with men and boys. *Monitor on Psychology, 50*, 34–39.

Parad, L., & Parad, H. (1968). A study of crisis oriented planned short –term treatment: Part II. *Social Casework, 49*(7), 418–426. doi:10.1177/104438946804900705

Parker, J.G. (2006, April). Watching the Clock. Safety and Health, 44-47.

Park, M., Chang, E. R., & You, S. (2015). Protective role of coping flexibility in PTSD and depressive symptoms following trauma. *Personality and Individual Differences, 82*, 102–106. doi:10.1016/j.paid.2015.03.007

Parra, A. (2013). Cognitive and Emotional Empathy in Relation to Five Paranormal/Anomalous Experiences. *North American Journal of Psychology, 15*(3), 405–612.

Pascoe, E. A., & Smart Richman, L. (2009). Perceived discrimination and health: A meta-analytic review. *Psychological Bulletin, 135*(4), 531–554. doi:10.1037/a0016059 PMID:19586161

Patton, C. L., Smith, S. F., & Lilienfeld, S. O. (2018). Psychopathy and heroism in first responders: Traits cut from the same cloth? *Personality Disorders, 9*, 354–368. PMID:29120196

Paulus, D. J., Vujanovic, A. A., Schuhmann, B. B., Smith, L. J., & Tran, J. (2017). Main and interactive effects of depression and posttraumatic stress in relation to alcohol dependence among urban male firefighters. *Psychiatry Research, 251*, 69–75. doi:10.1016/j.psychres.2017.02.011 PMID:28189939

Payne, M. (2006). *Narrative therapy: An introduction for counsellors* (2nd ed.). London, UK: Sage.

Peele, S. (1991). Out of the habit trap. In A. Monat & R. S. Lazarus (Eds.), *Stress and coping: An anthology* (3rd ed.; pp. 475–482). New York: Columbia University. doi:10.7312/mona92982-033

Perrott, T. (2016). Beyond 'Token' Firefighters: Exploring Women's Experiences of Gender and Identity at Work. *Sociological Research Online*, *21*(1), 1–14. doi:10.5153ro.3832

Petersen, K. U., Hansen, J., Ebbehoej, N. E., & Bonde, J. P. (2018, November). Infertility in a Cohort of Male Danish Firefighters: A Register-Based Study. *American Journal of Epidemiology*, 19. PMID:30452532

Peters, T., & Austin, N. (1985). *A Passion for Excellence – The Leadership Difference*. Random House, Inc.

Pfeiffer, P. N., Heisler, M., Piette, J. D., Rogers, M. A., & Valenstein, M. (2011). Efficacy of peer support interventions for depression: A meta-analysis. *General Hospital Psychiatry*, *33*(1), 29–36. doi:10.1016/j.genhosppsych.2010.10.002 PMID:21353125

Phillips, C. J., LeardMann, C. A., Gumbs, G. R., & Smith, B. (2010). Risk factors for posttraumatic stress disorder among deployed US male marines. *BMC Psychiatry*, *10*(52), 1–11. PMID:20579379

Pierce, H., & Lilly, M. M. (2012). Duty-related trauma exposure in 911 telecommunicators: Considering the risk for posttraumatic stress. *Journal of Traumatic Stress*, *25*(2), 211–215. doi:10.1002/jts.21687 PMID:22467384

Pierce, H., & Lilly, M. M. (2012). Duty-related trauma exposure in 911 telecommunicators: Considering the risk for posttraumatic stress. *Journal of Traumatic Stress*, *25*(2), 211–215. PMID:22467384

Pietrzak, R. H., Goldstein, R. B., Southwick, S. M., & Grant, B. F. (2011). Prevalence and Axis I comorbidity of full and partial posttraumatic stress disorder in the United States: Results from Wave 2 of the National Epidemiologic Survey on Alcohol and Related Conditions. *Journal of Anxiety Disorders*, *25*(3), 456–465. doi:10.1016/j.janxdis.2010.11.010 PMID:21168991

Pietrzak, R. H., Schechter, C. B., Bromet, E. J., Katz, C. L., Reissman, D. B., Ozbay, F., ... Southwick, S. M. (2012). The burden of full and subsyndromal posttraumatic stress disorder among police involved in the World Trade Center rescue and recovery effort. *Journal of Psychiatric Research*, *46*(7), 835–842. doi:10.1016/j.jpsychires.2012.03.011 PMID:22464942

Pirrallo, R. G., Levine, R., & Dickison, P. D. (2005). Behavioral health risk factors of U.S. emergency medical technicians: The LEADS project. *Prehospital and Disaster Medicine*, *20*(4), 235–242. doi:10.1017/S1049023X00002594 PMID:16128471

Polak, A. R., Witteveen, A. B., Reitsma, J. B., & Olff, M. (2012). The role of executive function in PTSD: A systematic review. *Journal of Affective Disorders*, *141*(1), 11–21. doi:10.1016/j.jad.2012.01.001 PMID:22310036

PoliceOne. (2017, January 30). *VA cops decompress in "quiet rooms."* Retrieved from https://www.policeone.com/health-fitness/articles/284889006-Va-cops-decompress-in-quiet-rooms/

Poplin, G. S., Harris, R. B., Pollack, K. M., Peate, W. F., & Burgess, J. L. (2011). Beyond the fireground: Injuries in the fire service. *Injury Prevention*, *18*(4), 228–233. doi:10.1136/injuryprev-2011-040149 PMID:22117024

Poston, W. (2012). Substance use issues among male career firefighters. *Journal of Substance Abuse Treatment*, *43*(3), e24. doi:10.1016/j.jsat.2012.08.115

Prati, G., & Pietrantoni, L. (2010). The relation of perceived and received social support to mental health among first responders: A meta-analytic review. *Journal of Community Psychology*, *38*(3), 403–417. doi:10.1002/jcop.20371

Price, M. (2017). Psychiatric disability in law enforcement officers. *Behavioral Sciences & the Law*, *35*(2), 113–123. doi:10.1002/bsl.2278 PMID:28303590

Puttonen, S., Harma, M., & Hublin, C. (2010). Shift work and cardiovascular disease - pathways from circadian stress to morbidity. *Scandinavian Journal of Work, Environment & Health*, *36*(2), 96–108. doi:10.5271jweh.2894 PMID:20087536

Pyle, S., Graham, R., Suminski, R., Poston, W. S. C., Haddock, C. K., & Glaros, A. (2009). Depressive symptoms, self-rated mental health, daily functioning and job satisfaction among firefighters. *International Fire Service Journal of Leadership and Management*, *3*(1), 19–24.

Quick, J., & Tetrick, L. E. (2003). *Handbook of occupational health psychology*. Washington, DC: American Psychological Association.

Rajaratnam, S. M., Barger, L. K., Lockley, S. W., Shea, S. A., Wang, W., Landrigan, C. P., ... Epstein, L. J. (2011). Sleep disorders, health, and safety in police officers. *Journal of the American Medical Association*, *306*(23), 2567–2578. PMID:22187276

Rallings, M. (2000). *Police and trauma: A prospective examination of the psychological effects of occupational exposure to traumatic events* (Doctoral dissertation). Retrieved from WorldCat.

Ramanujam, P., Guluma, K. Z., Castillo, E. M., Chacon, M., Jensen, M. B., Patel, E., ... Dunford, J. V. (2008). Accuracy of stroke recognition by emergency medical dispatchers and paramedics—San Diego experience. *Prehospital Emergency Care*, *12*(3), 307–313. doi:10.1080/10903120802099526 PMID:18584497

Rameshbabu, A., Reddy, D. M., & Fleming, R. (2013). Correlates of negative physical health in call center shift workers. *Applied Ergonomics*, *44*(3), 350–354. doi:10.1016/j.apergo.2012.09.002 PMID:23040668

Ramey, S. L., Perkhounkova, Y., Hein, M., Chung, S. J., & Anderson, A. A. (2017). Evaluation of stress experienced by emergency telecommunications personnel employed in a large metropolitan police department. *Workplace Health & Safety*, *65*(7), 287–294. doi:10.1177/2165079916667736 PMID:27941089

Rand, K. L., & Cheavens, J. S. (2009). Hope Theory. In S. J. Lopez & C. R. Snyder (Eds.), *The Oxford Handbook of Positive Psychology* (2nd ed.; pp. 323–333). New York: Oxford University Press.

Regehr, C., Goldberg, G., Glancy, G. D., & Knott, T. (2002). Posttraumatic symptoms and disability in paramedics. *Canadian Journal of Psychiatry*, *47*(10), 953–958. doi:10.1177/070674370204701007 PMID:12553131

Regehr, C., Hill, J., & Glancy, G. D. (2000). Individual predictors of traumatic reactions in firefighters. *The Journal of Nervous and Mental Disease*, *188*(6), 333–339. doi:10.1097/00005053-200006000-00003 PMID:10890341

Regehr, C., Hill, J., Goldberg, G., & Hughes, J. (2003). Postmortem inquiries and trauma responses in paramedics and firefighters. *Journal of Interpersonal Violence*, *18*(6), 607–622. doi:10.1177/0886260503251131

Regel, S. (2007). Post-trauma support in the workplace: The current status and practice of critical incident stress management (CISM) and psychological debriefing (PD) within organizations in the UK. *Occupational Medicine*, *57*(6), 411–416. doi:10.1093/occmed/kqm071 PMID:17728314

Regel, S. (2010). Does psychological debriefing work? *Healthcare Counseling and Psychotherapy Journal.*, *10*(2), 14–18.

Reivich, K. J., Seligman, M. E., & McBride, S. (2011). Master resilience training in the US Army. *The American Psychologist*, *66*(1), 25–34. doi:10.1037/a0021897 PMID:21219045

Renaud, E. F. (2008). The attachment characteristics of combat veterans with PTSD. *Traumatology*, *14*(3), 1–12. doi:10.1177/1534765608319085

Repper, J., & Carter, T. (2011). A review of the literature on peer support in mental health services. *Journal of Mental Health (Abingdon, England)*, *20*(4), 392–411. doi:10.3109/09638237.2011.583947 PMID:21770786

Resick, P. A., Monson, C. M., & Chard, K. M. (2016). *Cognitive processing therapy for PTSD: A comprehensive manual*. Boston: Guilford Press.

Reskin, B. F., & Bielby, D. D. (2005). A sociological perspective on gender and career outcomes.(wages, working hours). *The Journal of Economic Perspectives*, *19*(1), 71–86.

Richards, D. (2001). A field study of critical incident stress debriefing versus critical incident stress management. *Journal of Mental Health (Abingdon, England)*, *10*(3), 351–362. doi:10.1080/09638230124190

Richardson, D. C., Griffin, N. K., Zaki, L., Stephenson, A., Yan, J., Curry, T., & Devlin, J. T. (2018). Measuring narrative engagement: The heart tells the story. *bioRxiv*, 35–48. doi:10.1101/351148

Richmond, R. L., Wodak, A., Kehoe, L., & Heather, N. (1998). How healthy are the police? A survey of life-style factors. *Addiction (Abingdon, England)*, *93*(11), 1729–1737. doi:10.1046/j.1360-0443.1998.9311172910.x PMID:9926535

Richmond, R., Heather, N., Holt, P., & Hu, W. (1993). *Workplace policies and programs for tobacco, alcohol and other drug abuse in Australia: National campaign against drug abuse (National Campaign Against Drug Abuse Monograph No. 24)*. Canberra: Australian Government Publishing Services.

Roberts, A. (2005). Bridging the Past and Present to the Future of Crisis Intervention and Crisis Management. In A. Roberts (Ed.), *Crisis Intervention Handbook: Assessment, Treatment and Research* (3rd ed.). New York: Oxford University Press.

Robinson, H. M., Sigman, M. R., & Wilson, J. P. (1997). Duty-related stressors and PTSD symptoms in suburban police officers. *Psychological Reports*, *81*(3), 835–845. doi:10.2466/pr0.1997.81.3.835 PMID:9400075

Robinson, R., & Mitchell, J. (1993). Evaluation of psychological debriefings. *Journal of Traumatic Stress*, *6*, 367–382.

Rock, P. L., Roiser, J. P., Riedel, W. J., & Blackwell, A. D. (2014). Cognitive impairment in depression: A systematic review and meta-analysis. *Psychological Medicine*, *44*(10), 2029–2040. doi:10.1017/S0033291713002535 PMID:24168753

Rodin, J., & Salovey, P. (1989). Health psychology. *Annual Review of Psychology*, *40*(1), 533–579. doi:10.1146/annurev.ps.40.020189.002533 PMID:2648984

Rodríguez Vega, B., Bayón Pérez, C., PalaoTarrero, A., & Fernández Liria, A. (2014). Mindfulness-based narrative therapy for depression in cancer patients. *Clinical Psychology & Psychotherapy*, *21*(5), 411–419. doi:10.1002/cpp.1847 PMID:23716367

Rodriguez, L. M., Overup, C. S., & Neighbors, C. (2013). Perceptions of partner's problematic alcohol use affect relationship outcomes beyond partner self-reported drinking: Alcohol use in committed romantic relationships. *Psychology of Addictive Behaviors*, *27*, 627–638. PMID:23438240

Rosell, E., Miller, K., & Barber, K. (1995). Firefighting Women and Sexual Harassment. *Public Personnel Management*, *24*(3), 339–350.

Rose, R. D., Buckey, J. C. Jr, Zbozinek, T. D., Motivala, S. J., Glenn, D. E., Cartreine, J. A., & Craske, M. G. (2013). A randomized controlled trial of a self-guided, multimedia, stress management and resilience training program. *Behaviour Research and Therapy*, *51*(2), 106–112. doi:10.1016/j.brat.2012.11.003 PMID:23262118

Rose, S. C., Bisson, J., Churchill, R., & Wessely, S. (2002). Psychological debriefing for preventing post traumatic stress disorder (PTSD). *Cochrane Database of Systematic Reviews*, (2): CD000560. doi:10.1002/14651858.CD000560 PMID:12076399

Roskies, E. (1991). Stress management: A new approach to treatment. In A. Monat & R. S. Lazarus (Eds.), *Stress and coping: An anthology* (3rd ed.; pp. 411–431). New York: Columbia University Press. doi:10.7312/mona92982-031

Ross, J. M., Karney, B. R., Nguyen, T. P., & Bradbury, T. N. (2018). Communication that is maladaptive for middle-class couples is adaptive for socioeconomically disadvantaged couples. *Journal of Personality and Social Psychology*; advance online publication. doi:10.1037/pspi0000158 PMID:30321045

Rothbaum, B. O., & Foa, E. B. (1993). Subtypes of posttraumatic stress disorder and duration of symptoms. *Posttraumatic stress disorder: DSM-IV and beyond*, 23-35.

Roth, S., & Cohen, L. J. (1986). Approach, avoidance, and coping with stress. *The American Psychologist*, *41*(7), 813–819. doi:10.1037/0003-066X.41.7.813 PMID:3740641

Royle, L., Keenan, P., & Farrell, D. (2009). Issues of stigma for first responders accessing support for post traumatic stress. *International Journal of Emergency Mental Health*, *11*(2), 79–86. PMID:19927494

Roysircar, G. (2009a, August). *Resilience and self-care of Katrina responders: Outcomes and evaluations*. Paper presented at the annual conference of the American Psychological Association, Toronto, Canada.

Roysircar, G. (2012). Development of the Disaster Response Competencies Questionnaire (DRCQ): A pilot study. Grant application to the National Science Foundation, Arlington, VA.

Roysircar, G. (2018). Chapter 2: Counselor role and functions, professional ethics, stress, and self-care. In E. Ginter, G. Roysircar, & L. Gerstein (Eds.), Theories and strategies of counseling and psychotherapy: Relevance across cultures and settings (pp. 22-47). Thousand Oaks, CA: SAGE.

Roysircar, G., Pignatiello, V., Lanza, A., & Irigoyen, J. (2015, August). *A qualitative study of a disaster counseling model*. Paper presented at the annual conference of the American Psychological Association, Montreal, Canada.

Roysircar, G. (2008). *Building community resilience in Mississippi: Self-care for disaster response workers and caregivers (Grantor: Foundation of the Mid-South in partnership with the America Red Cross)*. Keene, NH: Antioch University New England, Multicultural Center for Research and Practice.

Roysircar, G. (2009b). The big picture of social justice advocacy: Counselor, heal society and thyself. *Journal of Counseling and Development*, *87*(3), 288–295. doi:10.1002/j.1556-6678.2009.tb00109.x

Roysircar, G. (2010). *Development of the Disaster Response Competencies Questionnaire (DRCQ): A Pilot Study. (Faculty Mini Grant, Antioch University New England)*. Keene, NH: Antioch University New England, Multicultural Center for Research and Practice.

Roysircar, G., Colvin, K. F., Afolayan, A. G., Thompson, A., & Robertson, T. W. (2017). Haitian children's resilience and vulnerability assessed with House-Tree-Person (HTP) drawings. *Traumatology*, *23*(1), 68–81. doi:10.1037/trm0000090

Roysircar, G., Geisinger, K., & Thompson, A. (2019). Haitian children's disaster trauma: Validation of pictorial assessment of resilience and vulnerability. *The Journal of Black Psychology*. doi:10.1177/0095798419838126

Roysircar, G., Podkova, M., & Pignatiello, V. (2013). Crisis intervention, social class, and counseling: Macrolevel disaster effects. In W. M. Liu (Ed.), *The Oxford Handbook of social class in counseling* (pp. 144–163). New York, NY: Oxford University Press. doi:10.1093/oxfordhb/9780195398250.013.0009

Roysircar, G., Thompson, A., & Geisinger, K. (in press). Mothers' and children's trauma coping among the poor in Haiti: Mixed methods study of community-level research. *The American Psychologist*.

Rudofossi, D. C. (1998). *The impact of trauma and loss on affective profiles of police officers*. Academic Press.

Ruggero, C. J., Kotov, R., Callahan, J. L., Kilmer, J. N., Luft, B. J., & Bromet, E. J. (2013). PTSD symptom dimensions and their relationship to functioning in World Trade Center responders. *Psychiatry Research, 210*(3), 1049–1055. PMID:24064462

Rutter, M. (1985). Resilience in the face of adversity: Protective factors and resistance to psychiatric disorder. *The British Journal of Psychiatry, 147*(6), 598–611. doi:10.1192/bjp.147.6.598 PMID:3830321

Ruzek, J. I., Brymer, M. J., Jacobs, A. K., Layne, C. M., Vernberg, E. M., & Watson, P. J. (2007). Psychological first aid. *Journal of Mental Health Counseling, 29*(1), 17–49. doi:10.17744/mehc.29.1.5racqxjueafabgwp

Rzeszutek, M., Partyka, M., & Golab, A. (2015). Temperament traits, social support, and secondary traumatic stress disorder symptoms in a sample of trauma therapists. *Professional Psychology, Research and Practice, 46*(4), 213–220. doi:10.1037/pro0000024

Sack, D. (2017, January 31). *Trauma and first responders: When the helpers need help*. Retrieved from https://www.psychologytoday.com/us/blog/where-science-meets-the-steps/201701/trauma-and-first-responders-when-the-helpers-need-help

Sadri, G., & Robertson, I. T. (1993). Self-efficacy and Work-related Behaviour: A Review and Meta-analysis. *Applied Psychology, 42*(2), 139–152. doi:10.1111/j.1464-0597.1993.tb00728.x

Salmon, T. S. (1919). War neuroses and their lesson. *New York Medical Journal, 108*, 993–994.

Salovey, P., Mayor, J. D., Goldman, S. L., Turvey, C., & Palfai, T. P. (2002). Emotional attention, clarity, and repair: exploring emotional intelligence using the trait meta-mood scale. In J. W. Pennebaker (Ed.), *Emotion, disclosure, and health* (pp. 125–154). Washington, DC: American Psychological Association.

Sampson, R. J., Raudenbush, S. W., & Earls, F. (1997). Neighborhoods and violent crime: A multilevel study of collective efficacy. *Science, 277*(5328), 918–924. doi:10.1126cience.277.5328.918 PMID:9252316

Samuels, S. (2018). *COPLINE: National law enforcement officers hotline*. Retrieved from http://www.copline.org

Santiago, P. N., Ursano, R. J., Gray, C. L., ... Fullerton, C. S. (2013). A systematic review of PTSD prevalence and trajectories of DSM-5 defined trauma exposed populations: Intentional and non-intentional traumatic events. *PLoS One, 8*(4), e59236. doi:10.1371/journal.pone.0059236 PMID:23593134

Schafer, I., & Najavits, L. M. (2007). Clinical challenges in the treatment of patients with posttraumatic stress disorder and substance abuse. *Current Opinion in Psychiatry, 20*(6), 614–618. PMID:17921765

Schetter, C. D. (2017). Moving research on health and close relationships forward—a challenge and an obligation: Introduction to the Special Issue. *The American Psychologist, 72*(6), 511–516. doi:10.1037/amp0000158 PMID:28880098

Schlosser, L. Z., & McAleer, G. (2017). *Opioid use disorders among police and public safety personnel: What law enforcement leaders need to know*. Retrieved from: http://www.policechiefmagazine.org/opioid-use-among-police-personnel/?ref=279dcb8fe44480f796646d6de97346de

Schlosser, L. Z., & Kudrick, A. A. Jr. (2019, May). You have to see the psych: Reducing the stigma of mental health treatment among police personnel. *The Police Chief, 86*(5), 50–56.

Schnider, K. R., Elhai, J. D., & Gray, M. J. (2007). Coping style use predicts posttraumatic stress and complicated grief symptom severity among college students reporting a traumatic loss. *Journal of Counseling Psychology, 54*(3), 344–350. doi:10.1037/0022-0167.54.3.344

Schnurr, P. P., Friedman, M. J., & Bernardy, N. C. (2002). Research on posttraumatic stress disorder: Epidemiology, pathophysiology, and assessment. *Journal of Clinical Psychology, 58*(8), 877–889. doi:10.1002/jclp.10064 PMID:12115712

Schockley, K. M., DeNunzio, M. M., Shen, W., Arvan, M. L., & Knudsen, E. A. (2017). Disentangling the relationship between gender and work-family conflict: An integration of theoretical perspectives using meta-analytic methods. *The Journal of Applied Psychology, 102*(12), 1601–1635. doi:10.1037/apl0000246 PMID:28749157

Schuettler, D., & Boals, A. (2011). The path to posttraumatic growth versus posttraumatic stress disorder: Contributions of event centrality and coping. *Journal of Loss and Trauma, 16*(2), 180–194. doi:10.1080/15325024.2010.519273

Scott, G., Clawson, J. J., Gardett, I., Broadbent, M., Williams, N., Fivaz, C., ... Olola, C. (2017). 9-1-1 triage of non-traumatic chest pain: Association with hospital diagnosis. *Prehospital Emergency Care, 21*(4), 525–534. doi:10.1080/10903127.2017.1302530 PMID:28409655

Scott, G., Clawson, J., Fivaz, M. C., McQueen, J., Gardett, M. I., Schultz, B., ... Olola, C. (2016, February). Using on-scene EMS responders' assessment and electronic patient care records to evaluate the suitability of EMD-triaged, low-acuity calls for secondary nurse triage in 911 centers. *Prehospital and Disaster Medicine, 31*(1), 46–57. doi:10.1017/S1049023X15005567 PMID:26758527

Scott, J. C., Matt, G. E., Wrocklage, K. M., Crnich, C., Jordan, J., Southwick, S. M., & ... . (2015). A quantitative meta-analysis of neurocognitive functioning in PTSD. *Psychological Bulletin, 141*(1), 105–140. doi:10.1037/a0038039 PMID:25365762

Scott, T. (2007). Expression of humour by emergency personnel involved in sudden deathwork. *Mortality, 12*(4), 350–364. doi:10.1080/13576270701609766

Segal, Z. V., Teasdale, J. D., Williams, J. M., & Gemar, M. C. (2002). The mindfulness-based cognitive therapy adherence scale: Inter-rater reliability, adherence to protocol and treatment distinctiveness. *Clinical Psychology & Psychotherapy, 9*(2), 131–138. doi:10.1002/cpp.320

Seligman, M. E. P., & Csikszentmihalyi, M. (2000). Positive psychology: An introduction. *The American Psychologist, 55*(1), 5–14. doi:10.1037/0003-066X.55.1.5 PMID:11392865

Sells, D., Davidson, L., Jewell, C., Falzer, P., & Rowe, M. (2006). The treatment relationship in peer-based and regular case management for clients with severe mental illness. *Psychiatric Services (Washington, D.C.), 57*(8), 1179–1184. doi:10.1176/ps.2006.57.8.1179 PMID:16870970

Senge, P. (1994). *The Fifth Discipline – The Art & Practice of The Learning Organization*. Doubleday Dell Publishing.

Sequeira, H., Hot, P., Silvert, L., & Delplanque, S. (2009). Electrical autonomic correlates of emotion. *International Journal of Psychophysiology, 71*(1), 50–56. doi:10.1016/j.ijpsycho.2008.07.009 PMID:18723054

Shakespeare-Finch, J., Rees, A., & Armstrong, D. (2015). Social support, self-efficacy, trauma and well-being in emergency medical dispatchers. *Social Indicators Research, 123*(2), 549–565. doi:10.100711205-014-0749-9

Shapiro, F. (2017). *Eye movement desensitization and processing (EMDR) therapy*. Boston, MA: Guilford Press.

Shapiro, J., & Galowitz, P. (2016). Peer support for clinicians: A programmatic approach. *Academic Medicine, 91*(9), 1200–1204. doi:10.1097/ACM.0000000000001297 PMID:27355784

Shapiro, S., Brown, K., & Biegel, G. (2007). Teaching self-care to caregivers: Effects of mindfulness-based stress reduction on the mental health of therapists in training. *Training and Education in Professional Psychology, 1*(2), 105–115. doi:10.1037/1931-3918.1.2.105

Shay, J. (2012). Moral injury. *Intertexts, 16*(1), 57–66.

Sheehan, D. C., Everly, G. S., & Langlieb, A. (2004). Current best practices coping with major critical incidents. *FBI L. Enforcement Bulletin, 73*(9), 1–13.

Shellenbarger, S. (2014, Jun 24). Work & family: Better responses to criticism at work - nobody likes negative feedback from the boss; taking it well requires humility and self-awareness. *Wall Street Journal.* Retrieved from https://libcatalog.atu.edu:443/login?url=https://search.proquest.com/docview/1539355996?accountid=8364

Shin, L. M., Rauch, S. L., & Pitman, R. K. (2006). Amygdala, medial prefrontal cortex, and hippocampal function in PTSD. *Annals of the New York Academy of Sciences, 1071*(1), 67–79. doi:10.1196/annals.1364.007 PMID:16891563

Simms, L. J., Watson, D., & Doebbeling, B. N. (2002). Confirmatory factor analyses of posttraumatic stress symptoms in deployed and nondeployed veterans of the Gulf War. *Journal of Abnormal Psychology, 111*(4), 637–647. doi:10.1037/0021-843X.111.4.637 PMID:12428777

Simons, J. S., Gaher, R. M., Jacobs, G. A., Meyer, D., & Johnson-Jimenez, E. (2005). Associations between alcohol use and PTSD symptoms among American Red Cross disaster relief workers responding to the 9/11/2001 attacks. *The American Journal of Drug and Alcohol Abuse, 31*(2), 285–304. doi:10.1081/ADA-47937 PMID:15912717

Simpson, R. J., & Guy, K. (2010). Coupling aging immunity with a sedentary lifestyle: Has the damage already been done? A mini-review. *Gerontology, 56*(5), 449–458. doi:10.1159/000270905 PMID:20029165

Simpson, T. L., Stappenbeck, C. A., Luterek, J. A., Lehavot, K., & Kaysen, D. L. (2014). Drinking motives moderate daily relationships between PTSD symptoms and alcohol use. *Journal of Abnormal Psychology, 123*(1), 237–247. doi:10.1037/a0035193 PMID:24661174

Sinden, K., Macdermid, J., Buckman, S., Davis, B., Matthews, T., & Viola, C. (2013). A qualitative study on the experiences of female firefighters. *Work (Reading, Mass.), 45*(1), 97–105. PMID:23241712

Singer, T. (2006). The neuronal basis and ontogeny of empathy and mind reading: Review of literature and implications for future research. *Neuroscience and Biobehavioral Reviews, 30*(6), 855–863. doi:10.1016/j.neubiorev.2006.06.011 PMID:16904182

Skogstad, M., Skorstad, M., Lie, A., Conradi, H. S., Heir, T., & Weisæth, L. (2013). Work-related post-traumatic stress disorder. *Occupational Medicine, 63*(3), 175–182. doi:10.1093/occmed/kqt003 PMID:23564090

Slaikeu, K. A. (1984). *Crisis intervention: A handbook for practice and research.* Boston, MA: Allyn and Bacon, Inc.

Sloan, D. M., Marx, B. P., Bovin, M. J., Feinstein, B. A., & Gallagher, M. W. (2012). Written exposure as an intervention for PTSD: A randomized clinical trial with motor vehicle accident survivors. *Behaviour Research and Therapy, 50*(10), 627–635. doi:10.1016/j.brat.2012.07.001 PMID:22863540

Sloan, D. M., Marx, B. P., Lee, D. J., & Resick, P. A. (2018). A brief exposure-based treatment vs cognitive processing therapy for posttraumatic stress disorder: A randomized noninferiority clinical trial. *JAMA Psychiatry, 75*(3), 233–239. doi:10.1001/jamapsychiatry.2017.4249 PMID:29344631

Sloan, P. (1988). Post-traumatic stress in survivors of an airplane crash-landing: A clinical and exploratory research intervention. *Journal of Traumatic Stress, 1*(2), 211–229. doi:10.1002/jts.2490010208

Smith, B. W., Epstein, E. M., Ortiz, J. A., Christopher, P. J., & Tooley, E. M. (2013). The foundations of resilience: What are the critical resources for bouncing back from stress? In *Resilience in children, adolescents, and adults* (pp. 167–187). New York, NY: Springer. doi:10.1007/978-1-4614-4939-3_13

Smith, B. W., Ortiz, J. A., Steffen, L. E., Tooley, E. M., Wiggins, K. T., Yeater, E. A., ... Bernard, M. L. (2011). Mindfulness is associated with fewer PTSD symptoms, depressive symptoms, physical symptoms, and alcohol problems in urban firefighters. *Journal of Consulting and Clinical Psychology*, *79*(5), 613–617. doi:10.1037/a0025189 PMID:21875175

Smith, E. M., North, C. S., McCool, R. E., & Shea, J. M. (1990). Acute postdisaster psychiatric disorders: Identification of persons at risk. *The American Journal of Psychiatry*, *147*(2), 202–206. doi:10.1176/ajp.147.2.202 PMID:2301660

Smith, J. L. (2015). Self-compassion and resilience in senior living residents. *Seniors Housing & Care Journal*, *23*(1), 17–31. doi:10.7748/ns.2017.e10671

Smith, L. J., Gallagher, M. W., Tran, J. K., & Vujanovic, A. A. (2018). Posttraumatic stress, alcohol use, and alcohol use motives in firefighters: The role of sleep disturbance. *Comprehensive Psychiatry*, *87*, 64–71. doi:10.1016/j.comppsych.2018.09.001 PMID:30219373

Smith, L. J., Paulus, D. J., Gallagher, M. W., Norman, S. B., Tran, J. K., & Vujanovic, A. A. (2018). Perceived stress and probable alcohol misuse in firefighters: The role of posttraumatic stress. *International Journal of Stress Management*; advance online publication. doi:10.1037tr0000118

Snyder, C. R. (2000). *Handbook of hope: Theory, measures, and applications*. San Diego, CA: Academic Press.

Snyder, C. R. (2002). Hope Theory: Rainbows in the Mind. *Psychological Inquiry*, *13*(4), 249–275. doi:10.1207/S15327965PLI1304_01

Sofianopoulos, S., Williams, B., Archer, F., & Thompson, B. (2011). The exploration of physical fatigue, sleep and depression in paramedics: A pilot study. *Australasian Journal of Paramedicine*, *9*(1). doi:10.33151/ajp.9.1.37

Solomon, E. P., & Heide, K. M. (2005). The biology of trauma: Implications for treatment. *Journal of Interpersonal Violence*, *20*(1), 51–60. doi:10.1177/0886260504268119 PMID:15618561

Solomon, Z., & Benbenishty, R. (1986). The role of proximity, immediacy, and expectancy in frontline treatment of combat stress reaction among Israelis in the Lebanon War. *The American Journal of Psychiatry*, *143*(5), 613–617. doi:10.1176/ajp.143.5.613 PMID:3963249

Soo, J., Webber, M. P., Gustave, J., Lee, R., Hall, C. B., Cohen, H. W., ... Prezant, D. J. (2011). Trends in probable PTSD in firefighters exposed to the World Trade Center disaster, 2001-2010. *Disaster Medicine and Public Health Preparedness*, *5*(S2Suppl 2), S197–S203. doi:10.1001/dmp.2011.48 PMID:21900417

Soteriades, E. S., Hauser, R., Kawachi, I., Christiani, D. C., & Kales, S. N. (2008). Obesity and risk of job disability in male firefighters. *Occupational Medicine*, *58*(4), 245–250. doi:10.1093/occmed/kqm153 PMID:18204003

Soteriades, E. S., Hauser, R., Kawachi, I., Liarokapis, D., Christiani, D. C., & Kales, S. N. (2005). Obesity and cardiovascular disease risk factors in firefighters: A prospective cohort study. *Obesity Research*, *13*(10), 1756–1763. doi:10.1038/oby.2005.214 PMID:16286523

Southwick, S. M., Pietrzak, R. H., Charney, D. S., & Krystal, J. H. (2015). Resilience: The role of accurate appraisal, thresholds, and socioenvironmental factors. *Behavioral and Brain Sciences*, , 38. PMID:26786005

Spielberger, C. D., Westberry, L. G., Grier, K. S., & Greenfield, G. (1981). *The police stress survey: Sources of stress in law enforcement*. National Institute of Justice.

Sprigg, C. A., Armitage, C. J., & Hollis, K. (2007). Verbal abuse in the National Health Service: Impressions of the prevalence, perceived reasons for and relationships with staff psychological well-being. *Emergency Medicine Journal*, *24*(4), 281–282. PMID:17384383

Staff. (2001, May 21). Aviation Workplace Safety Lags Other Industries. *Air Safety Week*.

Stajkovic, A. D., & Luthans, F. (1998). Social cognitive theory and self-efficacy: Goin beyond traditional motivational and behavioral approaches. *Organizational Dynamics*, *26*(4), 62–74. doi:10.1016/S0090-2616(98)90006-7

Standard of Care. (2019). In *Nolo*. Retrieved from https://www.nolo.com/dictionary/standard-of-care-term.html

Stanley, E. A., Schaldach, J. M., Kiyonaga, A., & Jha, A. P. (2011). Mindfulness-based mind fitness training: A case study of a high-stress predeployment military cohort. *Cognitive and Behavioral Practice*, *18*(4), 566–576. doi:10.1016/j.cbpra.2010.08.002

Stanley, I. H., Boffa, J. W., Hom, M. A., Kimbrel, N. A., & Joiner, T. E. (2017). Differences in psychiatric symptoms and barriers to mental health care between volunteer and career firefighters. *Psychiatry Research*, *247*, 236–242. doi:10.1016/j.psychres.2016.11.037 PMID:27930964

Stanley, I. H., Boffa, J. W., Tran, J. K., Schmidt, N. B., Joiner, T. E., & Vujanovic, A. A. (2019). Posttraumatic stress disorder symptoms and mindfulness facets in relation to suicide risk among firefighters. *Journal of Clinical Psychology*, 1–14. PMID:30672591

Stanley, I. H., Hom, M. A., Chu, C., Dougherty, S. P., Gallyer, A. J., Spencer-Thomas, S., ... Joiner, T. E. (2018). Perceptions of belongingness and social support attenuate PTSD symptom severity among firefighters: A multistudy investigation. *Psychological Services*. doi:10.1037er0000240 PMID:29595287

Stanley, I. H., Hom, M. A., Hagan, C. R., & Joiner, T. E. (2015). Career prevalence and correlates of suicidal thoughts and behaviors among firefighters. *Journal of Affective Disorders*, *187*, 163–171. PMID:26339926

Stanley, I. H., Hom, M. A., & Joiner, T. E. (2016). A systematic review of suicidal thoughts and behaviors among police officers, firefighters, EMTs, and paramedics. *Clinical Psychology Review*, *44*, 25–44. doi:10.1016/j.cpr.2015.12.002 PMID:26719976

Stanley, I. H., Hom, M. A., Spencer-Thomas, S., & Joiner, T. E. (2017). Suicidal thoughts and behaviors among women firefighters: An examination of associated features and comparison of pre-career and career prevalence rates. *Journal of Affective Disorders*, *221*, 107–114. doi:10.1016/j.jad.2017.06.016 PMID:28641147

Steenkamp, M. M., Litz, B. T., Hoge, C. W., & Marmar, C. R. (2015). Psychotherapy for military-related PTSD: A review of randomized clinical trials. *JAMA Psychiatry*, *314*(5), 489–500. doi:10.1001/ jama.2015.8370 PMID:26241600

Stephan, R. A., Alhassoon, O. M., Allen, K. E., Wollman, S. C., Hall, M., Thomas, W. J., ... Grant, I. (2017). Meta-analyses of clinical neuropsychological tests of executive dysfunction and impulsivity in alcohol use disorder. *The American Journal of Drug and Alcohol Abuse*, *43*(1), 24–43. doi:10.1080/00952990.2016.1206113 PMID:27712350

Sterud, T., Hem, E., Ekeberg, O., & Lau, B. (2007). Occupational stress and alcohol use: A study of two nationwide samples of operational police and ambulance personnel in Norway. *Journal of Studies on Alcohol and Drugs*, *68*(6), 896–904. doi:10.15288/jsad.2007.68.896 PMID:17960308

Stewart, S. H., Mitchell, T. L., Wright, K. D., & Loba, P. (2004). The relations of PTSD symptoms to alcohol use and coping drinking in volunteers who responded to the Swissair Flight 111 airline disaster. *Journal of Anxiety Disorders*, *18*(1), 51–68. PMID:14725868

Stierlin, E. (1909). *Psycho-neuropathology as a result of a Mining Disaster March 10, 1906*. Zurich: University of Zurich.

Stinson, P. M., & Liederbach, J. (2013). *Fox in the henhouse: A study of police officers arrested for crimes associated with domestic or family violence*. Bowling Green State University Criminal Justice Faculty Publications. Retrieved from https://scholarworks.bgsu.edu/crim_just_pub/6

Stinson, P. M., Liederbach, J., Brewer, S. L., & Todak, N. E. (2014). Drink, drive, go to jail? A study of police officers arrested for drunk driving. *Journal of Criminal Justice*, *37*, 356–376.

Stinson, P. M. Sr, Liederbach, J., & Freiburger, T. L. (2012). Off-duty and under arrest: A study of the crimes perpetuated by off-duty police. *Criminal Justice Policy Review*, *23*(2), 139–163. doi:10.1177/0887403410390510

Stinson, P. M., Todak, N. E., & Dodge, M. (2015). An exploration of crime by policewomen. *Police Practice and Research*, *16*(1), 79–93. doi:10.1080/15614263.2013.846222

Stirman, S. W., Gutiérrez-Colina, A., Toder, K., Esposito, G., Barg, F., Castro, F., ... Crits-Christoph, P. (2013). Clinicians' Perspectives on Cognitive Therapy in Community Mental Health Settings: Implications for Training and Implementation. *Administration and Policy in Mental Health*, *40*(4), 274–285. doi:10.100710488-012-0418-8 PMID:22426739

Substance Abuse and Mental Health Services Administration. (2018). *First responders: Behavioral health concerns, emergency response, and trauma*. Washington, DC: SAMHSA.

Suinn, R. M. (1997). Mental practice in sport psychology: Where have we been, where do we go? *Clinical Psychology: Science and Practice*, *4*(3), 189–207. doi:10.1111/j.1468-2850.1997.tb00109.x

Suls, J., & Fletcher, B. (1985). The relative efficacy of avoidant and nonavoidant coping strategies: A meta-analysis. *Health Psychology*, *4*(3), 249–288. doi:10.1037/0278-6133.4.3.249 PMID:4029107

Takamatsu, H., Noda, A., Kurumaji, A., Murakami, Y., Tatsumi, M., Ichise, R., & Nishimura, S. (2003). A PET study following treatment with a pharmacological stressor, FG7142, in conscious rhesus monkeys. *Brain Research*, *980*(2), 275–280. doi:10.1016/S0006-8993(03)02987-1 PMID:12867268

Tangherlini, T. R. (2000). Heroes and lies: Storytelling tactics among paramedics. *Folklore*, *111*(1), 43–66. doi:10.1080/001558700360889

Taylor, G. T. (2000). Recent developments in alexithymia theory and research. *Canadian Journal of Psychiatry*, *45*(2), 134–142. doi:10.1177/070674370004500203 PMID:10742872

Teasdale, J. D., Segal, Z., & Williams, J. M. G. (1995). How does cognitive therapy prevent depressive relapse and why should attentional control (mindfulness) training help? *Behaviour Research and Therapy*, *33*(1), 25–39. doi:10.1016/0005-7967(94)E0011-7 PMID:7872934

Tedeschi, R. G., & Calhoun, L. G. (1996). The posttraumatic growth inventory: Measuring the positive legacy of trauma. *Journal of Traumatic Stress*, *9*, 455–471. doi:10.1002/jts.2490090305 PMID:8827649

Tedeschi, R. G., & Kilmer, R. P. (2005). Assessing strengths, resilience, and growth to guide clinical interventions. *Professional Psychology, Research and Practice*, *36*(3), 230–237. doi:10.1037/0735-7028.36.3.230

Terpstra, J., & Schaap, D. (2013). Police culture, stress conditions and working styles. *European Journal of Criminology*, *10*(1), 59–73. doi:10.1177/1477370812456343

Territo, L., & Vetter, H. J. (1981). *Stress and Police Personnel*. Allyn and Bacon, Inc.

Thackray, R. I. (1981). The stress of boredom and monotony: A consideration of the evidence. *Psychosomatic Medicine*, *43*(2), 165–176. PMID:7267937

Tobin, M. I. (1997). *Perceptions of uncontrollability, unpredictability, and life-threat, in the development of crime-related PTSD symptomology* (Doctoral dissertation). Retrieved from ProQuest dissertations and theses database. (Order No. AAM9639151)

Toch, H. (2002). *Stress in policing*. American Psychological Association. doi:10.1037/10417-000

Todorova, I. L. G., Falcón, L., Lincoln, A. K., & Price, L. L. (2010). Perceived discrimination, psychological distress and health. *Sociology of Health & Illness*, *32*(6), 843–861. doi:10.1111/j.1467-9566.2010.01257.x PMID:20649891

Tomaka, J., Magoc, D., Morales-Monks, S. M., & Reyes, A. C. (2017). Posttraumatic stress symptoms and alcohol-related outcomes among municipal firefighters. *Journal of Traumatic Stress*, *30*(4), 416–424. PMID:28699663

Tompkins, M., Morin, W., Campbell, A., Hudson, D., Sumwalt, R., Johnson, J., ... Bracken, J. (1996). *Air Line Pilots Association: Critical Incident Response Program Manual*. Herndon, VA: ALPA.

Trachik, B., Marks, M. R., Bowers, C., Scott, G., Olola, C., & Gardett, I. (2015). Is dispatching a traffic accident as stressful as being in one? Acute stress disorder, secondary traumatic stress, and occupational burnout in 911 emergency dispatchers. *Annals of Emergency Dispatch & Response*, *3*(1), 27–38.

Trachik, B., Marks, M., Bowers, C., Scott, G., Olola, C., & Gardett, I. (2015). Is dispatching to a traffic accident as stressful as being in one? Acute stress disorder, secondary traumatic stress, and occupational burnout in 911 emergency dispatchers. *Annals of Emergency Dispatch and Response*, *3*(1), 27–38.

Tracy, S. J., & Tracey, K. (1998). Emotion labor at 911: A case study and theoretical critique. *Journal of Applied Communication Research*, *26*(4), 390–411. doi:10.1080/00909889809365516

Training & Development. (1998). *Leadership Lessons from the Magic Kingdom*. Author.

Training & Development. (1998). *The Teaching Organization*. Author.

Transformational leadership or effective managerial practices? (1998). *Group & Organization Management*, *23*(3), 220-237.

Traut, C. A., Larsen, R., & Feimer, S. H. (2009). Hanging on or fading out? Job satisfaction and the long-term worker. *Public Personnel Management*, *29*(3), 343–351. doi:10.1177/009102600002900304

Trippany, R. L., Kress, V. E. W., & Wilcoxon, S. A. (2004). Preventing vicarious trauma: What counselors should know when working with trauma survivors. *Journal of Counseling and Development*, *82*(1), 31–37. doi:10.1002/j.1556-6678.2004.tb00283.x

Troxell, R. M. (2008). *Indirect exposure to the trauma of others: The experiences of 911 telecommunicators* (Doctoral dissertation). Retrieved from ProQuest dissertations and theses database. (UMI number: 3335425)

Tsismenakis, A. J., Christophi, C. A., Burress, J. W., Kinney, A. M., Kim, M., & Kales, S. N. (2009). The obesity epidemic and future emergency responders. *Obesity (Silver Spring, Md.)*, *17*(8), 1648–1649. doi:10.1038/oby.2009.63 PMID:19300435

Tuckey, M. R. (2007). Issues in the debriefing debate for the emergency services. *Clinical Psychology: Science and Practice*, *14*(2), 106–116. doi:10.1111/j.1468-2850.2007.00069.x

Tuckey, M. R., & Scott, J. E. (2013). Group critical incident stress Debriefing with emergency services personnel: A randomized controlled trial. *Anxiety, Stress, and Coping*, *27*(1), 38–54. PMID:23799773

Tuckey, M. R., Winwood, P. C., & Dollard, M. F. (2012). Psychosocial culture and pathways to psychological injury within policing. *Police Practice and Research*, *13*(3), 224–240.

Tugade, M. M., & Fredrickson, B. L. (2004). Resilient Individuals Use Positive Emotions to Bounce Back From Negative Emotional Experiences. *Journal of Personality and Social Psychology*, *86*(2), 320–333. doi:10.1037/0022-3514.86.2.320 PMID:14769087

Turner, K. D., Lilly, M. M., Gamez, A. M., & Kressler, K. (2019). Impact of work-related factors on stress and health among 9-1-1 call-takers and dispatchers in California. *Journal of Emergency Dispatch;* Advanced online publication.

Turns, B., & Macey, P. (2015). Cinema narrative therapy: Utilizing family films to externalize children's 'problems'. *Journal of Family Therapy*, *37*(4), 590–606. doi:10.1111/1467-6427.12098

U.S. Commission on Civil Rights. (1981). *Who is guarding the guardians?* Washington, DC: U.S. Commission on Civil Rights.

U.S. Department of Homeland Security (USDHS). (2017). *Emergency services sector profile.* Washington, DC: Author.

U.S. Department of Labor. (2007). *2007 census of fatal occupational injuries (revised data).* Author.

U.S. Department of Transportation (USDOT). (2007). *National EMS scope of practice model* (DOT HS Publication No. 810-657). Retrieved from http://www.ems.gov/education/EMSScope.pdf

Uhernik, J. A., & Husson, M. A. (2009). Psychological first aid: An evidence informed approach for acute disaster behavioral health response. *Compelling counseling interventions. VISTAS*, *200*(9), 271–280.

Ujevic, R. M., Prizmic, J., Barisin, A. B., Maras, M., & Luetic, L. (2018). Is there a difference in job satisfaction at emergency medicine service (EMS) team and EMS dispatchers? *Resuscitation*, *130S*, e140.

United Nations Department of Safety and Security CISMU Staff. (2007a). *UNDSS CISMU Certification Training For Counselors. DSS Newsletter*. New York: United Nations Secretariat, Department of Safety and Security.

United Nations Department of Safety and Security CISMU Staff. (2007b). *New crisis and stress management training program launched. I Seek (May 2, 2007)*. New York: United Nations Secretariat.

United Nations Department of Safety and Security CISMU Staff. (2007c). *Certification training in Crisis and Stress Management. New York: UN Department of Safety and Security, Consultative Working Group on Stress in Collaboration with the International Critical Incident Stress Foundation, the American Academy of Experts in Traumatic Stress and the Comite National de L'urgence Medico-Psychologigue*. New York: United Nations, Department of Safety and Security.

United States Department of Labor, Bureau of Labor Statistics. (2008a). *Fatal Occupational Injuries Resulting from Transportation incidents and Homicides, All United States*. Washington, DC: US Department of Labor.

United States Department of Labor, Bureau of Labor Statistics. (2008b). *Fatal Occupational injuries by event or exposure, 2007-2008*. Washington, DC: US Department of Labor.

United States Department of Labor, Bureau of Labor Statistics. (2009). National Census of Fatal Occupational Injuries in 2008. Bureau of Labor Statistics News.

Ursano, R. J., & McCarroll, J. E. (1990). The nature of a traumatic stressor: Handling dead bodies. *The Journal of Nervous and Mental Disease*, *178*(6), 396–398. doi:10.1097/00005053-199006000-00010 PMID:2348196

Ursin, H., & Eriksen, H. (2004). The cognitive activation theory of stress. *Psychoneuroendocrinology*, *29*(5), 567–592. doi:10.1016/S0306-4530(03)00091-X PMID:15041082

US Department of Veterans Affairs. (2018). *PTSD: National Center for PTSD*. Retrieved from https://www.ptsd.va.gov/understand/common/common_adults.asp

US Fire Administration. (n.d.). *Firefighter Fatality Search Results*. Retrieved from https://apps.usfa.fema.gov/firefighter-fatalities/fatalityData/list?deathYear=2018&offset=0&max=10

Usher, L., Friedhoff, S., Cochran, S., & Pandya, A. (2016). *Preparing for the unimaginable: How chiefs can safeguard officer mental health before and after mass casualty events*. Washington, DC: U. S. Department of Justice Office of Community Oriented Policing Services.

Vallieres, A., Azaiez, A., Moreau, V., LeBlanc, M., & Morin, C. M. (2014). Insomnia in shift work. *Sleep Medicine*, *15*(12), 1440–1448. doi:10.1016/j.sleep.2014.06.021 PMID:25277664

Van der Kolk, B. A., & Saporta, J. (1993). Biological response to psychic trauma. In J. P. Wilson & B. Raphael (Eds.), *International handbook of traumatic stress syndromes* (pp. 25–33). Boston, MA: Springer. doi:10.1007/978-1-4615-2820-3_2

van der Kolk, B., McFarlane, A., & Weisaeth, L. (1996). *Traumatic stress*. New York, NY: Guildford Press.

Van Emmerick, A. A. P., Kamphuis, J. H., Hulsbosch, A. M., & Emmelkamp, P. M. G. (2002). Single session debriefing following psychotrauma, help or harm: A metaanalysis. *Lancet*, *360*, 766–771. PMID:12241834

Van Emmerik, A. A., Kamphuis, J. H., Hulsbosch, A. M., & Emmelkamp, P. M. (2002). Single session debriefing after psychological trauma: A meta-analysis. *Lancet*, *360*(9335), 766–771. doi:10.1016/S0140-6736(02)09897-5 PMID:12241834

Van Orden, K. A., Witte, T. K., Cukrowicz, K. C., Braithwaite, S. R., Selby, E. A., & Joiner, T. E. (2010). The interpersonal theory of suicide. *Psychological Review*, *117*(2), 575–600. doi:10.1037/a0018697 PMID:20438238

VanRaalte, R. C. (1979). Alcohol as a problem among officers. *The Police Chief*, *46*(2), 38–39.

Vargas de Barros, V., Martins, L. F., Saitz, R., Bastos, R. R., & Ronzani, T. M. (2013). Mental health conditions, individual and job characteristics and sleep disturbances among firefighters. *Journal of Health Psychology*, *18*(3), 350–358. doi:10.1177/1359105312443402 PMID:22517948

Vasterling, J. J., Duke, L. M., Brailey, K., Constans, J. I., Allain, A. N. Jr, & Sutker, P. B. (2002). Attention, learning, and memory performances and intellectual resources in Vietnam veterans: PTSD and no disorder comparisons. *Neuropsychology*, *16*(1), 5–14. doi:10.1037/0894-4105.16.1.5 PMID:11853357

Violanti, J. M. (1993). What does high stress police training teach recruits? An analysis of coping. *Journal of Criminal Justice*, *21*(4), 411–417. doi:10.1016/0047-2352(93)90022-F

Violanti, J. M. (1997). Residuals of police occupational trauma. *Australasian Journal of Disaster and Trauma Studies*.

Violanti, J. M. (1999). Alcohol abuse in policing: Prevention strategies. *FBI Law Enforcement Bulletin*, *68*, 16–18.

Violanti, J. M. (2004). Predictors of police suicide ideation. *Suicide & Life-Threatening Behavior*, *34*(3), 277–283. doi:10.1521uli.34.3.277.42775 PMID:15385182

Violanti, J. M. (2010). Dying for work. Stress and health in policing. *Gazette*, *72*(1), 20–21.

Violanti, J. M. (2010). Police suicide: A national comparison with firefighter and military personnel. *Policing: An International Journal of Police Strategies & Management*, *33*(2), 270–286. doi:10.1108/13639511011044885

Violanti, J. M. (2014). *Dying for the job: police work exposure and health*. Springfield, IL: Charles C Thomas Publishers.

Violanti, J. M. (2014). *Dying for the job: Police work exposure and health*. Springfield, IL: Charles C. Thomas.

Violanti, J. M., Andrew, M. E., Mnatsakanova, A., Hartley, T. A., Fekedulegn, D., & Burchfiel, C. M. (2016). Correlates of hopelessness in the high suicide risk police occupation. *Police Practice and Research*, *17*(5), 408–419. doi:10.1080/15614263.2015.1015125 PMID:26752981

Violanti, J. M., Burchfiel, C. M., Miller, D. B., Andrew, M. E., Dorn, J., Wactawski-Wende, J., & Sharp, D. S. (2006). The buffalo cardio-metabolic occupational police stress (BCOPS) pilot study: Methods and participant characteristics. *Annals of Epidemiology*, *16*(2), 148–156. doi:10.1016/j.annepidem.2005.07.054 PMID:16165369

Violanti, J. M., & Drylie, J. J. (2008). *Copicide: Concepts, cases, and controversies of suicide by cop*. Springfield, IL: Charles C. Thomas Publisher, LTD.

Violanti, J. M., Marshall, J. R., & Howe, B. (1985). Stress, coping, and alcohol use: The police connection. *Journal of Police Science and Administration.*

Violanti, J. M., & Paton, D. (1999). *Police trauma: Psychological aftermath of civilian combat*. Charles C Thomas Publisher.

Violanti, J. M., Robinson, C. F., & Shen, R. (2013). Law enforcement suicide: A national analysis. *International Journal of Emergency Mental Health and Human Resilience*, *15*(4), 289–297. PMID:24707591

Violanti, J. M., Slaven, J. E., Charles, L. E., Burchfiel, C. M., Andrew, M. E., & Homish, G. G. (2011). Police and alcohol use: A descriptive analysis and associations with stress outcomes. *American Journal of Criminal Justice*, *36*(4), 344–356.

Virgili, M. (2015). Mindfulness-based interventions reduce psychological distress in working adults: A meta-analysis of intervention studies. *Mindfulness*, *6*(2), 326–337. doi:10.100712671-013-0264-0

Viswesvaran, C., Sanchez, J. I., & Fisher, J. (1999). The role of social support in the process of work stress: A meta-analysis. *Journal of Vocational Behavior*, *54*(2), 314–334. doi:10.1006/jvbe.1998.1661

Vogel, D. L., Wester, S. R., Wei, M., & Boysen, G. A. (2005). The Role of Outcome Expectations and Attitudes on Decisions to Seek Professional Help. *Journal of Counseling Psychology*, *52*(4), 459–470. doi:10.1037/0022-0167.52.4.459

Vogel, J. M., Cohen, A. J., Habib, M. S., & Massey, B. D. (2004). In the wake of terrorism: Collaboration between a psychiatry department and a center for emergency medical services (EMS) to support EMS workers and their families. *Families, Systems & Health*, *22*(1), 35–46. doi:10.1037/1091-7527.22.1.35

Vogt, J., & Leonhardt, J. (Eds.). (2006). *Critical Incident Stress Management in Aviation*. Hampshire, UK: Ashgate Publishing Limited.

Vogt, J., Leonhardt, J., Koper, B., & Pennig, S. (2004). Economic Evaluation of CISM – A Pilot Study. *International Journal of Emergency Mental Health*, *6*(4), 185–196. PMID:15635899

Vogt, J., Pennig, S., & Leonhardt, J. (2007). Critical Incident Stress Management in air traffic control and its benefits. *Air Traffic Control Quarterly*, *15*(2), 127–156. doi:10.2514/atcq.15.2.127

Von Brachel, R., Teismann, T., Feider, L., & Margraf, J. (2019). Suicide ideation as a predictor of treatment outcomes in cognitive-behavioral therapy for unipolar mood disorders. *International Journal of Clinical and Health Psychology*, *19*(1), 80–84. doi:10.1016/j.ijchp.2018.09.002 PMID:30619501

Vorster, C., & Phipps, W. D. (2009). Narrative therapy: A return to the intrapsychic perspective? *South African Journal of Psychology. Suid-Afrikaanse Tydskrif vir Sielkunde*, *39*(1), 32–45. doi:10.1177/008124630903900103

Vujanovic, B.-M., Bonn-Miller, M. O., & Petry, N. M. (2016). Co-occurring posttraumatic stress and substance use: Emerging research on correlates, mechanisms, and treatments-Introduction to the special issue. *Psychology of Addictive Behaviors*, *30*(7), 713–719. doi:10.1037/adb0000222 PMID:27786510

Wagner, D., Heinrichs, M., & Ehlert, U. (1998). Prevalence of symptoms of posttraumatic stress disorder in German professional firefighters. *The American Journal of Psychiatry*, *155*(12), 1727–1732. doi:10.1176/ajp.155.12.1727 PMID:9842783

Wagner, S., & O'Neill, M. (2012). Job, Life, and Relationship Satisfaction for Paid-Professional Firefighters. *Journal of Loss and Trauma*, *17*(5), 423–438. doi:10.1080/15325024.2011.650129

Walker, S., Alpert, G. P., & Kenney, D. J. (2001, July). Early warning systems: Responding to the problem police officer. *National Institute of Justice Research in Brief, 1–8*. Retrieved from https://www.ncjrs.gov/pdffiles1/nij/grants/188565.pdf

Walker, S. (2003). *Early intervention systems for law enforcement agencies (United States Department of Justice, Office of Community Oriented Policing Services)*. Washington, DC: Police Executive Research Forum.

Walker, S., Milligan, S. O., & Berke, A. (2006). *Strategies for intervening with officers through early intervention systems: A guide for front-line supervisors (United States Department of Justice, Office of Community Oriented Policing Services)*. Washington, DC: Police Executive Research Forum.

Waters, J. A., & Ussery, W. (2007). Police stress: History, contributing factors, symptoms, and interventions. *Policing: An International Journal of Police Strategies & Management*, *30*(2), 169–188. doi:10.1108/13639510710753199

Watson, A. C., Corrigan, P., Larson, J. E., & Sells, M. (2007). Self-stigma in people with mental illness. *Schizophrenia Bulletin*, *33*(6), 1312–1318. doi:10.1093chbulbl076 PMID:17255118

Weathers, F. W., Litz, B. T., Keane, T. M., Palmieri, P. A., Marx, B. P., & Schnurr, P. P. (2013). *The PTSD Checklist for DSM-5 (PCL-5)*. Academic Press.

Weathers, F., Litz, B., Herman, D., Huska, J., & Keane, T. (1993). *The PTSD Checklist (PCL): Reliability, validity, and diagnostic utility*. Paper presented at the Annual Convention of the International Society for Traumatic Stress Studies, San Antonio, TX.

Weathers, F. W., Bovin, M. J., Lee, D. J., Sloan, D. M., Schnurr, P. P., Kaloupek, D. G., ... Marx, B. P. (2017). The Clinician-Administered PTSD Scale for DSM–5 (CAPS-5): Development and Initial Psychometric Evaluation in Military Veterans. *Psychological Assessment*, *30*(3), 383–395. doi:10.1037/pas0000486 PMID:28493729

Weaver, M. D., Patterson, P. D., Fabio, A., Moore, C. G., Freiberg, M. S., & Songer, T. J. (2015). An observational study of shift length, crew familiarity, and occupational injury and illness in emergency medical services workers. *Occupational and Environmental Medicine*, *72*(11), 798–804. doi:10.1136/oemed-2015-102966 PMID:26371071

Wee, D. F., Mills, D. M., & Koelher, G. (1999). The effects of Critical Incident Stress Debriefing on emergency medical services personnel following the Los Angeles civil disturbance. *International Journal of Emergency Mental Health*, *1*, 33–38. PMID:11227752

Weinberger, A. H., Maciejewski, P. K., McKee, S. A., Reutenauer, E. L., & Mazure, C. M. (2009). Gender differences in associations between lifetime alcohol, depression, panic disorder, and posttraumatic stress disorder and tobacco withdrawal. *The American Journal on Addictions*, *18*(2), 140–147. PMID:19283566

Weinberg, M., Gil, S., & Gilbar, O. (2014). Forgiveness, coping, and terrorism: Do tendency to forgive and coping strategies associate with the level of posttraumatic symptoms of injured victims of terror attacks? *Journal of Clinical Psychology*, *70*(7), 693–703. doi:10.1002/jclp.22056 PMID:24353169

Weiss, D. S., Brunet, A., Best, S. R., Metzler, T. J., Liberman, A., Pole, N., & Marmar, C. R. (2010). Frequency and severity approaches to indexing exposure to trauma: The critical incident history questionnaire for police officers. *Journal of Traumatic Stress*, *23*(6), 734–743. doi:10.1002/jts.20576 PMID:21171134

Wells, T. S., Bagnell, M. E., Miller, S. C., Smith, T. C., Gackstetter, G. D., & Boyko, E. J. (2014). U.S. Naval and Marine Corps occupations, posttraumatic stress disorder, depression risk, and absenteeism. *Journal of Workplace Behavioral Health*, *29*(2), 91–112. doi:10.1080/15555240.2014.899187

Wessely, S., & Deahl, M. (2003). Psychological debriefing is a waste of time. *The British Journal of Psychiatry*, *183*(1), 12–14. doi:10.1192/bjp.183.1.12 PMID:12835237

Western Management Consultants. (1996). *The Medical Services Branch CISM Evaluation Report*. Edmonton, Canada: WMC.

Wester, S. R., Arndt, D., Sedivy, S. K., & Arndt, L. (2010). Male police officers and stigma associated with counseling: The role of anticipated risks, anticipated benefits and gender role conflict. *Psychology of Men & Masculinity*, *11*(4), 286–302. doi:10.1037/a0019108

Westphal, G. (2009). Law Enforcement Healthy Marriage and Family Project. *The Police Chief*, *76*, 48–50.

White, E. K., & Honig, A. L. (1995). Law enforcement families. In M. I. Kurke & E. M. Scrivner (Eds.), *Police psychology into the 21st century* (pp. 189–206). Hillsdale, NJ: Lawrence Erlbaum Associates.

White, M. (1995). *Re-authoring lives: Interviews and essays*. Adelaide, South Australia, Australia: Dulwich Centre.

White, M. (2007). *Maps of narrative practice*. New York, NY: Norton.

Wiegand, D. M. (2013). *Evaluation of job stress and work-related health concerns of a telephone call center*. Retrieved from: http://www.cdc.gov/niosh/hhe/reports/pdfs/2012-0211-3197. pdf

Williams, D. R., Neighbors, H. W., & Jackson, J. S. (2003). Racial/Ethnic discrimination and health: Findings from community studies. *American Journal of Public Health*, *93*(2), 200–208. doi:10.2105/AJPH.93.2.200 PMID:12554570

Williams, V., Ciarrochi, J., & Deane, F. P. (2010). On being mindful, emotionally aware, and more resilient: Longitudinal pilot study of police recruits. *Australian Psychologist*, *45*(4), 274–282. doi:10.1080/00050060903573197

Women in Military Service for America Memorial Foundation, Inc. (2010). *Statistics on Women in the Military*. Washington, DC: Women in Military Service for America Memorial Foundation.

Woodhouse, S., Ayers, S., & Field, A. P. (2015). The relationship between adult attachment style and post-traumatic stress symptoms: A meta-analysis. *Journal of Anxiety Disorders*, *35*, 103–117. doi:10.1016/j.janxdis.2015.07.002 PMID:26409250

Wu, D., Yin, H., Xu, S., & Zhao, Y. (2011). Risk factors for posttraumatic stress reactions among Chinese students following exposure to a snowstorm disaster. *BMC Public Health*, *11*(1), 96. doi:10.1186/1471-2458-11-96 PMID:21314959

Yi, J. P., Vitaliano, P. P., Smith, R. E., Yi, J. C., & Weinger, K. (2008). The role of resilience on psychological adjustment and physical health in patients with diabetes. *British Journal of Health Psychology*, *13*(2), 311–325. doi:10.1348/135910707X186994 PMID:17535497

Yip, J., Zeig-Owens, R., Hall, C. B., Webber, M. P., Olivieri, B., Schwartz, T., ... Prezant, D. J. (2016). Health conditions as mediators of the association between World Trade Center exposure and health-related quality of life in firefighters and EMS workers. *Journal of Occupational and Environmental Medicine*, *58*(2), 200–206. doi:10.1097/JOM.0000000000000597 PMID:26849265

Yip, J., Zeig-Owens, R., Webber, M. P., Kablanian, A., Hall, C. B., Vossbrinck, M., ... Prezant, D. J. (2016). World Trade Center-related physical and mental health burden among New York City Fire Department emergency medical service workers. *Occupational and Environmental Medicine*, *73*(1), 13–20. doi:10.1136/oemed-2014-102601 PMID:25876606

Yun, J. A., Ahn, Y. S., Jeong, K. S., Joo, E. J., & Choi, K. S. (2015). The relationship between chronotype and sleep quality in Korean firefighters. *Clinical Psychopharmacology and Neuroscience*, *13*(2), 201–208. doi:10.9758/cpn.2015.13.2.201 PMID:26243849

Zlotnick, C., Franklin, C. L., & Zimmerman, M. (2002). Does "subthreshold" posttraumatic stress disorder have any clinical relevance? *Comprehensive Psychiatry*, *43*(6), 413–419. doi:10.1053/comp.2002.35900 PMID:12439826

About the Contributors

Clint Bowers, PhD, is a Pegasus Professor of Psychology and Director of the RETRO laboratory at the University of Central Florida. His recent research is in the area of technology-based training. Current research projects include the development and evaluation of game-based learning technologies across a variety of domains. He has published numerous refereed journal articles and book chapters in the area of training and has edited three books related to training and technology.

Deborah Beidel, Ph.D., ABPP, is Trustee Chair and Pegasus Professor of Psychology and Medical Education. She is the author of over 300 scientific publications including journal articles, book chapters and books on the treatment of anxiety disorders and post-traumatic stress disorder. Dr. Beidel is the Director of UCF RESTORES, a clinical research center dedicated to trauma and PTSD. The recipient of over $31 million dollars in federal research funding, her recent work focuses on developing effective treatments for PTSD for veterans, active duty personnel, first responders and survivors of mass shootings, utilizing technology to enhance effective treatments and translate them into standard clinical practice.

Madeline Marks, M.S., is a doctoral student in the clinical psychology program and member of the RETRO laboratory at the University of Central Florida. Current research projects include the development and evaluation of game-based learning technologies across a variety of domains, which include military and first responder populations.

* * *

Eamonn Arble is an assistant professor of psychology at Eastern Michigan University. He has worked extensively with coauthor Dr. Arnetz in the development, assessment, and implementation of first responder interventions.

Bengt Arnetz is a professor and chair in the Department of Family Medicine, in the College of Human Medicine, at Michigan State University. He has worked extensively with coauthor Dr. Arble in the development, assessment, and implementation of first responder interventions.

Brooke Bartlett is a third-year doctoral student and teaching fellow in the clinical psychology program and a graduate research assistant in the Trauma and Stress Studies Center (TaSSC) at the University of Houston. She received a B.A. in psychology from the University of California, Irvine in 2011, a M.A. in psychology from Boston University in 2013, and a M.A. in clinical psychology from the University of

Houston in 2018. From 2013-2016, Brooke worked with Dr. Karen Mitchell as a Psychology Research Technician in the National Center for PTSD - Women's Health Sciences Division, VA Boston Healthcare System and Boston University School of Medicine exploring multiple research questions surrounding etiology and risk factors for eating disorders and PTSD among veterans and active duty military members. Her current research interests focus on the etiology and treatment of trauma-related pathology (e.g., PTSD, suicidality, substance use), with a focus on risk and resilience factors (e.g., distress tolerance, emotion regulation), particularly among first responder and veteran populations

Daniel Blumberg is a licensed clinical psychologist who has spent the past 30 years providing all facets of clinical and consulting psychological services to numerous local, state, and federal law enforcement agencies. He specializes in employment-related psychological evaluations, psycho- educational training, and management consultation. In addition to his expertise in workplace stress prevention and trauma recovery, Dr. Blumberg is an authority on undercover police operations and the selection, training and supervision of undercover operatives. His training program on successful hiring of public safety personnel has received widespread praise. Dr. Blumberg is an Associate Professor in the Department of Undergraduate Psychology at Alliant International University's San Diego Campus where he teaches a variety of psychology and forensic psychology courses. His research interests include police integrity, emotional intelligence, and programs to improve relations between the police and the community.

Emily Brucia earned her Ph.D. in Clinical Psychology at Palo Alto University in 2018 and she is currently the Posttraumatic Stress Disorder (PTSD) and Returning Veterans Clinical Psychology Postdoctoral Fellow at the San Francisco Veterans Affairs (VA) Health Care System, where she provides brief and long-term, individual and group evidence-based treatment for mixed era Veterans with PTSD and complex/developmental trauma. In this role she also teaches and serves as a clinical supervisor for psychology trainees and psychiatry residents. She completed her predoctoral internship at the VA Northern California Health Care System and she previously trained with the Berkeley Police Department Mobile Crisis Team. Dr. Brucia is currently participating in The Leadership Program in Integrative Healthcare at Duke University and she serves as Vice President of the Board of Trustees for the First Responder Support Network, a residential treatment program for first responders with posttraumatic stress reactions as well as their families. Her research interests include early intervention, risk and protective factors, and posttraumatic resilience.

Jaysyn Carson is a retired twenty-seven-year veteran with the Fairfax County Police Department and currently the departments Director of Incident Support Services. He holds a Bachelor's degree in Business Management and an Associate's Degree in Criminal Justice. During his career he has served as a detective in the department's Gang Investigations Unit and supervised the specialty units of Organized Crimes and Narcotics, and the Major Crimes Division. He was also the Assistant Commander of the Regional Intelligence Center and the Assistant Commander of the Peer Support Team / Incident Support Services. Jay spent the last twenty-one years as a member of the department's Peer Support Team and ended his law enforcement career as one of the team's two commanders. As team commander, his enthusiasm, position and experience afforded him the opportunity to be instrumental in producing and directing a suicide prevention film that has been recognized at the national level. Subsequently, he constructed a survey with department psychologists to identify possible contributants to the suicide rate within first responders. In concert with these projects, he organized and began development of a comprehensive wellness program. This program was in part a culmination of Jay's focus on the role of stress and trauma as it relates to the suicide rate among first responders. The goals include changing the culture, reducing stigma, enhancing physical and mental health, preventing suicide, and lessening trauma reactions. These goals will be achieved with progressive policy changes and research-driven education and training. Jay currently travels, teaching federal, state, and local jurisdictions about changing the culture, reducing stigma, understanding and normalizing the effects of trauma, and addressing suicide in first responders.

Matthew Cordova, Ph.D, is a Staff Psychologist in Behavioral Medicine at the VA Northern California Health Care System and an Associate Professor at Palo Alto University. He teaches and supervises graduate students, predoctoral interns, and postdoctoral fellows and has published numerous articles and book chapters on traumatic stress and early intervention. He holds a BS from UC Davis and a PhD from the University of Kentucky; he completed an internship at the VA Palo Alto and a postdoctoral fellowship at Stanford University.

Zena Dadouch is a fourth year doctoral student in the Clinical Psychology Program at Northern Illinois University. She earned her B.A. in Psychology in 2015 from the University of California, Berkeley. Her undergraduate research experiences incorporated survivor guilt and PTSD in children and mother survivors of domestic violence, as well as sexual assault. She worked as a research assistant at the University of California, San Francisco and the San Francisco General Hospital. Zena earned her M.A. at Northern Illinois University in 2019. Zena is originally from Damascus, Syria, where she grew up, and her research interests in trauma originated from the war that has been going on in Syria since 2011. After coming to the U.S. to pursue her education, her passion for studying survivors of trauma, particularly refugees of war, has grown. Zena is now interested in examining risk and resiliency factors for well-being particularly in specialized groups (e.g., 9-1-1 telecommunicators, journalists) after exposure to trauma as well as culturally-specific trauma-treatments for minorities and refugees.

Amanda DeDiego received her PhD in Counselor Education from the University of Tennessee in 2016. Prior to this, she received her MS in Community Counseling from the University of North Georgia. She is currently an Assistant Professor of Counseling at the University of Wyoming and a National Certified Counselor. Her clinical work and research includes first responder populations in addition to focus on counselor training and development.

Isabel Farrell received her PhD in Counselor Education from the University of Tennessee in 2018. Prior to this, she received her MS in Counseling Psychology from Northeastern State University. She is currently an Assistant Professor of Counseling at Wake Forest University. Her clinical work includes bilingual Latinx communities and domestic violence and sexual assault survivors. Her research focus is on bilingual counseling, cultural identity, social justice and professional legislative advocacy.

Angelique Finestone is a Ph.D. student at Palo Alto University/ Pacific Graduate School of Psychology studying Clinical Psychology, emphasizing in Adult Trauma. Angelique's career goals include working with first responders pre- and post- trauma to increase well-being and resilience, manage work-related stress, and provide treatment to those with post traumatic symptoms. Her passion for working with first responder communities was influenced by her family's involvement in law enforcement and her recognition for an increased demand of mental health support.

Isabel Gardett is the Director of Academics, Research, and Communications at the International Academies of Emergency Dispatch.

Lisa Berg Garmezy, Ph.D., graduated from Pennsylvania State University in 1986 with a doctorate in Clinical Psychology. Her experience includes twenty-two years of full-time employment with the Houston Police Department Psychological Services Division. Through the American Red Cross, the Texas Psychological Association, and in the past, the National Organization for Victim Assistance, she has provided disaster mental health services at national emergencies including the September 11 terrorist attacks, hurricanes and recent wildfires. Enhancing mental health by strengthening community institutions is a particular interest.

Luciano Giromini, PhD, is assistant professor in the Department of Psychology at the University of Turin. He specializes in personality assessment, statistics, and psychometrics and has taught these subjects at universities in Italy and California. He is co-author of the Inventory of Problems - 29 (www.iop-test.com), a world-wide utilized, malingering-related test, and his neuro-physiological studies on the Rorschach have been published in several high quality, peer-reviewed journals. He has received several internationally recognized awards and acknowledgments, including a Mary Cerney Award (issued by the Society for Personality Assessment) and an "Alien of Extraordinary Ability in Personality Assessment" U.S. Visa (issued by the U.S. Citizenship and Immigration Service).

Bernardo Gonzalez acquired a doctorate degree in Organizational Leadership from Nova Southeastern University. He also possesses an Educational Specialist and Graduate Degrees in Education and Criminal Justice Studies. Dr. Gonzalez recently served as a strategic business partner to C-level executives, senior government officials, and other stakeholders on the design, implementation, and optimization of enterprise leadership, organizational development, and operational readiness programs. Dr. Gonzalez directed cross-functional leadership and consulting teams across program lifecycle from initial situational assessment through analysis, development, and implementation of strategic roadmaps and measurement systems, and organization-level change management. Dr. Gonzalez retired from the Miami-Dade Police Department after 28 years of honorable service. During his tenure, he was promoted to an executive leadership role directing the training and education vision for a 4,700-employee police department, as well as the leadership and overall responsibility of the Miami-Dade Police Institute, shaping and executing the full lifecycle of enterprise professional development programs.

Mario Gonzalez is a Firefighter/Chaplain Mario Gonzalez and was hired by Miami-Dade Fire Rescue (MDFR) in August of 1992. In his 27 years at MDFR, Mario has been an agent of hope and change both inside and outside the Department. For 25 years alongside his wife Jean, and his three children Jordan, Julianne and James, the Gonzalez family lived on the Campus of His House Children's Home, an organization founded and directed by his wife Jean. During their time at His House, over 10,000 children, inclusive of the over 500 evacuated orphans due to the devastating earthquake in Haiti, passed through their doors. As a firefighter, Mario served honorably as a tailboard in some of the busiest houses in the County. He was officially recognized as a Chaplain in January 2011. He was instrumental in the creation of the Department's Critical Incident and Chaplaincy Peer Support Teams, designing programs with the focus on peer support, training, and educational awareness of firefighter mental health issues. Firefighter Gonzalez wrote and co-produced four mental health videos that have been seen all over the world covering the subjects of suicide prevention, PTSD, and firefighter resiliency beyond the call. His impact and influence on MDFR as it pertains to mental health is unprecedented and the Department is a much better organization as a result of his efforts.

Suzy Gulliver is a licensed Clinical Psychologist focused on health risk behaviors including addictions. She is Director of the Warriors Research Institute of Baylor Scott& White Health, and a Professor of Psychiatry at Texas A&M College of Medicine Health Sciences Center. She has adapted multiple individual and group cognitive behavioral treatment programs to special populations including pregnant women, anxiety disordered alcoholics, and firefighters suffering from acute stress disorders. One of her treatment protocols (Broad Spectrum Treatment) is featured as an evidence-based CBT manual for addiction by SAMSHA. Dr. Gulliver is the chief Behavioral Health consultant to the International Association of Firefighters, having devoted over 20 years to research and clinical work with Fire Service.

Marie G. Gumá MS. PsyD (ABD) Marie was born in Caracas, Venezuela. Her family moved to Miami, Florida when she was 3 years old. From a very early age Marie knew she wanted to study psychology and work in the helping profession. She attended Barry University where she majored in psychology. Marie obtained her Master of Science and Doctoral coursework in Clinical Psychology at Carlos Albizu University graduating Cum Laude and a member of the Honor Society (PSI CHI). Marie is a well-known and experienced professional in the substance abuse community in South Florida. She began her career providing psychological therapy to the underprivileged youth in Miami-Dade County. After 8 years of practicing in the public sector, Marie opened a private practice office in Coral Gables. In 2010, she was exposed to the world of substance abuse and business development when she was asked to become the department head of a detox unit at Mercy Hospital in Miami, Florida. She has spent years building relationships nationally as an executive in the substance abuse field and has created a name for herself due to her professionalism, ethics, experience and passion. When Marie introduced substance abuse treatment to the First Responder industry, her second life-calling and passion awoke. Since 2011, Marie has been an advocate, educator, resource and clinical consultant for many South Florida Fire and Police Departments. In November of 2017, Marie attended the Clinician Awareness Program hosted by the Florida Firefighters Safety and Health Collaborative (FFSHC) in Coral Springs/Parkland. Marie helps to manage the Clinician Awareness Trainings in the state of Florida for the FFSHC. She is also a proud and active member of the Clinical Response Team for Coral Springs Parkland. She holds high standards for herself and the organizations she relates to. Her clinical background and first responder industry exposure has helped to develop her vision and enthusiasm for this industry.

Brittany Hollerbach is a Project Coordinator at the Institute for Biobehavioral Health Research, part of the National Development and Research Institutes, Inc. She currently works on studies being conducted by the Center for Fire, Rescue, and EMS Health Research and the Center for Military and Veteran's Health Research. Her current work focuses on firefighter health and a military PTSD clinical trial. Brittany is a doctoral candidate at Kansas State University and has been working on both military and firefighter projects with NDRI since she started her master's degree. She has an interest in firefighter health in general and female firefighter health specifically, given her background as a former firefighter.

She also has experience teaching at the fire academy and is well-connected to the fire service community in Kansas City. Brittany also has extensive experience working with military personnel through the ATHIS study, a cluster randomized clinical trial being conducted in the US Army by IBHR/NDRI and Kansas State University investigators.

Jennifer Kelly, Ph.D., ABPP, is a New Jersey licensed psychologist and board certified in Police & Public Safety Psychology by the American Board of Professional Psychology. Dr. Kelly's clinical practice involves a variety of police and public safety psychological services including conducting post-offer pre-employment psychological evaluations, fitness for duty evaluations, and specialty assignment examinations. To date, she has been retained to carry out psychological evaluations by more than 120 municipalities and public safety departments. Dr. Kelly offers treatment services to public safety agencies including critical incident debriefings of public safety employees, EAP services, as well as annual wellness sessions. She has published in the area of psychological treatment with public safety personnel and wellness programming within police agencies. Dr. Kelly is currently a member-at-large on the Council of Organizations in Police Psychology and a member of the International Association of Chiefs of Police, Police Psychological Services Section.

Allyssa Lanza is a licensed clinical psychologist practicing in Maryland and Virginia with a focus on treating trauma disorders.

Antoine Lebeaut is a first-year doctoral student in the clinical psychology program and a graduate research assistant in the Trauma and Stress Studies Center (TaSSC) at the University of Houston. He received his B.A. in psychology from Franklin & Marshall College in 2015. Following graduation, Antoine completed a research assistantship with Dr. Dean McKay at Fordham University, exploring the etiology and maintenance of comorbid OCD and PTSD. Recently, he was a research assistant at Rutgers University Behavioral Health Care, working with Dr. Steven Silverstein on a study evaluating the effectiveness of a novel behavioral intervention for children with externalizing behaviors and with Dr. Judy Thompson on a study investigating the efficacy of a visual remediation intervention for schizophrenia. Antoine's current research interests involve identifying risk factors that influence the transition from trauma exposure to PTSD and improving the efficacy of treatment for trauma-related disorders.

Michelle Lilly is an Associate Professor of Clinical Psychology at Northern Illinois University (NIU). She completed her undergraduate training at Brown University before earning her doctorate in clinical psychology at University of Michigan in 2008. Throughout her professional career, Dr. Lilly has studied the psychological and physical impact of violence and trauma. Her dissertation focused on how world views and coping affect risk for posttraumatic stress disorder (PTSD) and depression in female survivors of domestic violence. Early in her career at NIU, she became involved in research with 9-1-1 telecommunicators and has continued to focus on this understudied population. Dr. Lilly's research on mental and physical health in the 9-1-1 industry has been used to argue for job reclassification for 9-1-1 telecommunicators across the nation. In addition, she is a licensed clinical psychologist in the state of Illinois.

Marie Macedonia is a psychologist who specializes in the treatment of co-occurring disorders. She works in a community mental health care center in Nashua, New Hampshire. Her practice of self-care includes reading, spending time with her family, and gardening.

Andrea McGrath is a doctoral student in the Counselor Education and Supervision program at the University of Wyoming. She received a Master's degree in Counseling Psychology from the University of Denver. She is a Licensed Professional Counselor and Licensed Addiction Counselor. Her clinical focus is adult mental health and substance use treatment. Her research interests include substance use and co-occurring disorders, underserved populations, and counselors in recovery from substance use.

Jill Milloy, Ph.D., has been a Licensed Clinical Psychologist since 1996. She has worked with law enforcement for over 20 years, and has been with the Fairfax County Police Department for the past 8 years. She provides evidence-based wellness, prevention and psycho-educational trainings as well as psychotherapy, individual and group crisis intervention, and consultation. She is trained in evidence-based Cognitive-Behavioral treatments for issues to include mood and anxiety disorders, Posttraumatic Stress Disorder, early interventions for critical incidents, and is a trainer for Stress First Aid from the National Center for Posttraumatic Stress Disorder. As a psychologist working with the Fairfax County Police Department, Dr. Milloy responds to emerging needs within law enforcement and other public safety agencies. She collaborated on a suicide prevention video that has been recognized at the national level and a subsequent survey to identify possible contributors to the suicide rate among first responders. These efforts have influenced the design and implementation of a comprehensive wellness program. Dr. Milloy developed training for self-care strategies for law enforcement recruits; the formation of supportive groups (e.g., Veterans, Cancer); and, co-researched and designed a pilot intervention program to promote wellness for specialty units as well as measuring the efficacy of the program. She consults with various departments regarding behavioral health issues, supports officers during times of injury and investigation, and consults on work performance issues. She has extensive training and experience responding to critical incidents for local and federal public safety agencies and trains law enforcement departments and other agencies on issues including behavioral health, Posttraumatic Stress Disorder, crisis negotiation, suicide prevention, wellness and prevention, and mindfulness and psychological resilience.

Colby Mills, Ph.D., is a clinical and police psychologist in Northern Virginia. He provides a wide array of services to public safety agencies, including psychotherapy, consultation, training, and critical incident response. Most of his work is with the Fairfax County (VA) Police Department, where he has been a contracted police psychologist since 2011. He has also provided consultations to the Major Cities Chiefs Association, the National EMS Management Association, and U.S. Immigration and Customs Enforcement. Dr. Mills has lectured on law enforcement psychology at Marymount University and George Mason University. Dr. Mills is trained in Prolonged Exposure, Cognitive Processing Therapy, and Stress First Aid, among other modalities. He is a member of Division 18 of the American Psychological Association.

Jeffrey T. Mitchell holds an M.A. in counseling psychology from Loyola University in Baltimore, Maryland, and a Ph.D. in human development from the University of Maryland at College Park. Dr. Mitchell is a Clinical Professor of Emergency Health Services at the University of Maryland, Baltimore County (UMBC). He serves on the Graduate Faculty of UMBC. He is a certified trauma specialist, Co Founder and past president of the International Critical Stress Foundation, Inc., and served as the clinical director of the Howard County Critical Incident Stress Management Team for 27 years. Dr. Mitchell is a member of the International Journal of Emergency Mental Health's editorial board. He also serves on the editorial review board for the Journal of the American Medical Association (JAMA) and the Journal of Disaster Medicine. He is an adjunct faculty member at the Federal Emergency Management Agency's Emergency Management Institute in Emmitsburg, Maryland. Previously, he served as an elementary school teacher, an emergency medical technician, a paramedic, a firefighter, and a regional coordinator for the Maryland Institute for Emergency Medical Services Systems (MIEMSS). He specializes in crisis intervention, stress management, and disaster psychology. He teaches an annual introductory stress management program for the Maryland State Police recruits. Dr. Mitchell is the author of 25 books and more than 275 articles on crisis intervention and stress management. He has taught stress and crisis intervention courses in all fifty states and in 32 other nations. His work is recognized and utilized by the United Nations and he is a member of the working group on stress in the United Nations' Department of Safety and Security. He was awarded the Bronze Medal from the Austrian Red Cross for his crisis intervention work after the disastrous Kaprun train tunnel fire in Austria in the year 2000. He has provided Critical Incident Stress Management support services at over 60 major disasters including the Oklahoma City Bombing, the attacks on America on September 11, 2001, and the El Salvador Earthquake in 1986. He provided support services to members of the Critical Incident Response Team for the Connecticut State Police in the aftermath of the horrific shootings of young school children and school personnel in Newtown. He provided support to the teachers and staff of the Marjory Stoneman Douglas High School in Parkland, Florida.

Kimberly Neisler joined UCF RESTORES in 2019 after retiring as the Fire Chief of the Maitland Fire Rescue Department where she served nearly 37 years. She has been involved in programs relating to First Responder stress management throughout her career. During her tenure as Fire Chief, she was tasked with establishing the Central Florida Regional Fire Rescue Behavioral Health Collaborative to provide a means for sharing resources for Peer Support. She serves as the Fire/EMS Outreach Coordinator for UCF RESTORES. Kimberly holds degrees in EMS, Nursing, and Fire Science. She previously served as an RN/Clinical Educator for Valencia State College's Paramedic program.

Christopher Olola, PhD, is the Director of Biomedical Informatics and Research at the Academics, Research & Communications (ARC) Department of the International Academies of Emergency Dispatch (IAED). Chris has over 27 years of informatics, academic and clinical research experience, including five years as a regional clinical data coordinator for the severe malaria in African children (SMAC) network project, with the Kenya Medical Research Institute/Wellcome Trust Research Labs. Chris received his Ph.D in Biomedical informatics (Public Health Informatics emphasis), from the University of Utah in 2009. His doctorate research focused on the adoption of American Society for Testing and Materials Continuity of Care Record (CCR) standard -- E2369-05, to advance continuity of care in the United States healthcare community. Dr. Olola has published widely and he is an Editor-in-Chief (emeritus) of the IAED's scientific peer-reviewed journal; Annals of Emergency Dispatch & Response - AEDR (www.aedrjournal.org), and founder member of the Kenya Health Informatics Association-KeHIA (www.kehia.org) and Editor-in-Chief of KeHIA Journal.

Konstantinos Papazoglou, PhD, CPsych (Supervised Practice), is a Clinical and Forensic Psychologist and has recently been accepted a Postdoctoral Fellowship position at Yale School of Medicine. He completed his doctoral degree (PhD) in psychology (clinical - forensic area) as Vanier Scholar at the University of Toronto (UofT). He is a former Police Major of the Hellenic Police Force and European Police College and he holds a master's degree in applied psychology from New York University (NYU) as Onassis Scholar. Currently, his research work focuses on stress, trauma and suicide prevention, and resilience promotion among police officers. Towards this direction he has established research collaboration with many law enforcement agencies in US, Canada, and Europe (e.g., Police Training Institute – Illinois State Police, State Police of Kentucky, National Police of Finland). He has published more than 40 scholarly articles in peer-reviewed journals and book chapters. In addition, he presented his research work (more than 100 presentations) in many scientific venues (e.g., American Psychological Association, Academy of Criminal Justice Sciences, International Society for Traumatic Stress Studies) and received many awards (e.g., American Psychological Association – Criminal Justice Section Outstanding Doctoral Research Award; American Psychological Foundation – Levinson Scholarship Award; American Psychological Association – Police and Public Safety Section - Outstanding Doctoral Research Award in Police and Public Safety; American Security Today – Homeland Security Platinum Award). Further, he conducted workshops and presented to numerous government agencies in US, Canada, and Europe (e.g., Federal Police University of Germany, Police University College of Finland, Trainer the Trainers Seminar – European Police College, Canada Department of National Defense – Research Centre, Ontario Ministry of Community Safety and Correctional Services, etc.). Konstantinos is a member of the research advisory team in Badge of Life Canada and a doctoral representative of the American Psychological Association – Police and Public Safety Section. Moreover, he is a co-moderator of the European Medical and Psychology Experts Network (EMPEN), an official network of police health professionals established and sponsored by the European Police College (CEPOL). He currently works as a Clinical and Forensic Psychologist (Supervised Practice) with the Ontario Ministry of Community Safety and Correctional Services providing clinical services (assessment and treatment) to criminal justice offenders.

Diana Robinson is a third-year doctoral student in the clinical psychology program at Northern Illinois University. She earned her B.A. in Psychology in 2014 from California State University, San Bernardino (CSUSB). Her undergraduate research focused on intimate partner violence and sexual assault prevention education. After receiving her B.A., Diana continued her education and earned her M.A. in General Experimental Psychology in 2017 from CSUSB. Her Master's thesis focused on female-perpetrated intimate partner violence among college women. Diana's overarching research interests are interpersonal violence, trauma, and resiliency. Specifically, her interests include identifying and understanding cognitive and behavioral factors that contribute to intimate partner violence and sexual assault (e.g., emotion regulation, attachment insecurity, substance use), as well as the psychosocial factors that lead to the positive and/or negative trajectory of recovery from such traumas (e.g., factors contributing to resilience vs. posttraumatic stress).

Nancy Rosado, a retired NYPD sergeant and Clinical Social Worker, serves as the Outreach Consultant for UCF RESTORES. Ms. Rosado has an extensive history in law enforcement, including being among the first police officers to respond to the attack on 9/11. Since her retirement from NYPD and after her move to Orlando, Florida. Ms. Rosado has served as an advocate for many underrepresented populations, including the Latino, LGBTQ+ and first responder communities, including advocating for culturally competent training for local officials following the Pulse Nightclub shooting and advocating for a standard of care for first responders.

Gargi Roysircar, EdD, retired full professor, Antioch University New England, founded in 2000 the Antioch Multicultural Center for Research and Practice, the first community outreach and research center in the nation that engaged in international work domestically and globally. She provides mental health service, including assessment, in U.S. refugee and immigrant communities and in international disaster settings. Dr. Roysircar does research on disaster trauma and resilience, immigrant mental health, multicultural competencies, and training in culturally informed practices, authoring more than 100 journal articles and chapters. She is an APA Fellow (in Divs. 17, 45, 52, 56) and served on the APA Task Force for the APA 2017 Multicultural Guidelines: An Ecological Approach to Context, Identity, and Intersectionality http://www.apa.org/about/policy/multicultural-guidelines.aspx/. The American Psychological Foundation awarded Dr. Roysircar a grant for: Developing and implementing an integrated system for providing resilience-based trauma assessment and counseling to Palestinian children in the West Bank (2015). Dr. Roysircar was the first woman and Asian editor of the Journal of Multicultural Counseling and Development (2004-2011). In 2019, APA awarded her the International Humanitarian Award in recognition of her "sustained and enduring humanitarian services to underserved populations." Dr. Roysircar received the APA Div. 35 Psychology of Women Strickland Daniel Mentoring Award (2016); the American Counseling Association's Research Award (2007, for the article: Development of counseling trainees' multicultural awareness through mentoring ESL students. Journal of Multicultural Counseling and Development, 33(1), 17-36), and the Extended Research Award (2002); and APA Div. 17 Society of Counseling Psychology Best Practice Award (2012) and SERD Community Advocacy Award (2006). Dr. Roysricar was the first recipient of Antioch University's Horace Mann Spirit of Service Award (2011), and served as the lead delegate of the Multicultural Counseling Delegation to Sao Paulo and Rio de Janeiro, Brazil, for People to People Ambassador Programs (2011). Dr. Roysircar recently co-authored: "Theories and Strategies of Counseling and Psychotherapy: Relevance across Cultures and Settings" (2018, SAGE). Dr. Roysircar's instrument, Multicultural Counseling Inventory, is the most frequently cited instrument among published multicultural competency scales. Her article (Sodowsky et al., 1998), which uses the MCI instrument, was ranked 13th over the past decades among 25 most cited articles of the Journal of Counseling Psychology. Dr. Roysircar is ranked in productivity ratings of authors in multicultural/cross-cultural journals. Dr. Roysircar has provided mental health counseling in earthquake-destroyed Haiti; tsunami-affected fishing communities in Southern India; Hurricanes Katrina and Rita-affected communities and first responders in the United States Gulf Coast; flood-ravaged city of Villahermosa, Tabasco, Mexico; and in South African HIV/AIDS orphanages. Dr. Roysircar's 44-year teaching career has been spent in three countries across three continents. Dr. Roysircar serves on the Board of Trustees of Apple Hill Center for Chamber Music and Playing for Peace Society, Nelson, NH.

Greg Scott is Operations Research Analyst at the International Academies of Emergency Dispatch.

Lia Smith is a third-year doctoral student in the clinical psychology program, teaching fellow, and the research program coordinator in the Trauma and Stress Studies Center (TaSSC) at the University of Houston.She received a B.A. in psychology from Wheaton College in 2013. While there, she also earned a certificate in Human Needs and Global Resources for her research with trauma-exposed women and children in Huánuco, Peru. Most recently, Lia studied biopsychosocial mechanisms related to alcohol and nicotine dependence with Dr. Andrea King at the University of Chicago. She also was a behavioral health intern with Dr. Karla Torres at Lawndale Christian Health Center, an inner-city primary care clinic on Chicago's west side. Lia received her M.A. in clinical psychology from the University of Houston in 2018. Her current research interests focus on the risk and resilience processes at the intersection of addictions, trauma, and health disparities.

Renee Thornton is an organizational psychologist with a specialty in resilience who has spent nearly 20 years providing workforce development and human resources consulting services in the public and private sectors. Her specialty is translating research into performance management tools that improve cultural wellness and efficiency. Dr. Thornton is the creator of the virtual wellness program, The HE-ROES Project, and is currently working on the development of a Resilience Certification program for first response organizations seeking to set an excellence standard in public safety and service. She is the founder of the Command Post, a nonprofit organization providing advocacy to law enforcement agencies through research, training, and communication. Her research interests include resilience, leadership, and the performance management of first-response organizations.

Edward Trefts is a Research and Technical Writer at the International Academies of Emergency Dispatch.

Anka Vujanovic is an Associate Professor of Psychology and licensed clinical psychologist. She is the Director of the Trauma and Stress Studies Center and Co-Director of the Trauma and Anxiety Clinic of Houston. Dr. Vujanovic received a doctoral degree in clinical psychology from the University of Vermont in 2009, upon completing the pre-doctoral clinical psychology internship program at the Alpert Medical School of Brown University. Dr. Vujanovic's research program is focused on three interwoven lines of inquiry: (1) investigation of etiological and maintenance processes related to PTSD; (2) exploration of clinically significant correlates of trauma exposure and PTSD (e.g., suicidality); and (3) examination of biopsychosocial mechanisms underlying the comorbidity of PTSD and substance use disorders. The overarching aim of this program is to expand upon our understanding of the etiology, course, and phenomenology of PTSD/subclinical posttraumatic stress and related conditions so as to improve extant treatment approaches and develop novel intervention strategies.

William Walsh of the Voorhees Police Department began his career as a police dispatcher at the age of 16 and continued in the field by serving as a police officer assigned to various roles and functions during his tenure as an officer since 2003. Lt. Walsh has led the Department's Community Affairs Bureau and is currently responsible for leading the Patrol Bureau. Lt. Walsh has a passion for not only helping the community, but also his fellow first responders through his work with officer health and wellness initiatives. Lt. Walsh has earned a master's degree from Fairleigh Dickinson University, and holds several graduate certificates including a certificate in Police Leadership from Temple University. Lt. Walsh is an adjunct instructor at Rowan College at Gloucester County and the Gloucester County Police Academy. He developed and instructs the Officer Health and Wellness course at Gloucester County Police Academy's Supervision School and has presented on this and related topics to numerous law enforcement and corrections agencies, unions, the College and University Police and Investigators Conference, and the National Park Service. Lt. Walsh has presented at the International Association of Chiefs of Police.

Maya Zegel a clinical psychology doctoral student at the University of Houston and a graduate research assistant in the Trauma and Stress Studies Center. She received her B.A. in psychology from Boston University in 2016. After graduation, Maya worked at McLean Hospital in the Functional Integration of Addiction Research Laboratory and the Behavioral Psychopharmacology Research Laboratory.

Index

Ensure Quality Research is Introduced to the Academic Community

Become an Evaluator for IGI Global Authored Book Projects

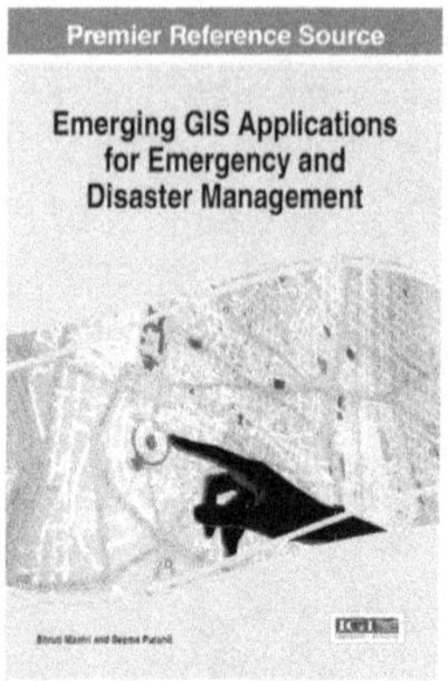

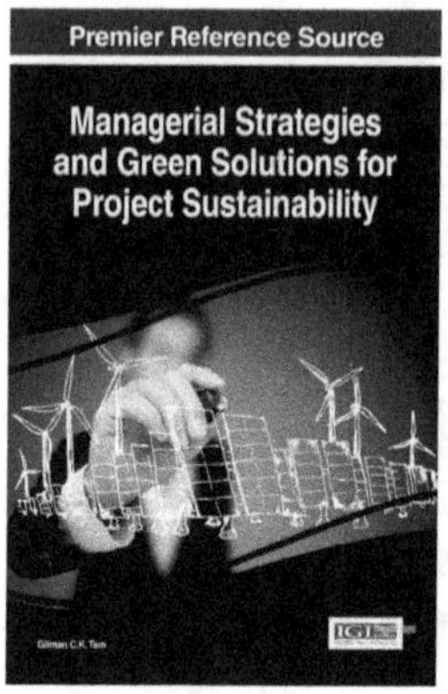

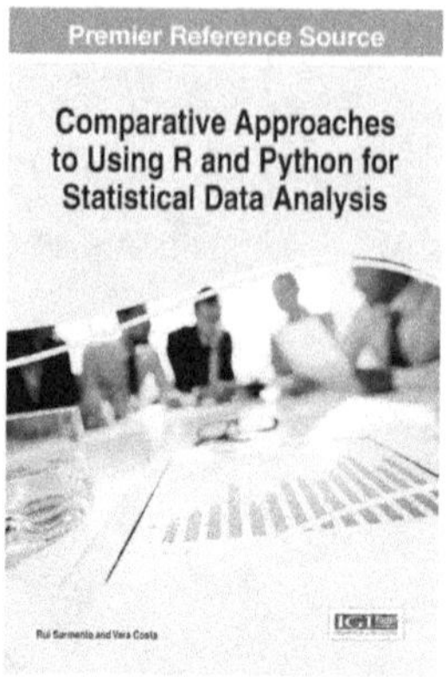

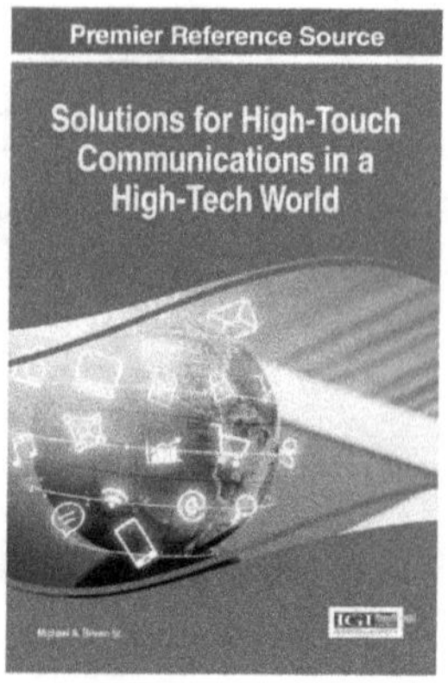

The overall success of an authored book project is dependent on quality and timely manuscript evaluations.

Applications and Inquiries may be sent to:
development@igi-global.com

Applicants must have a doctorate (or equivalent degree) as well as publishing, research, and reviewing experience. Authored Book Evaluators are appointed for one-year terms and are expected to complete at least three evaluations per term. Upon successful completion of this term, evaluators can be considered for an additional term.

If you have a colleague that may be interested in this opportunity, we encourage you to share this information with them.

www.ingramcontent.com/pod-product-compliance
Lightning Source LLC
LaVergne TN
LVHW060409300926
849162LV00006B/1383